Taylor's Handbook of Clinical Nursing Skills

Second Edition

Pamela Lynn, MSN, RN

Instructor
Frances M. Maguire School of Nursing
and Health Professions
Gwynedd Mercy University
Gwynedd Valley, Pennsylvania

Wolters Kluwer

Philadelphia • Baltimore • New York • London
Buenos Aires • Hong Kong • Sydney • Tokyo

Publisher: Lisa McAllister
Executive Editor: Sherry Dickinson
Product Developmental Editor: Christine Abshire
Editorial Assistant: Dan Reilly
Marketing Manager: Dean Karampelas
Production Project Manager: Cynthia Rudy
Design Coordinator: Holly Reid McLaughlin
Illustration Coordinator: Jennifer Clements
Manufacturing Coordinator: Karin Duffield
Production Services: Aptara, Inc.

2nd Edition

Copyright © 2015 by Wolters Kluwer

9 8 7 6 5 4 3 2 1

Printed in China

Library of Congress Cataloging-in-Publication Data

Lynn, Pamela (Pamela Barbara), 1961- author.
 Taylor's handbook of clinical nursing skills / Pamela Lynn. — Second edition.
  p. ; cm.
 Handbook of clinical nursing skills
 Abridgement of: Taylor's clinical nursing skills : a nursing process approach / Pamela Lynn.
4th ed. 2015.
 Includes bibliographical references.
 ISBN 978-1-4511-9363-3 (alk. paper)
 I. Lynn, Pamela (Pamela Barbara), 1961- Taylor's clinical nursing skills. Abridgement of (work):
II. Title. III. Title: Handbook of clinical nursing skills.
 [DNLM: 1. Nursing Process–Handbooks. 2. Clinical Medicine–methods–Handbooks.
3. Nursing Care–methods–Handbooks. WY 49]
 RT51
 610.73—dc23
                                                                        2014021540

CCS0814

With love, to John, Jenn, and Anna.
You fill every day with joy!

Contributors and Reviewers

**CONTRIBUTOR TO
PREVIOUS EDITION**

Lynn Burbank, RN, CPNP, MSN
Learning Resource Coordinator
Dixon School of Nursing
Abington Memorial Hospital
Abington, Pennsylvania
Medications

REVIEWERS

**Kamomilani Anduha Wong,
MSN, FNP-BC, APRN**
Assistant Professor
College of Nursing and Health
    Sciences
Hawaii Pacific University
Kaneohe, Hawaii

**Jennifer Douglas Pearce, MSN,
RN, CNE**
Professor
University of Cincinnati Blue
    Ash College
Blue Ash, Ohio

**David Dunham, DHEd, MS,
CRNI, RN**
Associate Professor
Director, Clinical Laboratories
College of Nursing and Health
    Sciences
Hawaii Pacific University
Kaneohe, Hawaii

Kimbra Gabhart, MSN-BC
ADN Nursing Faculty
Elizabethtown Community and
    Technical College
Elizabethtown, Kentucky

**Freda Lynn McAllister, RN,
BSN, MSN**
Nursing Program Head
Dabney S. Lancaster Community
    College
Clifton Forge, Virginia

**Diane McPhillips, RN, MSN,
CNE, CNS**
Associate Professor
University of Cincinnati Blue
    Ash College
Cincinnati, Ohio

Delia G. Meyer, MSN, RN, CE
Instructor
Ila Faye Miller School of Nursing
University of the Incarnate Word
San Antonio, Texas

Michelle Natrop, MSN
Normandale Community College
Bloomington, Minnesota

Linda Lee Phelps, MSN, RN
Assistant Professor—Adjunct
    Faculty
Ivy Tech Community College
Indianapolis, Indiana

**Milena P. Staykova, EdD,
FNP-BC**
Assistant Professor
Jefferson College of Health
    Sciences
Roanoke, Virginia

Amber Young-Brice, MSN, RN
Clinical Instructor
Marquette University
Milwaukee, Wisconsin

Preface

Taylor's Handbook of Clinical Nursing Skills is a quick-reference guide to basic and advanced nursing skills. It outlines step-by-step instructions and reinforces the cognitive and technical knowledge needed to perform skills safely and effectively. The convenient handbook format is helpful for student review in the lab or clinical setting and as a reference for graduate nurses in practice.

LEARNING EXPERIENCE

This text and the entire Taylor Suite have been created with the student's experience in mind. Care has been taken to appeal to all learning styles. The student-friendly writing style ensures that students will comprehend and retain information. The extensive art program enhances understanding of important actions. In addition, each element of the Taylor Suite, which is described later in the Preface, coordinates the information to provide a consistent and cohesive learning experience.

ORGANIZATION

In general, the content of this book provides streamlined skills consistent with those in *Taylor's Clinical Nursing Skills*, 4th Edition. Skills are organized alphabetically, based on the main word(s) of the skill, allowing the user to access the information about the desired skill quickly and easily.

FEATURES

- **Step-by-step skills.** Each skill is presented in a concise, straightforward, and simplified two-column format to facilitate competent performance of nursing skills.
- The **nursing process** framework is used to integrate related nursing responsibilities for each of the five steps.*
- **Scientific rationales** accompany each nursing action to promote a deeper understanding of the basic principles supporting nursing care.
- **Documentation guidelines** direct students and graduate nurses in accurate documentation of the skill and their findings.
- **Delegation considerations** assist students and graduate nurses in developing the critical decision-making skills necessary to transfer responsibility for the performance of an activity to another individual and to ensure safe and effective nursing care. Delegation decision-making information is provided in each skill, using delegation guidelines based on American Nurses Association (ANA) and National Council of State Boards of Nursing (NCSBN) principles and recommendations (Appendix A).
- **Photos.** Key steps are clarified and reinforced with pictures.
- **General considerations**, which explain the varying needs of patients across the lifespan and in various settings, are available on thePoint.

TAYLOR SUITE RESOURCES

From traditional texts to video and interactive products, the Taylor Fundamentals/Skills Suite is tailored to fit every learning style. This integrated suite of products offers students a seamless learning experience not found elsewhere. The following products accompany *Taylor's Handbook of Clinical Nursing Skills:*

- ***Fundamentals of Nursing: The Art and Science of Person-Centered Nursing Care,* 8th Edition,** by Carol Taylor, Carol Lillis, and Pamela Lynn. This traditional Fundamentals text promotes nursing as an evolving art and science, directed to human health and well-being. It challenges students to focus on the four blended skills of nursing care, which prepare students to combine the highest level of scientific knowledge and technologic skill with responsible, caring practice. The text includes engaging features to promote critical thinking and comprehension.
- ***Taylor's Clinical Nursing Skills,* 4th Edition,** by Pamela Lynn, covers all of the Skills and Guidelines for Nursing Care identified in Fundamentals of Nursing, Eighth Edition—plus additional skills—at the basic, intermediate, and advanced levels, each following the nursing process format. Features include Skill Variations, which present alternate techniques; Documentation Guidelines and Samples; Unexpected Situations and Associated Interventions; Delegation Considerations; and Special Considerations.
- ***Taylor's Video Guide to Clinical Nursing Skills.*** With more than 12 hours of video footage, this updated series follows nursing students and their instructors as they perform a range of essential nursing procedures. Institutions can purchase the videos on enhanced DVD or access them online.

Contact your sales representative or check out LWW.com/Nursing for more details and ordering information.

Guide to Icons Used in This Book

IDENTIFY THE PATIENT

 Identifying the patient ensures the right patient receives the right treatment or intervention and helps prevent errors. The patient should be identified using at least two methods (TJC, 2013) whenever you are administering medications or blood products, taking blood samples and other specimens for clinical testing, or providing any other treatments or procedures. For example:

• Check the patient's name and identification number, birth date, or social security number on the patient's identification band. This is the most reliable method.
• Ask the patient to state his or her name. This requires a response from the patient. Be aware that illness and strange surroundings often cause patients to be confused.

DO NOT USE the name on the door or over the bed (these may be inaccurate) or the patient's room number.**

PERFORM HAND HYGIENE

 Hand hygiene is the most effective way to help prevent the spread of organisms. The term hand hygiene applies to either the use of antiseptic hand rubs, including alcohol-based products; handwashing with soap and water; or surgical hand antisepsis. The Centers for Disease Control (CDC), the government agency responsible for investigating, preventing, and controlling disease, issued guidelines for hand hygiene in health care settings.

If the health care worker's hands are not visibly soiled, alcohol-based handrubs are recommended because they save time, are more accessible and easy to use, and reduce bacterial count on the hands. The following are clinical situations when an alcohol-based handrub can be used to decontaminate hands:

• Before direct contact with patients
• After direct contact with a patient's skin
• After contact with body fluids, mucous membranes, nonintact skin, and wound dressings if hands are not visibly soiled
• After removing gloves
• Before inserting urinary catheters, peripheral vascular catheters, or invasive devices that do not require surgical placement
• Before donning sterile gloves prior to an invasive procedure (e.g., inserting a central intravascular catheter)

- If moving from a contaminated body site to a clean body site during patient care
- After contact with objects (including equipment) located in the patient's environment

Handwashing with either antimicrobial soap or non-antimicrobial soap and water is required if a health care worker's hands are visibly soiled or contaminated with blood or body fluids. Handwashing is also required before eating and after using the restroom. Handwashing is also required if exposure to certain organisms, such as *Clostridium difficile*, is known or suspected.***

Pamela Lynn, MSN, RN

*Material related to nursing diagnoses from *Nursing Diagnoses—Definitions and Classification 2012–2014*. Copyright © 2014, 2009, 2007, 2005, 2003, 2001, 1998, 1996, 1994 by NANDA International. Used by arrangement with Wiley-Blackwell-Publishing, a company of John Wiley & Sons, Inc. To make safe and effective judgments using NANDA-I nursing diagnoses, it is essential that nurses refer to the definitions and defining characteristics of the diagnoses listed in this work.

**Source for Patient Identification Guidelines: The Joint Commission (TJC). (2013). *National patient safety goals*. Available http://www.jointcommission.org/standards_information/npsgs.aspx.

***Source for Hand Hygiene Guidelines: Joint Commission. [2013]. *National patient safety goals*. Available http://www.jointcommission.org/standards_information/npsgs.aspx; Centers for Disease Control and Prevention (CDC). (2002). Guideline for hand hygiene in health-care settings. *Morbidity and Mortality Weekly Report 2002, 51*(RR16), 1–45; Centers for Disease Control and Prevention. [2013]. *Hand hygiene in healthcare settings*. Available http://www.cdc.gov/handhygiene/; and Institute for Healthcare Improvement (IHI). (2011). *How-to guide: Improving hand hygiene*. Available http://www.IHI.org.

Acknowledgments

This edition is the work of many talented people. I would like to acknowledge the hard work of all who have contributed to the completion of this project. Thanks to Carol Taylor and Carol Lillis for offering generous support and encouragement. You have been excellent mentors.

The work of this book was skillfully coordinated by my dedicated Product Developmental Editor, Christine Abshire, in the Nursing Education division of Wolters Kluwer. I am grateful to you for your patience, support, unending encouragement, and total commitment. My thanks to Sherry Dickinson, Executive Editor, for her hard work and guidance throughout the project. Thank you to the members of the Production Department, who patiently pulled everything together to form a completed book: Cindy Rudy, Production Project Manager; Holly Reid McLaughlin, Design Coordinator; and Jennifer Clements, Illustration Coordinator.

A special thanks to my colleagues at Gwynedd Mercy University, who offer unending support and professional guidance.

Finally, I would like to gratefully acknowledge my family, for their love, understanding, and encouragement. Their support was essential during the long hours of research and writing.

Pamela Lynn, MSN, RN

Contents

SKILL 1 ASSISTING A PATIENT WITH AMBULATION

Walking exercises most of the body's muscles and increases joint flexibility. It improves respiratory and gastrointestinal function. Ambulating also reduces the risk for complications of immobility. However, even a short period of immobility can decrease a person's tolerance for ambulating. If necessary, make use of appropriate equipment and assistive devices to aid in patient movement and handling.

DELEGATION CONSIDERATIONS

Assisting a patient with ambulation may be delegated to nursing assistive personnel (NAP) or to unlicensed assistive personnel (UAP), as well as to licensed practical/vocational nurses (LPNs/LVNs). The decision to delegate must be based on careful analysis of the patient's needs and circumstances, as well as the qualifications of the person to whom the task is being delegated. Refer to the Delegation Guidelines in Appendix A.

EQUIPMENT

- Gait belt, as necessary
- Nonskid shoes or slippers
- Nonsterile gloves and/or other PPE, as indicated
- Stand-assist device as necessary, if available
- Additional staff for assistance as needed

ASSESSMENT

- Assess the patient's ability to walk and the need for assistance. Review the patient's record for conditions that may affect ambulation.
- Perform a pain assessment before initiating the activity. If the patient reports pain, administer the prescribed medication in sufficient time to allow for the full effect of the analgesic.
- Take vital signs and assess the patient for dizziness or light-headedness with position changes.

NURSING DIAGNOSIS

- Impaired Physical Mobility
- Activity Intolerance
- Risk for Falls
- Impaired Walking

OUTCOME IDENTIFICATION AND PLANNING

- Patient ambulates safely, without falls or injury.
- Patient demonstrates improved muscle strength and joint mobility.
- Patient's level of independence increases.
- Patient remains free of complications of immobility.

IMPLEMENTATION

ACTION	RATIONALE
1. Review the medical record and nursing plan of care for conditions that may influence the patient's ability to move and ambulate. Assess for tubes, IV lines, incisions, or equipment that may alter the procedure for ambulation. Identify any movement limitations.	Reviewing the medical record and plan of care validates the correct patient and correct procedure. Checking for equipment and limitations reduces the risk for patient injury.
2. Perform hand hygiene. Put on PPE, as indicated.	Hand hygiene and PPE prevent the spread of microorganisms. PPE is required based on transmission precautions.
3. Identify the patient. Explain the procedure to the patient. Ask the patient to report any feelings of dizziness, weakness, or shortness of breath while walking. Decide how far to walk.	Patient identification validates the correct patient and correct procedure. Discussion and explanation help allay anxiety and prepare the patient for what to expect.
4. Place the bed in the lowest position.	Proper bed height ensures safety when getting the patient out of bed.
5. Encourage the patient to make use of a stand-assist aid, either freestanding or attached to the side of the bed, if available, to move to the side of the bed. Assist the patient to the side of the bed, if necessary.	Use of assistive devices encourages independence, reduces strain for staff, and decreases risk for patient injury.
6. Have the patient sit on the side of the bed for several minutes and assess for dizziness or light-headedness. Have the patient stay sitting until he or she feels secure.	Having the patient sit at the side of the bed minimizes the risk for blood pressure changes (orthostatic hypotension) that can occur with position change. Allowing the patient to sit until he or she feels secure reduces anxiety and helps prevent injury.

ACTION	RATIONALE
7. Assist the patient to put on footwear and a robe, if desired.	Doing so ensures safety and patient warmth.
8. Wrap the gait belt around the patient's waist, based on assessed need and facility policy.	Gait belts improve the caregiver's grasp, reducing the risk of musculoskeletal injuries to staff and the patient. The belt also provides a firmer grasp for the caregiver if the patient should lose his or her balance.
9. Encourage the patient to make use of the stand-assist device. Assist the patient to stand, using the gait belt, if necessary. Assess the patient's balance and leg strength. If the patient is weak or unsteady, return the patient to the bed or assist to a chair.	Use of gait belt prevents injury to the nurse and to the patient. Assessing balance and strength helps to identify the need for additional assistance to prevent falling.
10. If you are the only person assisting, position yourself to the side and slightly behind the patient. Support the patient by the waist or transfer belt (Figure 1).	Positioning to the side and slightly behind the patient encourages the patient to stand and walk erect. It also places the nurse in a safe position if the patient should lose his or her balance or begin to fall.

FIGURE 1 Nurse positioned to the side and slightly behind the patient while walking, supporting the patient by the gait belt or waist.

ACTION	RATIONALE
• When two caregivers assist, position yourself to the side and slightly behind the patient, supporting the patient by the waist or gait belt. Have the other caregiver carry or manage equipment or provide additional support from the other side.	Gait belts improve the caregiver's grasp, reducing the risk of musculoskeletal injuries to staff and the patient, and allow for a firmer grasp for the caregiver if the patient should lose his or her balance.
• Alternately, when two caregivers assist, stand at the patient's sides (one nurse on each side) with near hands grasping the gait belt and far hands holding the patient's lower arm or hand.	
11. Take several steps forward with the patient. Continue to assess the patient's strength and balance. Remind the patient to stand erect.	Taking several steps with the patient and standing erect promote good balance and stability. Continued assessment helps maintain patient safety.
12. Continue with ambulation for the planned distance and time. Return the patient to the bed or chair based on the patient's tolerance and condition. Remove gait belt.	Ambulation as prescribed promotes activity and prevents fatigue.
13. Ensure the patient is comfortable, with the side rails up and the bed in the lowest position, as necessary. Place call bell and other essential items within reach.	Proper positioning with raised side rails and proper bed height provide for patient comfort and safety. Having the call bell and other essential items within reach promotes safety.
14. Clean transfer aids per facility policy, if not indicated for single patient use. Remove gloves and any other PPE, if used. Perform hand hygiene.	Proper cleaning of equipment between patient use prevents the spread of microorganisms. Removing PPE properly reduces the risk for infection transmission and contamination of other items. Hand hygiene prevents the spread of microorganisms.

EVALUATION

- Patient ambulates safely for the prescribed distance and time and remains free from falls or injury.
- Patient exhibits increasing muscle strength, joint mobility, and independence.
- Patient remains free of any signs and symptoms of immobility.

DOCUMENTATION

- Document the activity, any other pertinent observations, the patient's tolerance of the procedure, and the distance walked. Document the use of transfer aids and the number of staff required for transfer.

SKILL 2 | ASSISTING A PATIENT WITH AMBULATION USING A CANE

Canes are useful for patients who can bear weight but need support for balance. They are also useful for patients who have decreased strength in one leg. Canes provide an additional point of support during ambulation. Canes are made of wood or metal and often have a rubberized cap on the tip to prevent slipping. Canes come in three variations: single-ended canes with half-circle handles (recommended for patients requiring minimal support and for those who will be using stairs frequently); single-ended canes with straight handles (recommended for patients with hand weakness because the handgrip is easier to hold, but not recommended for patients with poor balance); canes with three (tripod) or four prongs (quad cane) or legs to provide a wide base of support (recommended for patients with poor balance). The cane should rise from the floor to the height of the person's waist, and the elbow should be flexed about 30 degrees when holding the cane. The patient holds the cane in the hand opposite the weak or injured leg.

DELEGATION CONSIDERATIONS

Patient teaching regarding use of a cane cannot be delegated to nursing assistive personnel (NAP) or to unlicensed assistive personnel (UAP). Reinforcement or implementation of the use of a cane may be delegated to NAP or UAP. Assisting a patient with ambulation using a cane may be delegated to licensed practical/vocational nurses (LPNs/LVNs). The decision to delegate must be based on careful analysis of the patient's needs and circumstances, as well as the qualifications of the person to whom the task is being delegated. Refer to the Delegation Guidelines in Appendix A.

EQUIPMENT

- Cane of appropriate size with rubber tip
- Nonskid shoes or slippers
- Nonsterile gloves and/or other PPE, as indicated
- Stand-assist aid, if necessary and available
- Gait belt, based on assessment

ASSESSMENT

- Assess the patient's upper body strength, ability to bear weight and to walk, and the need for assistance.
- Review the patient's record for conditions that may affect ambulation.
- Perform a pain assessment before initiating the activity. If the patient reports pain, administer the prescribed medication in sufficient time to allow for the full effect of the analgesic.
- Take vital signs and assess the patient for dizziness or light-headedness with position changes.
- Assess the patient's knowledge regarding the use of a cane.

NURSING DIAGNOSIS

- Risk for Falls
- Impaired Walking
- Deficient Knowledge
- Activity Intolerance

OUTCOME IDENTIFICATION AND PLANNING

- Patient ambulates safely without falls or injury.
- Patient demonstrates proper use of the cane.
- Patient demonstrates increased muscle strength, joint mobility, and independence.
- Patient exhibits no evidence of injury from use of the cane.

IMPLEMENTATION

ACTION	RATIONALE
1. Review the medical record and nursing plan of care for conditions that may influence the patient's ability to move and ambulate. Assess for tubes, IV lines, incisions, or equipment that may alter the procedure for ambulation.	Review of the medical record and plan of care validates the correct patient and correct procedure. Identification of equipment and limitations helps reduce the risk for injury.
2. Perform hand hygiene. Put on PPE, as indicated.	Hand hygiene and PPE prevent the spread of microorganisms. PPE is required based on transmission precautions.

ACTION	RATIONALE

3. Identify the patient. Explain the procedure to the patient. Tell the patient to report any feelings of dizziness, weakness, or shortness of breath while walking. Decide how far to walk.

Patient identification validates the correct patient and correct procedure. Discussion and explanation help allay anxiety and prepare the patient for what to expect.

4. Place the bed in the lowest position, if the patient is in bed.

Proper bed height ensures safety when getting the patient out of bed.

5. Encourage the patient to make use of a stand-assist aid, either freestanding or attached to the side of the bed, if available, to move to the side of the bed.

Use of assistive devices encourages independence, reduces strain for staff, and decreases risk for patient injury.

6. Assist the patient to the side of the bed, if necessary. Have the patient sit on the side of the bed. Assess for dizziness or light-headedness. Have the patient stay seated until he or she feels secure.

Having the patient sit on the side of the bed minimizes the risk for blood pressure changes (orthostatic hypotension) that can occur with position change. Assessing patient complaints helps prevent injury.

7. Assist the patient to put on footwear and a robe, if desired.

Doing so ensures safety and warmth.

8. Wrap the gait belt around the patient's waist, based on assessed need and facility policy.

Gait belts improve the caregiver's grasp, reducing the risk of musculoskeletal injuries to staff and the patient and provide firmer grasp for the caregiver if patient should lose his or her balance.

9. Encourage the patient to make use of the stand-assist device to stand with weight evenly distributed between the feet and the cane.

A stand-assist device reduces strain for the caregiver and decreases the risk for patient injury. Evenly distributed weight provides a broad base of support and balance.

ACTION	RATIONALE

10. Have the patient hold the cane on his or her stronger side, close to the body, while the nurse stands to the side and slightly behind the patient (Figure 1).

Holding the cane on the stronger side helps to distribute the patient's weight away from the involved side and prevents leaning. Positioning to the side and slightly behind the patient encourages the patient to stand and walk erect. It also places the nurse in a safe position if the patient should lose his or her balance or begin to fall.

FIGURE 1 The nurse stands slightly behind the patient. The cane is held on the patient's stronger side, close to the body.

11. Tell the patient to advance the cane 4 to 12 inches (10 to 30 cm) and then, while supporting his or her weight on the stronger leg and the cane, advance the weaker foot forward, parallel with the cane.

Moving in this manner provides support and balance.

12. While supporting his or her weight on the weaker leg and the cane, have the patient advance the stronger leg forward ahead of the cane (heel slightly beyond the tip of the cane).

Moving in this manner provides support and balance.

13. Tell the patient to move the weaker leg forward until it is even with the stronger leg, and then advance the cane again.

This motion provides support and balance.

ACTION	RATIONALE
14. Continue with ambulation for the planned distance and time. Return the patient to the bed or chair based on the patient's tolerance and condition. Remove gait belt.	Continued ambulation promotes activity. Adhering to the planned distance and time prevents the patient from becoming fatigued.
15. Ensure the patient is comfortable, with the side rails up and the bed in the lowest position, as necessary. Place call bell and other essential items within reach.	Proper positioning with raised side rails and proper bed height provides for patient comfort and safety. Having the call bell and other essential items within reach promotes safety.
16. Clean transfer aids per facility policy, if not indicated for single patient use. Remove gloves and any other PPE, if used. Perform hand hygiene.	Proper cleaning of equipment between patient use prevents the spread of microorganisms. Removing PPE properly reduces the risk for infection transmission and contamination of other items. Hand hygiene prevents the spread of microorganisms.

EVALUATION

• Patient uses the cane to ambulate safely and is free from falls or injury.
• Patient demonstrates proper use of the cane.
• Patient exhibits increased muscle strength, joint mobility, and independence.
• Patient experiences no injury related to cane use.

DOCUMENTATION

• Document the activity, any other pertinent observations, the patient's ability to use the cane, the patient's tolerance of the procedure, and the distance walked. Document the use of transfer aids and the number of staff required for transfer.

SKILL 3 | ASSISTING A PATIENT WITH AMBULATION USING CRUTCHES

Crutches enable a patient to walk and remove weight from one or both legs. The patient uses the arms to support the body weight. Crutches can be used for the short or the long term. This section will discuss short-term crutch use. Crutches must be fitted to each person. Have the patient stand up straight with the palm of the hand pressed against the body under the arm. The hand should fit between the top of the crutches and the armpit. When using crutches, the elbow should be slightly bent at about 30 degrees and the hands, not the armpits, should support the patient's weight. Weight on the armpits can cause nerve damage. If anything needs to be carried, it is best to use a backpack (University of Iowa Hospitals and Clinics, 2008). A physical therapist usually teaches the procedure for crutch walking, but it is important for the nurse to be knowledgeable about the patient's progress and the gait being taught. Be prepared to guide the patient at home or in the hospital after the initial teaching is completed. Remind the patient that the support of body weight should be primarily on the hands and arms while using the crutches. There are a number of different ways to walk using crutches, based on how much weight the patient is allowed to bear on one or both legs.

DELEGATION CONSIDERATIONS

Patient teaching regarding use of crutches cannot be delegated to nursing assistive personnel (NAP) or unlicensed assistive personnel (UAP). Reinforcement or implementation of the use of crutches may be delegated to NAP or UAP. Assisting a patient with ambulation using crutches may be delegated to licensed practical/vocational nurses (LPNs/LVNs). The decision to delegate must be based on careful analysis of the patient's needs and circumstances, as well as the qualifications of the person to whom the task is being delegated. Refer to the Delegation Guidelines in Appendix A.

EQUIPMENT

- Crutches with axillary pads, handgrips, and rubber suction tips
- Nonskid shoes or slippers
- PPE, as indicated
- Stand-assist device, as necessary, if available
- Gait belt, based on assessment

ASSESSMENT

- Review the patient's record and nursing plan of care to determine the reason for using crutches and instructions for weight bearing. Check for specific instructions from physical therapy.
- Perform a pain assessment before the time for the activity. If the patient reports pain, administer the prescribed medication in sufficient time to allow for the full effect of the analgesic.
- Determine the patient's knowledge regarding the use of crutches and assess the patient's ability to balance on the crutches.

- Assess for muscle strength in the legs and arms.
- Determine the appropriate gait for the patient to use.

NURSING DIAGNOSIS
- Impaired Walking
- Deficient Knowledge
- Risk for Falls

OUTCOME IDENTIFICATION AND PLANNING
- Patient ambulates safely without experiencing falls or injury.
- Patient demonstrates proper crutch-walking technique.
- Patient demonstrates increased muscle strength and joint mobility.
- Patient exhibits no evidence of injury related to crutch use.

IMPLEMENTATION

ACTION	RATIONALE
1. Review the medical record and nursing plan of care for conditions that may influence the patient's ability to move and ambulate. Assess for tubes, IV lines, incisions, or equipment that may alter the procedure for ambulation. Assess the patient's knowledge and previous experience regarding the use of crutches. Determine that the appropriate size crutch has been obtained.	Reviewing the medical record and plan of care validates the correct patient and correct procedure. Assessment helps identify problem areas to minimize the risk for injury.
2. Perform hand hygiene. Put on PPE, if indicated.	Hand hygiene and PPE prevent the spread of microorganisms. PPE is required based on transmission precautions.
3. Identify the patient. Explain the procedure to the patient. Tell the patient to report any feelings of dizziness, weakness, or shortness of breath while walking. Decide how far to walk.	Patient identification validates the correct patient and correct procedure. Discussion and explanation help allay anxiety and prepare the patient for what to expect.
4. Place the bed in the lowest position, if the patient is in bed.	Proper bed height ensures safety when getting the patient out of bed.

ACTION	RATIONALE
5. Encourage the patient to make use of a stand-assist aid, either free-standing or attached to the side of the bed, if available, to move to the side of the bed.	Use of assistive devices encourages independence, reduces strain for staff, and decreases risk for patient injury.
6. Assist the patient to the side of the bed, if necessary. Have the patient sit on the side of the bed. Assess for dizziness or light-headedness. Have the patient stay seated until he or she feels secure.	Having the patient sit on the side of the bed minimizes the risk for blood pressure changes (orthostatic hypotension) that can occur with position change. Assessing patient complaints helps prevent injury.
7. Assist the patient to put on footwear and a robe, if desired.	Doing so ensures safety and warmth.
8. Wrap the gait belt around the patient's waist, based on assessed need and facility policy.	Gait belts improve the caregiver's grasp, reducing the risk of musculoskeletal injuries to staff and the patient and provide for a firmer grasp if patient should lose his or her balance.
9. Assist the patient to stand erect, face forward in the tripod position (Figure 1). This means the patient holds	Positioning the crutches in this manner provides a wide base of support to increase stability and balance.

FIGURE 1 Assisting the patient to stand erect facing forward in the tripod position.

ACTION	RATIONALE

the crutches 12 inches in front of, and 12 inches to the side of, each foot.

10. For the four-point gait:

   a. Have the patient move the right crutch forward 12 inches and then move the left foot forward to the level of the right crutch.

   b. Then have the patient move the left crutch forward 12 inches and then move the right foot forward to the level of the left crutch.

This movement ensures stability and safety.

11. For the three-point gait:

   a. Have the patient move the affected leg and both crutches forward about 12 inches.

   b. Have the patient move the stronger leg forward to the level of the crutches.

Patient bears weight on the stronger leg.

12. For the two-point gait:

   a. Have the patient move the left crutch and the right foot forward about 12 inches at the same time.

   b. Have the patient move the right crutch and left leg forward to the level of the left crutch at the same time.

Patient bears partial weight on both feet.

13. For the swing-to gait:

   a. Have the patient move both crutches forward about 12 inches.

   b. Have the patient lift the legs and swing them to the crutches, supporting his or her body weight on the crutches.

Swing-to gait provides mobility for patients with weakness or paralysis of the hips or legs.

ACTION	RATIONALE
14. Continue with ambulation for the planned distance and time. Return the patient to the bed or chair based on the patient's tolerance and condition. Remove gait belt.	Continued ambulation promotes activity. Adhering to the planned distance and time prevents the patient from becoming fatigued.
15. Ensure the patient is comfortable, with the side rails up and the bed in the lowest position, as necessary. Place call bell and other essential items within reach.	Proper positioning with raised side rails and proper bed height provide for patient comfort and safety. Having the call bell and other essential items within reach promotes safety.
16. Clean transfer aids per facility policy, if not indicated for single patient use. Remove gloves and any other PPE, if used. Perform hand hygiene.	Proper cleaning of equipment between patient use prevents the spread of microorganisms. Removing PPE properly reduces the risk for infection transmission and contamination of other items. Hand hygiene prevents the spread of microorganisms.

EVALUATION

- Patient demonstrates correct use of crutches to ambulate safely and without injury.
- Patient demonstrates increased muscle strength and joint mobility.
- Patient exhibits no evidence of injury related to crutch use.

DOCUMENTATION

- Document the activity, any other pertinent observations, the patient's ability to use the crutches, the patient's tolerance of the procedure, and the distance walked. Document the use of transfer aids and number of staff required for transfer.

SKILL 4 | ASSISTING A PATIENT WITH AMBULATION USING A WALKER

A walker is a lightweight metal frame with four legs. Walkers provide stability and security for patients with insufficient strength and balance to use other ambulatory aids. There are several kinds of walkers; the choice of which to use is based on the patient's arm strength and balance. Regardless of the type used, the patient stands between the back legs of the walker with arms relaxed at the side; the top of the walker should line up with the crease on the inside of the patient's wrist. When the patient's hands are placed on the grips, elbows should be flexed about 30 degrees (Mayo Clinic, 2011). Usually, the legs of the walker can be adjusted to the appropriate height.

DELEGATION CONSIDERATIONS

Patient teaching regarding use of a walker cannot be delegated to nursing assistive personnel (NAP) or to unlicensed assistive personnel (UAP). Reinforcement or implementation of ambulation using a walker may be delegated to NAP or UAP. Assisting a patient with ambulation using a walker may be delegated to licensed practical/vocational nurses (LPNs/LVNs). The decision to delegate must be based on careful analysis of the patient's needs and circumstances, as well as the qualifications of the person to whom the task is being delegated. Refer to the Delegation Guidelines in Appendix A.

EQUIPMENT

- Walker, adjusted to the appropriate height
- Nonskid shoes or slippers
- Nonsterile gloves and/or other PPE, as indicated
- Additional staff for assistance, as needed
- Stand-assist device, as necessary, if available
- Gait belt, based on assessment

ASSESSMENT

- Assess the patient's ability to walk and the need for assistance.
- Review the patient's record for conditions that may affect ambulation.
- Perform a pain assessment before the time for the activity. If the patient reports pain, administer the prescribed medication in sufficient time to allow for the full effect of the analgesic.
- Take vital signs and assess the patient for dizziness or light-headedness with position changes.
- Assess the patient's knowledge regarding the use of a walker.
- Ensure that the walker is at the appropriate height for the patient.

NURSING DIAGNOSIS

- Risk for Falls
- Impaired Walking
- Deficient Knowledge
- Activity Intolerance

OUTCOME IDENTIFICATION AND PLANNING

- Patient ambulates safely with the walker and is free from falls or injury.
- Patient demonstrates proper use of the walker and states the need for the walker.
- Patient demonstrates increasing muscle strength, joint mobility, and independence.
- Patient remains free of complications of immobility.

IMPLEMENTATION

ACTION	RATIONALE
1. Review the medical record and nursing plan of care for conditions that may influence the patient's ability to move and ambulate, and for specific instructions for ambulation, such as distance. Assess for tubes, IV lines, incisions, or equipment that may alter the procedure for ambulation. Assess the patient's knowledge and previous experience regarding the use of a walker. Identify any movement limitations.	Reviewing the medical record and plan of care validates the correct patient and correct procedure. Checking for equipment and limitations helps minimize the risk for injury.
2. Perform hand hygiene. Put on PPE, if indicated.	Hand hygiene and PPE prevent the spread of microorganisms. PPE is required based on transmission precautions.
3. Identify the patient. Explain the procedure to the patient. Tell the patient to report any feelings of dizziness, weakness, or shortness of breath while walking. Decide how far to walk.	Patient identification validates the correct patient and correct procedure. Discussion and explanation help allay anxiety and prepare the patient for what to expect.
4. Place the bed in the lowest position, if the patient is in bed.	Proper bed height ensures safety when getting the patient out of bed.

ACTION	RATIONALE
5. Encourage the patient to make use of a stand-assist aid, either free-standing or attached to the side of the bed, if available, to move to the side of the bed.	Use of assistive devices encourages independence, reduces strain for staff, and decreases risk for patient injury.
6. Assist the patient to the side of the bed, if necessary. Have the patient sit on the side of the bed. Assess for dizziness or light-headedness. Have the patient stay seated until he or she feels secure.	Having the patient sit on the side of the bed minimizes the risk for blood pressure changes (orthostatic hypotension) that can occur with position change. Assessing patient complaints helps prevent injury.
7. Assist the patient to put on footwear and a robe, if desired.	Doing so ensures safety and warmth.
8. Wrap the gait belt around the patient's waist, based on assessed need and facility policy.	Gait belts improve the caregiver's grasp, reducing the risk of musculoskeletal injuries to staff and the patient and provide for a firmer grasp if patient should lose his or her balance.
9. Place the walker directly in front of the patient. Ask the patient to push him- or herself off the bed or chair; make use of the stand-assist device, or assist the patient to stand. Once the patient is standing, have him or her hold the walker's handgrips firmly and equally. Stand slightly behind the patient, on one side.	Proper positioning with the walker ensures balance. Standing within the walker and holding the handgrips firmly provide stability when moving the walker and helps ensure safety. Positioning to the side and slightly behind the patient encourages the patient to stand and walk erect. It also places the nurse in a safe position if the patient should lose his or her balance or begin to fall.
10. Have the patient move the walker forward 6 to 8 inches and set it down, making sure all four feet of the walker stay on the floor. Then, tell the patient to step forward with either foot into the walker, supporting him- or herself on his or her arms. Follow through with the other leg.	Having all four feet of the walker on the floor provides a broad base of support. Moving the walker and stepping forward moves the center of gravity toward the walker, ensuring balance and preventing tipping of the walker.

ACTION	RATIONALE

11. Move the walker forward again, and continue the same pattern. Continue with ambulation for the planned distance and time (Figure 1). Return the patient to the bed or chair based on the patient's tolerance and condition, ensuring that the patient is comfortable. Remove gait belt.

Moving the walker promotes activity. Continuing for the planned distance and time prevents the patient from becoming fatigued.

FIGURE 1 Assisting the patient to walk with the walker.

12. Ensure the patient is comfortable, with the side rails up and the bed in the lowest position, as necessary. Place call bell and other essential items within reach.

Proper positioning with raised side rails and proper bed height provides for patient comfort and safety. Having the call bell and other essential items within reach promotes safety.

13. Clean transfer aids per facility policy, if not indicated for single patient use. Remove gloves and any other PPE, if used. Perform hand hygiene.

Proper cleaning of equipment between patient use prevents the spread of microorganisms. Removing PPE properly reduces the risk for infection transmission and contamination of other items. Hand hygiene prevents the spread of microorganisms.

EVALUATION
- Patient uses the walker to ambulate safely and remains free of injury.
- Patient exhibits increased muscle strength, joint mobility, and independence.
- Patient demonstrates independent walker use.
- Patient exhibits no evidence of complications of immobility.

DOCUMENTATION
- Document the activity, any other pertinent observations, the patient's ability to use the walker, the patient's tolerance of the procedure, and the distance walked. Document the use of transfer aids and number of staff required for transfer.

SKILL 5 | REMOVING PERIPHERAL ARTERIAL CATHETERS

Arterial catheters, which are used for intensive and continuous cardiac monitoring and intra-arterial access, are ideally placed in the radial, brachial, or dorsalis pedis sites in adults to reduce the risk of infection (O'Grady et al., 2011), although the femoral site can be used as well. As soon as the arterial catheter is no longer needed or has become ineffective, it should be removed (O'Grady et al.). Consult facility policy to determine whether nurses are permitted to perform this procedure. Two nurses should be at the bedside until bleeding is controlled, and are available to give emergency medications, if necessary. The patient should be kept NPO until the catheter is removed in case of nausea with a vasovagal response.

DELEGATION CONSIDERATIONS

Removal of an arterial catheter is not delegated to nursing assistive personnel (NAP), unlicensed assistive personnel (UAP), or licensed practical/vocational nurses (LPN/LVNs).

EQUIPMENT

- Sterile gloves
- Clean gloves
- Goggles or face shield
- Sterile gauze pads
- Waterproof protective pad
- Sterile suture removal set
- Transparent dressing
- Hypoallergenic tape
- For femoral catheter: small sandbag (5 to 10 pounds), wrapped in a towel or pillowcase, based on facility policy
- Emergency medications (e.g., atropine, for a vasovagal response with femoral catheter removal) for emergency response, per facility policy and guidelines
- Indelible pen

ASSESSMENT

- Review the patient's medical record and plan of care for information about discontinuation of the arterial catheter.
- Assess the patient's coagulation status, including laboratory studies, to reduce the risk of complications secondary to impaired clotting ability.
- Assess the patient's understanding of the procedure. Inspect the site for leakage, bleeding, or hematoma.
- Assess skin color and temperature and assess distal pulses for strength and quality. Mark distal pulses with an "X" for easy identification after the procedure.
- Assess the patient's blood pressure; systolic blood pressure should be less than 180 mm Hg before the catheter is removed.

NURSING DIAGNOSIS

- Risk for Injury
- Impaired Skin Integrity
- Risk for Infection
- Anxiety

OUTCOME IDENTIFICATION AND PLANNING

- Catheter is removed intact and without injury to the patient.
- Site remains clean and dry, without evidence of infection, bleeding, or hematoma.

IMPLEMENTATION

ACTION	RATIONALE
1. Verify the order for removal of the arterial catheter in the patient's medical record.	This ensures that the correct intervention is performed on the correct patient.
2. Gather all equipment.	Assembling equipment provides for an organized approach to the task.
3. Perform hand hygiene and put on PPE, if indicated.	Hand hygiene and PPE prevent the spread of microorganisms. PPE is required based on trans-mission precautions.
4. Identify the patient.	Identifying the patient ensures the right patient receives the intervention and helps prevent errors.

ACTION	RATIONALE
5. Close the curtains around the bed and close the door to the room, if possible. Explain the procedure to the patient.	This ensures the patient's privacy. Explanation relieves anxiety and facilitates cooperation.
6. Maintain an IV infusion of normal saline via another venous access during the procedure, as per medical orders or facility guidelines.	IV access may be needed in case of hypotension or bradycardia.
7. If the bed is adjustable, raise it to a comfortable working height, usually elbow height of the caregiver (VISN 8 Patient Safety Center, 2009).	Having the bed at the proper height prevents back and muscle strain.
8. Put on clean gloves, goggles, and gown.	These prevent contact with blood and body fluids.
9. If the catheter being removed is in a femoral site, use Doppler ultrasound to locate the femoral artery 1 to 2 inches above the entrance site of the femoral catheter. Mark with an "X" using an indelible pen.	This ensures accurate location of the femoral artery.
10. Turn off the monitor alarms and then turn off the flow clamp to the flush solution. Carefully remove the dressing over the insertion site. Remove any sutures using the suture removal kit; make sure all sutures have been removed.	These measures help prepare for withdrawal of the catheter.
11. **Withdraw the catheter using a gentle, steady motion. Keep the catheter parallel to the blood vessel during withdrawal. Watch for hematoma formation during catheter removal by gently palpating surrounding tissue. If hematoma starts to form, reposition your hands until optimal pressure is obtained to prevent further leakage of blood.**	Using a gentle, steady motion parallel to the blood vessel reduces the risk for traumatic injury.

ACTION	RATIONALE
12. **Immediately after with-drawing the catheter, apply pressure 1 or 2 inches above the site at the previously marked spot with a sterile 4 × 4 gauze pad. Maintain pressure for at least 10 min-utes, or per facility policy (longer if bleeding or oozing persists).** Apply additional pressure to a femoral site or if the patient has a coagulation abnormality or is receiving anticoagulants (INS, 2011).	If sufficient pressure is not applied, a large, painful hematoma may form.
13. **Assess distal pulses every 3 to 5 minutes while pres-sure is being applied.** Note: Dorsalis pedis and posterior tibial pulses should be mark-edly weaker from baseline if sufficient pressure is applied to the femoral artery.	Assessment of distal pulses determines blood flow to the extremity. Pulses should return to baseline after pressure is released.
14. Cover the site with an appro-priate dressing and secure the dressing with tape. If stipulated by facility policy, make a pressure dressing for a femoral site by folding four sterile 4 × 4 gauze pads in half, and then applying the dressing.	Sufficient pressure is needed to prevent continued bleeding and hematoma formation.
15. Cover the dressing with a tight adhesive bandage, per facility policy. Remove gog-gles and gloves. If the cath-eter was in a femoral site, use these additional interven-tions: Cover the bandage with a sandbag, depending on facility policy. Maintain the patient on bed rest, with the head of the bed elevated less than 30 degrees, for 6 hours with the sandbag in	Sufficient pressure is needed to prevent continued bleeding and hematoma formation. Removing PPE properly reduces the risk for infection transmis-sion and contamination of other items. Raising the head increases intra-abdominal pressure, which could lead to bleeding from the site.

ACTION	RATIONALE

place. Instruct the patient not to lift his or her head while on bed rest. Use logrolling to assist the patient in using the bedpan, if needed.

16. Lower the bed height. Remove additional PPE. Perform hand hygiene. Send specimens to the laboratory immediately.

Lowering the bed promotes patient safety. Removing PPE properly reduces the risk for infection transmission and contamination of other items. Hand hygiene prevents transmission of microorganisms. Specimens must be processed in a timely manner to ensure accuracy.

17. Observe the site for bleeding. Assess circulation in the extremity distal to the site by evaluating color, pulses, and sensation. Repeat this assessment every 15 minutes for the first 1 hour, every 30 minutes for the next 2 hours, hourly for the next 2 hours, then every 4 hours, or according to facility policy.

Continued assessment allows for early detection and prompt intervention should problems arise.

EVALUATION
- Patient exhibits an arterial catheter site that is clean and dry without evidence of injury, infection, bleeding, or hematoma.
- Patient demonstrates intact peripheral circulation and verbalizes a reduction in anxiety.

DOCUMENTATION
- Document the time the catheter was removed and how long pressure was applied. Document site assessment every 5 minutes while pressure is being applied (second nurse can do this). Document assessment of peripheral circulation, appearance of site, type of dressing applied, the timed assessments, patient's response, and any medications given.

Massage has many benefits, including general relaxation and increased circulation. Massage can help alleviate pain. A back massage can be incorporated into the patient's bath, as part of care before bedtime, or at any time to promote increased patient comfort. Some nurses do not always give back massages to patients because they do not think they have sufficient time. However, giving a back massage provides an opportunity for the nurse to observe the skin for signs of breakdown. It also improves circulation; decreases pain, symptom distress, and anxiety; improves sleep quality; and provides a means of communicating with the patient through the use of touch. A back massage also provides cutaneous stimulation as a method of pain relief.

Because some patients consider the back massage a luxury and may be reluctant to accept it, communicate its importance and value to the patient. An effective back massage should take 4 to 6 minutes to complete. A lotion is usually applied; warm it before applying to the back. Be aware of the patient's medical diagnosis when considering giving a back massage. A back massage is contraindicated, for example, when the patient has had back surgery or has fractured ribs. Position the patient on the abdomen or, if this is contraindicated, on the side for a back massage.

DELEGATION CONSIDERATIONS

Providing a back massage may be delegated to nursing assistive personnel (NAP) or to unlicensed assistive personnel (UAP), as well as to licensed practical/vocational nurses (LPN/LVNs). The decision to delegate must be based on careful analysis of the patient's needs and circumstances, as well as the qualifications of the person to whom the task is being delegated. Refer to the Delegation Guidelines in Appendix A.

EQUIPMENT

- Pain assessment tool and pain scale
- Powder, if not contraindicated
- Bath blanket
- Towel
- Nonsterile gloves, if indicated
- Additional PPE, as indicated

ASSESSMENT

- Review the patient's medical record and plan of care for information about the patient's status and contraindications to back massage. Question the patient about any conditions that might require modifications or that might contraindicate a massage.
- Inquire about any allergies, such as to lotions or scents. Ask if the patient has any preferences for lotion or has his or her own lotion.
- Assess the patient's level of pain. Check the patient's medication administration record for the time an analgesic was last administered.

If appropriate, administer an analgesic early enough so that it has time to take effect.

NURSING DIAGNOSIS

• Acute Pain
• Chronic Pain
• Disturbed Sleep Pattern

OUTCOME IDENTIFICATION AND PLANNING

• Patient reports increased comfort and/or decreased pain, and that the patient is relaxed.
• Patient displays decreased anxiety and improved relaxation.
• Patient verbalizes an understanding of the reasons for back massage.

IMPLEMENTATION

ACTION	RATIONALE
1. Perform hand hygiene and put on PPE, if indicated.	Hand hygiene and PPE prevent the spread of microorganisms. PPE is required based on transmission precautions.
2. Identify the patient.	Identifying the patient ensures the right patient receives the intervention and helps prevent errors.
3. Offer a back massage to the patient and explain the procedure.	Explanation encourages patient understanding and cooperation and reduces apprehension.
4. Put on gloves, if indicated.	Gloves are not usually necessary. Gloves prevent contact with blood and body fluid.
5. Close the room door and/or the curtain around the bed.	Closing the door or curtain provides privacy, promotes relaxation, and reduces noise and stimuli that may aggravate pain and reduce comfort.
6. Assess the patient's pain, using an appropriate assessment tool and measurement scale.	Accurate assessment is necessary to guide treatment and pain relief interventions and to evaluate the effectiveness of pain control measures.

ACTION	RATIONALE
7. Raise the bed to a comfortable working position, usually elbow height of the caregiver (VISN 8 Patient Safety Center, 2009), and lower the side rail.	Having the bed at the proper height prevents back and muscle strain.
8. Assist the patient to a comfortable position, preferably the prone or side-lying position. Remove the covers and move the patient's gown just enough to expose the patient's back from the shoulders to sacral area. Drape the patient, as needed, with the bath blanket.	This position exposes an adequate area for massage. Draping the patient provides privacy and warmth.
9. Warm the lubricant or lotion in the palm of your hand, or place the container in small basin of warm water. **During massage, observe the patient's skin for reddened or open areas. Pay particular attention to the skin over bony prominences.**	Cold lotion causes chilling and discomfort. Pressure may interfere with circulation and lead to pressure ulcers.
10. Using light, gliding strokes (*effleurage*), apply lotion to patient's shoulders, back, and sacral area.	Effleurage relaxes the patient and lessens tension.
11. Place your hands beside each other at the base of the patient's spine and stroke upward to the shoulders and back downward to the buttocks in slow, continuous strokes. Continue for several minutes.	Continuous contact is soothing and stimulates circulation and muscle relaxation.
12. Massage the patient's shoulders, entire back, areas over iliac crests, and sacrum with circular stroking motions. **Keep your hands in contact with the patient's skin.** Continue for several minutes, applying additional lotion, as necessary.	A firm stroke with continuous contact promotes relaxation.

ACTION	RATIONALE
13. Knead the patient's skin by gently alternating grasping and compression motions (*pétrissage*).	Kneading increases blood circulation.
14. Complete the massage with additional long, stroking movements that eventually become lighter in pressure.	Long, stroking motions are soothing and promote relaxation; continued stroking with gradual lightening of pressure helps extend the feeling of relaxation.
15. Use the towel to pat the patient dry and to remove excess lotion.	Drying provides comfort and reduces the feeling of moisture on the back.
16. Remove gloves, if worn. Reposition patient's gown and covers. Raise side rail and lower bed. Assist patient to a position of comfort.	Repositioning bedclothes, linens, and the patient helps to promote patient comfort and safety.
17. Remove additional PPE, if used. Perform hand hygiene.	Removing PPE properly reduces the risk for infection transmission and contamination of other items. Hand hygiene prevents transmission of microorganisms.
18. Evaluate the patient's response to this intervention. Reassess level of discomfort or pain using original assessment tools. Reassess and alter plan of care, as appropriate.	Reassessment allows for individualization of the patient's plan of care and promotes optimal patient comfort.

EVALUATION

- Patient reports increased comfort and/or decreased pain.
- Patient displays decreased anxiety and improved relaxation.
- Patient verbalizes an understanding of the reasons for back massage.

DOCUMENTATION

- Document pain assessment and other significant assessments. Document massage use, length of time of massage, and patient response. Record alternative treatments to consider, if appropriate.

Bandages are used to apply pressure over an area, immobilize a body part, prevent or reduce edema, and secure splints and dressings. Bandages can be elasticized or made of gauze, flannel, or muslin. In general, narrow bandages are used to wrap feet, the lower legs, hands, and arms, and wider bandages are used for the thighs and trunk. A roller bandage is a continuous strip of material wound on itself to form a roll. The free end is anchored and the roll is passed or rolled around the body part, maintaining equal tension with all turns. The bandage is unwound gradually and only as needed. The bandage should overlap itself evenly and by one-half to two-thirds the width of the bandage. The figure-eight turn consists of oblique overlapping turns that ascend and descend alternately. It is used around the knee, elbow, ankle, and wrist.

DELEGATION CONSIDERATIONS

The application of a figure-eight bandage may not be delegated to nursing assistive personnel (NAP) or to unlicensed assistive personnel (UAP). The application of a figure-eight bandage may be delegated to licensed practical/vocational nurses (LPN/LVNs). The decision to delegate must be based on careful analysis of the patient's needs and circumstances, as well as the qualifications of the person to whom the task is being delegated. Refer to the Delegation Guidelines in Appendix A.

EQUIPMENT

- Elastic or other bandage of the appropriate width
- Tape, pins, or self-closures
- Gauze pads
- Nonsterile gloves and/or other PPE, as indicated

ASSESSMENT

- Review the medical record and nursing plan of care and assess the situation to determine the need for a bandage.
- Assess the affected limb for pain and edema.
- Perform a neurovascular assessment of the affected extremity. Assess body parts distal to the site for evidence of cyanosis, pallor, coolness, numbness, tingling, and swelling and absent or diminished pulses. Assess the distal circulation of the extremity after the bandage is in place and at least every 4 hours thereafter.

NURSING DIAGNOSIS

- Impaired Physical Mobility
- Risk for Peripheral Neurovascular Dysfunction
- Risk for Impaired Skin Integrity

OUTCOME IDENTIFICATION AND PLANNING

- Bandage is applied correctly without injury or complications.
- Patient maintains circulation to the affected part and remains free of neurovascular complications.

IMPLEMENTATION

ACTION	RATIONALE
1. Review the medical record and nursing plan of care to determine the need for a figure-eight bandage.	Reviewing the medical record and plan of care validates the correct patient and correct procedure and reduces risk for injury.
2. Perform hand hygiene. Put on PPE, as indicated.	Hand hygiene and PPE prevent the spread of microorganisms. PPE is required based on transmission precautions.
3. Identify the patient. Explain the procedure to the patient.	Patient identification validates the correct patient and correct procedure. Discussion and explanation help allay anxiety and prepare the patient for what to expect.
4. Close the curtains around the bed and close the door to the room, if possible. Place the bed at an appropriate and comfortable working height, usually elbow height of the caregiver (VISN 8 Patient Safety Center, 2009).	Closing the door or curtains provides privacy. Proper bed height helps reduce back strain.
5. Assist the patient to a comfortable position, with the affected body part in a normal functioning position.	Keeping the body part in a normal functioning position promotes circulation and prevents deformity and discomfort.
6. Hold the bandage roll with the roll facing upward in one hand while holding the free end of the roll in the other hand. Make sure to hold the bandage roll so it is close to the affected body part.	Proper handling of the bandage allows application of even tension and pressure.

ACTION	RATIONALE

7. Wrap the bandage around the limb twice, below the joint, to anchor it (Figure 1).

Anchoring the bandage ensures that it will stay in place.

FIGURE 1 Wrapping the bandage around the patient's limb twice, below the joint, to anchor it.

8. Use alternating ascending and descending turns to form a figure eight (Figure 2). Overlap each turn of the bandage by one-half to two-thirds the width of the strip (Figure 3).

Making alternating ascending and descending turns helps to ensure the bandage will stay in place on a moving body part.

FIGURE 2 Using alternating ascending and descending turns to form a figure eight.

FIGURE 3 Overlapping each turn of the bandage by one-half to two-thirds the width of the strip.

9. Unroll the bandage as you wrap, not before wrapping.

Unrolling the bandage with wrapping prevents uneven pressure, which could interfere with blood circulation.

10. **Wrap firmly, but not tightly. Assess the patient's comfort as you wrap. If the patient reports tingling, itching, numbness, or pain, loosen the bandage.**

Firm wrapping is necessary to provide support and prevent injury, but wrapping too tightly interferes with circulation. Patient complaints are helpful indicators of possible circulatory compromise.

11. After the area is covered, wrap the bandage around the limb twice, above the joint, to anchor it. Secure the end

Anchoring at the end ensures the bandage will stay in place. Metal clips can cause injury.

ACTION	RATIONALE

of the bandage with tape, pins, or self-closures. Avoid metal clips.

12. Place the bed in the lowest position, with the side rails up. Make sure the call bell and other necessary items are within easy reach.

Repositioning the bed and having items nearby ensure patient safety.

13. Remove PPE, if used. Perform hand hygiene.

Removing PPE properly reduces the risk for infection transmission and contamination of other items. Hand hygiene prevents the spread of microorganisms.

14. Elevate the wrapped extremity for 15 to 30 minutes after application of the bandage.

Elevation promotes venous return and reduces edema.

15. Assess the distal circulation after the bandage is in place.

Elastic may tighten as it is wrapped. Frequent assessment of distal circulation ensures patient safety and prevents injury.

16. Lift the distal end of the bandage and assess the skin for color, temperature, and integrity. Assess for pain and perform a neurovascular assessment of the affected extremity after applying the bandage and at least every 4 hours, thereafter, or per facility policy.

Assessment aids in prompt detection of compromised circulation and allows for early intervention for skin irritation and other complications.

EVALUATION

- Patient exhibits a bandage that is applied correctly, without causing injury or neurovascular compromise.
- Patient demonstrates proper alignment of the bandaged body part.
- Patient remains free of evidence of complications.
- Patient demonstrates an understanding of signs and symptoms to report immediately.

DOCUMENTATION

- Document the time, date, and site that the bandage was applied and the size of the bandage used. Include the skin assessment and care provided before application. Document the patient's response to the bandage and the neurovascular status of the extremity.

Some patients must remain in bed as a part of their therapeutic regimen, but can still bathe themselves. Other patients are not on bed rest, but require total or partial assistance with bathing in bed due to physical limitations, such as fatigue or limited range of motion. A bed bath may be considered a partial bed bath if the patient is well enough to perform most of the bath, and the nurse needs to assist with washing areas that the patient cannot reach easily. A partial bath may also refer to bathing only those body parts that absolutely have to be cleaned, such as the perineal area, and any soiled body parts. Perform bathing in a matter-of-fact and dignified manner. If this approach is followed, patients generally do not find care by a person of the opposite gender to be offensive or embarrassing. Make any necessary adaptations for individual patients. For example, if the patient is confused and becomes agitated as a result of overstimulation when bathing, reduce the stimuli. Turn down the lights and play soft music and/or warm the room before giving the patient a bath (Johnson, 2011). This skill reviews providing a bed bath using water and cleanser. Refer to the Skill Variation at the end of the skill for guidelines to use a disposable bathing system.

DELEGATION CONSIDERATIONS

The implementation of a shower or tub bath may be delegated to nursing assistive personnel (NAP) or to unlicensed assistive personnel (UAP), as well as to licensed practical/vocational nurses (LPN/LVNs). The decision to delegate must be based on careful analysis of the patient's needs and circumstances, as well as the qualifications of the person to whom the task is being delegated. Refer to the Delegation Guidelines in Appendix A.

EQUIPMENT

- Washbasin and warm water or disposable bathing system
- Personal hygiene supplies (deodorant, lotion, and others)
- Skin-cleaning agent
- Emollient and skin barrier, as indicated
- Towels (2)
- Washcloths (2)
- Bath blanket
- Gown or pajamas
- Bedpan or urinal
- Laundry bag
- Nonsterile gloves; other PPE, as indicated

ASSESSMENT

- Assess the patient's knowledge of hygiene practices and bathing preferences: frequency, time of day, and type of hygiene products.
- Assess for any physical-activity limitations.
- Assess the patient's ability to bathe him- or herself.
- Assess the patient's skin for dryness, redness, or areas of breakdown.

NURSING DIAGNOSIS

- Bathing Self-Care Deficit
- Impaired Skin Integrity
- Risk for Infection
- Risk for Impaired Skin Integrity

OUTCOME IDENTIFICATION AND PLANNING

- The patient will be clean and fresh.
- The patient regains feelings of control by assisting with the bath.
- The patient verbalizes positive body image.
- The patient demonstrates understanding about the need for cleanliness.

IMPLEMENTATION

ACTION	RATIONALE
1. Review the patient's health record for any limitations in physical activity.	Identifying limitations prevents patient discomfort and injury.
2. Perform hand hygiene and 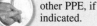 put on gloves and/or other PPE, if indicated.	Hand hygiene and PPE prevent the spread of microorganisms. PPE is required based on transmission precautions.
3. Identify the patient. Discuss the procedure with the patient and assess the patient's ability to assist in the bathing process, as well as personal hygiene preferences.	Identifying the patient ensures the right patient receives the intervention and helps prevent errors. Discussion promotes reassurance and provides knowledge about the procedure. Dialogue encourages patient participation and allows for individualized nursing care.
4. Assemble equipment on overbed table within reach.	Organization facilitates performance of the task.
5. Close the curtains around the bed and close the door to the room, if possible. Adjust the room temperature, if necessary.	This ensures the patient's privacy and lessens the risk for loss of body heat during the bath.
6. Adjust the bed to a comfortable working height; usually elbow height of the caregiver (VISN 8 Patient Safety Center, 2009).	Having the bed at the proper height prevents back and muscle strain.

ACTION	RATIONALE
7. Remove sequential compression devices and antiembolism stockings from lower extremities according to agency protocol.	Most manufacturers and agencies recommend removal of these devices before the bath to allow for assessment.
8. Put on gloves. Offer patient bedpan or urinal.	Gloves are necessary for potential contact with blood or body fluids. Voiding or defecating before the bath lessens the likelihood that the bath will be interrupted, because warm bath water may stimulate the urge to void.
9. Remove gloves and perform hand hygiene.	Hand hygiene deters the spread of microorganisms.
10. Put on a clean pair of gloves. Lower side rail nearest to you and assist patient to side of bed where you will work. Have patient lie on his or her back.	Gloves prevent transmission of microorganisms. Having the patient positioned near the nurse and lowering the side rail prevent unnecessary stretching and twisting of muscles on the part of the nurse.
11. Loosen top covers and remove all except the top sheet. Place bath blanket over patient and then remove top sheet while patient holds bath blanket in place. If linen is to be reused, fold it over a chair. Place soiled linen in laundry bag. Take care to prevent linen from coming in contact with your clothing.	The patient is not exposed unnecessarily, and warmth is maintained. If a bath blanket is unavailable, the top sheet may be used in its place.
12. Remove patient's gown and keep bath blanket in place. If patient has an IV line and is not wearing a gown with snap sleeves, remove gown from other arm first. Lower the IV container and pass gown over the tubing and	This provides uncluttered access during the bath and maintains warmth of the patient. IV fluids must be maintained at the prescribed rate.

ACTION	RATIONALE
the container. **Rehang the container and check the drip rate.**	
13. **Raise side rails.** Fill basin with a sufficient amount of comfortably warm water (100°F to 120°F–125°F). Add the skin cleanser, if appropriate, according to manufacturer's directions. Change as necessary throughout the bath. Lower side rail nearest to you when you return to the bedside to begin the bath.	Side rails maintain patient safety. Adjusting the water temperature to 100°F to less than 120°F to 125°F decreases risk of burns and drying of the skin. The lower temperature is recommended for children and adults over 65 years of age (Burn Foundation, 2012). Warm water is comfortable and relaxing for the patient. It also stimulates circulation and provides for more effective cleansing.
14. Put on gloves, if necessary. If desired, fold the washcloth like a mitt on your hand so that there are no loose ends.	Gloves are necessary if there is potential contact with blood or body fluids. Having loose ends of cloth drag across the patient's skin is uncomfortable. Loose ends cool quickly and feel cold to the patient.
15. Lay a towel across the patient's chest and on top of bath blanket.	This prevents chilling and keeps the bath blanket dry.
16. **With no cleanser on the washcloth, wipe one eye from the inner part of the eye, near the nose, to the outer part. Rinse or turn the cloth before washing the other eye.**	Soap is irritating to the eyes. Moving from the inner to the outer aspect of the eye prevents carrying debris toward the nasolacrimal duct. Rinsing or turning the washcloth prevents spreading organisms from one eye to the other.
17. Bathe patient's face, neck, and ears. Apply appropriate emollient.	Use of emollients is recommended to restore and maintain skin integrity (Voegeli, 2010).
18. Expose patient's far arm and place towel lengthwise under it. Using firm strokes, wash hand, arm, and axilla, lifting the arm as necessary to access axillary region. Rinse, if necessary, and dry. Apply appropriate emollient.	The towel helps to keep the bed dry. Washing the far side first eliminates contaminating a clean area once it is washed. Gentle friction stimulates circulation and muscles and helps remove dirt, oil, and organisms. Long, firm strokes are relaxing and

ACTION	RATIONALE
	more comfortable than short, uneven strokes. Rinsing is necessary when using some cleansing products. Use of emollients is recommended to restore and maintain skin integrity (Voegeli, 2010).
19. Place a folded towel on the bed next to the patient's hand and put basin on it. Soak the patient's hand in basin. Wash, rinse if necessary, and dry hand. Apply appropriate emollient.	Placing the hand in the basin of water is an additional comfort measure for the patient. It facilitates thorough washing of the hands and between the fingers and aids in removing debris from under the nails. Use of emollients is recommended to restore and maintain skin integrity (Voegeli, 2010).
20. Repeat Actions 18 and 19 for the arm nearest you. An option for the nurse who is shorter or susceptible to back strain might be to bathe one side of the patient first and then move to the other side of the bed to complete the bath.	
21. Spread a towel across patient's chest. Lower bath blanket to patient's umbilical area. Wash, rinse, if necessary, and dry chest. Keep chest covered with towel between the wash and rinse. Pay special attention to the folds of skin under the breasts. Apply appropriate emollient.	Exposing, washing, rinsing, and drying one part of the body at a time avoids unnecessary exposure and chilling. Areas of skin folds may be sources of odor and skin breakdown if not cleaned and dried properly. Use of emollients is recommended to restore and maintain skin integrity (Voegeli, 2010).
22. Lower bath blanket to the perineal area. Place a towel over patient's chest.	Keeping the bath blanket and towel in place avoids exposure and chilling.
23. Wash, rinse, if necessary, and dry abdomen. Carefully inspect and clean umbilical area and any abdominal folds or creases. Apply appropriate emollient.	Skin-fold areas may be sources of odor and skin breakdown if not cleaned and dried properly. Use of emollients is recommended to restore and maintain skin integrity (Voegeli, 2010).

ACTION	RATIONALE

24. Return bath blanket to original position and expose far leg. Place towel under far leg. Using firm strokes, wash, rinse, if necessary, and dry leg from ankle to knee and knee to groin. Apply appropriate emollient.

The towel protects linens and prevents the patient from feeling uncomfortable from a damp or wet bed. Washing from ankle to groin with firm strokes promotes venous return. Use of emollients is recommended to restore and maintain skin integrity (Voegeli, 2010).

25. Wash, rinse if necessary, and dry the foot. Pay particular attention to the areas between toes. Apply appropriate emollient.

Drying of the feet is important to prevent irritation, possible skin breakdown, and infections (National Institute on Aging, 2012). Use of emollients is recommended to restore and maintain skin integrity (Voegeli, 2010).

26. Repeat Actions 24 and 25 for the other leg and foot.

27. Make sure patient is covered with bath blanket. Change water and washcloth at this point or earlier, if necessary.

The bath blanket maintains warmth and privacy. Clean, warm water prevents chilling and maintains patient comfort.

28. Assist patient to a prone or side-lying position. Put on gloves, if not applied earlier. Position bath blanket and towel to expose only the back and buttocks.

Positioning the towel and bath blanket protects the patient's privacy and provides warmth. Gloves prevent contact with body fluids.

29. Wash, rinse, if necessary, and dry back and buttocks area. **Pay particular attention to cleansing between gluteal folds, and observe for any redness or skin breakdown in the sacral area.**

Fecal material near the anus may be a source of microorganisms. Prolonged pressure on the sacral area or other bony prominences may compromise circulation and lead to development of decubitus ulcer.

30. If not contraindicated, give patient a backrub, as described in Skill 6. Alternatively, back massage may be given after perineal care. Apply appropriate emollient and/or skin barrier product.

A backrub improves circulation to the tissues and is an aid to relaxation. A backrub may be contraindicated in patients with cardiovascular disease or musculoskeletal injuries. Use of emollients is recommended to restore and maintain skin integrity (Voegeli, 2010). Skin barriers

ACTION	RATIONALE
	protect the skin from damage caused by excessive exposure to water and irritants, such as urine and feces.
31. Raise the side rail. Refill basin with clean water. Discard washcloth and towel. Remove gloves and put on clean gloves.	The washcloth, towel, and water are contaminated after washing the patient's gluteal area. Changing to clean supplies decreases the spread of organisms from the anal area to the genitals.
32. Clean perineal area or set patient up so that he or she can complete perineal self-care. If the patient is unable to do so, lower the side rail and complete perineal care. Follow the guidelines in the accompanying Skill Variation. Apply skin barrier, as indicated. Raise side rail, remove gloves, and perform hand hygiene.	Providing perineal self-care may decrease embarrassment for the patient. Effective perineal care reduces odor and decreases the risk for infection through contamination. Skin barriers protect the skin from damage caused by excessive exposure to water and irritants, such as urine and feces.
33. Help patient put on a clean gown and assist with the use of other personal toiletries, such as deodorant or cosmetics.	This provides for the patient's warmth and comfort.
34. Protect pillow with towel and groom patient's hair.	
35. **When finished, make sure the patient is comfortable, with the side rails up and the bed in the lowest position.**	Proper positioning with raised side rails and proper bed height provide for patient comfort and safety.
36. Change bed linens, as described in Skills 11 and 12. Dispose of soiled linens according to facility policy. Clean bath basin according to facility policy before returning to storage at bedside. Remove gloves and any other PPE, if used. Perform hand hygiene.	Proper disposal of linens and cleaning of bath basin reduces the risk for transmission of microorganisms. Removing PPE properly reduces the risk for infection transmission and contamination of other items. Hand hygiene prevents the spread of microorganisms.

EVALUATION

- Patient is clean.
- Patient demonstrates some feeling of control in his or her care.
- Patient verbalizes an improved body image.
- Patient verbalizes the importance of cleanliness.

DOCUMENTATION

- Record any significant observations and communication. Document the condition of the patient's skin. Record the procedure, amount of assistance given, and patient participation. Document the application of skin care products, such as a skin barrier.

SKILL VARIATION | **Performing Perineal Cleansing**

Perineal care may be carried out while the patient remains in bed. Perform perineal cleaning in a matter-of-fact and dignified manner. If this approach is followed, patients generally do not find care by a person of the opposite gender to be offensive or embarrassing. When performing perineal care, follow these guidelines:

1. Perform hand hygiene and put on PPE, if indicated.

2. Identify the patient.

3. Explain what you are going to do and the reason for doing it to the patient.
4. Assemble necessary equipment on the bedside stand or overbed table.
5. Close the curtains around the bed and close the door to the room, if possible.
6. Put on gloves. Cover the patient with a bath blanket

and remove top linens to expose only the perineal area. Wash and rinse the groin area (both male and female patients):

- **For a female patient,** spread the labia and move the washcloth from the pubic area toward the anal area to prevent carrying organisms from the anal area back over the genital area (Figure A). Always proceed from the least contaminated area to the most contaminated area. Use a clean portion of the washcloth for each stroke. Rinse the washed areas well with plain water.
- **For a male patient,** clean the tip of the penis first, moving the washcloth in a circular motion from the meatus outward. Wash the shaft of the penis using downward strokes toward the pubic area (Figure B). Always proceed from the least contaminated area to the most contaminated

continued on page 40

Performing Perineal Cleansing *continued*

FIGURE A Performing female perineal care.

FIGURE B Performing male perineal care.

area. Rinse the washed areas well with plain water. In an *uncircumcised male patient* (teenage or older), retract the foreskin (prepuce) while washing the penis. **It is not recommended to retract the foreskin for cleaning during infancy and childhood, because injury and scarring could occur (MedlinePlus, 2012).**

• Pull the *uncircumcised male patient's* foreskin back into place over the glans penis to prevent constriction of the penis, which may result in edema and tissue injury. Wash and rinse the male patient's scrotum. Handle the scrotum, which houses the testicles, with care because the area is sensitive.

7. Dry the cleaned areas and apply an emollient, as indicated. Apply skin barrier (protectant) to area, as indicated. Avoid the use of powder. Powder may become a medium for bacteria growth.

Performing Perineal Cleansing *continued*

8. Turn the patient on his or her side and continue cleansing the anal area. Continue in the direction of least contaminated to most contaminated area. In the female, cleanse from the vagina toward the anus. In both female and male patients, change the wash-cloth with each stroke until the area is clean. Rinse and dry the area. Apply skin barrier (protectant) to area, as indicated.

9. Remove gloves and perform hand hygiene. Continue with additional care as necessary.

SKILL VARIATION | **Giving a Bath Using a Disposable Self-contained Bathing System**

A disposable bathing system is packaged with 8 to 10 premoistened disposable washcloths. If more than 8 cloths are available in the package, use a separate cloth for hands and feet. When giving a bath with a disposable system, follow these guidelines:

1. Warm the unopened package in the microwave, according to manufacturer's directions or remove package from storage warmer.

2. Perform hand hygiene and put on PPE, if indicated.

3. Identify the patient.

4. Explain what you are going to do and the reason for doing it to the patient.

5. Assemble necessary equipment on the bedside stand or overbed table.

6. Close the curtains around the bed and close the door to the room, if possible.

7. Put on gloves. Cover the patient with a bath blanket and remove top linens. Remove patient's gown and keep the bath blanket in place.

8. Remove first cloth from the package. Wipe one eye from the inner part of the eye, near the nose, to the outer part. Use a different part of the cloth for the other eye.

9. Bathe the face, neck, and ears. Allow the skin to air dry for approximately 30 seconds, according to manufacturer's directions. Air drying allows the emollient ingredient of the cleanser to remain on the skin. Alternately, dry the skin with a towel, based on the product used. Apply appropriate emollient. Dispose of cloth in trash receptacle.

continued on page 42

Giving a Bath Using a Disposable Self-contained Bathing System *continued*

10. Expose the patient's far arm. Remove another cloth. Using firm strokes, wash hand, arm, and axilla. Allow the skin to air dry for approximately 30 seconds, according to manufacturer's directions. Air drying allows the emollient ingredient of the cleanser to remain on the skin. Alternately, dry the skin with a towel, based on the product used. Apply appropriate emollient. Dispose of cloth in trash receptacle. Cover arm with blanket.

11. Repeat for nearer arm with a new cloth. Cover arm with blanket.

12. Expose the patient's chest. Remove new cloth and cleanse chest. Allow the skin to air dry for approximately 30 seconds, according to manufacturer's directions. Cover chest with a towel. Expose patient's abdomen. Cleanse abdomen. Allow the skin to air dry for approximately 30 seconds, according to manufacturer's directions. Air drying allows the emollient ingredient of the cleanser to remain on the skin. Alternately, dry the skin with a towel, based on the product used. Apply appropriate emollient. Dispose of cloth in trash receptacle. Cover patient's body with blanket.

13. Expose far leg. Remove new cloth and cleanse leg and foot. Allow the skin to air dry for approximately 30 seconds, according to manufacturer's directions. Air drying allows the emollient ingredient of the cleanser to remain on the skin. Alternately, dry the skin with a towel, based on the product used. Apply appropriate emollient. Dispose of cloth in trash receptacle. Cover patient's leg with blanket.

14. Repeat for nearer leg with a new cloth. Cover leg with blanket.

15. Assist patient to prone or side-lying position. Put on gloves, if not applied earlier. Position blanket to expose back and buttocks. Remove a new cloth and cleanse back and buttocks area. Allow the skin to air dry for approximately 30 seconds, according to manufacturer's directions. Air drying allows the emollient ingredient of the cleanser to remain on the skin. Alternately, dry the skin with a towel, based on the product used. Apply appropriate emollient. Dispose of cloth in trash receptacle. If not contraindicated, give the patient a back massage. Apply skin barrier, as indicated. Cover patient with blanket.

16. Remove gloves and put on clean gloves. Remove last cloth and cleanse the perineal area. Refer to the guidelines in the previous Skill Variation. Dispose of

Giving a Bath Using a Disposable Self-contained Bathing System   *continued*

cloth in trash receptacle. Apply skin barrier, as indicated.

17. Remove gloves. Assist the patient to put on a clean gown. Perform hand hygiene. Assist with the use of other personal toiletries.

18. Change bed linens as described in Skills 11 and 12. Dispose of soiled linens according to facility policy.

19. Remove gloves and additional PPE, if used. Perform hand hygiene.

SKILL 9   ASSISTING WITH A SHOWER OR TUB BATH

A shower may be the preferred method of bathing for patients who are ambulatory and able to tolerate the activity. Tub baths may be an option, particularly in long-term care or other community-based settings, depending on facility policy. Make any necessary adaptations for individual patients. For example, if the patient is confused and becomes agitated as a result of overstimulation when bathing, reduce the stimuli. Turn down the lights and play soft music and/or warm the room before taking the patient into it (Johnson, 2011). Bathing is performed in a matter-of-fact and dignified manner. If this approach is followed, patients generally do not find care by a person of the opposite gender to be offensive or embarrassing.

DELEGATION CONSIDERATIONS

The implementation of a shower or tub bath may be delegated to nursing assistive personnel (NAP) or unlicensed assistive personnel (UAP), as well as to licensed practical/vocational nurses (LPN/LVNs). The decision to delegate must be based on careful analysis of the patient's needs and circumstances, as well as the qualifications of the person to whom the task is being delegated. Refer to the Delegation Guidelines in Appendix A.

EQUIPMENT

- Personal hygiene supplies (deodorant, lotion, and others)
- Skin-cleaning agent
- Emollient and skin barrier, as indicated
- Towels and washcloths
- Robe and slippers or nonskid socks
- Gown or pajamas, or clothing
- Laundry bag
- Shower or tub chair, as needed
- Nonsterile gloves, as indicated
- Additional PPE, as indicated

ASSESSMENT

- Assess the patient's knowledge of hygiene practices and bathing preferences: frequency, time of day, and type of hygiene products.
- Assess for any physical-activity limitations.
- Assess the patient's ability to bathe him- or herself.
- Assess the patient's skin for dryness, redness, or areas of break-down, and gather any other appropriate supplies that may be needed as a result of the assessment.

NURSING DIAGNOSIS

- Bathing Self-Care Deficit
- Risk for Infection
- Risk for Impaired Skin Integrity
- Deficient Knowledge

OUTCOME IDENTIFICATION AND PLANNING

- Patient will be clean and fresh, and without injury.
- Patient regains feelings of control by assisting with the bath.
- Patient verbalizes positive body image.
- Patient demonstrates understanding about the need for cleanliness.

IMPLEMENTATION

ACTION	RATIONALE
1. Review the patient's health record for any limitations in physical activity. Check presence of medical order for clearing the patient to shower, if required by facility policy.	Identifying limitations prevents patient discomfort and injury. In some settings, a medical order is required for showering.
2. Check to see that the bathroom is available, clean, and safe. Make sure showers and tubs have mats or nonskid strips to prevent patients from falling. Place a mat or towel on floor in front of shower or tub. Put a shower or tub chair in place, as appropriate. Place 'occupied' sign on door of room.	A clean bathroom prevents transmission of microorganisms. Mats and nonskid materials prevent patients from slipping and falling. Having a place for a weak or physically disabled patient to sit in a shower prevents falls; warm water could cause vasodilation and pooling of blood in lower extremities, contributing to light-headedness or dizziness. Use of sign allows others to be aware of use of room and ensures patient privacy.

ACTION	RATIONALE

3. Gather necessary hygienic and toiletry items, and linens. Place within easy reach of shower or tub.

Bringing everything to the bathing location conserves time and energy. Arranging items nearby is convenient, saves time, and avoids unnecessary reaching and possible falls.

4. Perform hand hygiene.

Hand hygiene prevents the spread of microorganisms.

5. Identify the patient. Discuss the procedure with the patient and assess the patient's ability to assist in the bathing process, as well as personal hygiene preferences.

Identifying the patient ensures the right patient receives the intervention and helps prevent errors. Discussion promotes reassurance and provides knowledge about the procedure. Dialogue encourages patient participation and allows for individualized nursing care.

6. Assist patient to bathroom to void or defecate, if appropriate.

Voiding or defecating before the bath lessens the likelihood that the bath will be interrupted, because warm bath water may stimulate the urge to void.

7. Assist the patient to put on a robe and slippers or nonskid socks. Cover IV access site(s) according to facility policy.

This ensures the patient's privacy, prevents chilling, and decreases the risk for slipping and falling. Coverage of IV site prevents loosening of dressings from exposure to moisture, and maintains integrity of IV access.

8. Assist the patient to the shower or tub.

This prevents accidental falls.

9. Close the curtains around the shower or tub, as appropriate and close the door to the bathroom. Adjust the room temperature, if necessary.

Shower: Turn shower on. Check to see that the water temperature is safe and comfortable.

This ensures the patient's privacy and lessens the risk for loss of body heat during the bath. Adjusting the water temperature to 100°F to less than 120°F to 125°F decreases risk of burns and drying of the skin. The lower temperature is recommended for children and adults over 65 years

ACTION	RATIONALE

Tub: Fill tub halfway with water. Check to see that the water temperature is safe and comfortable.

Water temperature should be 100°F to less than 120°F to 125°F.

of age (Burn Foundation, 2012). Warm water is relaxing, stimulates circulation, and provides for more effective cleansing.

10. Explain the use of the call device and ensure that it is within reach of the shower or tub.

Use of the call device allows the patient to call for help if necessary.

11. Put on gloves, as indicated. Help the patient get in and out of the shower or tub, as necessary. Use safety bars. For a tub: Have the patient grasp the handrails at the side of the tub, or place a chair at the side of the tub. The patient sits on the chair and eases to the edge of the tub. After putting both feet into the tub, have the patient reach to the opposite side and ease down into the tub. The patient may kneel first in the tub and then sit in it.

Gloves are required if contact with blood or body fluids is anticipated. Gloves prevent the transmission of microorganisms.

This prevents slipping and falling.

12. If necessary, use a hydraulic lift, when available, to lower patients who are unable to maneuver safely or completely bear their own weight. Some community-based settings have walk-in tubs available.

This prevents slipping and falling and prevents strain and injury to patients and nurses.

13. Adjust water temperature if appropriate, based on patient preference. Keep room door unlocked. Remain in room with patient to offer assistance, as appropriate. If assistance is needed with bathing, put on gloves. Otherwise, check on patient every 5 minutes.

These actions promote safety. Health personnel should be able to enter with ease if the patient needs help. Gloves are required if contact with blood or body fluids is anticipated. Gloves prevent the transmission of microorganisms.

ACTION	RATIONALE
Never leave young children or confused patients alone in the bathroom.	
14. Assist patient out of shower or tub when bathing is complete. Obtain the assistance of additional personnel as appropriate. Use safety bars. For a tub: Drain the water from the tub. Have the patient grasp the handrails at the side of the tub. Assist the patient to the edge of the tub. Have the patient ease to a chair placed at the side of the tub, then remove feet out of tub. The patient may kneel first in the tub and then move to the side of the tub.	This prevents slipping and falling. Use of additional personnel prevents strain and injury to patients and nurses.
15. If necessary, use a hydraulic lift, when available, to raise patients who are unable to maneuver safely or completely bear their own weight.	This prevents slipping and falling and prevents strain and injury to patients and nurses.
16. Put on gloves, as indicated. Assist the patient with drying, application of emollients, and dressing as appropriate or necessary. Remove cover from IV access site.	Gloves are required if contact with blood or body fluids is anticipated. Gloves prevent the transmission of microorganisms. Prevents chilling and promotes patient comfort. Use of emollients is recommended to restore and maintain skin integrity (Voegeli, 2010).
17. Remove gloves, if used. Assist patient to room and into a position of comfort.	Removing gloves properly reduces risk for infection transmission and contamination of other items. Promotes patient comfort and safety.
18. Clean shower or tub according to facility policy. Dispose of soiled linens according to facility policy. Remove 'occupied' sign from door of bathroom.	Reduces risk for infection transmission and contamination of other items. Allows others to make use of room.

ACTION	RATIONALE
19. Perform hand hygiene.	Hand hygiene prevents the spread of microorganisms.

EVALUATION

The expected outcomes are met when the patient is clean; demonstrates some feeling of control in his or her care; verbalizes an improved body image; and verbalizes the importance of cleanliness.

DOCUMENTATION

• Record any significant observations and communication. Document the condition of the patient's skin. Record the procedure, amount of assistance given, and patient participation. Document the application of skin care products, such as an emollient.

SKILL 10 ASSISTING WITH A SITZ BATH

Sitz baths are a method of applying tepid or warm water to the perineal or rectal areas by sitting in a basin filled with this water. A sitz bath can help relieve pain and discomfort in the perineal area, such as after childbirth or surgery, and can increase circulation to the tissues, promoting healing.

DELEGATION CONSIDERATIONS

Assisting with a sitz bath may be delegated to nursing assistive personnel (NAP) or to unlicensed assistive personnel (UAP), as well as to licensed practical/vocational nurses (LPN/LVNs). The decision to delegate must be based on careful analysis of the patient's needs and circumstances, as well as the qualifications of the person to whom the task is being delegated. Refer to the Delegation Guidelines in Appendix A.

EQUIPMENT

• Clean gloves
• Additional PPE, as indicated
• Towel
• Adjustable IV pole
• Disposable sitz bath bowl with water bag

ASSESSMENT

• Review any orders related to the sitz bath.

- Determine patient's ability to ambulate to the bathroom and maintain a sitting position for 15 to 20 minutes.
- Prior to the sitz bath, inspect perineal/rectal area for swelling, drainage, redness, warmth, and tenderness. Assess bladder fullness and encourage patient to void before sitz bath.

NURSING DIAGNOSIS

- Acute Pain
- Risk for Infection
- Impaired Tissue Integrity

OUTCOME IDENTIFICATION AND PLANNING

- Patient states an increase in comfort.
- Patient experiences a decrease in healing time.
- Patient maintains normal body temperature and remains free of any signs and symptoms of infection.
- Patient exhibits signs and symptoms of healing.

IMPLEMENTATION

ACTION	RATIONALE
1. Review the medical order for the application of a sitz bath, including frequency and length of time for the application. Gather necessary supplies.	Reviewing the order and plan of care validates the correct patient and correct procedure. Preparation promotes efficient time management and an organized approach to the task.
2. Perform hand hygiene and put on PPE, if indicated.	Hand hygiene and PPE prevent the spread of microorganisms. PPE is required based on transmission precautions.
3. Identify the patient.	Identifying the patient ensures the right patient receives the intervention and helps prevent errors.
4. Close the curtains around the bed and close the door to the room, if possible.	This ensures the patient's privacy.
5. Put on gloves. Assemble equipment either at the bedside if using a bedside commode or in the bathroom.	Gloves prevent exposure to blood and body fluids. Organization facilitates performance of task.

ACTION	RATIONALE
6. Raise lid of toilet or commode. Place bowl of sitz bath, with drainage ports to rear and infusion port in front, in the toilet. Fill bowl of sitz bath about halfway full with tepid to warm water (98°F–115°F [37°C–46°C]).	Sitz bath will not drain appropriately if placed in toilet backwards. Tepid water can promote relaxation and help with edema; warm water can help with circulation.
7. Clamp tubing on bag. Fill bag with same temperature water as mentioned above. Hang bag above patient's shoulder height on the IV pole.	If bag is hung lower, the flow rate will not be sufficient and water may cool too quickly.
8. Assist patient to sit on toilet or commode. The patient should be able to sit in the basin or tub with the feet flat on the floor without any pressure on the sacrum or thighs. Wrap a blanket around the shoulders and provide extra draping, if needed. Insert tubing into the infusion port of the sitz bath. Slowly unclamp tubing and allow the sitz bath to fill.	Excessive pressure on the sacrum or thighs could cause tissue injury. Blanket and draping protects from chilling and exposure. If tubing is placed into the sitz bath before the patient sits on the toilet, the patient may trip over tubing. Filling the sitz bath ensures that the tissue is submerged in water.
9. Clamp tubing once sitz bath is full. Instruct patient to open clamp when water in bowl becomes cool. **Ensure that call bell is within reach. Instruct patient to call if he or she feels light-headed or dizzy or has any problems. Instruct the patient not to try standing without assistance.**	Cool water may produce hypothermia. Patient may become light-headed due to vasodilation, so call bell should be within reach.
10. Remove gloves and perform hand hygiene.	Hand hygiene deters the spread of microorganisms.
11. When patient is finished (in about 15–20 minutes, or prescribed time), put on clean gloves. Assist the patient to stand and gently	Gloves prevent contact with blood and body fluids. Patient may be light-headed and dizzy due to vasodilation. Patient should not stand alone, and

ACTION	RATIONALE
pat perineal area dry. Remove gloves. Assist patient to bed or chair. Ensure that call bell is within reach.	bending over to dry self may cause patient to fall.
12. Put on gloves. Empty and disinfect sitz bath bowl according to agency policy.	Proper equipment cleaning deters the spread of microorganisms.
13. Remove gloves and any additional PPE, if used. Perform hand hygiene.	Removing PPE properly reduces the risk for infection transmission and contamination of other items. Hand hygiene prevents the spread of microorganisms.

EVALUATION
- Patient tolerates sitz bath without incident.
- Patient verbalizes a decrease in pain or discomfort.
- Patient remains free of any signs and symptoms of infection.
- Patient demonstrates signs of healing.

DOCUMENTATION
- Document administration of the sitz bath, including water temperature and duration. Document patient response, and assessment of perineum before and after administration.

SKILL 11 MAKING AN OCCUPIED BED

If the patient cannot get out of bed, the linens may need to be changed with the patient still in the bed. This is termed an "occupied" bed. The following procedure explains how to make the bed using a fitted bottom sheet. Some facilities do not provide fitted bottom sheets, or sometimes a fitted bottom sheet may not be available. If this is the case, refer to the Skill Variation for using a flat bottom sheet instead of a fitted sheet, located at the end of Skill 12, Making an Unoccupied Bed.

DELEGATION CONSIDERATIONS

The making of an occupied bed may be delegated to nursing assistive personnel (NAP) or to unlicensed assistive personnel (UAP), as well as to licensed practical/vocational nurses (LPN/LVNs).The decision to delegate must be based on careful analysis of the patient's needs and circumstances, as well as the qualifications of the person to whom the task is being delegated. Refer to the Delegation Guidelines in Appendix A.

EQUIPMENT

- One large flat sheet
- One fitted sheet
- Drawsheet (optional)
- Blankets
- Bedspread
- Pillowcases
- Linen hamper or bag
- Bedside chair
- Protective pad (optional)
- Disposable gloves
- Additional PPE, as indicated

ASSESSMENT

- Assess the patient's preferences regarding linen changes.
- Assess for any precautions or activity restrictions for the patient.
- Check the bed for any patient belongings that may have accidentally been placed or fallen there, such as eyeglasses or prayer cloths.
- Note the presence and position of any tubes or drains that the patient may have.

NURSING DIAGNOSIS

- Risk for Impaired Skin Integrity
- Impaired Physical Mobility
- Impaired Bed Mobility

OUTCOME IDENTIFICATION AND PLANNING

- The bed linens are applied without injury to the patient or nurse.
- The patient participates in moving from side to side.
- The patient verbalizes feelings of increased comfort.

IMPLEMENTATION

ACTION	RATIONALE
1. Check health care record for limitations on patient's physical activity.	This facilitates patient cooperation, determines level of activity, and promotes patient safety.
2. Perform hand hygiene. Put on PPE, as indicated.	Hand hygiene and PPE prevent the spread of microorganisms. PPE is required based on transmission precautions.
3. Identify the patient. Explain what you are going to do.	Patient identification validates the correct patient and correct procedure. Discussion and explanation allay anxiety and prepare the patient for what to expect.

ACTION	RATIONALE
4. Assemble equipment on overbed table within reach.	Organization facilitates performance of task.
5. Close the curtains around the bed and close the door to the room, if possible.	This ensures the patient's privacy.
6. Adjust the bed to a comfortable working height, usually elbow height of the caregiver (VISN 8 Patient Safety Center, 2009).	Having the bed at the proper height prevents back and muscle strain.
7. Lower side rail nearest you, leaving the opposite side rail up. Place bed in flat position unless contraindicated.	Having the mattress flat makes it easier to prepare a wrinkle-free bed.
8. Put on gloves. Check bed linens for patient's personal items. **Disconnect the call bell or any tubes/drains from bed linens.**	Gloves prevent the spread of microorganisms. It is costly and inconvenient when personal items are lost. Disconnecting tubes from linens prevents discomfort and accidental dislodging of the tubes.
9. Place a bath blanket over the patient. Have the patient hold on to the bath blanket while you reach under it and remove top linens. Leave top sheet in place if a bath blanket is not used. Fold linen that is to be reused over the back of a chair. Discard soiled linen in laundry bag or hamper. **Do not place on floor or furniture. Do not hold soiled linens against your uniform.**	The blanket provides warmth and privacy. Placing linens directly into the hamper helps prevent the spread of microorganisms. The floor is heavily contaminated; soiled linen will further contaminate furniture. Soiled linen contaminates the nurse's uniform, and this may spread organisms to another patient.
10. If possible, and another person is available to assist, grasp mattress securely and shift it up to head of bed.	This allows more foot room for the patient.
11. Assist patient to turn toward opposite side of the bed, and reposition pillow under patient's head.	This allows the bed to be made on the vacant side.

ACTION	RATIONALE

12. Loosen all bottom linens from head, foot, and side of bed.

This facilitates removal of linens.

13. Fan-fold or roll soiled linens as close to the patient as possible.

This makes it easier to remove linens when the patient turns to the other side.

14. Use clean linen and make the near side of the bed. Place the bottom sheet with its centerfold in the center of the bed. Open the sheet and fan-fold to the center, positioning it under the old linens. Pull the bottom sheet over the corners at the head and foot of the mattress.

Opening linens on the bed reduces strain on the nurse's arms and diminishes the spread of microorganisms. Centering the sheet ensures sufficient coverage for both sides of the mattress. Positioning under the old linens makes it easier to remove linens.

15. If using, place the drawsheet with its centerfold in the center of the bed and positioned so it will be located under the patient's midsection. Open the drawsheet and fan-fold it to the center of the mattress. Tuck the drawsheet securely under the mattress. If a protective pad is used, place it over the drawsheet in the proper area and open to the centerfold. Not all facilities use drawsheets routinely. The nurse may decide to use one.

If the patient soils the bed, drawsheet and pad can be changed without the bottom and top linens on the bed. A drawsheet can aid in moving the patient in bed.

16. Raise side rail. Assist patient to roll over the folded linen in the middle of the bed toward you. Reposition pillow and bath blanket or top sheet. Move to other side of the bed and lower side rail.

This ensures patient safety. The movement allows the bed to be made on the other side. The bath blanket provides warmth and privacy.

17. Loosen and remove all bottom linen. Discard soiled linen in laundry bag or hamper. **Do not place on floor or furniture. Do not hold soiled linens against your uniform.**

Placing linens directly into the hamper helps prevent the spread of microorganisms. The floor is heavily contaminated; soiled linen will further contaminate furniture. Soiled

ACTION	RATIONALE
	linen contaminates the nurse's uniform, and this may spread organisms to another patient.
18. Ease clean linen from under the patient. Pull the bottom sheet taut and secure at the corners at the head and foot of the mattress. Pull the drawsheet tight and smooth. Tuck the drawsheet securely under the mattress.	This removes wrinkles and creases in the linens, which are uncomfortable to lie on.
19. Assist patient to turn back to the center of bed. Remove pillow and change pillowcase. Open each pillowcase in the same manner as you opened other linens. Gather the pillowcase over one hand toward the closed end. Grasp the pillow with the hand inside the pillowcase. Keep a firm hold on the top of the pillow and pull the cover onto the pillow. Place the pillow under the patient's head.	Opening linens by shaking them causes organisms to be carried on air currents.
20. Apply top linen, sheet, and blanket, if desired, so that it is centered. Fold the top linens over at the patient's shoulders to make a cuff. Have patient hold on to top linen and remove the bath blanket from underneath.	This allows bottom hems to be tucked securely under the mattress and provides for privacy.
21. Secure top linens under foot of mattress and miter corners. (Refer to Skill Variation in Skill 12.) Loosen top linens over patient's feet by grasping them in the area of the feet and pulling gently toward foot of bed.	This provides for a neat appearance. Loosening linens over the patient's feet gives more room for movement.

ACTION	RATIONALE
22. Return patient to a position of comfort. Remove your gloves. Raise side rail and lower bed. Reattach call bell.	Promotes patient comfort and safety. Removing gloves properly reduces the risk for infection transmission and contamination of other items.
23. Dispose of soiled linens according to agency policy.	Deters the spread of microorganisms.
24. Remove any other PPE, if used. Perform hand hygiene.	Removing PPE properly reduces the risk for infection transmission and contamination of other items. Hand hygiene prevents the spread of microorganisms.

EVALUATION

- The bed linens are changed, with the patient and nurse remaining free of injury.
- Patient assists in moving from side to side.
- Patient verbalizes feelings of increased comfort.

DOCUMENTATION

- Changing of bed linens does not require documentation. The use of a specialty bed, or bed equipment, such as Balkan frame or foot cradle, should be documented. Document any significant observations and communication.

SKILL 12 MAKING AN UNOCCUPIED BED

Usually bed linens are changed after the bath, but some agencies change linens only when soiled. If the patient can get out of bed, the nurse should make the bed while it is unoccupied to decrease stress on the patient and the nurse. The following procedure explains how to make the bed using a fitted bottom sheet. Some facilities do not provide fitted bottom sheets, or sometimes a fitted bottom sheet may not be available. If this is the case, refer to the accompanying Skill Variation for using a flat bottom sheet, instead of a fitted sheet.

DELEGATION CONSIDERATIONS

The making of an unoccupied bed may be delegated to nursing assistive personnel (NAP) or to unlicensed assistive personnel (UAP), as well as to licensed practical/vocational nurses (LPN/LVNs). The decision to delegate must be based on careful analysis of the patient's needs and circumstances, as well as the qualifications of the person to whom the task is being delegated. Refer to the Delegation Guidelines in Appendix A.

EQUIPMENT

- One large flat sheet
- One fitted sheet
- Drawsheet (optional)
- Blankets
- Bedspread
- Pillowcases
- Linen hamper or bag
- Bedside chair
- Waterproof protective pad (optional)
- Disposable gloves
- Additional PPE, as indicated

ASSESSMENT

- Assess the patient's preferences regarding linen changes.
- Assess for any physical activity limitations.
- Check for any patient belongings that may have accidentally been placed in the bed linens, such as eyeglasses or prayer cloths.

NURSING DIAGNOSIS

- Risk for Impaired Skin Integrity
- Risk for Activity Intolerance
- Impaired Physical Mobility

OUTCOME IDENTIFICATION AND PLANNING

- The bed linens will be changed without injury to the nurse or patient.

IMPLEMENTATION

ACTION	RATIONALE
1. Perform hand hygiene. Put on PPE, as indicated.	Hand hygiene and PPE prevent the spread of microorganisms. PPE is required based on transmission precautions.
2. Explain to the patient what you are going to do and the reason for doing it, if the patient is present in room.	Explanation facilitates cooperation.
3. Assemble necessary equipment to the bedside stand or overbed table.	Arranging items nearby is convenient, saves time, and avoids unnecessary stretching and twisting of muscles on the part of the nurse.

ACTION	RATIONALE
4. Adjust the bed to a comfortable working height, usually elbow height of the caregiver (VISN 8 Patient Safety Center, 2009). Drop the side rails.	Having the bed at the proper height prevents back and muscle strain. Having the side rails down reduces strain on the nurse while working.
5. Disconnect call bell or any tubes from bed linens.	Disconnecting devices prevents damage to the devices.
6. Put on gloves. Loosen all linen as you move around the bed, from the head of the bed on the far side to the head of the bed on the near side.	Gloves prevent the spread of microorganisms. Loosening the linen helps prevent tugging and tearing on linen. Loosening the linen and moving around the bed systematically reduce strain caused by reaching across the bed.
7. Fold reusable linens, such as sheets, blankets, or spread, in place on the bed in fourths and hang them over a clean chair.	Folding saves time and energy when reusable linen is replaced on the bed. Folding linens while they are on the bed reduces strain on the nurse's arms. Some facilities change linens only when soiled.
8. Snugly roll all the soiled linen inside the bottom sheet and place directly into the laundry hamper. **Do not place on floor or furniture. Do not hold soiled linens against your uniform.**	Rolling soiled linens snugly and placing them directly into the hamper helps prevent the spread of microorganisms. The floor is heavily contaminated; soiled linen will further contaminate furniture. Soiled linen contaminates the nurse's uniform, and this may spread organisms to another patient.
9. If possible, shift mattress up to head of bed. If mattress is soiled, clean and dry according to facility policy before applying new sheets.	This allows more foot room for the patient.
10. Remove your gloves, unless indicated for transmission-based precautions. Place the bottom sheet with its center-fold in the center of the bed. Open the sheet and fan-fold to the center.	Gloves are not necessary to handle clean linen. Removing gloves properly reduces the risk for infection transmission and contamination of other items. Opening linens on the bed reduces strain on the nurse's arms and diminishes the spread of microorganisms. Centering

ACTION	RATIONALE
	the sheet ensures sufficient coverage for both sides of the mattress.
11. Pull the bottom sheet over the corners at the head and foot of the mattress. (See accompanying Skill Variation for using a flat bottom sheet, instead of a fitted sheet.)	Making the bed on one side and then completing the bedmaking on the other side saves time. Having bottom linens free of wrinkles reduces patient discomfort.
12. If using, place the drawsheet with its center fold in the center of the bed and positioned so it will be located under the patient's midsection. Open the drawsheet and fan-fold to the center of the mattress. If a protective pad is used, place it over the drawsheet in the proper area and open to the center fold. Not all facilities use drawsheets routinely. The nurse may decide to use one. In some institutions, the protective pad doubles as a drawsheet. Tuck the drawsheet securely under the mattress.	If the patient soils the bed, drawsheet and pad can be changed without the bottom and top linens on the bed. Having all bottom linens in place before tucking them under the mattress avoids unnecessary moving about the bed. A drawsheet can aid moving the patient in bed.
13. Move to the other side of the bed to secure bottom linens. Pull the bottom sheet tightly and secure over the corners at the head and foot of the mattress. Pull the drawsheet tightly and tuck it securely under the mattress.	This removes wrinkles from the bottom linens, which can cause patient discomfort and promote skin breakdown.
14. Place the top sheet on the bed with its center fold in the center of the bed and with the hem even with the head of the mattress. Unfold the top sheet. Follow same procedure with top blanket or spread, placing the upper edge about 6 inches below the top of the sheet.	Opening linens by shaking them spreads organisms into the air. Holding linens overhead to open them causes strain on the nurse's arms.

ACTION	RATIONALE
15. Tuck the top sheet and blanket under the foot of the bed on the near side. Miter the corners. (See accompanying Skill Variation.)	This saves time and energy and keeps the top linen in place.
16. Fold the upper 6 inches of the top sheet down over the spread and make a cuff.	This makes it easier for the patient to get into bed and pull up the covers.
17. Move to the other side of the bed and follow the same procedure for securing top sheets under the foot of the bed and making a cuff.	Working on one side of the bed at a time saves energy and is more efficient.
18. Place the pillows on the bed. Open each pillowcase in the same manner as you opened other linens. Gather the pillowcase over one hand toward the closed end. Grasp the pillow with the hand inside the pillowcase. Keep a firm hold on the top of the pillow and pull the cover onto the pillow. Place the pillow at the head of the bed.	Opening linens by shaking them causes organisms to be carried on air currents. Covering the pillow while it rests on the bed reduces strain on the nurse's arms and back.
19. Fan-fold or pie-fold the top linens.	Having linens opened makes it more convenient for the patient to get into bed.
20. Secure the signal device on the bed, according to facility policy.	The patient will be able to call for assistance as necessary. Promotes patient comfort and safety.
21. Raise side rail and lower bed.	Promotes patient comfort and safety.
22. Dispose of soiled linen according to facility policy.	Deters the spread of microorganisms.
23. Remove any other PPE, if used. Perform hand hygiene.	Removing PPE properly reduces the risk for infection transmission and contamination of other items. Hand hygiene prevents the spread of microorganisms.

EVALUATION

• The bed linens are changed without any injury to the patient or nurse.

DOCUMENTATION

Changing of bed linens does not require documentation. The use of a specialty bed, or bed equipment, such as Balkan frame or foot cradle, should be documented.

SKILL VARIATION   Making a Bed With a Flat Bottom Sheet

1. Perform hand hygiene and put on PPE, if indicated.

2. Explain what you are going to do and the reason for doing it to the patient, if the patient is present in room.

3. Assemble necessary equipment on the bedside stand or overbed table. Two large flat sheets are needed.

4. Raise bed to a comfortable working position, usually elbow height of the caregiver (VISN 8 Patient Safety Center, 2009). Disconnect call bell or any tubes from bed linens.

5. Put on gloves. Loosen all linen as you move around the bed, from the head of the bed on the far side to the head of the bed on the near side.

6. Fold reusable linens, such as sheets, blankets, or spread, in place on the bed in fourths and hang them over a clean chair.

7. Snugly roll all the soiled linen inside the bottom sheet and place directly into the laundry hamper. Do not place on floor or furniture. Do not hold soiled linens against your uniform.

8. If possible, shift mattress up to head of bed.

9. Remove your gloves. Place the bottom sheet with its centerfold in the center of the bed and high enough to be able to tuck it under the head of the mattress. Open the sheet and fan-fold to the center.

10. If using, place the drawsheet with its centerfold in the center of the bed and positioned so it will be located under the patient's midsection. Open the drawsheet and fan-fold it to the center of the mattress. If a protective pad is used, place it over the drawsheet in the proper area and open it to the centerfold.

11. Tuck the bottom sheet securely under the head of the mattress on one side of the bed, making a corner. Corners are usually mitered. Grasp the side

continued on page 62

Making a Bed With a Flat Bottom Sheet *continued*

FIGURE A Grasping the side edge of the sheet and lifting up to form a triangle.

FIGURE C Tucking sheet under mattress.

FIGURE D Placing top of triangular fold over mattress side.

FIGURE E Tucking end of triangular linen fold under mattress to complete mitered corner.

edge of the sheet about 18 inches down from the mattress top (Figure A). Lay the sheet on top of the mattress to form a triangular, flat fold (Figure B). Tuck the portion of the sheet that is hanging loose below the mattress under the mattress without pulling on the triangular fold (Figure C). Pick the top of the triangle fold and place it over the side of the mattress (Figure D). Tuck this loose portion of the sheet under the mattress. Continue tucking the remaining bottom sheet and drawsheet securely under the mattress (Figure E). Move to

FIGURE B Laying sheet on top of the bed to make triangular, flat fold.

the other side of the bed to secure bottom linens. Pull the sheets across the mattress from the centerfold. Secure the bottom of the sheet under the head of the bed and miter the corner. Pull the remainder of the sheet and the drawsheet tightly and tuck under the mattress, starting at the

Making a Bed With a Flat Bottom Sheet *continued*

FIGURE F Tucking sheet snugly under mattress.

head of the bed and moving toward the foot (Figure F).

12. Place the top sheet on the bed with its centerfold in the center of the bed and with the hem even with the head of the mattress. Unfold the top sheet. Follow same procedure with top blanket or spread, placing the upper edge about 6 inches below the top of the sheet.

13. Tuck the top sheet and blanket under the foot of the bed on the near side. Miter the corners.

14. Fold the upper 6 inches of the top sheet down over the spread and make a cuff.

15. Move to the other side of the bed and follow the same procedure for securing top sheets under the foot of the bed and making a cuff.

16. Place the pillows on the bed. Open each pillowcase in the same manner as you opened other linens. Gather the pillowcase over one hand toward the closed end. Grasp the pillow with the hand inside the pillowcase. Keep a firm hold on the top of the pillow and pull the cover onto the pillow. Place the pillow at the head of the bed.

17. Fan-fold or pie-fold the top linens. Remove gloves.

18. Secure the signal device on the bed according to facility policy.

19. Adjust bed to low position. Raise rail.

20. Dispose of soiled linen according to agency policy. Perform hand hygiene.

SKILL 13 USING A BED SCALE

Obtaining a patient's weight is an important component of assessment. In addition to providing baseline information of the patient's overall status, weight is a valuable indicator of nutritional status and fluid balance. Changes in a patient's weight can provide clues to underlying problems, such as nutritional deficiencies or fluid excess or deficiency, or indicate the development of new problems, such as fluid overload. Weight also can be used to evaluate a patient's response to treatment. For example, if a patient is receiving nutritional supplementation, obtaining daily or biweekly weights is used to determine achievement of the expected outcome (i.e., weight gain).

Typically, the nurse will measure weight by having the patient stand on an upright scale. However, doing so requires that the patient is mobile and can maintain his or her balance. Chair scales are available for patients who are unable to stand. For patients who are confined to the bed, have limited mobility, or cannot maintain a balanced upright or standing position for a short period of time, a bed scale can be used. With a bed scale, the nurse places the patient in a sling and raises the patient above the bed. To ensure safety, a second nurse should be on hand to assist with weighing the patient. Many facilities are providing beds for patient use with built-in scales. The following procedure explains how to weigh the patient with a portable bed scale.

DELEGATION CONSIDERATIONS

Measurement of body weight may be delegated to nursing assistive personnel (NAP) or unlicensed assistive personnel (UAP), as well as to licensed practical/vocational nurses (LPN/LVNs). The decision to delegate must be based on careful analysis of the patient's needs and circumstances, as well as the qualifications of the person to whom the task is being delegated. Refer to the Delegation Guidelines in Appendix A.

EQUIPMENT

- Bed scale with sling
- Cover for sling
- Sheet or bath blanket
- PPE, as indicated

ASSESSMENT

- Assess the patient's ability to stand for a weight measurement. If the patient cannot stand, assess the patient's ability to sit in a chair or to lie still for a weight measurement.
- Assess the patient for pain. If necessary, give medication for pain or sedation before placing the patient on a bed scale.
- Assess for the presence of any material, such as tubes, drains, or IV tubing, which could become entangled in the scale or pulled during the weighing procedure.

NURSING DIAGNOSIS

- Risk for Injury
- Impaired Physical Mobility
- Imbalanced Nutrition: Less Than Body Requirements
- Imbalanced Nutrition: More Than Body Requirements

OUTCOME IDENTIFICATION AND PLANNING

- Patient's weight is assessed accurately and without injury.
- Patient experiences minimal discomfort.

IMPLEMENTATION

ACTION	RATIONALE

1. Check the medical order or nursing plan of care for frequency of weight measurement. More frequent measurement of the patient's weight may be appropriate based on nursing judgment. Obtain the assistance of a second caregiver, based on the patient's mobility and ability to cooperate with the procedure.

This provides for patient safety and appropriate care.

2. Perform hand hygiene and put on PPE, if indicated.

Hand hygiene and PPE prevent the spread of microorganisms. PPE is required based on transmission precautions.

3. Identify the patient.

Identifying the patient ensures that the right patient receives the intervention and helps prevent errors.

4. Close the curtains around the bed and close the door to room if possible. Discuss the procedure with the patient and assess the patient's ability to assist with the procedure.

This ensures the patient's privacy. Explanation relieves anxiety and facilitates cooperation.

5. Place a cover over the sling of the bed scale.

Using a cover deters the spread of microorganisms.

6. Attach the sling to the bed scale. Lay the sheet or bath blanket in the sling. Turn on the scale. **Balance the scale so that weight reads 0.0.**

Scale will add the sling into the weight unless it is zeroed with the sling, blanket, and cover.

7. Adjust the bed to a comfortable working position, usually elbow height of the caregiver (VISN 8, 2009). Position one caregiver on each side of the bed, if two caregivers are present. Raise

Having the bed at the proper height prevents back and muscle strain. Having one caregiver on each side of the bed provides for patient safety and appropriate care. Side rail assists patient with movement. Blanket maintains

ACTION	RATIONALE

side rail on the opposite side of the bed from where the scale is located, if not already in place. Cover the patient with the sheet or bath blanket. Remove other covers and any pillows.

patient's dignity and provides warmth.

8. Turn the patient onto his or her side facing the side rail, keeping his or her body covered with the sheet or blanket. Remove the sling from the scale. Place the cover on the sling. Roll the cover and sling lengthwise. Place rolled sling under the patient, making sure the patient is centered in the sling.

Rolling the patient onto his or her side facilitates placing the patient onto the sling. Blanket maintains patient's dignity and provides warmth.

9. Roll the patient back over the sling and onto the other side. Pull the sling through, as if placing the sheet under the patient, unrolling the sling as it is pulled through.

This facilitates placing the patient onto the sling.

10. Roll the scale over the bed so that the arms of the scale are directly over the patient. **Spread the base of the scale.** Lower the arms of the scale and place the arm hooks into the holes on the sling.

By spreading the base, you are giving the scale a wider base, thus preventing the scale from toppling over with the patient. Hooking sling to scale provides secure attachment to the scale and prevents injury.

11. Once the scale arms are hooked onto the sling, gradually elevate the sling so that the patient is lifted up off of the bed (Figure 1).

The scale must be hanging free to obtain an accurate weight. Any tubing that is hanging off the scale will add weight to the patient.

FIGURE 1 Using a bed scale.

ACTION	RATIONALE
Assess all tubes and drains, making sure that none have tension placed on them as the scale is lifted. Once the sling is no longer touching the bed, ensure that nothing else is hanging onto the sling (e.g., ventilator or IV tubing). If any tubing is connected to the patient, raise it up so that it is not adding any weight to the patient.	
12. Note the weight reading on the scale. Slowly and gently, lower the patient back onto the bed. Disconnect the scale arms from the sling. Close the base of the scale and pull it away from the bed.	Lowering the patient slowly does not alarm the patient. Closing the base of the scale facilitates moving the scale.
13. Raise the side rail. Turn the patient to the side rail. Roll the sling up against the patient's backside.	Raising the side rail is a safety measure.
14. Raise the other side rail. Roll the patient back over the sling and up facing the other side rail. Remove the sling from the bed. Remove gloves, if used. Raise the remaining side rail.	The patient needs to be removed from the sling before it can be removed from the bed.
15. Cover the patient and help him or her to a position of comfort. Place the bed in the lowest position.	Ensures patient comfort and safety.
16. Remove the disposable cover from the sling and discard in the appropriate receptacle.	Using a cover deters the spread of microorganisms.
17. Remove additional PPE, if used. Clean equipment based on facility policy. Perform hand hygiene.	Removing PPE properly reduces the risk for infection transmission and contamination of other items. Cleaning equipment prevents transmission of microorganisms. Hand hygiene deters the spread of microorganisms.

ACTION	RATIONALE
18. Replace the scale and sling in the appropriate spot. Plug the scale into the electrical outlet.	Scale should be ready for use at any time.

EVALUATION

• The expected outcome is met when the patient is weighed accurately without injury using the bed scale.

DOCUMENTATION

• Document weight, unit of measurement, and scale used.

SKILL 14 | ASSISTING WITH THE USE OF A BEDPAN

Patients who cannot get out of bed because of physical limitations or medical orders need to use a bedpan or urinal for voiding. Male patients confined to bed usually prefer to use the urinal for voiding (see Skill 174) and the bedpan for defecation; female patients usually prefer to use the bedpan for both. Many patients find it difficult and embarrassing to use the bedpan. When a patient uses a bedpan, promote comfort and normalcy and respect the patient's privacy as much as possible. Be sure to maintain a professional manner. In addition, provide skin care, perineal hygiene, and hand hygiene after bedpan use.

Regular bedpans have a rounded, smooth upper end and a tapered, open lower end. The upper end fits under the patient's buttocks toward the sacrum, with the open end toward the foot of the bed. A special bedpan called a *fracture bedpan* is frequently used for patients with fractures of the femur or lower spine. Smaller and flatter than the ordinary bedpan, this type of bedpan is helpful for patients who cannot easily raise themselves onto the regular bedpan. The fracture pan has a shallow, narrow upper end with a flat wide rim, and a deeper, open lower end. The upper end fits under the patient's buttocks toward the sacrum, with the deeper, open lower end toward the foot of the bed.

DELEGATION CONSIDERATIONS

Assisting a patient with the use of a bedpan may be delegated to nursing assistive personnel (NAP) or to unlicensed assistive personnel (UAP), as well as to licensed practical/vocational nurses (LPN/LVNs). The decision to delegate must be based on careful analysis of the patient's needs and circumstances, as well as the qualifications of the person to

whom the task is being delegated. Refer to the Delegation Guidelines in Appendix A.

EQUIPMENT

- Bedpan (regular or fracture)
- Toilet tissue
- Disposable clean gloves
- Additional PPE, as indicated
- Cover for bedpan or urinal (disposable waterproof pad or cover)
- Disposable washcloths and skin cleanser
- Moist towelettes, skin cleanser and water, or hand sanitizer

ASSESSMENT

- Assess the patient's normal elimination habits.
- Determine why the patient needs to use a bedpan (e.g., a medical order for strict bed rest or immobilization).
- Assess the patient's degree of limitation and ability to help with activity. Assess for activity limitations, such as hip surgery or spinal injury, which would contraindicate certain actions by the patient.
- Check for the presence of drains, dressings, intravenous fluid infusion sites/equipment, traction, or any other devices that could interfere with the patient's ability to help with the procedure or that could become dislodged.
- Assess the characteristics of the urine and the patient's skin.

NURSING DIAGNOSIS

- Impaired Physical Mobility
- Impaired Urinary Elimination
- Toileting Self-Care Deficit

OUTCOME IDENTIFICATION AND PLANNING

- Patient is able to void with assistance.
- Patient maintains continence.
- Patient demonstrates how to use the bedpan with assistance.
- Patient maintains skin integrity.

IMPLEMENTATION

ACTION	RATIONALE
1. Review the patient's medical record for any limitations in physical activity. (See Skill Variation: Assisting With Use of a Bedpan When the Patient Has Limited Movement.) Gather equipment.	Activity limitations may contraindicate certain actions by the patient. Assembling equipment provides for an organized approach to the task.

ACTION	RATIONALE
2. Perform hand hygiene and put on PPE, if indicated.	Hand hygiene and PPE prevent the spread of microorganisms. PPE is required based on transmission precautions.
3. Identify the patient.	Identifying the patient ensures the right patient receives the intervention and helps prevent errors.
4. Assemble equipment on chair next to bed within reach.	Arranging items nearby is convenient, saves time, and avoids unnecessary stretching and twisting of muscles on the part of the nurse.
5. Close curtains around the bed and close the door to the room, if possible. Discuss the procedure with the patient and assess the patient's ability to assist with the procedure, as well as personal hygiene preferences.	This ensures the patient's privacy. Discussion promotes reassurance and provides knowledge about the procedure. Dialogue encourages patient participation and allows for individualized nursing care.
6. Unless contraindicated, apply powder to the rim of the bedpan. Place bedpan and cover on chair next to bed. Put on gloves.	Powder helps keep the bedpan from sticking to the patient's skin and makes it easier to remove. Powder is not applied if the patient has respiratory problems, is allergic to powder, or if a urine specimen is needed (could contaminate the specimen). The bedpan on the chair allows for easy access. Gloves prevent contact with blood and body fluids.
7. Adjust the bed to a comfortable working height, usually elbow height of the caregiver (VISN 8 Patient Safety Center, 2009). Place the patient in a supine position, with the head of the bed elevated about 30 degrees, unless contraindicated.	Having the bed at the proper height prevents back and muscle strain. Supine position is necessary for correct placement of patient on bedpan.

ACTION	RATIONALE
8. Fold top linen back just enough to allow placement of bedpan. If no waterproof pad is on the bed and time allows, consider placing a waterproof pad under patient's buttocks before placing the bedpan.	Folding back the linen in this manner minimizes unnecessary exposure while still allowing the nurse to place the bedpan. The waterproof pad will protect the bed should there be a spill.
9. Ask the patient to bend the knees. Have the patient lift his or her hips upward. Assist the patient, if necessary, by placing your hand that is closest to the patient palm up, under the lower back, and assist with lifting. Slip the bedpan into place with other hand.	The nurse uses less energy when the patient can assist by placing some of his or her weight on the heels.
10. **Ensure that the bedpan is in the proper position and the patient's buttocks are resting on the rounded shelf of the regular bedpan or the shallow rim of the fracture bedpan.**	Having the bedpan in the proper position prevents spills onto the bed, ensures patient comfort, and prevents injury to the skin from a misplaced bedpan.
11. Raise head of bed as near to sitting position as tolerated, unless contraindicated. Cover the patient with bed linens.	This position makes it easier for the patient to void or defecate, avoids strain on the patient's back, and allows gravity to aid in elimination. Covering promotes warmth and privacy.
12. **Place call bell and toilet tissue within easy reach. Place the bed in the lowest position.** Leave patient if it is safe to do so. Use side rails appropriately.	Falls can be prevented if the patient does not have to reach for items he or she needs. Placing the bed in the lowest position promotes patient safety. Leaving the patient alone, if possible, promotes self-esteem and shows respect for privacy. Side rails assist the patient in repositioning.
13. Remove gloves and additional PPE, if used. Perform hand hygiene.	Proper removal of PPE prevents transmission of microorganisms. Hand hygiene deters the spread of microorganisms.

Removing the Bedpan

14. Perform hand hygiene and put on gloves and additional PPE, as indicated. Adjust the bed to a comfortable working height, usually elbow height of the caregiver (VISN 8 Patient Safety Center, 2009). Have a receptacle, such as plastic trash bag, handy for discarding tissue.

15. Lower the head of the bed, if necessary, to about 30 degrees. Remove bedpan in the same manner in which it was offered, being careful to hold it steady. Ask the patient to bend the knees and lift the buttocks up from the bedpan. Assist the patient, if necessary, by placing your hand that is closest to the patient palm up, under the lower back, and assist with lifting. Place the bedpan on the bedside chair and cover it.

16. If patient needs assistance with hygiene, wrap tissue around the hand several times, and wipe patient clean, using one stroke from the pubic area toward the anal area. Discard tissue. Use warm, moist disposable washcloth and skin cleanser to clean perineal area. Place patient on his or her side and spread buttocks to clean anal area.

17. Do not place toilet tissue in the bedpan if a specimen is required or if output is being

Hand hygiene deters the spread of microorganisms. Gloves prevent exposure to blood and body fluids. Having the bed at the proper height prevents back and muscle strain. Proper disposal of soiled tissue prevents transmission of microorganisms.

Holding the bedpan steady prevents spills. The nurse uses less energy when the patient can assist by placing some of his or her weight on the heels. Covering the bedpan helps to prevent the spread of microorganisms.

Cleaning area from front to back minimizes fecal contamination of the vagina and urinary meatus. Cleaning the patient after he or she has used the bedpan prevents offensive odors and skin irritation.

Mixing toilet tissue with a specimen makes laboratory examination more difficult and

ACTION	RATIONALE
recorded. Place toilet tissue in appropriate receptacle.	interferes with accurate output measurement.
18. Return the patient to a comfortable position. Make sure the linens under the patient are dry. Replace or remove pad under the patient, as necessary. Remove your gloves and ensure that the patient is covered.	Positioning helps to promote patient comfort. Removing contaminated gloves prevents spread of microorganisms.
19. Raise side rail. Lower bed height and adjust head of bed to a comfortable position. Reattach call bell.	These actions promote patient safety.
20. Offer patient supplies to wash and dry his or her hands, assisting as necessary.	Washing hands after using the urinal helps prevent the spread of microorganisms.
21. Put on clean gloves. Empty and clean the bedpan, measuring urine in graduated container, as necessary. Discard trash receptacle with used toilet paper per facility policy.	Gloves prevent exposure to blood and body fluids. Cleaning reusable equipment helps prevent the spread of microorganisms.
22. Remove additional PPE, if used. Perform hand hygiene.	Removing PPE properly reduces the risk for infection transmission and contamination of other items. Hand hygiene prevents the spread of microorganisms.

EVALUATION

- Patient voids using the bedpan.
- Patient does not experience episodes of incontinence.
- Patient demonstrates measures to assist with using the bedpan.
- Patient does not experience impaired skin integrity.

DOCUMENTATION

- Document the patient's tolerance of the activity. Record the amount of urine voided on the intake and output record, if appropriate. Document any other assessments, such as unusual urine characteristics or alterations in the patient's skin.

Patients who are unable to lift themselves onto the bedpan or who have activity limitations that prohibit the required actions can be assisted onto the bedpan in an alternate manner using these actions:

1. Review patient's chart for any limitations in physical activity. Gather equipment.

2. Put on PPE, as indicated and perform hand hygiene. Check the patient's identification band.

3. Place bedpan and cover on chair next to bed. Close curtains around the bed and close the door to the room, if possible.

4. Discuss procedure with the patient and assess the patient's ability to assist with the procedure, as well as personal hygiene preferences.

5. Unless contraindicated, apply powder to the rim of the bedpan.

6. Adjust the bed to a comfortable working height, usually elbow height of the caregiver (VISN 8 Patient Safety Center, 2009). Place the patient in a supine position, with the head of the bed elevated about 30 degrees, unless contraindicated. Put on disposable gloves.

7. Fold top linen just enough to turn the patient, while minimizing exposure. If no waterproof pad is on the bed and time allows, consider placing a waterproof pad under patient's buttocks before placing bedpan.

8. Assist the patient to roll to the opposite side or turn the patient into a side-lying position.

9. Hold the bedpan firmly against the patient's buttocks, with the upper end of the bedpan under the patient's buttocks toward the sacrum, and down into the mattress.

10. Keep one hand against the bedpan. Apply gentle pressure to ensure the bedpan remains in place as you assist the patient to roll back onto the bedpan.

11. Ensure that the bedpan is in the proper position and the patient's buttocks are resting on rounded shelf of the regular bedpan or the shallow rim of the fracture bedpan.

12. Raise the head of bed as near to sitting position as tolerated, unless contraindicated. Cover the patient with bed linens.

13. Place call bell and toilet tissue within easy reach. Place the bed in the lowest position. Leave the patient if it is safe to do so. Use side rails appropriately.

Assisting With Use of a Bedpan When the Patient Has Limited Movement *continued*

14. Remove gloves, and PPE, if used. Perform hand hygiene.

15. To remove the bedpan, perform hand hygiene and put on disposable gloves, and additional PPE, as indicated. Raise the bed to a comfortable working height. Have a receptacle handy for discarding tissue.

16. Lower the head of the bed. Grasp the closest side of the bedpan. Apply gentle pressure to hold the bedpan flat and steady. Assist the patient to roll to the opposite side or turn the patient into a side-lying position with the assistance of a second caregiver. Remove the bedpan and set on chair. Cover the bedpan.

17. If patient needs assistance with hygiene, wrap tissue around the hand several times, and wipe patient clean, using one stroke from the pubic area toward the anal area. Discard tissue. Use warm, moist disposable washcloth and skin cleanser to clean perineal area. Place the patient on his or her side and spread buttocks to clean anal area.

18. Return the patient to a comfortable position. Make sure the linens under the patient are dry and that the patient is covered.

19. Remove your gloves. Offer the patient supplies to wash and dry his or her hands, assisting as necessary.

20. Raise side rail. Lower bed height and adjust head of bed to a comfortable position. Reattach call bell.

21. Put on clean gloves. Empty and clean the bedpan, measuring urine in graduated container, as necessary. Remove gloves and additional PPE, if used. Perform hand hygiene.

SKILL 15 | ADMINISTERING A CONTINUOUS CLOSED BLADDER OR CATHETER IRRIGATION (CBI)

Bladder irrigation is not recommended unless obstruction is anticipated, as might occur with bleeding after prostate or bladder surgery (SUNA, 2010, p.9). Sediment or debris, as well as blood clots, might block the catheter, preventing the flow of urine out of the catheter. Indwelling catheters sometimes require continuous irrigation, or flushing, with solution to restore or maintain the patency of the drainage system. Catheter irrigation should be avoided unless necessary to relieve or prevent obstruction (Herter & Wallace Kazer, 2010). If obstruction is anticipated, continuous irrigation is suggested to prevent obstruction (SUNA).

Irrigations might also be used to instill medications that will act directly on the bladder wall. Irrigating a catheter through a closed system is preferred to opening the catheter because opening the catheter could lead to contamination and infection. A triple-lumen or three-way catheter is used for a continuous irrigation in order to maintain a closed system.

DELEGATION CONSIDERATIONS

The administration of continuous closed bladder irrigation is not delegated to nursing assistive personnel (NAP) or to unlicensed assistive personnel (UAP). Depending on the state's nurse practice act and the organization's policies and procedures, administration of continuous closed bladder irrigation may be delegated to licensed practical/vocational nurses (LPN/ LVNs). The decision to delegate must be based on careful analysis of the patient's needs and circumstances, as well as the qualifications of the person to whom the task is being delegated. Refer to the Delegation Guidelines in Appendix A.

EQUIPMENT

- Sterile irrigating solution (at room temperature or warmed to body temperature)
- Sterile tubing with drip chamber and clamp for connection to irrigating solution
- IV pole
- IV pump (if bladder is being irrigated with a solution containing medication)

- Three-way indwelling catheter in place in patient's bladder
- Indwelling catheter drainage setup (tubing and collection bag)
- Alcohol or other disinfectant swab
- Bath blanket
- Disposable gloves
- Additional PPE, as indicated

ASSESSMENT

- Assess the catheter to ensure that it has an irrigation port (if the patient has an indwelling catheter already in place).
- Assess the characteristics of urine present in tubing and drainage bag.
- Review the patient's medical record for, and ask the patient about, any allergies to medications.
- Assess the bladder for fullness either by palpation or with a handheld bladder ultrasound device.
- Assess for signs of adverse effects, which may include pain, bladder spasm, bladder distension/fullness, or lack of drainage from the catheter.

NURSING DIAGNOSIS

- Impaired Urinary Elimination
- Risk for Infection

OUTCOME IDENTIFICATION AND PLANNING

- Patient exhibits free-flowing urine through the catheter. Initially, clots or debris may be noted. These should decrease over time, with the patient ultimately exhibiting urine that is free of clots or debris.
- The continuous bladder irrigation continues without adverse effect.
- Drainage is greater than the hourly amount of irrigation solution being placed in the bladder.
- Patient exhibits no signs and symptoms of infection.

IMPLEMENTATION

ACTION	RATIONALE
1. Confirm the order for catheter irrigation in the medical record, including type and amount of solution and infusion parameters. If irrigation is to be implemented via gravity infusion, calculate the drip rate. Often, orders are to infuse to keep the urine clear of blood.	Verifying the medical order ensures that the correct intervention is administered to the right patient. Solution must be administered via gravity at the appropriate rate as prescribed.
2. Gather equipment.	Assembling equipment provides for an organized approach to the task.
3. Perform hand hygiene and put on PPE, if indicated.	Hand hygiene and PPE prevent the spread of microorganisms. PPE is required based on transmission precautions.
4. Identify the patient.	Identifying the patient ensures the right patient receives the intervention and helps prevent errors.
5. Close the curtains around the bed and close the door to the room, if possible. Discuss the procedure with the patient.	This ensures the patient's privacy. Discussion promotes reassurance and provides knowledge about the procedure. Dialogue encourages patient participation and allows for individualized nursing care.
6. Assemble equipment on overbed table within reach.	Arranging items nearby is convenient, saves time, and avoids unnecessary stretching and twisting of muscles on the part of the nurse.

ACTION	RATIONALE
7. Adjust the bed to a comfortable working height, usually elbow height of the caregiver (VISN 8 Patient Safety Center, 2009).	Having the bed at the proper height prevents back and muscle strain.
8. Empty the catheter drainage bag and measure the amount of urine, noting the amount and characteristics of the urine.	Emptying the drainage bag allows for accurate assessment of drainage after the irrigation solution is instilled. Assessment of urine provides baseline for future comparison.
9. Assist the patient to a comfortable position and expose the irrigation port on the catheter setup. Place waterproof pad under the catheter and aspiration port.	This provides adequate visualization. Waterproof pad protects the patient and bed from leakage.
10. Prepare sterile irrigation bag for use as directed by manufacturer. Clearly label the solution as 'Bladder Irrigant.' Include the date and time on the label. Hang bag on IV pole 2.5 to 3 feet above the level of the patient's bladder. Secure tubing clamp and insert sterile tubing with drip chamber to container using aseptic technique. Release clamp and remove protective cover on end of tubing without contaminating it. Allow solution to flush tubing and remove air. Clamp tubing and replace end cover.	Proper labeling provides accurate information for caregivers. Sterile solution not used within 24 hours of opening should be discarded. Aseptic technique prevents contamination of solution irrigation system. Priming the tubing before attaching irrigation clears air from the tubing that might cause bladder distention.
11. Put on gloves. **Cleanse the irrigation port on the catheter with an alcohol swab. Using aseptic technique, attach irrigation tubing to irrigation port of three-way indwelling catheter.**	Aseptic technique prevents the spread of microorganisms into the bladder.
12. Check the drainage tubing to make sure clamp, if present, is open.	An open clamp prevents accumulation of solution in the bladder.

ACTION	RATIONALE
13. **Release clamp on irrigation tubing and regulate flow at determined drip rate, according to the ordered rate.** If the bladder irrigation is to be done with a medicated solution, use an electronic infusion device to regulate the flow.	This allows for continual gentle irrigation without causing discomfort to the patient. An electronic infusion device regulates the flow of the medication.
14. Remove gloves. Assist the patient to a comfortable position. Cover the patient with bed linens. Place the bed in the lowest position.	Positioning and covering provide warmth and promote comfort and safety.
15. Assess the patient's response to the procedure, and the quality and amount of drainage.	Assessment is necessary to determine the effectiveness of the intervention and to detect adverse effects.
16. Remove equipment. Remove gloves and additional PPE, if used. Perform hand hygiene.	Proper disposal of equipment prevents transmission of microorganisms. Removing PPE properly reduces the risk for infection transmission and contamination of other items. Hand hygiene prevents the spread of microorganisms.
17. As irrigation fluid container nears empty, clamp the administration tubing. Do not allow drip chamber to empty. Disconnect empty bag and attach a new full irrigation solution bag.	This eliminates the need to separate tubing from the catheter and clear air from the tubing. Opening the drainage system provides access for microorganisms.
18. Put on gloves and empty drainage collection bag as each new container is hung and recorded.	Gloves protect against exposure to blood, body fluids, and microorganisms.

EVALUATION

- Urine flows freely through the catheter.
- Patient should exhibit urine that is clear, without evidence of clots or debris.
- Continuous bladder irrigation is administered without adverse effect.

- Drainage is greater than the hourly amount of irrigation solution being instilled in bladder.
- Patient exhibits no signs and symptoms of infection.

DOCUMENTATION

- Document baseline assessment of the patient. Document the amount and type of irrigation solution used and the patient's tolerance of the procedure. Record urine amount emptied from the drainage bag before the procedure and the amount of irrigant used on intake and output record. Record the amount of urine and irrigant emptied from the drainage bag. **Subtract the amount of irrigant instilled from the total volume of drainage to obtain the volume of urine output.**

SKILL 16	ASSESSING BLADDER VOLUME USING AN ULTRASOUND BLADDER SCANNER

A portable bladder ultrasound scanner is an accurate, reliable, and non-invasive device used to assess bladder volume. Bladder scanners do not pose a risk for the development of a urinary tract infection, unlike intermittent catheterization, which is also used to determine bladder volume. They are used when there is urinary frequency, absent or decreased urine output, bladder distention, or inability to void, and when establishing intermittent catheterization schedules. Protocols can be established to guide the decision to catheterize a patient. Some scanners offer the ability to print the scan results for documentation purposes.

Results are most accurate when the patient is in the supine position during the scanning. The device must be programmed for the gender of the patient by pushing the correct button on it. If a female patient has had a hysterectomy, the male button is pushed (Altschuler & Diaz, 2006). A postvoid residual (PVR) volume less than 50 mL indicates adequate bladder emptying. A PVR of greater than 150 mL is often recommended as the guideline for catheterization, because residual urine volumes of greater than 100 mL have been associated with the development of urinary tract infections (NKUDIC, 2012).

DELEGATION CONSIDERATIONS

The assessment of bladder volume using an ultrasound bladder scanner is not delegated to nursing assistive personnel (NAP) or to unlicensed assistive personnel (UAP). Depending on the state's nurse practice act and the organization's policies and procedures, this procedure may be delegated to licensed practical/vocational nurses (LPN/LVNs). The decision to delegate must be based on careful analysis of the patient's needs and circumstances, as well as the qualifications of the person to whom the task is being delegated. Refer to the Delegation Guidelines in Appendix A.

EQUIPMENT

- Bladder scanner
- Ultrasound gel or bladder scan gel pad
- Alcohol wipe or other sanitizer recommended by the scanner
- manufacturer and/or facility policy
- Clean gloves
- Additional PPE, as indicated
- Paper towel or washcloth

ASSESSMENT

- Assess the patient for the need to check bladder volume, including signs of urinary retention, measurement of PVR volume, verification that the bladder is empty, identification of obstruction in an indwelling catheter, and evaluation of bladder distension to determine if catheterization is necessary.

NURSING DIAGNOSIS

- Impaired Urinary Elimination
- Urinary Retention

OUTCOME IDENTIFICATION AND PLANNING

- Volume of urine in the bladder will be accurately measured.
- Patient's urinary elimination will be maintained, with a urine output of at least 30 mL/hour.
- Patient's bladder will not be distended.

IMPLEMENTATION

ACTION	RATIONALE
1. Verify medical order, if required by facility. Many facilities allow the use of a bladder scanner as a nursing judgment. Review the patient's medical record for any limitations in physical activity. Gather equipment.	Reviewing the medical record and plan of care validates the correct patient and correct procedure. Physical limitations may require adaptations in performing the skill. Assembling equipment provides for an organized approach to the task.
2. Perform hand hygiene and put on PPE, if indicated.	Hand hygiene and PPE prevent the spread of microorganisms. PPE is required based on transmission precautions.
3. Identify the patient.	Identifying the patient ensures the right patient receives the intervention and helps prevent errors.

ACTION	RATIONALE
4. Close the curtains around the bed and close the door to the room, if possible. Discuss the procedure with the patient and assess the patient's ability to assist with the procedure, as well as personal hygiene preferences.	This ensures the patient's privacy. Discussion promotes reassurance and provides knowledge about the procedure. Dialogue encourages patient participation and allows for individualized nursing care.
5. Adjust the bed to a comfortable working height, usually elbow height of the caregiver (VISN 8 Patient Safety Center, 2009). Place the patient in a supine position. Drape patient. Stand on the patient's right side if you are right-handed, patient's left side if you are left-handed.	Having the bed at the proper height prevents back and muscle strain. Proper positioning allows accurate assessment of bladder volume. Keeping the patient covered as much as possible promotes patient comfort and privacy. Positioning allows for ease of use of dominant hand for the procedure.
6. Put on clean gloves.	Gloves prevent contact with blood and body fluids.
7. Press the ON button. Wait until the device warms up. Press the SCAN button to turn on the scanning screen.	Many devices require a few minutes to prepare the internal programs.
8. Press the appropriate gender button. The appropriate icon for male or female will appear on the screen.	The device must be programmed for the gender of the patient by pushing the correct button on it. If a female patient has had a hysterectomy, the male button is pushed (Altschuler & Diaz, 2006).
9. Clean the scanner head with the appropriate cleaner.	Cleaning the scanner head deters transmission of microorganisms.
10. Gently palpate the patient's symphysis pubis. Place a generous amount of ultrasound gel or gel pad midline on the patient's abdomen, about 1 to 1.5 inches above the symphysis pubis.	Palpation identifies the proper location and allows for correct placement of the scanner head over the patient's bladder.

ACTION	RATIONALE

11. Place the scanner head on the gel or gel pad, **with the directional icon on the scanner head toward the patient's head (Figure 1). Aim the scanner head toward the bladder (point the scanner head slightly downward toward the coccyx) (Patraca, 2005).** Press and release the scan button.

Proper placement allows for accurate reading of urine in the bladder.

FIGURE 1 Positioning the scanner head with directional icon toward the patient's bladder.

12. Observe the image on the scanner screen. **Adjust the scanner head to center the bladder image on the crossbars (Figure 2).**

This action allows for accurate reading of urine in the bladder.

FIGURE 2 Centering the image on the crossbars. (From Patraca, K. (2005). Measure bladder volume without catheterization. *Nursing, 35*(4), 4.)

13. Press and hold the DONE button until it beeps. Read the volume measurement on the screen. Print the results, if required, by pressing PRINT.

This action provides for accurate documentation of reading.

ACTION	RATIONALE
14. Use a washcloth or paper towel to remove remaining gel from the patient's skin. Alternately, gently remove gel pad from patient's skin. Return the patient to a comfortable position. Remove your gloves and ensure that the patient is covered.	Removal of the gel promotes patient comfort. Removing contaminated gloves prevents spread of microorganisms.
15. Lower bed height and adjust head of bed to a comfortable position. Reattach call bell, if necessary.	These actions promote patient safety.
16. Remove additional PPE, if used. Perform hand hygiene.	Removing PPE properly reduces the risk for infection transmission and contamination of other items. Hand hygiene prevents the spread of microorganisms.

EVALUATION

- Volume of urine in the bladder is accurately measured.
- Patient's urinary elimination is maintained, with a urine output of at least 30 mL/hour.
- Patient's bladder is not distended.

DOCUMENTATION

- Document the assessment data that led to the use of the bladder scanner, relevant symptoms, the urine volume measured, and the patient's response.

SKILL 17 OBTAINING A CAPILLARY BLOOD SAMPLE FOR GLUCOSE TESTING

Blood glucose monitoring provides information about how the body is controlling glucose metabolism. Controlling the patient's blood glucose levels is an important part of care for patients with many conditions, including diabetes, seizures, enteral and parenteral feeding, liver disease, pancreatitis, head injury, stroke, alcohol and drug intoxication, sepsis, and in patients prescribed corticosteroids (American Diabetes Association, 2013). Point-of-care testing (testing done at the bedside, where samples are not sent to the laboratory) provides a convenient, rapid, and accurate measurement of blood glucose (American Diabetes Association, 2013). This type of testing is used by patients with diabetes as an important part of disease management to monitor blood glucose and adjust lifestyle interventions and treatment (U.S. FDA, 2013). Blood samples are commonly obtained from the edges of the fingers for adults, but samples can be obtained from the palm of the hand, forearm, upper arm, calf, and anterior thigh, depending on the time of testing and monitor used (U.S. FDA, 2013). Avoid fingertips, because they are more sensitive. Rotate sites to prevent skin damage. **It is important to be familiar with and follow the manufacturer's guidelines and facility policy and procedure to ensure accurate results.** Normal fasting glucose for adults is less than 110 mg/dL (LeFever Kee, 2013).

DELEGATION CONSIDERATIONS

Obtaining a capillary blood sample for glucose testing may be delegated to nursing assistive personnel (NAP) or to unlicensed assistive personnel (UAP), as well as licensed practical/vocational nurses (LPN/LVNs). The decision to delegate must be based on careful analysis of the patient's needs and circumstances, as well as the qualifications of the person to whom the task is being delegated. Refer to the Delegation Guidelines in Appendix A.

EQUIPMENT

- Blood glucose meter
- Sterile lancet
- Cotton balls or gauze squares
- Testing strips for meter
- Nonsterile gloves
- Additional PPE, as indicated
- Skin cleanser and water or alcohol swab

ASSESSMENT

- Assess the patient's history for indications necessitating the monitoring of blood glucose levels, such as high-carbohydrate feedings, history of diabetes mellitus, or corticosteroid therapy.
- Assess for signs and symptoms of hypoglycemia and hyperglycemia.
- Assess the patient's knowledge about monitoring blood glucose.
- Inspect the area of the skin to be used for testing. Avoid bruised and open areas.

NURSING DIAGNOSIS

- Risk for Unstable Blood Glucose Level
- Deficient Knowledge
- Anxiety

OUTCOME IDENTIFICATION AND PLANNING

- Patient's blood glucose level is measured accurately without adverse effect.
- Patient remains free of injury.

• Patient demonstrates a blood glucose level within acceptable parameters.
• Patient demonstrates the ability to participate in monitoring.
• Patient verbalizes increased comfort with the procedure.

IMPLEMENTATION

ACTION	RATIONALE
1. Check the patient's medical record or nursing plan of care for monitoring schedule. You may decide that additional testing is indicated based on nursing judgment and the patient's condition.	This confirms scheduled times for checking blood glucose. Independent nursing judgment may lead to the decision to test more frequently, based on the patient's condition.
2. Gather equipment. Check expiration date on blood test strips.	This provides an organized approach to the task. Blood test strips that are past expiration date could cause inaccurate results and should not be used.
3. Perform hand hygiene and put on PPE, if indicated.	Hand hygiene and PPE prevent the transmission of microorganisms. PPE is required based on transmission precautions.
4. Identify the patient. Explain the procedure to the patient and instruct the patient about the need for monitoring blood glucose.	Identifying the patient ensures the right patient receives the intervention and helps prevent errors. Explanation helps to alleviate anxiety and facilitate cooperation.
5. Close curtains around the bed and close the door to the room, if possible.	Closing the curtain or door provides for patient privacy.
6. Turn on the monitor.	The monitor must be on for use.
7. Enter the patient's identification number or scan their identification bracelet, if required, according to facility policy.	Use of identification number allows for electronic storage and accurate identification of patient data.
8. Put on nonsterile gloves.	Gloves protect the nurse from exposure to blood or body fluids.
9. Prepare lancet using aseptic technique.	Aseptic technique maintains sterility.

ACTION	RATIONALE
10. Remove test strip from the vial. **Recap container immediately.** Test strips also come individually wrapped. **Check that the code number for the strip matches the code number on the monitor screen.**	Immediate recapping protects strips from exposure to humidity, light, and discoloration. Matching code numbers on the strip and glucose monitor ensures that the machine is calibrated correctly.
11. Insert the strip into the meter according to directions for that specific device. Alternately, strip may be placed in meter after collection of sample on test strip, depending on meter in use.	Correctly inserted strip allows meter to read blood glucose level accurately.
12. **Have the patient wash hands with skin cleanser and warm water and dry thoroughly. Alternately, cleanse the skin with an alcohol swab. Allow skin to dry completely.**	Washing with skin cleanser and water or alcohol cleanses the puncture site. Warm water also helps to cause vasodilation. Alcohol can interfere with accuracy of results if not completely dried.
13. Choose a skin site free of lesions and calluses. Make sure there is no edema, and that the site is warm (Van Leeuwen et al., 2011).	Areas with lesions are not suitable for capillary sampling. Calluses, edema, and vasoconstriction (cool to palpation) interfere with the ability to obtain a blood sample.
14. Hold lancet perpendicular to skin and pierce site with lancet (Figure 1).	Holding lancet in proper position facilitates proper skin penetration.

FIGURE 1 Piercing patient's finger with lancet.

15. Wipe away first drop of blood with gauze square or cotton ball if recommended by manufacturer of monitor.	Manufacturers recommend discarding the first drop of blood, which may be contaminated by serum or cleansing product, producing an inaccurate reading.

ACTION	RATIONALE
16. Encourage bleeding by lowering the hand, making use of gravity. Lightly stroke the finger, if necessary, until a sufficient amount of blood has formed to cover the sample area on the strip, based on monitor requirements (check instructions for monitor). Take care not to squeeze the finger, not to squeeze at puncture site, or not to touch puncture site or blood.	An appropriate-sized droplet facilitates accurate test results. Squeezing can cause injury to the patient and alter the test result (Ferguson, 2005).
17. Gently touch a drop of blood to the test strip without smearing it (Figure 2). Depending on meter in use, insert strip into meter after collection of sample on test strip.	Smearing blood on the strip may result in inaccurate test results.

FIGURE 2 Applying blood to test strip.

ACTION	RATIONALE
18. Press time button if directed by manufacturer.	Correct timing produces accurate results.
19. Apply pressure to puncture site with a cotton ball or dry gauze. **Do not use alcohol wipe.**	Pressure causes hemostasis. Alcohol stings and may prolong bleeding.
20. Read blood glucose results and document appropriately at bedside. Inform patient of test result.	Timing depends on type of meter.
21. Turn off meter, remove test strip, and dispose of supplies appropriately. Place lancet in sharps container.	Proper disposal prevents exposure to blood and accidental needlestick.

ACTION	RATIONALE
22. Remove gloves and any other PPE, if used. Perform hand hygiene.	Removing PPE properly reduces the risk for infection transmission and contamination of other items. Hand hygiene reduces the transmission of microorganisms.

EVALUATION

- Patient's blood glucose level is measured accurately without adverse effect.
- Patient's blood glucose level is within acceptable limits.
- Patient participates in monitoring.
- Patient verbalizes comfort with the procedure.

DOCUMENTATION

- Document blood glucose level on a flow sheet in the medical record, according to facility policy. Document pertinent patient assessments, any intervention related to glucose level, and any patient teaching. Report abnormal results and/or significant assessments to primary care provider.

SKILL 18   ASSESSING BLOOD PRESSURE BY AUSCULTATION

Blood pressure refers to the force of the blood against arterial walls. Systolic pressure is the highest point of pressure on arterial walls when the ventricles contract and push blood through the arteries at the beginning of systole. When the heart rests between beats during diastole, the pressure drops. The lowest pressure present on arterial walls during diastole is the diastolic pressure (Taylor et al., 2015). Blood pressure, measured in millimeters of mercury (mm Hg), is recorded as a fraction. The numerator is the systolic pressure; the denominator is the diastolic pressure.

Take routine measurements after the patient has rested for a minimum of 5 minutes. In addition, make sure the patient does not have any caffeine or nicotine 30 minutes before measuring blood pressure. Use of a cuff of the correct size for the patient, correct limb placement, recommended deflation rate, and correct interpretation of the sounds heard are necessary to ensure accurate blood pressure measurement (Hinkle & Cheever, 2014; Pickering et al., 2004).

Various sites can be used to assess blood pressure. The brachial artery and the popliteal artery are used most commonly. This skill discusses using the brachial artery site to obtain a blood pressure measurement. The skill begins with the procedure for estimating systolic pressure. Estimation of systolic pressure prevents inaccurate readings in the presence of an auscultatory gap (a pause in the auscultated sounds). To identify the first Korotkoff sound accurately, the cuff must be inflated to a pressure above the point at which the pulse can no longer be felt.

DELEGATION CONSIDERATIONS

The assessment of brachial artery blood pressure may be delegated to nursing assistive personnel (NAP) or to unlicensed assistive personnel (UAP), as well as to licensed practical/vocational nurses (LPN/LVNs). The decision to delegate must be based on careful analysis of the patient's needs and circumstances, as well as the qualifications of the person to whom the task is being delegated. Refer to the Delegation Guidelines in Appendix A.

EQUIPMENT

- Stethoscope
- Sphygmomanometer
- Blood pressure cuff of appropriate size
- Pencil or pen, paper or flow sheet
- Alcohol swab
- PPE, as indicated

ASSESSMENT

- Assess the brachial pulse, or the pulse appropriate for the site being used.
- Assess for an intravenous infusion or breast or axilla surgery on the side of the body corresponding to the arm used. Assess for the presence of a cast, arteriovenous shunt, or injured or diseased limb. If any of these conditions are present, do not use the affected arm to monitor blood pressure.
- Assess the size of the limb so that the appropriate-sized blood pressure cuff can be used. The correct cuff should have a bladder length that is 80% of the arm circumference and a width that is at least 40% of the arm circumference: a length to width ratio of 2:1.
- Assess for factors that could affect blood pressure reading, such as the patient's age, exercise, position, weight, fluid balance, smoking, and medications.
- Note baseline or previous blood pressure measurements. Assess the patient for pain.
- If the patient reports pain, give pain medication as ordered before assessing blood pressure. If the blood pressure is taken while the patient is in pain, make a notation concerning the pain if the blood pressure is elevated.

NURSING DIAGNOSIS

- Decreased Cardiac Output
- Ineffective Health Maintenance
- Risk for Falls

OUTCOME IDENTIFICATION AND PLANNING

• Patient's blood pressure is measured accurately without injury.

IMPLEMENTATION

ACTION	RATIONALE
1. Check the medical order or nursing care plan for frequency of blood pressure measurement. More frequent measurement may be appropriate based on nursing judgment.	Provides for patient safety.
2. Perform hand hygiene and put on PPE, if indicated.	Hand hygiene and PPE prevent the spread of microorganisms. PPE is required based on transmission precautions.
3. Identify the patient.	Identifying the patient ensures the right patient receives the intervention and helps prevent errors.
4. Close the curtains around the bed and close the door to the room, if possible. Discuss the procedure with the patient and assess the patient's ability to assist with the procedure. Validate that the patient has relaxed for several minutes.	This ensures the patient's privacy. Explanation relieves anxiety and facilitates cooperation. Activity immediately before measurement can result in inaccurate results.
5. Put on gloves, if indicated.	Gloves prevent contact with blood and body fluids. Gloves are usually not required for measurement of blood pressure, unless contact with blood or body fluids is anticipated.
6. Select the appropriate arm for application of the cuff.	Measurement of blood pressure may temporarily impede circulation to the extremity.
7. Have the patient assume a comfortable lying or sitting position with the forearm supported at the level of the heart and the palm of the	The position of the arm can have a major influence when the blood pressure is measured; if the upper arm is below the level of the right atrium, the readings will

ACTION	RATIONALE
hand upward. If the measurement is taken in the supine position, support the arm with a pillow. In the sitting position, support the arm yourself or by using the bedside table. If the patient is sitting, have the patient sit back in the chair so that the chair supports his or her back. In addition, make sure the patient keeps the legs uncrossed.	be too high. If the arm is above the level of the heart, the readings will be too low (Pickering et al., 2004). If the back is not supported, the diastolic pressure may be elevated falsely; if the legs are crossed, the systolic pressure may be elevated falsely (Pickering et al., 2004). This position places the brachial artery on the inner aspect of the elbow so that the bell or diaphragm of the stethoscope can rest on it easily. This sitting position ensures accuracy.
8. Expose the brachial artery by removing garments, or move a sleeve, if it is not too tight, above the area where the cuff will be placed.	Clothing over the artery interferes with the ability to hear sounds and can cause inaccurate blood pressure readings. A tight sleeve would cause congestion of blood and possibly inaccurate readings.
9. Palpate the location of the brachial artery. **Center the bladder of the cuff over the brachial artery, about midway on the arm, so that the lower edge of the cuff is about 2.5 to 5 cm (1 to 2 inches) above the inner aspect of the elbow. Line the artery marking on the cuff up with the patient's brachial artery.** The tubing should extend from the edge of the cuff nearer the patient's elbow (Figure 1).	Pressure in the cuff applied directly to the artery provides the most accurate readings. If the cuff gets in the way of the stethoscope, readings are likely to be inaccurate. A cuff placed upside down with the tubing toward the patient's head may give a false reading.

FIGURE 1 Placing blood pressure cuff. *(Photo by B. Proud.)*

ACTION	RATIONALE
10. Wrap the cuff around the arm smoothly and snugly, and fasten it. Do not allow any clothing to interfere with the proper placement of the cuff.	A smooth cuff and snug wrapping produce equal pressure and help promote an accurate measurement. A cuff wrapped too loosely results in an inaccurate reading.
11. Check that the needle on the aneroid gauge is within the zero mark. If using a mercury manometer, check to see that the manometer is in the vertical position and that the mercury is within the zero level with the gauge at eye level.	If the needle is not in the zero area, the blood pressure reading may not be accurate. Tilting a mercury manometer, inaccurate calibration, or improper height for reading the gauge can lead to errors in determining the pressure measurements.

Estimating Systolic Pressure

ACTION	RATIONALE
12. Palpate the pulse at the brachial or radial artery by pressing gently with the fingertips.	Palpation allows for measurement of the approximate systolic reading.
13. Tighten the screw valve on the air pump.	The bladder within the cuff will not inflate with the valve open.
14. **Inflate the cuff while continuing to palpate the artery. Note the point on the gauge where the pulse disappears.**	The point where the pulse disappears provides an estimate of the systolic pressure. To identify the first Korotkoff sound accurately, the cuff must be inflated to a pressure above the point at which the pulse can no longer be felt.
15. Deflate the cuff and wait 1 minute.	Allowing a brief pause before continuing permits the blood to refill and circulate through the arm.

Obtaining Blood Pressure Measurement

ACTION	RATIONALE
16. Assume a position that is no more than 3 feet away from the gauge.	A distance of more than about 3 feet can interfere with accurate readings of the numbers on the gauge.
17. Place the stethoscope earpieces in your ears. Direct the earpieces forward into the canal and not against the ear itself.	Proper placement blocks extraneous noise and allows sound to travel more clearly.

ACTION	RATIONALE
18. Place the bell or diaphragm of the stethoscope firmly but with as little pressure as possible over the brachial artery. Do not allow the stethoscope to touch clothing or the cuff.	Having the bell or diaphragm directly over the artery allows more accurate readings. Heavy pressure on the brachial artery distorts the shape of the artery and the sound. Placing the bell or diaphragm away from clothing and the cuff prevents noise, which would distract from the sounds made by blood flowing through the artery.
19. Pump the pressure 30 mm Hg above the point at which the systolic pressure was palpated and estimated. Open the valve on the manometer and allow air to escape slowly (allowing the gauge to drop 2 to 3 mm per second).	Increasing the pressure above the point where the pulse disappeared ensures a period before hearing the first sound that corresponds with the systolic pressure. It prevents misinterpreting phase II sounds as phase I sounds.
20. **Note the point on the gauge at which the first faint, but clear, sound appears that slowly increases in intensity. Note this number as the systolic pressure. Read the pressure to the closest 2 mm Hg.**	Systolic pressure is the point at which the blood in the artery is first able to force its way through the vessel at a similar pressure exerted by the air bladder in the cuff. The first sound is phase I of Korotkoff sounds.
21. Do not reinflate the cuff once the air is being released to recheck the systolic pressure reading.	Reinflating the cuff while obtaining the blood pressure is uncomfortable for the patient and can cause an inaccurate reading. Reinflating the cuff causes congestion of blood in the lower arm, which lessens the loudness of Korotkoff sounds.
22. **Note the point at which the sound completely disappears. Note this number as the diastolic pressure. Read the pressure to the closest 2 mm Hg.**	The point at which the sound disappears corresponds to the beginning of phase V Korotkoff sounds and is generally considered the diastolic pressure reading (Pickering et al., 2004).
23. Allow the remaining air to escape quickly. Repeat any suspicious reading, but wait at least 1 minute. Deflate the cuff	False readings are likely to occur if there is congestion of blood in the limb while obtaining repeated readings.

ACTION	RATIONALE
completely between attempts to check the blood pressure.	
24. When measurement is completed, remove the cuff. Remove gloves, if worn. Cover the patient and help him or her to a position of comfort.	Removing PPE properly reduces the risk for infection transmission and contamination of other items. Ensures patient comfort.
25. Clean the diaphragm of the stethoscope with the alcohol wipe. Clean and store the sphygmomanometer, according to facility policy.	Appropriate cleaning deters the spread of microorganisms. Equipment should be left ready for use.
26. Remove additional PPE, if used. Perform hand hygiene.	Removing PPE properly reduces the risk for infection transmission and contamination of other items. Hand hygiene deters the spread of microorganisms.

EVALUATION

• Patient's blood pressure is measured accurately without injury and with minimal patient discomfort.

DOCUMENTATION

• Record the findings on paper, flow sheet, or computerized record. Report abnormal findings to the appropriate person. Identify arm used and site of assessment if other than brachial.

SKILL 19 ASSESSING SYSTOLIC BLOOD PRESSURE USING A DOPPLER ULTRASOUND

Blood pressure can be measured with a Doppler ultrasound device, which amplifies sound. It is especially useful if the sounds are indistinct or inaudible with a regular stethoscope. This method provides only an estimate of systolic blood pressure.

DELEGATION CONSIDERATIONS

The assessment of brachial artery blood pressure may be delegated to nursing assistive personnel (NAP) or to unlicensed assistive personnel

(UAP), as well as to licensed practical/vocational nurses (LPN/LVNs). The decision to delegate must be based on careful analysis of the patient's needs and circumstances, as well as the qualifications of the person to whom the task is being delegated. Refer to the Delegation Guidelines in Appendix A.

EQUIPMENT

- Stethoscope
- Sphygmomanometer
- Blood pressure cuff of appropriate size
- Pencil or pen, paper or flow sheet
- Alcohol swab
- PPE, as indicated

ASSESSMENT

- Assess the brachial pulse, or the pulse appropriate for the site being used.
- Assess for an intravenous infusion or breast or axilla surgery on the side of the body corresponding to the arm used. Assess for the presence of a cast, arteriovenous shunt, or injured or diseased limb. If any of these conditions are present, do not use the affected arm to monitor blood pressure.
- Assess the size of the limb so that the appropriate-sized blood pressure cuff can be used. The correct cuff should have a bladder length that is 80% of the arm circumference and a width that is at least 40% of the arm circumference: a length to width ratio of 2:1.
- Assess for factors that could affect blood pressure reading, such as the patient's age, exercise, position, weight, fluid balance, smoking, and medications. Assess the patient for pain.
- Assess the situation to determine the appropriateness and necessity for using a Doppler device to obtain systolic blood pressure measurement.

NURSING DIAGNOSIS

- Decreased Cardiac Output
- Ineffective Health Maintenance
- Risk for Falls

OUTCOME IDENTIFICATION AND PLANNING

- Patient's systolic blood pressure is measured accurately without injury.

IMPLEMENTATION

ACTION	RATIONALE
1. Check the medical order or nursing care plan for frequency of blood pressure measurement. More frequent measurement may be appropriate based on	Provides for patient safety. Using a Doppler device provides measurement of only the systolic blood pressure and is often used only in an emergency situation.

ACTION	RATIONALE
nursing judgment. Assess the situation to determine the appropriateness and necessity for using a Doppler device to obtain systolic blood pressure measurement.	
2. Perform hand hygiene and put on PPE, if indicated.	Hand hygiene and PPE prevent the spread of microorganisms. PPE is required based on transmission precautions.
3. Identify the patient.	Identifying the patient ensures the right patient receives the intervention and helps prevent errors.
4. Close the curtains around the bed and close the door to the room, if possible. Discuss the procedure with the patient and assess patient's ability to assist with the procedure. Validate that the patient has relaxed for several minutes.	This ensures the patient's privacy. Explanation relieves anxiety and facilitates cooperation. Activity immediately before measurement can result in inaccurate results.
5. Put on gloves, if indicated.	Gloves prevent contact with blood and body fluids. Gloves are usually not required for measurement of blood pressure, unless contact with blood or body fluids is anticipated.
6. Select the appropriate arm for application of the cuff.	Measurement of blood pressure may temporarily impede circulation to the extremity.
7. Have the patient assume a comfortable lying or sitting position with the forearm supported at the level of the heart and the palm of the hand upward. If the measurement is taken in the supine position, support the arm with a pillow. In the sitting position, support the arm yourself or by using the bedside table.	Arm position can have a major influence when the blood pressure is measured; if the upper arm is below the level of the right atrium, the readings will be too high. If the arm is above the level of the heart, the readings will be too low (Pickering et al., 2004).

ACTION	RATIONALE
8. Expose the brachial artery by removing garments, or move a sleeve, if it is not too tight, above the area where the cuff will be placed.	Clothing over the artery interferes with the ability to hear sounds and can cause inaccurate blood pressure readings. A tight sleeve would cause congestion of blood and possibly inaccurate readings.
9. Palpate the location of the brachial artery. **Center the bladder of the cuff over the brachial artery, about midway on the arm, so that the lower edge of the cuff is about 2.5 to 5 cm (1 to 2 inches) above the inner aspect of the elbow. Line the artery marking on the cuff up with the patient's brachial artery.** The tubing should extend from the edge of the cuff nearer the patient's elbow.	Pressure in the cuff applied directly to the artery provides the most accurate readings. If the cuff gets in the way of the stethoscope, readings are likely to be inaccurate. A cuff placed upside down with the tubing toward the patient's head may give a false reading.
10. Wrap the cuff around the arm smoothly and snugly, and fasten it. Do not allow any clothing to interfere with the proper placement of the cuff.	A smooth cuff and snug wrapping produce equal pressure and help promote an accurate measurement. A cuff wrapped too loosely results in an inaccurate reading.
11. Check that the needle on the aneroid gauge is within the zero mark. If using a mercury manometer, check to see that the manometer is in the vertical position and that the mercury is within the zero level with the gauge at eye level.	If the needle is not in the zero area, the blood pressure reading may not be accurate. Tilting a mercury manometer, inaccurate calibration, or improper height for reading the gauge can lead to errors in determining the pressure measurements.
12. Place a small amount of conducting gel over the artery.	Conduction gel is necessary to provide conduction of sound from artery to Doppler.
13. Hold the Doppler device in your nondominant hand. Using your dominant hand, place the Doppler tip in the gel. Adjust the volume as	Locates arterial pulse for measurement.

ACTION	RATIONALE

needed. Move the Doppler tip around until you hear the pulse.

14. Once the pulse is found using the Doppler device, close the valve to the sphygmomanometer. Tighten the screw valve on the air pump. **Inflate the cuff while continuing to use the Doppler device on the artery. Note the point on the gauge where the pulse disappears (Figure 1).**

The point where the pulse disappears provides a measurement of the systolic pressure.

FIGURE 1 Inflating cuff while listening to artery pulsations. *(Photo by B. Proud.)*

15. Open the valve on the manometer and allow air to escape quickly. Repeat any suspicious reading, but wait at least 1 minute between readings to allow normal circulation to return in the limb. Deflate the cuff completely between attempts to check the blood pressure.

Allowing a brief pause before continuing permits the blood to refill and circulate through the arm.

16. Remove the Doppler tip and turn off the Doppler device. Wipe excess gel off the patient's skin with tissue. Remove the cuff.

Removing gel from the patient's skin promotes patient comfort.

17. Wipe any gel remaining on the Doppler probe off with a tissue. Clean the Doppler device according to facility policy or manufacturer's recommendations.

Appropriate cleaning deters the spread of microorganisms. Equipment should be left ready for use.

ACTION	RATIONALE
18. Remove gloves, if worn. Cover the patient and help him or her to a position of comfort.	Removing PPE properly reduces the risk for infection transmission and contamination of other items. Ensures patient comfort.
19. Remove additional PPE, if used. Perform hand hygiene.	Removing PPE properly reduces the risk for infection transmission and contamination of other items. Hand hygiene deters the spread of microorganisms.
20. Return the Doppler device to the charge base, as necessary, and store according to facility policy.	Equipment should be left ready for use.

EVALUATION

• Systolic blood pressure is measured accurately without injury and with minimal patient discomfort.

DOCUMENTATION

• Record the findings on paper, flow sheet, or computerized record. Report abnormal findings to the appropriate person. Identify arm used and site of assessment if other than brachial.

SKILL 20   ASSESSING BLOOD PRESSURE USING AN AUTOMATIC ELECTRONIC BLOOD PRESSURE MONITOR

Automatic, electronic equipment is often used to monitor blood pressure in acute care settings, during anesthesia, postoperatively, or any time frequent assessments are necessary. This unit determines blood pressure by analyzing the sounds of blood flow or measuring oscillations. The machine can be set to take and record blood pressure readings at preset intervals. Irregular heart rates, excessive patient movement, and environmental noise can interfere with the readings. Because electronic equipment is more sensitive to outside interference, these readings are susceptible to error. The cuff is applied in the same manner as the auscultatory method, with the microphone or pressure sensor positioned directly over the artery. When using an automatic blood pressure device for serial readings, check the cuffed limb frequently. Incomplete deflation of the cuff between measurements can lead to inadequate arterial perfusion and venous drainage, compromising the circulation in the limb (Bern et al., 2007; Pickering et al., 2004).

DELEGATION CONSIDERATIONS

The assessment of brachial artery blood pressure may be delegated to nursing assistive personnel (NAP) or unlicensed assistive personnel (UAP), as well as to licensed practical/vocational nurses (LPN/LVNs). The decision to delegate must be based on careful analysis of the patient's needs and circumstances, as well as the qualifications of the person to whom the task is being delegated. Refer to the Delegation Guidelines in Appendix A.

EQUIPMENT

- Stethoscope
- Sphygmomanometer
- Blood pressure cuff of appropriate size
- Pencil or pen, paper or flow sheet
- Alcohol swab
- PPE, as indicated

ASSESSMENT

- Assess the brachial pulse, or the pulse appropriate for the site being used.
- Assess for an intravenous infusion or breast or axilla surgery on the side of the body corresponding to the arm used. Assess for the presence of a cast, arteriovenous shunt, or injured or diseased limb. If any of these conditions are present, do not use the affected arm to monitor blood pressure.
- Assess the size of the limb so that the appropriate-sized blood pressure cuff can be used. The correct cuff should have a bladder length that is 80% of the arm circumference and a width that is at least 40% of the arm circumference: a length to width ratio of 2:1.
- Assess for factors that could affect blood pressure reading, such as the patient's age, exercise, position, weight, fluid balance, smoking, and medications.
- Note baseline or previous blood pressure measurements. Assess the patient for pain.
- If the patient reports pain, give pain medication as ordered before assessing blood pressure. If the blood pressure is taken while the patient is in pain, make a notation concerning the pain if the blood pressure is elevated.

NURSING DIAGNOSIS

- Decreased Cardiac Output
- Ineffective Health Maintenance
- Risk for Falls

OUTCOME IDENTIFICATION AND PLANNING

- Patient's blood pressure is measured accurately without injury.

IMPLEMENTATION

ACTION	RATIONALE
1. Check the medical order or nursing care plan for frequency of blood pressure measurement. More frequent measurement may be appropriate based on nursing judgment.	Provides for patient safety.
2. Perform hand hygiene and put on PPE, if indicated.	Hand hygiene and PPE prevent the spread of microorganisms. PPE is required based on transmission precautions.
3. Identify the patient.	Identifying the patient ensures the right patient receives the intervention and helps prevent errors.
4. Close the curtains around the bed and close the door to the room, if possible. Discuss the procedure with the patient and assess patient's ability to assist with the procedure. Validate that the patient has relaxed for several minutes.	This ensures the patient's privacy. Explanation relieves anxiety and facilitates cooperation. Activity immediately before measurement can result in inaccurate results.
5. Select the appropriate arm for application of the cuff.	Measurement of blood pressure may temporarily impede circulation to the extremity.
6. Have the patient assume a comfortable lying or sitting position with the forearm supported at the level of the heart and the palm of the hand upward. If the measurement is taken in the supine position, support the arm with a pillow. In the sitting position, support the arm yourself or by using the bedside table. If the patient is sitting, have the patient	Arm position can have a major influence when the blood pressure is measured; if the upper arm is below the level of the right atrium, the readings will be too high. If the arm is above the level of the heart, the readings will be too low (Pickering et al., 2004). If the back is not supported, the diastolic pressure may be elevated falsely; if the legs are crossed, the systolic pressure may be elevated falsely

ACTION	RATIONALE
sit back in the chair so that the chair supports his or her back. In addition, make sure the patient keeps the legs uncrossed.	(Pickering et al., 2004). This position places the brachial artery on the inner aspect of the elbow so that the bell or diaphragm of the stethoscope can rest on it easily. This sitting position ensures accuracy.
7. Expose the brachial artery by removing garments, or move a sleeve, if it is not too tight, above the area where the cuff will be placed.	Clothing over the artery interferes with the ability to hear sounds and can cause inaccurate blood pressure readings. A tight sleeve would cause congestion of blood and possibly inaccurate readings.
8. Palpate the location of the brachial artery. **Center the bladder of the cuff over the brachial artery, about midway on the arm, so that the lower edge of the cuff is about 2.5 to 5 cm (1 to 2 inches) above the inner aspect of the elbow. Line the artery marking on the cuff up with the patient's brachial artery.** The tubing should extend from the edge of the cuff nearer the patient's elbow.	Pressure in the cuff applied directly to the artery provides the most accurate readings. If the cuff gets in the way of the stethoscope, readings are likely to be inaccurate. A cuff placed upside down with the tubing toward the patient's head may give a false reading.
9. Wrap the cuff around the arm smoothly and snugly, and fasten it. Do not allow any clothing to interfere with the proper placement of the cuff (Figure 1).	A smooth cuff and snug wrapping produce equal pressure and help promote an accurate measurement. A cuff wrapped too loosely results in an inaccurate reading.

FIGURE 1 Electronic blood pressure device. *(Photo by B. Proud.)*

ACTION	RATIONALE
10. Turn on the machine. **If the machine has different settings for infants, children and adults, select the appropriate setting.** Push the start button. Instruct the patient to hold the limb still.	Turning on the device allows for blood pressure measurement. Improper setting on the device and movement of limb can lead to errors in determining the pressure measurements.
11. Wait until the machine beeps and the blood pressure reading appears. Remove the cuff from the patient's limb and clean and store the equipment.	Machine signals when measurement is completed. Proper cleaning prevents the transmission of microorganisms.
12. Remove additional PPE, if used. Perform hand hygiene.	Removing PPE properly reduces the risk for infection transmission and contamination of other items. Hand hygiene deters the spread of microorganisms.

EVALUATION

• Patient's blood pressure is measured accurately without injury and with minimal patient discomfort.

DOCUMENTATION

• Record the findings on paper, flow sheet, or computerized record. Report abnormal findings to the appropriate person. Identify arm used and site of assessment if other than brachial.

SKILL 21 OBTAINING AN ARTERIAL BLOOD SAMPLE FROM AN ARTERIAL CATHETER

Obtaining an arterial blood sample requires percutaneous puncture of the brachial, radial, or femoral artery. However, an arterial blood sample can also be obtained from an arterial catheter. Arterial catheters are used for hemodynamic monitoring, blood gas analysis and obtaining blood samples. A pressure monitoring system transmits pressures from the intravascular space or cardiac chambers through a catheter and fluid-filled tubing to a pressure transducer, which converts the physiologic signal from the patient to a pressure tracing and digital value. Patency of the system and prevention of backflow of blood through the catheter and tubing is maintained by using a continuous flush solution under pressure (Morton & Fontaine, 2013).

The procedure below describes obtaining a sample from an open, stopcock system. For information on obtaining an arterial blood sample from a closed reservoir system, please see the Skill Variation at the end of this skill.

DELEGATION CONSIDERATIONS

Obtaining an arterial blood sample from an arterial catheter is not delegated to nursing assistive personnel (NAP), unlicensed assistive personnel (UAP), or licensed practical/vocational nurses (LPN/LVNs).

EQUIPMENT

- Arterial blood gas (ABG) syringe with needleless cannula, rubber cap for ABG syringe hub, and ice-filled plastic bag or cup, if ABG is ordered
- Gloves
- Goggles
- Additional PPE, as indicated
- Vacutainer with needleless luer adapter and appropriate blood collection tubes for ordered tests

- Two additional blood collection tubes, for discard blood volume
- Alcohol swabs or chlorhexidine, per facility policy
- Waterproof protective pad
- Sterile cap for arterial catheter stopcock
- Label with patient identification information
- Blank labels (2)
- Biohazard bag
- Bath blanket

ASSESSMENT

- Review the patient's medical record and plan of care for information about the patient's need for an arterial blood sample.
- Assess the patient's cardiac status, including heart rate, blood pressure, and auscultation of heart sounds.
- Assess the patient's respiratory status, including respiratory rate, excursion, lung sounds, and use of oxygen, if ordered.
- Check the patency and functioning of the arterial catheter.
- Assess the patient's understanding about the need for specimen collection.

NURSING DIAGNOSIS

- Impaired Gas Exchange
- Decreased Cardiac Output
- Excess Fluid Volume

OUTCOME IDENTIFICATION AND PLANNING

- Specimen is obtained without compromise to the patency of the arterial catheter.
- Patient experiences minimal discomfort and anxiety.
- Patient remains free from infection.
- Patient demonstrates an understanding about the need for the specimen collection.

IMPLEMENTATION

ACTION	RATIONALE
1. Verify the order for laboratory testing in the patient's medical record.	This ensures that the correct intervention is performed on the correct patient.
2. Gather all equipment.	Assembling equipment provides for an organized approach to the task.
3. Perform hand hygiene and put on PPE, if indicated.	Hand hygiene and PPE prevent the spread of microorganisms. PPE is required based on transmission precautions.
4. Identify the patient.	Identifying the patient ensures the right patient receives the intervention and helps prevent errors.
5. Close curtains around the bed and close the door to the room, if possible. Explain the procedure to the patient.	This ensures the patient's privacy. Explanation relieves anxiety and facilitates cooperation.
6. Assemble equipment on overbed table within reach.	Arranging items nearby is convenient, saves time, and avoids unnecessary stretching and twisting of muscles on the part of the nurse.
7. Compare specimen label with patient identification bracelet. Label should include patient's name and identification number, time specimen was collected, route of collection, identification of the person obtaining the sample, and any other information required by facility policy.	Verifying the patient's identity validates that the correct procedure is being done on the correct patient, and the specimen is accurately labeled.
8. Use blank labels to label the two blood sample collection tubes to be used for discard blood sample and discard flush.	Labeling of discard tubes prevents accidental confusion with blood specimen tubes.

ACTION	RATIONALE
9. Assist the patient to a comfortable position that provides easy access to the sampling site. Use the bath blanket to cover any exposed area other than the sampling site. Place a waterproof pad under the site.	Patient positioning and use of a bath blanket provide for comfort and warmth. Waterproof pad protects underlying surfaces.
10. Put on gloves and goggles or face shield.	Gloves and goggles (or face shield) prevent contact with blood and body fluids.
11. Temporarily silence the arterial pressure monitor alarms.	The integrity of the system is being altered, which will cause the system to sound an alarm. Facility policy may require the alarm be left on.
12. Locate the stopcock nearest the arterial line insertion site. Remove the nonvented cap from the stopcock. Use the alcohol swab or chlorhexidine to scrub the sampling port on the stopcock. Allow to air dry.	Removal of stopcock cap allows access for blood sampling. Cleansing sampling port reduces the risk of contamination.
13. Attach the needleless luer adapter to the Vacutainer. Connect the needleless adapter of the Vacutainer to the sampling port of the stopcock. Turn off the stopcock to the flush solution. Insert the labeled blood sample tube for the discard sample into the Vacutainer. Follow facility policy for the volume of discard blood to collect (usually 5 to 10 mL).	A sufficient amount of discard volume needs to be withdrawn before obtaining the blood sample to be tested in the laboratory. This sample is discarded because it is diluted with flush solution, possibly leading to inaccurate test results. If an insufficient amount of discard volume is withdrawn, the specimen may be diluted and contaminated with flush solution. If an excessive amount of discard volume is withdrawn, the patient may experience an iatrogenic (treatment-induced) blood loss.
14. Remove the discard syringe and dispose of appropriately, according to facility policy.	Proper disposal reduces the risk of accidental blood exposure and transmission of microorganisms.

ACTION	RATIONALE
15. Insert each blood sample collection tube into the Vacutainer, keeping the stopcock turned off to the flush solution. For each additional sample required, repeat this procedure. If coagulation tests are included in the required tests, obtain blood for this from the final sample. Apply the rubber cap to the ABG syringe hub, if necessary.	Turning the stopcock off to the flush solution allows for sampling and prevents dilution from the flush device. The Vacutainer is a nonvented system, preventing backflow of blood from the patient. Obtaining coagulation samples last prevents dilution from the flush device. The rubber cap on the ABG syringe hub prevents entry of air into the blood sample.
16. After obtaining the final blood sample, turn off the stopcock to the Vacutainer. Activate the in-line flushing device.	Turning the stopcock off and in-line flushing clears the tubing to maintain the integrity of the system and prevent clotting and infection.
17. Turn off the stopcock to the patient. Attach a labeled discard blood sample tube to the Vacutainer. Activate the in-line flushing device.	Turning the stopcock off and in-line flushing clears the stopcock sampling port to maintain the integrity of the system and prevent clotting and infection.
18. Turn off the stopcock to the sampling port. Remove the Vacutainer. Place a new sterile nonvented cap on the blood sampling port of the stopcock.	Capping the port maintains system integrity system and reduces the risk for contamination and infection.
19. Remove gloves. Reactivate the monitor alarms. Record date and time the samples were obtained on the labels, as well as the required information to identify the person obtaining the samples. If ABG was collected, record oxygen flow rate (or room air) on label. Apply labels to the specimens, according to facility policy. Place in biohazard bags; place ABG sample in bag with ice.	Removing gloves properly reduces the risk for infection transmission and contamination of other items. Reactivating the system ensures proper functioning. Proper labeling prevents error. Recording oxygen flow rate ensures accurate interpretation of results of ABG. Use of a biohazard bag prevents contact with blood and body fluids. Ice maintains integrity of the sample.
20. Check the monitor for return of the arterial waveform and pressure reading.	This ensures proper functioning and integrity of the system.

ACTION	RATIONALE
21. Return the patient to a comfortable position. Lower bed height, if necessary, and adjust head of bed to a comfortable position.	Repositioning promotes patient comfort. Lowering the bed promotes patient safety.
22. Remove goggles and additional PPE, if used. Perform hand hygiene. Send specimens to the laboratory immediately.	Removing PPE properly reduces the risk for infection transmission and contamination of other items. Hand hygiene prevents transmission of microorganisms. Specimens must be processed in a timely manner to ensure accuracy.

EVALUATION

- Specimen is obtained without compromise to the patency of the arterial catheter.
- Patient experiences minimal discomfort and anxiety.
- Patient remains free from infection.
- Patient demonstrates an understanding about the need for the specimen collection.

DOCUMENTATION

- Document any pertinent assessments, the laboratory specimens obtained, date and time specimens were obtained, and disposition of specimens.

SKILL VARIATION **Obtaining an Arterial Blood Sample From a Closed Reservoir System**

1. Verify the order for laboratory testing in the patient's medical record. Gather all equipment (including additional syringes to collect blood samples, based on samples ordered).

2. Perform hand hygiene. Put on PPE, as indicated.

3. Check the patient's identification. Assemble equipment on overbed table within reach. Compare the specimen label with the patient's identification.

continued on page 110

Obtaining an Arterial Blood Sample From a Closed Reservoir System *continued*

4. Explain the procedure to the patient. Close curtains around the bed and close the door to the room, if possible.

5. If the bed is adjustable, raise it to a comfortable working height.

6. Assist the patient to a comfortable position that provides easy access to the sampling site. Use the bath blanket to cover any exposed area other than the sampling site. Place a waterproof pad under the site.

7. Put on gloves and goggles or face shield.

8. Locate the closed-system reservoir and blood-sampling site. Temporarily silence monitor alarms.

9. Clean the sampling site with an alcohol swab or chlorhexidine.

10. Holding the reservoir upright, grasp the flexures, and slowly fill the reservoir with blood over a 3- to 5-second period. If you feel resistance, reposition the extremity and check the catheter site for obvious problems (e.g., kinking of the tubing). Then continue with blood withdrawal.

11. Turn off the one-way valve to the reservoir by turning the handle perpendicular to the tubing. Using a syringe with attached cannula, insert the cannula into the sampling site. Slowly fill the syringe. Then grasp the cannula near the sampling site and remove the syringe and cannula as one unit. Repeat the procedure, as needed, to fill the required number of syringes. If coagulation tests have been ordered, obtain blood for those tests from the final syringe.

12. After filling the syringes, turn the one-way valve to its original position, parallel to the tubing. Push down evenly on the plunger until the flexures lock in place in the fully closed position and all fluid has been re-infused. The fluid should be re-infused over a 3- to 5-second period. Activate the fast-flush release.

13. Clean the sampling site with an alcohol swab or chlorhexidine. Reactivate the monitor alarms. Transfer blood samples to the appropriate specimen tubes, if necessary. Record on the labels the date and time the samples were obtained, as well as the required information to identify the person obtaining the samples. Apply labels to the specimens according to facility policy. Place in biohazard bags; place ABG sample in bag with ice. Remove gloves.

14. Check the monitor for return of the arterial waveform and pressure reading.

15. Remove any remaining equipment. Remove goggles and additional PPE, if used. Perform hand hygiene. Send specimens to the laboratory immediately.

Venipuncture involves piercing a vein with a needle to obtain a venous blood sample, which is collected in a syringe or tube. The superficial veins of the arm in the antecubital fossa are typically used for venipuncture (Malarkey & McMorrow, 2012), which include the basilic, median cubital, and cephalic veins (Figure 1). However, venipuncture can be performed on a vein in the dorsal forearm, the dorsum of the hand, or another accessible location.

When performing a venipuncture, remember the following:

- Do not use the inner wrist because of the high risk for damage to underlying structures.
- Avoid areas that are edematous, paralyzed, burned, scarred, have a tattoo, or are on the same side as a mastectomy, arteriovenous shunt, or graft.
- Avoid an extremity affected by a cerebrovascular accident, areas of infection, or areas with abnormal skin conditions.
- Do not draw blood from the same extremity being used for administration of intravenous medications, fluids, or blood transfusions. Some facilities will allow use of such sites as a 'last resort,' after the infusion has been held for a period of time. If necessary, choose a site distal to the intravenous access site. Check facility policy and procedure (Infusion Nurses Society [INS], 2011; Van Leeuwen et al., 2011).

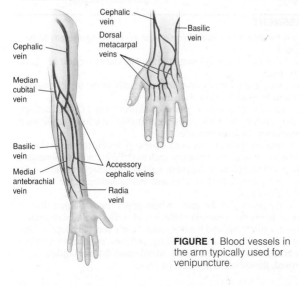

FIGURE 1 Blood vessels in the arm typically used for venipuncture.

Explanation and communication with patients about the need for venipuncture can reduce anxiety. It is important to explain carefully the information about the need for blood tests to ensure patient understanding.

Measures to reduce the risk of infection are an important part of venipuncture. Hand hygiene, aseptic technique, the use of personal protective equipment, and safe disposal of sharps are key to providing safe venipuncture (Adams, 2012; Lavery & Ingram, 2005).

DELEGATION CONSIDERATIONS

The use of venipuncture to obtain a blood sample may be delegated to nursing assistive personnel (NAP) or to unlicensed assistive personnel (UAP) in some settings, as well as to licensed practical/vocational nurses (LPN/LVNs). The decision to delegate must be based on careful analysis of the patient's needs and circumstances, as well as the qualifications of the person to whom the task is being delegated. Refer to the Delegation Guidelines in Appendix A.

EQUIPMENT

- Tourniquet
- Nonsterile gloves
- Additional PPE, as indicated
- Antimicrobial swab, such as chlorhexidine or alcohol
- Sterile needle, gauge appropriate to the vein and sampling needs, using the smallest possible
- Vacutainer needle adaptor
- Blood-collection tubes appropriate for ordered tests
- Appropriate label for specimen, based on facility policy and procedure
- Biohazard bag
- Gauze pads (2 × 2)
- Adhesive bandage

ASSESSMENT

- Review the patient's medical record for the blood specimens to be obtained.
- Ensure that the necessary computerized laboratory request has been completed.
- Assess the patient for any allergies, especially to the topical antimicrobial to be used for skin cleansing.
- Investigate for the presence of any conditions or use of medications that may prolong bleeding time, necessitating additional application of pressure to the puncture site.
- Ask the patient about any previous laboratory testing that he or she may have had, including any problems, such as difficulty with venipuncture, fainting, or complaints of dizziness, light-headedness, or nausea.
- Assess the patient's anxiety level and understanding of the reasons for the blood test.
- Assess the patency of the veins in both upper limbs. Palpate the veins to assess the condition of the vessel; vein should be straight, feel soft, cylindrical, and bounce when lightly pressed. Appropriate vessels will compress without rolling, and have rapid rebound filling after compression (Scales, 2008). Avoid veins that are tender, sclerosed, thrombosed, fibrosed, or hard.

NURSING DIAGNOSIS

- Deficient Knowledge
- Anxiety
- Risk for Injury
- Risk for Infection

OUTCOME IDENTIFICATION AND PLANNING

- Uncontaminated specimen will be obtained without the patient experiencing undue anxiety, injury, or infection.

IMPLEMENTATION

ACTION	RATIONALE
1. Gather the necessary supplies. Check product expiration dates. Identify ordered tests and select the appropriate blood-collection tubes.	Organization facilitates efficient performance of the procedure. Use of products that have not expired ensures proper functioning of equipment. Using correct bottles ensures accurate blood sampling.
2. Perform hand hygiene and put on PPE, if indicated.	Hand hygiene and PPE prevent the transmission of microorganisms. PPE is required based on transmission precautions.
3. Identify the patient.	Identifying the patient ensures the right patient receives the intervention and helps prevent errors.
4. Explain the procedure to the patient. Allow the patient time to ask questions and verbalize concerns about the venipuncture procedure.	Explanation provides reassurance and promotes cooperation.
5. Check the specimen label with the patient's identification bracelet. Label should include the patient's name and identification number, time specimen was collected, route of collection, identification of the person obtaining the sample, and any other information required by facility policy.	Confirmation of patient identification information ensures the specimen is labeled correctly for the right patient.

ACTION	RATIONALE
6. Assemble equipment on overbed table within reach.	Arranging items nearby is convenient, saves time, and avoids unnecessary stretching and twisting of muscles on the part of the nurse.
7. Close curtains around the bed and close the door to the room, if possible.	Closing the door or curtain provides for patient privacy.
8. Provide for good light. Artificial light is recommended.	Good lighting is necessary to perform the procedure properly.
Place a trash receptacle within easy reach.	Having the trash receptacle within easy reach allows for safe disposal of contaminated materials.
9. Assist the patient to a comfortable position, either sitting or lying. If the patient is lying in bed, raise the bed to a comfortable working height, usually elbow height of the caregiver (VISN 8 Patient Safety Center, 2009).	Proper positioning allows easy access to the site and promotes patient comfort and safety. Proper bed height helps reduce back strain while performing the procedure.
10. Determine the patient's preferred site for the procedure based on his or her previous experience. Expose the arm, supporting it in an extended position on a firm surface, such as a tabletop. Position self on the same side of the patient as the site selected. Apply a tourniquet to the upper arm on the chosen side approximately 3 to 4 inches above the potential puncture site. Apply sufficient pressure to impede venous circulation but not arterial blood flow.	Patient preference promotes patient participation in treatment and gives the nurse information that may aid in site selection (Lavery & Ingram, 2005). Positioning close to the chosen site reduces back strain. Use of a tourniquet increases venous pressure to aid in vein identification. Tourniquet should remain in place no more than 60 seconds to prevent injury (Fischbach & Dunning, 2009).
11. Put on gloves. Assess the veins using inspection and palpation to determine the best puncture site. Refer to the Assessment section above.	Gloves reduce transmission of microorganisms. Using the best site reduces the risk of injury to the patient. Observation and palpation allow for making distinction between other structures, such as tendons and arteries, in the area to avoid injury.

ACTION	RATIONALE

12. **Release the tourniquet. Check that the vein has decompressed.**

Releasing the tourniquet reduces the length of time the tourniquet is applied (Lavery & Ingram, 2005). Tourniquet should remain in place no more than 60 seconds to prevent injury, stasis, and hemoconcentration, which may alter results (Fischbach & Dunning, 2009). Thrombosed veins will remain firm and palpable and should not be used for venipuncture (Lavery & Ingram, 2005).

13. Attach the needle to the Vacutainer device. Place first blood-collection tube into the Vacutainer, but not engaged in the puncture device in the Vacutainer.

Device is prepared for use to ensure efficiency with the task.

14. **Clean the patient's skin at the selected puncture site with the antimicrobial swab. If using chlorhexidine, use a gentle back and forth motion or use the procedure recommended by the manufacturer. If using alcohol, wipe in a circular motion spiraling outward. Allow the skin to dry before performing the venipuncture. Do not wipe or blot. Allow to dry completely.**

Cleaning the patient's skin reduces the risk for transmission of microorganisms. Allowing the skin to dry maximizes antimicrobial action and prevents contact of the substance with the needle on insertion, thereby reducing the sting associated with insertion.

15. Alternately, for patients who bruise easily, are at risk for bleeding, or have fragile skin, **apply the chlorhexidine without scrubbing for at least 30 seconds. Allow to dry completely. Do not wipe or blot.**

Avoiding use of scrubbing decreases risk of injury. Application for a minimum of 30 seconds is necessary for chlorhexidine to be effective (Hadaway, 2006). Organisms on the skin can be introduced into the tissues or the bloodstream with the needle.

ACTION	RATIONALE

16. Reapply the tourniquet approximately 3 to 4 inches above the identified puncture site. Apply sufficient pressure to impede venous circulation but not arterial blood flow. **After disinfection, do not palpate the venipuncture site unless sterile gloves are worn.**

Use of a tourniquet increases venous pressure to aid in vein identification. Tourniquet should remain in place no more than 60 seconds to prevent injury, stasis, and hemoconcentration, which may alter results (Fischbach & Dunning, 2009).

17. Hold the patient's arm in a downward position with your nondominant hand. Align the needle and Vacutainer device with the chosen vein, holding the Vacutainer and needle in your dominant hand. Use the thumb or first finger of your nondominant hand to apply pressure and traction to the skin just below the identified puncture site.

Applying pressure helps immobilize and anchor the vein. Taut skin at entry site aids smooth needle entry.

18. **Inform the patient that he or she is going to feel a pinch.** With the bevel of the needle up, insert the needle into the vein at a 15-degree angle to the skin (Malarkey & McMorrow, 2012) (Figure 2).

Warning the patient prevents reaction related to surprise. Positioning the needle at the proper angle reduces the risk of puncturing through the vein.

FIGURE 2 Inserting the needle at a 15-degree angle, with the bevel up.

19. Grasp the Vacutainer securely to stabilize it in the vein with your nondominant

The collection tube is a vacuum; negative pressure within the tube pulls blood into the tube.

ACTION	RATIONALE
hand, and push the first collection tube into the puncture device in the Vacutainer, until the rubber stopper on the collection tube is punctured. You will feel the tube push into place on the puncture device. Blood will flow into the tube automatically.	
20. **Remove the tourniquet as soon as blood flows adequately into the tube.**	Tourniquet removal reduces venous pressure and restores venous return to help prevent bleeding and bruising (Van Leeuwen et al., 2011; Scales, 2008).
21. Continue to hold the Vacutainer in place in the vein and continue to fill the required tubes, removing one and inserting another. Gently rotate each tube as you remove it.	Filling the required tubes ensures that the sample is accurate. Gentle rotation helps to mix any additive in the tube with the blood sample.
22. After you have drawn all required blood samples, remove the last collection tube from the Vacutainer. **Place a gauze pad over the puncture site and slowly and gently remove the needle from the vein. Engage needle guard. Do not apply pressure to site until the needle has been fully removed.**	Slow, gentle needle removal prevents injury to the vein. Releasing the vacuum before withdrawing the needle prevents injury to the vein and hematoma formation. Use of a needle guard prevents accidental needlestick injuries.
23. Apply gentle pressure to the puncture site for 2 to 3 minutes or until bleeding stops.	Applying pressure to the site after needle removal prevents injury, bleeding, and extravasation into the surrounding tissue, which can cause a hematoma.
24. After bleeding stops, apply an adhesive bandage.	The bandage protects the site and aids in applying pressure.
25. Remove equipment and return the patient to a position of comfort. Raise side rail and lower bed.	Repositioning promotes patient comfort. Raising rails promotes safety.

ACTION	RATIONALE
26. Discard Vacutainer and needle in sharps container.	Proper disposal of equipment reduces transmission of microorganisms.
27. Remove gloves and perform hand hygiene.	Removing gloves properly reduces the risk for infection transmission and contamination of other items.
28. Place label on the container per facility policy. Place container in plastic, sealable biohazard bag.	Proper labeling ensures accurate reporting of results. Packaging the specimen in a biohazard bag prevents the person transporting the container from coming in contact with blood and body fluids.
29. Check the venipuncture site to see if a hematoma has developed.	Development of a hematoma requires further intervention.
30. Remove other PPE, if used. Perform hand hygiene.	Removing PPE properly reduces the risk for infection transmission and contamination of other items. Hand hygiene reduces the transmission of microorganisms.
31. Transport the specimen to the laboratory immediately. If immediate transport is not possible, check with laboratory personnel or policy manual whether refrigeration is contraindicated.	Timely transport ensures accurate results.

EVALUATION

- Uncontaminated blood specimen is obtained without adverse event.
- Patient states reason for blood test.
- Patient verbalizes minor, if any, complaint of pain at venipuncture site and minimal anxiety.
- Patient exhibits no signs and symptoms of injury at venipuncture site.

DOCUMENTATION

- Record the date, time, and site of the venipuncture; the name of the test(s); the time the sample was sent to the laboratory; the amount of blood collected, if required; and any significant assessments or patient reactions.

Normally bacteria-free, blood is susceptible to infection through infusion lines as well as from thrombophlebitis, surgical drains, infected shunts, and bacterial endocarditis due to prosthetic heart-valve replacements. Bacteria may also move into the bloodstream through the lymphatic system from an infection of a specific body site when the person's immune system cannot contain the infection at its source, such as the bladder or kidneys from a urinary tract infection. Patients with a compromised immune system are at higher risk for septicemia.

Blood cultures are performed to detect bacterial invasion (bacteremia) or fungi (fungemia) and the systemic spread of such an infection (septicemia) through the bloodstream. In this procedure, a venous blood sample is collected by venipuncture into two bottles (one set), one containing an anaerobic medium and the other an aerobic medium. The bottles are incubated, encouraging any organisms present in the sample to grow in the media. Ideally, two sets of cultures from two different venipuncture sites should be obtained. In the past, multiple sets of cultures were obtained at different time intervals. Currently, best practice is to draw blood one time, obtaining at least 30 mL of blood (for adults) from two different venipuncture sites. In general, no more than two to three sets of blood specimens over a 24-hour period should be collected (Malarkey & McMorrow, 2012; Myers III & Reyes, 2011).

The main problem encountered with blood-culture testing is that the specimen is easily contaminated with bacteria from the environment. Care must be taken to clean the skin at the venipuncture site properly to prevent contamination with skin flora, and aseptic technique must be used during the procedure. In addition, the access ports on the blood-culture bottles must be properly cleaned before use.

Refer to Skill 22 for additional considerations related to venipuncture and blood sample collection.

DELEGATION CONSIDERATIONS

The use of venipuncture to obtain a blood sample for blood culture may be delegated to nursing assistive personnel (NAP) or to unlicensed assistive personnel (UAP) in some settings, as well as to licensed practical/vocational nurses (LPN/LVNs). The decision to delegate must be based on careful analysis of the patient's needs and circumstances, as well as the qualifications of the person to whom the task is being delegated. Refer to the Delegation Guidelines in Appendix A.

EQUIPMENT

- Tourniquet
- Nonsterile gloves
- Additional PPE, as indicated

- Antimicrobial swabs, such as chlorhexidine, per facility policy, for cleaning skin and culture bottle tops

- Vacutainer needle adaptor
- Sterile butterfly needle, gauge appropriate to the vein and sampling needs, using the smallest possible, with extension tubing
- Two blood-culture collection bottles for each set being obtained; one anaerobic bottle and one aerobic bottle
- Appropriate label for specimen, based on facility policy and procedure
- Biohazard bag
- Nonsterile gauze pads (2 × 2)
- Sterile gauze pads (2 × 2)
- Adhesive bandage

ASSESSMENT

- Review the patient's medical record and the medical orders for the number and type of blood cultures to be obtained.
- Ensure that the appropriate computer laboratory request has been completed.
- Assess the patient for signs and symptoms of infection, including vital signs, and note any antibiotic therapy being administered.
- Inspect any invasive monitoring insertion sites or incisions for indications of infection.
- Assess the patient for any allergies, especially related to the topical antimicrobial used for skin cleansing.
- Assess for presence of any conditions or use of medications that may prolong bleeding time, necessitating additional application of pressure to the puncture site.
- Ask the patient about any previous laboratory testing that he or she may have had, including any problems, such as difficulty with venipuncture, fainting, or complaints of dizziness, light-headedness, or nausea.
- Assess the patient's anxiety level and understanding about the reasons for the blood test.
- Assess the patency of the veins in both upper limbs.
- Palpate the veins to assess the condition of the vessel; the vein should be straight, feel soft, cylindrical, and bounce when lightly pressed. Appropriate vessels will compress without rolling, and have rapid rebound filling after compression (Scales, 2008). Avoid veins that are tender, sclerosed, thrombosed, fibrosed, or hard.

NURSING DIAGNOSIS

- Deficient Knowledge
- Anxiety
- Risk for Injury
- Risk for Infection

OUTCOME IDENTIFICATION AND PLANNING

- Uncontaminated specimen will be obtained without the patient experiencing undue anxiety and injury.

IMPLEMENTATION

ACTION	RATIONALE
1. Gather the necessary supplies. Check product expiration dates. Identify ordered number of blood culture sets and select the appropriate blood-collection bottles (at least one anaerobic and one aerobic bottle). **If tests are ordered in addition to the blood cultures, collect the blood-culture specimens before other specimens.**	Organization facilitates efficient performance of the procedure. Use of products that have not expired ensures proper functioning of equipment. Using correct tubes ensures accurate blood sampling.
2. Perform hand hygiene and put on PPE, if indicated.	Hand hygiene and PPE prevent the transmission of microorganisms. PPE is required based on transmission precautions.
3. Identify the patient.	Identifying the patient ensures the right patient receives the intervention and helps prevent errors.
4. Explain the procedure. Allow the patient time to ask questions and verbalize concerns about the venipuncture procedure.	Explanation provides reassurance and promotes cooperation.
5. Check specimen label with the patient's identification bracelet. Label should include the patient's name and identification number, time specimen was collected, route of collection, identification of person obtaining the sample, and any other information required by facility policy.	Confirmation of patient identification information ensures the specimen is labeled correctly for the right patient.
6. Assemble equipment on overbed table within reach.	Arranging items nearby is convenient, saves time, and avoids unnecessary stretching and twisting of muscles on the part of the nurse.

ACTION	RATIONALE
7. Close curtains around the bed and close the door to the room, if possible.	Closing the door or curtain provides for patient privacy.
8. Provide for good light. Artificial light is recommended. Place a trash receptacle within easy reach.	Good lighting is necessary to perform the procedure properly. Having the trash receptacle in easy reach allows for safe disposal of contaminated materials.
9. Assist the patient to a comfortable position, either sitting or lying. If the patient is lying in bed, raise the bed to a comfortable working height, usually elbow height of the caregiver (VISN 8 Patient Safety Center, 2009).	Proper positioning allows easy access to the site and promotes patient comfort and safety. Proper bed height helps reduce back strain while performing the procedure.
10. Determine the patient's preferred site for the procedure based on his or her previous experience. Expose the arm, supporting it in an extended position on a firm surface, such as a tabletop. Position self on the same side of the patient as the site selected. Apply a tourniquet to the upper arm on the chosen side approximately 3 to 4 inches above the potential puncture site. Apply sufficient pressure to impede venous circulation, but not arterial blood flow.	Patient preference allows the patient to be involved in treatment and gives the nurse information that may aid in site selection (Lavery & Ingram, 2005). Positioning close to the chosen site reduces back strain. Use of a tourniquet increases venous pressure and distention to aid in vein identification. Tourniquet should remain in place no more than 60 seconds to prevent injury, stasis, and hemoconcentration, which may alter results (Fischbach & Dunning, 2009).
11. Put on nonsterile gloves. Assess the veins using inspection and palpation to determine the best puncture site. Refer to the Assessment section above.	Gloves reduce transmission of microorganisms. Using the best site reduces the risk of injury to the patient. Palpation allows for making a distinction between other structures, such as tendons and arteries, in the area to avoid injury.
12. **Release the tourniquet. Check that the vein has decompressed.**	Releasing the tourniquet reduces the length of time the tourniquet is applied. Tourniquet should

ACTION	RATIONALE
	remain in place no more than 60 seconds to prevent injury, stasis, and hemoconcentration, which may alter results (Fischbach & Dunning, 2009). Thrombosed veins will remain firm and palpable and should not be used for venipuncture (Lavery & Ingram, 2005).
13. Attach the butterfly needle extension tubing to the Vacutainer device.	Connection prepares device for use.
14. Move collection bottles to a location close to the arm, with bottles sitting upright on tabletop.	Bottles must be close enough to reach with extension tubing on butterfly needle to fill after venipuncture is completed. Bottles should remain upright to prevent backflow of contents to patient.
15. **Clean the patient's skin at the selected puncture site with the antimicrobial swab, according to facility policy. If using chlorhexidine, use a gentle back and forth motion or use the procedure recommended by the manufacturer. Do not wipe or blot. Allow to dry completely.**	Cleaning the patient's skin reduces the risk for transmission of microorganisms. Allowing the skin to dry maximizes antimicrobial action and prevents contact of the substance with the needle on insertion, thereby reducing the sting associated with insertion.
16. Alternately, for patients who bruise easily, are at risk for bleeding, or have fragile skin, **apply the chlorhexidine without scrubbing for at least 30 seconds. Allow to dry completely. Do not wipe or blot.**	Avoiding use of scrubbing decreases risk of injury. Application for a minimum of 30 seconds is necessary for chlorhexidine to be effective (Hadaway, 2006). Organisms on the skin can be introduced into the tissues or the bloodstream with the needle.
17. Using a new antimicrobial swab, clean the stoppers of the culture bottles with the appropriate antimicrobial, per facility policy. Cover bottle top with sterile gauze square, based on facility policy.	Cleaning the bottle top reduces the risk for transmission of microorganisms into the bottle. Covering the top reduces risk of contamination.

ACTION	RATIONALE

18. Reapply the tourniquet approximately 3 to 4 inches above the identified puncture site. Apply sufficient pressure to impede venous circulation, but not arterial blood flow. **After disinfection, do not palpate the venipuncture site unless sterile gloves are worn.**

Use of tourniquet increases venous pressure to aid in vein identification. Tourniquet should remain in place no more than 60 seconds to prevent injury, stasis, and hemoconcentration, which may alter results. Palpation is the greatest potential cause of blood culture contamination (Fischbach & Dunning, 2009).

19. Hold the patient's arm in a downward position with your nondominant hand. Align the butterfly needle with the chosen vein, holding the needle in your dominant hand. Use the thumb or first finger of your nondominant hand to apply pressure and traction to the skin just below the identified puncture site. **Do not touch the insertion site.**

Applying pressure helps immobilize and anchor the vein. Taut skin at the entry site aids smooth needle entry. Not touching the insertion site helps to prevent contamination.
Palpation is the greatest potential cause of blood culture contamination (Myers III & Reyes, 2011; Fischbach & Dunning, 2009).

20. **Inform the patient that he or she is going to feel a pinch.** With the bevel of the needle up, insert the needle into the vein at a 15-degree angle to the skin (Malarkey & McMorrow, 2012). You should see a flash of blood in the extension tubing close to the needle when the vein is entered.

Warning the patient prevents reaction related to surprise. Positioning the needle at the proper angle reduces the risk of puncturing through the vein. Flash of blood indicates entrance into the vein.

21. Grasp the butterfly needle securely to stabilize it in the vein with your nondominant hand, and push the Vacutainer onto the first collection bottle (anaerobic bottle), until the rubber stopper on the collection bottle is punctured. You will feel the bottle push into place on the puncture device. Blood will flow into the bottle automatically.

The collection bottle is a vacuum; negative pressure within the bottle pulls blood into the bottle.

ACTION	RATIONALE
22. **Remove the tourniquet as soon as blood flows adequately into the bottle.**	Tourniquet removal reduces venous pressure and restores venous return to help prevent bleeding and bruising (Van Leeuwen et al., 2011; Scales, 2008).
23. Continue to hold the butterfly needle in place in the vein. Once the first bottle is filled, remove it from the Vacutainer and insert the second bottle. After the blood culture specimens are obtained, continue to fill any additional required tubes, removing one and inserting another. Gently rotate each bottle and tube as you remove it.	Filling the required bottles ensures that the sample is accurate. Gentle rotation helps to mix any additive in the tube with the blood sample.
24. After you have drawn all required blood samples, remove the last collection tube from the Vacutainer. **Place a gauze pad over the puncture site and slowly and gently remove the needle from the vein. Engage needle guard. Do not apply pressure to the site until the needle has been fully removed.**	Slow, gentle needle removal prevents injury to the vein. Releasing the vacuum before withdrawing the needle prevents injury to the vein and hematoma formation. Use of a needle guard prevents accidental needlestick injuries.
25. Apply gentle pressure to the puncture site for 2 to 3 minutes or until bleeding stops.	Applying pressure to the site after needle removal prevents injury, bleeding, and extravasation into the surrounding tissue, which can cause a hematoma.
26. After bleeding stops, apply an adhesive bandage.	The bandage protects the site and aids in applying pressure.
27. Remove equipment and return patient to a position of comfort. Raise side rail and lower bed.	Repositioning promotes patient comfort. Raising rails promotes safety.
28. Discard Vacutainer and butterfly needle in sharps container.	Proper disposal of equipment reduces transmission of microorganisms.

ACTION	RATIONALE
29. Remove gloves and perform hand hygiene.	Removing gloves properly reduces the risk for infection transmission and contamination of other items. Hand hygiene reduces the transmission of microorganisms.
30. Place label on the container, per facility policy. Place containers in plastic, sealable biohazard bag. Refer to facility policy regarding the need for separate biohazard bags for blood culture specimens and other blood specimens.	Proper labeling ensures accurate reporting of results. Packaging the specimen in a biohazard bag prevents the person transporting the container from coming in contact with blood or body fluids. Some facility policies call for individual bagging.
31. Collect blood for second set of cultures from a second site, using the same technique.	Best practice involves drawing blood one time, obtaining at least 30 mL of blood (for adults) from two different venipuncture sites (Malarkey & McMorrow, 2012; Myers III & Reyes, 2011).
32. Check the venipuncture sites to see if a hematoma has developed.	Development of a hematoma requires further intervention.
33. Remove other PPE, if used. Perform hand hygiene.	Removing PPE properly reduces the risk for infection transmission and contamination of other items. Hand hygiene reduces the transmission of microorganisms.
34. Transport the specimen to the laboratory immediately. If immediate transport is not possible, check with laboratory personnel or policy manual as to appropriate handling.	Timely transport ensures accurate results.

EVALUATION

- Uncontaminated blood culture specimens are obtained without adverse event.
- Patient states reason for blood cultures.
- Patient verbalizes minor, if any, complaint of pain at venipuncture site.
- Patient reports decreased anxiety.
- Patient exhibits no signs and symptoms of injury at venipuncture site.

DOCUMENTATION

• Record the date, time, and site of the venipunctures; the name of the test(s); the time the sample was sent to the laboratory; the amount of blood collected, if required; and any significant assessments or patient reactions.

SKILL 24 OBTAINING AN ARTERIAL BLOOD SPECIMEN FOR BLOOD GAS ANALYSIS

Arterial blood gases (ABGs) are obtained to determine the adequacy of oxygenation and ventilation, to assess acid–base status, and to monitor the effectiveness of treatment. The most common site for sampling arterial blood is the radial artery. Other arteries may be used, but an advanced health care provider's order may be required to obtain the sample from another artery.

Analysis of ABG evaluates ventilation by measuring blood pH and the partial pressures of arterial oxygen (Pao_2) and partial pressure of arterial carbon dioxide ($Paco_2$). Blood pH measurement reveals the blood's acid–base balance. Pao_2 indicates the amount of oxygen that the lungs deliver to the blood, and $Paco_2$ indicates the lungs' capacity to eliminate carbon dioxide. ABG samples can also be analyzed for oxygen content and saturation, and for bicarbonate values. A respiratory technician or specially trained nurse can collect most ABG samples, but an advanced practice professional usually performs collection from the femoral artery, depending on facility policy. An Allen's test should always be performed before using the radial artery to determine whether the ulnar artery delivers sufficient blood to the hand and fingers, in case there is damage to the radial artery during the blood sampling.

DELEGATION CONSIDERATIONS

Obtaining an arterial blood specimen for blood gas analysis is not delegated to nursing assistive personnel (NAP) or to unlicensed assistive personnel (UAP). Depending on the state's nurse practice act and the organization's policies and procedures, obtaining an arterial blood specimen for blood gas analysis may be delegated to licensed practical/vocational nurses (LPN/LVNs). The decision to delegate must be based on careful analysis of the patient's needs and circumstances, as well as the qualifications of the person to whom the task is being delegated. Refer to the Delegation Guidelines in Appendix A.

EQUIPMENT

• ABG kit, *or* heparinized self-filling 10-mL syringe with 22-G, 1-inch needle attached
• Airtight cap for hub of syringe
• 2 × 2 gauze pad
• Band-Aid
• Antimicrobial swab, such as chlorhexidine

- Biohazard bag
- Appropriate label for specimen, based on facility policy and procedure
- Cup or bag of ice and water
- Nonsterile gloves
- Additional PPE, as indicated
- Rolled towel

ASSESSMENT

- Review the patient's medical record and plan of care for information about the need for an ABG specimen.
- Assess the patient's cardiac status, including heart rate, blood pressure, and auscultation of heart sounds.
- Assess the patient's respiratory status, including respiratory rate, excursion, lung sounds, and use of oxygen, including the amount being used, if ordered.
- Determine the adequacy of peripheral blood flow to the extremity to be used by performing the Allen's test (detailed below). If Allen's test reveals no or little collateral circulation to the hand, do not perform an arterial stick to that artery. Assess the patient's radial pulse. If unable to palpate the radial pulse, consider using the other wrist.
- Assess the patient's understanding about the need for specimen collection.
- Ask the patient if he or she has ever felt faint, sweaty, or nauseated when having blood drawn.

NURSING DIAGNOSIS

- Impaired Gas Exchange
- Risk for Injury
- Ineffective Airway Clearance
- Anxiety
- Decreased Cardiac Output

OUTCOME IDENTIFICATION AND PLANNING

- Blood sample is obtained from the artery without damage to the artery.
- Patient experiences minimal pain and anxiety during the procedure.
- Patient demonstrates an understanding of the need for the ABG specimen.

IMPLEMENTATION

ACTION	RATIONALE
1. Gather the necessary supplies. Check product expiration dates. Identify ordered arterial blood gas analysis. Check the chart to make sure	Organization facilitates efficient performance of the procedure. Use of products that have not expired ensures proper functioning of equipment. Suctioning may change the oxygen saturation

ACTION	RATIONALE
the patient has not been suctioned within the past 20 to 30 minutes. Check facility policy and/or procedure for guidelines on administering local anesthesia for arterial punctures. Administer anesthetic and allow sufficient time for full effect before beginning procedure.	and is a temporary change not to be confused with baseline for the patient. Arterial puncture is a source of pain and discomfort. Intradermal injection of lidocaine around the puncture site has been shown to decrease the incidence and severity of localized pain when used before arterial puncture (AACN, 2011).
2. Perform hand hygiene and put on PPE, if indicated.	Hand hygiene and PPE prevent the transmission of microorganisms. PPE is required based on transmission precautions.
3. Identify the patient.	Identifying the patient ensures the right patient receives the intervention and helps prevent errors.
4. Explain the procedure to the patient. Tell the patient you need to collect an arterial blood sample and the needlestick will cause some discomfort but that he or she must remain still during the procedure.	Explanation facilitates cooperation and provides reassurance for the patient.
5. Check specimen label with the patient's identification bracelet. Label should include patient's name and identification number, time specimen was collected, route of collection, identification of person obtaining the sample, amount of oxygen the patient is receiving, type of oxygen administration device, patients' body temperature, and any other information required by facility policy.	Confirmation of patient identification information ensures the specimen is labeled correctly for the right patient. Oxygen information and patient's body temperature are required for accurate analysis.

ACTION	RATIONALE
6. Assemble equipment on overbed table within reach.	Arranging items nearby is convenient, saves time, and avoids unnecessary stretching and twisting of muscles on the part of the nurse.
7. Close curtains around the bed and close the door to the room, if possible.	Closing the door or curtain provides for patient privacy.
8. Provide for good light. Artificial light is recommended. Place a trash receptacle within easy reach.	Good lighting is necessary to perform the procedure properly. Having the trash receptacle in easy reach allows for safe disposal of contaminated materials.
9. If the patient is on bed rest, ask him or her to lie in a supine position, with the head slightly elevated and the arms at the sides. Ask an ambulatory patient to sit in a chair and support the arm securely on an armrest or a table. Place a waterproof pad under the site and a rolled towel under the wrist.	Positioning the patient comfortably helps minimize anxiety. Using a rolled towel under the wrist provides for easy access to the insertion site.
10. **Perform Allen's test (Figure 1) before obtaining a specimen from the radial artery.**	Allen's testing assesses patency of the ulnar and radial arteries.
a. Have the patient clench the wrist to minimize blood flow into the hand.	
b. Using your index and middle fingers, press on the radial and ulnar arteries (Figure 1A). Hold this position for a few seconds.	
c. Without removing your fingers from the arteries, ask the patient to unclench the fist and hold the hand in a relaxed position (Figure 1B). The palm will be blanched because pressure from your fingers has impaired the normal blood flow.	

ACTION	RATIONALE

d. Release pressure on the ulnar artery (Figure 1C). If the hand becomes flushed, which indicates that blood is filling the vessels, it is safe to proceed with the radial artery puncture. This is considered a positive test. If the hand does not flush, perform the test on the other arm.

11. Put on nonsterile gloves. Locate the radial artery and lightly palpate it for a strong pulse.

Gloves reduce transmission of microorganisms. If you push too hard during palpation, the radial artery will be obliterated and hard to palpate.

12. **Clean the patient's skin at the puncture site with the antimicrobial swab, according to facility policy. If using chlorhexidine, use a gentle back and forth motion or use the procedure recommended by the manufacturer. Do not wipe or blot. Allow to dry completely. After disinfection, do not palpate the site unless sterile gloves are worn.**

Site cleansing prevents potentially infectious skin flora from being introduced into the vessel during the procedure. Palpation after cleansing contaminates the area.

FIGURE 1 Performing Allen's test. (**A**) Compressing the arteries with the patient's fist closed. (**B**) Maintaining compression as patient unclenches fist. (**C**) Compressing only the radial artery.

ACTION	RATIONALE
13. Alternately, for patients who bruise easily, are at risk for bleeding, or have fragile skin, **apply the chlorhexidine without scrubbing for at least 30 seconds. Allow to dry completely. Do not wipe or blot.**	Avoiding scrubbing decreases the risk of injury. Application for a minimum of 30 seconds is necessary for chlorhexidine to be effective (Hadaway, 2006). Organisms on the skin can be introduced into the tissues or the bloodstream with the needle.
14. Stabilize the hand with the wrist extended over the rolled towel, palm up. Palpate the artery above the puncture site with the index and middle fingers of your nondominant hand while holding the syringe over the puncture site with your dominant hand. **Do not directly touch the area to be punctured.**	Stabilizing the hand and palpating the artery with one hand while holding the syringe in the other provides better access to the artery. Palpating the area to be punctured would contaminate the clean area.
15. Hold the needle bevel up at a 45- to 60-degree angle at the site of maximal pulse impulse, with the shaft parallel to the path of the artery.	The proper angle of insertion ensures correct access to the artery. The artery is shallow and does not require a deeper angle to penetrate.
16. Puncture the skin and arterial wall in one motion. Watch for blood backflow in the syringe. Pulsating blood will flow into the syringe. Do not pull back on the plunger. Fill the syringe to the 5-mL mark.	The blood should enter the syringe automatically due to arterial pressure.
17. After collecting the sample, withdraw the syringe while your nondominant hand is beginning to place pressure proximal to the insertion site	If insufficient pressure is applied, a large, painful hematoma may form, hindering future arterial puncture at the site.

ACTION	RATIONALE
with the 2 × 2 gauze. **Press a gauze pad firmly over the puncture site until the bleeding stops—at least 5 minutes. If the patient is receiving anticoagulant therapy or has a blood dyscrasia, apply pressure for 10 to 15 minutes; if necessary, ask a coworker to hold the gauze pad in place while you prepare the sample for transport to the laboratory, but do not ask the patient to hold the pad.**	
18. When the bleeding stops and the appropriate time has lapsed, apply a small adhesive bandage or small pressure dressing (fold a 2 × 2 gauze into fourths and firmly apply tape, stretching the skin tight).	Applying a dressing also prevents arterial hemorrhage and extravasation into the surrounding tissue, which can cause a hematoma.
19. Once the sample is obtained, check the syringe for air bubbles. If any appear, remove them by holding the syringe upright and slowly ejecting some of the blood onto a 2 × 2 gauze pad.	Air bubbles can affect the laboratory values.
20. Engage the needle guard and remove the needle. Place the airtight cap on the syringe. Gently rotate the syringe. Do not shake.	Engaging the needle guard prevents accidental needlestick injury. Using an airtight cap prevents the sample from leaking and keeps air out of the syringe, because blood will continue to absorb oxygen and will give a false reading if allowed to have contact with air. Rotating the syringe ensures proper mixing of heparin in syringe with the sample; heparin prevents blood from clotting. Vigorous shaking may cause hemolysis.

ACTION	RATIONALE
21. Place label on the syringe per facility policy. Place syringe in plastic, sealable biohazard bag. Insert the syringe into a cup or bag of ice water.	Labeling ensures the specimen is the correct one for the right patient. Packaging the specimen in a biohazard bag prevents the person transporting the samples from coming in contact with blood. Ice prevents the blood from degrading.
22. Discard the needle in sharps container. Remove gloves and perform hand hygiene.	Proper disposal of equipment prevents accidental injury and reduces transmission of microorganisms. Removing gloves properly reduces the risk for infection transmission and contamination of other items. Hand hygiene reduces transmission of microorganisms.
23. Remove other PPE, if used. Perform hand hygiene.	Removing PPE properly reduces the risk for infection transmission and contamination of other items. Hand hygiene reduces the transmission of microorganisms.
24. Transport the specimen to the laboratory immediately.	Timely transport ensures accurate results.

EVALUATION
- Arterial blood specimen is obtained, and the patient reports minimal pain during the procedure.
- Site remains free of injury, without evidence of hematoma formation.
- Patient verbalizes an understanding of the rationale for the specimen collection.

DOCUMENTATION
- Document results of Allen's test, time the sample was drawn, arterial puncture site, amount of time pressure was applied to the site to control bleeding, type and amount of oxygen therapy that the patient was receiving, pulse oximetry values, respiratory rate, respiratory effort, patient's body temperature, and any other significant assessments.

SKILL 25 ADMINISTERING A BLOOD TRANSFUSION

A blood transfusion is the infusion of whole blood or a blood component such as plasma, red blood cells, cryoprecipitate, or platelets into the patient's venous circulation. A blood product transfusion is given when a patient's red blood cells, platelets, or coagulation factors decrease to levels that compromise a patient's health. Before a patient can receive a blood product, his or her blood must be typed to ensure that he or she receives compatible blood. Otherwise, a serious and life-threatening transfusion reaction may occur involving clumping and hemolysis of the red blood cells and, possibly, death. The nurse must also verify the infusion rate, based on facility policy or medical order. Follow the facility's policies and guidelines to determine if the transfusion should be administered by an electronic infusion device or by gravity.

DELEGATION CONSIDERATIONS

The administration of a blood transfusion is not delegated to nursing assistive personnel (NAP), to unlicensed assistive personnel (UAP), or to licensed practical/vocational nurses (LPN/LVNs).

EQUIPMENT

- Blood product
- Blood administration set (tubing with in-line filter, or add-on filter, and Y for saline administration)
- 0.9% normal saline for IV infusion
- IV pole
- Venous access; if peripheral site, preferably initiated with a 20-gauge catheter or larger
- Alcohol or other disinfectant wipes
- Clean gloves
- Additional PPE, as indicated
- Tape (hypoallergenic)
- Second registered nurse (or other licensed practitioner; e.g., a physician) to verify blood product and patient information

ASSESSMENT

- Obtain a baseline assessment of the patient, including vital signs, heart and lung sounds, and urinary output.
- Review the most recent laboratory values, in particular, the complete blood count (CBC).
- Ask the patient about any previous transfusions, including the number he or she has had and any reactions experienced during a transfusion.

- Inspect the IV insertion site, noting the gauge of the IV catheter. Blood or blood components may be transfused via a 14- to 24-gauge peripheral venous access device. Transfusion for neonate or pediatric patients is usually given using a 22- to 24-gauge peripheral venous access device (INS, 2011).

NURSING DIAGNOSIS

- Risk for Injury
- Excess Fluid Volume
- Ineffective Peripheral Tissue Perfusion

OUTCOME IDENTIFICATION AND PLANNING

- Patient will remain free of injury and any signs and symptoms of IV complications.
- The capped venous access device will remain patent.

IMPLEMENTATION

ACTION	RATIONALE
1. Verify the medical order for transfusion of a blood product. Verify the completion of informed consent documentation in the medical record. Verify any medical order for pre-transfusion medication. If ordered, administer medication at least 30 minutes before initiating transfusion.	Verification of order ensures the right patient receives the correct intervention. Premedication is sometimes administered to decrease the risk for allergic and febrile reactions for patients who have received multiple previous transfusions.
2. Gather all equipment.	Preparation promotes efficient time management and an organized approach to the task.
3. Perform hand hygiene and put on PPE, if indicated.	Hand hygiene and PPE prevent the spread of microorganisms. PPE is required based on transmission precautions.
4. Identify the patient.	Identifying the patient ensures the right patient receives the intervention and helps prevent errors.

ACTION	RATIONALE
5. Close the curtains around the bed and close the door to the room, if possible. Explain what you are going to do and why you are going to do it to the patient. Ask the patient about previous experience with a transfusion and any reactions. Advise the patient to report any chills, itching, rash, or unusual symptoms.	This ensures the patient's privacy. Explanation relieves anxiety and facilitates cooperation. Previous reactions may increase the risk for reaction to this transfusion. Any reaction to the transfusion necessitates stopping the transfusion immediately and evaluating the situation.
6. Prime blood administration set with the normal saline IV fluid. Refer to Skill 91.	Normal saline is the solution of choice for blood product administration. Solutions with dextrose may lead to clumping of red blood cells and hemolysis.
7. Put on gloves. If patient does not have a venous access in place, initiate peripheral venous access. (Refer to Skill 129.) Connect the administration set to the venous access device via the extension tubing. (Refer to Skill 129.) Infuse the normal saline per facility policy.	Gloves prevent contact with blood and body fluids. Infusion of fluid via venous access maintains patency until the blood product is administered. Start an IV before obtaining the blood product in case the initiation takes longer than 30 minutes. Blood must be stored at a carefully controlled temperature (4°C) and transfusion must begin within 30 minutes of release from the blood bank.
8. Obtain blood product from blood bank according to agency policy. Scan for bar codes on blood products if required.	Bar codes on blood products are currently being implemented in some agencies to identify, track, and assign data to transfusions as an additional safety measure.
9. Two nurses compare and validate the following information with the medical record, patient identification band, and the label of the blood product: • Medical order for transfusion of blood product • Informed consent • Patient identification number	Most states/agencies require two registered nurses to verify the following information: unit numbers match; ABO group and Rh type are the same; expiration date (after 35 days, red blood cells begin to deteriorate). Blood is never administered to a patient without an identification band. If clots or signs of contamination

ACTION	RATIONALE

- Patient name
- Blood group and type
- Expiration date
- Inspection of blood product for clots, clumping, gas bubbles

(clumping, gas bubbles) are present, return blood to the blood bank.

10. **Obtain baseline set of vital signs before beginning the transfusion.**

Any change in vital signs during the transfusion may indicate a reaction.

11. Put on gloves. If using an electronic infusion device, put the device on "hold." Close the roller clamp closest to the drip chamber on the saline side of the administration set. Close the roller clamp on the administration set below the infusion device. Alternately, if infusing via gravity, close the roller clamp on the administration set.

Gloves prevent contact with blood and body fluids. Stopping the infusion prevents blood from infusing to the patient before completion of preparations. Closing the clamp to saline allows blood product to be infused via electronic infusion device.

12. Close the roller clamp closest to the drip chamber on the blood product side of the administration set. Remove the protective cap from the access port on the blood container. Remove the cap from the access spike on the administration set. Using a pushing and twisting motion, insert the spike into the access port on the blood container, taking care not to contaminate the spike. Hang the blood container on the IV pole. Open the roller clamp on the blood side of the administration set. Squeeze drip chamber until the in-line filter is saturated. Remove gloves.

Filling the drip chamber prevents air from entering the administration set. The filter in the blood administration set removes particulate material formed during storage of blood. If the administration set becomes contaminated, the entire set would have to be discarded and replaced.

13. **Start administration slowly (no more than 25 to 50 mL for the first 15 minutes). Stay with the patient for**

Transfusion reactions typically occur during this period, and a slow rate will minimize the volume of red blood cells infused.

ACTION	RATIONALE
the first 5 to 15 minutes of transfusion. Open the roller clamp on the administration set below the infusion device. Set the flow rate and begin the transfusion. Alternately, start the flow of solution by releasing the clamp on the tubing and counting the drops. Adjust until the correct drop rate is achieved. Assess the flow of the blood and function of the infusion device. Inspect the insertion site for signs of infiltration.	Verifying the rate and device settings ensures the patient receives the correct volume of solution. If the catheter or needle slips out of the vein, the blood will accumulate (infiltrate) into the surrounding tissue.
14. Observe the patient for flushing, dyspnea, itching, hives or rash, or any unusual comments.	These signs and symptoms may be an early indication of a transfusion reaction.
15. After the observation period (5 to 15 minutes) increase the infusion rate to the calculated rate to complete the infusion within the prescribed time frame, no more than 4 hours.	If no adverse effects occurred during this time, the infusion rate is increased. If complications occur, they can be observed and the transfusion can be stopped immediately. Verifying the rate and device settings ensures the patient receives the correct volume of solution. Transfusion must be completed within 4 hours due to potential for bacterial growth in blood product at room temperature.
16. Reassess vital signs after 15 minutes. Obtain vital signs thereafter according to facility policy and nursing assessment.	Vital signs must be assessed as part of monitoring for possible adverse reaction. Facility policy and nursing judgment will dictate frequency.
17. Maintain the prescribed flow rate as ordered or as deemed appropriate based on the patient's overall condition, keeping in mind the outer limits for safe administration. Ongoing monitoring is crucial throughout the entire	Rate must be carefully controlled, and the patient's reaction must be monitored frequently.

ACTION	RATIONALE

duration of the blood transfusion for early identification of any adverse reactions.

18. **During transfusion, assess frequently for transfusion reaction. Stop blood transfusion if you suspect a reaction. Quickly replace the blood tubing with a new administration set primed with normal saline for IV infusion. Initiate an infusion of normal saline for IV at an open rate, usually 40 mL/hour. Obtain vital signs. Notify primary care provider and blood bank.**

If a transfusion reaction is suspected, the blood must be stopped. Do not infuse the normal saline through the blood tubing because you would be allowing more of the blood into the patient's body, which could complicate a reaction. Besides a serious life-threatening blood transfusion reaction, the potential for fluid–volume overload exists in older patients and patients with decreased cardiac function.

19. When transfusion is complete, close roller clamp on blood side of the administration set and open the roller clamp on the normal saline side of the administration set. Initiate infusion of normal saline. When all of blood has infused into the patient, clamp the administration set. Obtain vital signs. Put on gloves. Cap access site or resume previous IV infusion. (Refer to Skill 129 and Skill 128.) Dispose of blood-transfusion equipment or return to blood bank, according to facility policy.

Saline prevents hemolysis of red blood cells and clears remainder of blood in IV line.

Proper disposal of equipment reduces transmission of microorganisms and potential contact with blood and body fluids.

20. Remove equipment. Ensure patient's comfort. Remove gloves. Lower bed, if not in lowest position.

Promotes patient comfort and safety. Removing gloves properly reduces the risk for infection transmission and contamination of other items.

21. Remove additional PPE, if used. Perform hand hygiene.

Removing PPE properly reduces the risk for infection transmission and contamination of other items. Hand hygiene prevents transmission of microorganisms.

ACTION	RATIONALE
22. Monitor and assess the patient for one hour after the transfusion for signs and symptoms of delayed transfusion reaction. Provide patient education about signs and symptoms of delayed transfusion reactions.	Ensures early detection and prompt intervention. Delayed transfusion reactions can occur one to several days after transfusion.

EVALUATION

- Patient receives the blood transfusion without any evidence of a transfusion reaction or complication.
- Patient exhibits signs and symptoms of fluid balance, improved cardiac output, and enhanced peripheral tissue perfusion.
- The venous access device remains patent.

DOCUMENTATION

- Document that the patient received the blood transfusion; include the type of blood product. Record the patient's condition throughout the transfusion, including pertinent data, such as vital signs, lung sounds, and the subjective response of the patient to the transfusion. Document any complications or reactions and whether the patient had received the transfusion without any complications or reactions. Document the assessment of the IV site, and any other fluids infused during the procedure. Document transfusion volume and other IV fluid intake on the patient's intake and output record.

SKILL 26 APPLYING A CARDIAC MONITOR

Bedside cardiac monitoring provides continuous observation of the heart's electrical activity. It focuses on the detection of clinically significant dysrhythmias (Larson & Brady, 2008). Cardiac monitoring is used for patients with conduction disturbances and for those at risk for life-threatening arrhythmias, such as postoperative patients and patients who are sedated. As with other forms of electrocardiography (ECG), cardiac monitoring uses electrodes placed on the patient's chest to transmit electrical signals that are converted into a tracing of cardiac rhythm on an oscilloscope. Three-lead or five-lead systems may be used (Figure 1). The three-lead–wire monitoring system facilitates monitoring of the

FIGURE 1 Electrode positions for three-lead (*left*) and five-lead (*right*) systems.

Positions for the three-lead system:

RA (white electrode) below right clavicle, second ICS, right midclavicular line

LA (black electrode) below left clavicle, second ICS, left midclavicular line

LL (red electrode) left lower ribcage, eighth ICS, left midclavicular line

Positions for five-lead system:

RA (white electrode) below right clavicle, second ICS, right midclavicular line

RL (green electrode) right lower ribcage, eighth ICS, right midclavicular line

LA (black electrode) below left clavicle, second ICS, left midclavicular line

LL (red electrode) left lower ribcage, eighth ICS, left midclavicular line

Chest (brown electrode) any V lead position, usually V_1 (fourth ICS, right sternal border)

patient in any of the limb leads, as well as a modified version of any of the six chest leads (Morton & Fontaine, 2013). The five-lead–wire monitoring system facilitates monitoring of the patient in any one of the standard 12 leads.

Two types of monitoring may be performed: hardwire or telemetry. In hardwire monitoring, the patient is connected to a monitor at the bedside. The rhythm display appears at the bedside, but may also be transmitted to a console at a remote location. Telemetry uses a small transmitter connected to an ambulatory patient to send electrical signals to another location, where they are displayed on a monitor screen. Battery-powered and portable, telemetry frees patients from cumbersome wires and cables and lets them be comfortably mobile. Telemetry is especially useful for monitoring arrhythmias that occur during sleep, rest, exercise, or stressful situations. Wireless telemetry devices are also being introduced, using microchips to record patient data, eliminating the need for new leads each time the patient is moved to a different location. (Goulette, 2008)

Regardless of the type, cardiac monitors can display the patient's heart rate and rhythm, produce a printed record of cardiac rhythm, and sound an alarm if the heart rate exceeds or falls below specified limits. Monitors also recognize and count abnormal heartbeats as well as changes. Cardiac monitoring systems may incorporate computer systems that store, analyze and trend monitored data, automatic chart documentation, and wireless communication devices that provide data and alarms that can be carried by the nurse (Morton & Fontaine, 2013).

Gel foam electrodes are commonly used. Electrodes should be changed every 24 hours, or according to facility policy, to prevent skin irritation and maintain quality of data. Hypoallergenic electrodes are available for patients with hypersensitivity to tape or adhesive. Any loose or nonadhering electrode should be replaced immediately to prevent inaccurate or missing data.

DELEGATION CONSIDERATIONS

The application of a cardiac monitor is not delegated to nursing assistive personnel (NAP) or to unlicensed assistive personnel (UAP). Depending on the state's nurse practice act and the organization's policies and procedures, application of a cardiac monitor may be delegated to licensed practical/vocational nurses (LPN/LVNs).The decision to delegate must be based on careful analysis of the patient's needs and circumstances, as well as the qualifications of the person to whom the task is being delegated. Refer to the Delegation Guidelines in Appendix A.

EQUIPMENT

- Lead wires
- Pregelled (gel foam) electrodes (number varies from 3 to 5)
- Gauze pads
- Skin cleanser
- Patient cable for hardwire cardiac monitoring
- Transmitter, transmitter pouch, and telemetry battery pack for telemetry
- PPE, as indicated

ASSESSMENT

- Review the patient's medical record and plan of care for information about the patient's need for cardiac monitoring.
- Assess the patient's cardiac status, including heart rate, blood pressure, and auscultation of heart sounds.
- Inspect the patient's chest for areas of irritation, breakdown, or excessive hair that might interfere with electrode placement. Electrode sites must be dry, with minimal hair.
- The patient may be sitting or supine, in a bed or chair.

NURSING DIAGNOSIS

- Decreased Cardiac Output
- Excess Fluid Volume
- Deficient Knowledge

OUTCOME IDENTIFICATION AND PLANNING

- A clear waveform, free from artifact, is displayed on the cardiac monitor.
- Patient verbalizes an understanding of the reason for monitoring.
- Patient experiences reduced anxiety.

IMPLEMENTATION

ACTION	RATIONALE
1. Verify the order for cardiac monitoring on the patient's medical record.	This ensures that the correct intervention is performed on the correct patient.
2. Gather equipment.	Assembling equipment provides for an organized approach to the task.
3. Perform hand hygiene and put on PPE, if indicated.	Hand hygiene and PPE prevent the spread of microorganisms. PPE is required based on transmission precautions.
4. Identify the patient.	Identifying the patient ensures the right patient receives the intervention and helps prevent errors.
5. Close curtains around the bed and close the door to the room, if possible. Explain the procedure to the patient. Tell the patient that the monitoring records the heart's electrical activity. Emphasize that no electrical current will enter his or her body. Ask the patient about allergies to adhesive, as appropriate.	This ensures the patient's privacy. Explanation relieves anxiety and facilitates cooperation. Possible allergies may exist related to adhesive on ECG leads.
6. For hardwire monitoring, plug the cardiac monitor into an electrical outlet and turn it on to warm up the unit while preparing the equipment and the patient. For telemetry monitoring, insert a new battery into the	Proper setup ensures proper functioning. Not all models have a test button. Test according to manufacturer's directions.

ACTION	RATIONALE
transmitter. Match the poles on the battery with the polar markings on the transmitter case. Press the button at the top of the unit, test the battery's charge, and test the unit to ensure that the battery is operational.	
7. Insert the cable into the appropriate socket in the monitor.	Proper setup ensures proper functioning.
8. Connect the lead wires to the cable. In some systems, the lead wires are permanently secured to the cable. For telemetry, if the lead wires are not permanently affixed to the telemetry unit, attach them securely. If they must be attached individually, connect each one to the correct outlet.	Proper setup ensures proper functioning.
9. Connect an electrode to each of the lead wires, carefully checking that each lead wire is in its correct outlet.	Proper setup ensures proper functioning.
10. If the bed is adjustable, raise it to a comfortable working height, usually elbow height of the caregiver (VISN 8, 2009).	Having the bed at the proper height prevents back and muscle strain.
11. Expose the patient's chest and determine electrode positions, based on which system and leads are being used. (Refer to Figure 1.) If necessary, clip the hair from an area about 10 cm in diameter around each electrode site. Abrade the skin by gently rubbing the area with a gauze pad. Clean the area with skin cleanser and water and dry it completely.	These actions allow for better adhesion of the electrode and thus better conduction. Gentle abrasion removes dead skin cells. Cleaning skin removes oily residues. Alcohol, benzoin, and antiperspirant are not recommended to prepare the skin.

ACTION	RATIONALE
12. Remove the backing from the pregelled electrode. Check the gel for moistness. If the gel is dry, discard it and replace it with a fresh electrode. **Apply the electrode to the site and press firmly to ensure a tight seal.** Repeat with the remaining electrodes to complete the three-lead or five-lead system.	Gel acts as a conduit and must be moist and secured tightly.
13. When all the electrodes are in place, connect the appropriate lead wire to each electrode. Check waveform for clarity, position, and size. **To verify that the monitor is detecting each beat, compare the digital heart rate display with an auscultated count of the patient's heart rate.** If necessary, use the gain control to adjust the size of the rhythm tracing, and use the position control to adjust the waveform position on the monitor.	This ensures accuracy of reading.
14. Set the upper and lower limits of the heart rate alarm, based on the patient's condition or unit policy.	Setting the alarm allows for audible notification if the heart rate is beyond limits. The default setting for the monitor automatically turns on all alarms; limits should be set for each patient.
15. For telemetry, place the transmitter in the pouch in the hospital gown. If no pouch is available in the gown, use a portable pouch. Tie the pouch strings around the patient's neck and waist, making sure that the pouch fits snugly without causing discomfort. If no pouch is available, place the transmitter in the patient's bathrobe pocket.	Patient comfort leads to compliance.

ACTION	RATIONALE
16. To obtain a rhythm strip, press the RECORD key either at the bedside for monitoring or at the central station for telemetry. Label the strip with the patient's name and room number, date, time, and rhythm identification. Analyze the strip, as appropriate. Place the rhythm strip in the appropriate location in the patient's chart.	A rhythm strip provides a baseline for future comparison.
17. Return the patient to a comfortable position. Lower the bed height and adjust the head of bed to a comfortable position.	Repositioning promotes patient comfort. Lowering the bed promotes patient safety.
18. Remove additional PPE, if used. Perform hand hygiene.	Removing PPE properly reduces the risk for infection transmission and contamination of other items. Hand hygiene prevents transmission of microorganisms.

EVALUATION

- Cardiac monitoring waveform displays the patient's cardiac rhythm, with a waveform that is detecting each beat, and is appropriate for clarity, position, and size.
- Patient demonstrates no undue anxiety and remains free of complications or injury.

DOCUMENTATION

- Record the date and time that monitoring begins and the monitoring lead used in the medical record. Document a rhythm strip at least every 8 hours and with any changes in the patient's condition (or as stated by facility's policy). Label the rhythm strip with the patient's name and room number, date, and time.

Cardiopulmonary resuscitation (CPR), also known as basic life support, is used in any situation in which either breathing alone or breathing and a heartbeat are absent. It is a combination of chest compressions, which circulate blood, and mouth-to-mouth breathing, which supplies oxygen to the lungs. The brain is sensitive to hypoxia and will sustain irreversible damage after 4 to 6 minutes of no oxygen. The faster CPR is initiated, the greater the chance of survival.

If breathing alone or breathing and a heartbeat are absent, assess the victim for a response, activate the emergency response system, get an automated external defibrillator (AED) or defibrillator, and begin CPR with the CAB sequence (chest compressions, airway, breathing) and defibrillation (American Heart Association [AHA], 2011).

In the hospital setting, it is imperative that personnel be aware of the patient's stated instructions regarding any wish not to be resuscitated. This should be clearly expressed and documented in the patient's medical record.

Learning conventional CPR is still recommended for emergency interventions outside of health care facilities. However, the AHA alternately recommends that when a teen or an adult suddenly collapses, people near the victim should call 911 (to activate the emergency response system), and push hard and fast in the center of the victim's chest. Studies of real emergencies that have occurred in homes, at work, or in public locations, show that these two steps, called Hands-Only CPR, can be as effective as conventional CPR. Providing Hands-Only CPR to an adult who has collapsed from a sudden cardiac arrest can more than double that person's chance of survival (AHA, 2012).

DELEGATION CONSIDERATIONS

The initiation and provision of cardiopulmonary resuscitation is appropriate for all health care providers.

EQUIPMENT

- Personal protective equipment, such as a face shield or one-way valve mask and gloves, if available
- Ambu-bag and oxygen, if available

ASSESSMENT

- Assess the patient's vital parameters and determine the patient's level of responsiveness.
- Check for partial or complete airway obstruction.
- Assess for the absence or ineffectiveness of respirations.
- Assess for the absence of signs of circulation and pulses.

NURSING DIAGNOSIS

- Decreased Cardiac Output
- Impaired Gas Exchange
- Impaired Spontaneous Ventilation

OUTCOME IDENTIFICATION AND PLANNING

- CPR is performed effectively without adverse effect to the patient.
- Patient regains a pulse and respirations.
- Patient's heart and lungs maintain adequate function to sustain life.
- Advanced cardiac life support is initiated.
- Patient does not experience injury.

IMPLEMENTATION

ACTION	RATIONALE
1. Assess responsiveness. Look for breathing. If the patient is not responsive and is not breathing or not breathing normally, call for help, pull call bell, and call the facility emergency response number. Call for the automated external defibrillator (AED) or defibrillator, if available.	Assessing responsiveness prevents starting CPR on a conscious patient. Activating the emergency response system initiates a rapid response.
2. Put on gloves, if available. Position the patient supine on his or her back on a firm, flat surface, with arms alongside the body. If the patient is in bed, place a backboard or other rigid surface under the patient (often the footboard of the patient's bed). Position yourself at the patient's side.	Gloves prevent contact with blood and body fluids. The supine position is required for resuscitative efforts and evaluation to be effective. Backboard provides a firm surface on which to apply compressions. If the patient must be rolled, move as a unit so the head, shoulders, and torso move simultaneously without twisting.
3. Provide **defibrillation at the earliest possible moment, as soon as an AED becomes available.** Refer to Skill 47 and Skill 48.	The interval from collapse to defibrillation is one of the most important determinants of survival from sudden cardiac arrest (AHA, 2011).
4. Check for a pulse, palpating the carotid pulse. This assessment should take at least 5 seconds and no	Pulse assessment evaluates cardiac function. Delays in chest compressions should be minimized, so the health care

ACTION	RATIONALE

more than 10 seconds. If you do not definitely feel a pulse within 10 seconds, begin CPR using the compression:ventilation ratio of 30 compressions to 2 breaths, starting with chest compressions (CAB sequence).

provider should take no more than 10 seconds to check for a pulse. If it is not felt within that time period, chest compressions should be started (Neumar et al., 2010)

5. Position the heel of one hand in the center of the chest between the nipples, directly over the lower half of the sternum. Place the heel of the other hand directly on top of the first hand. Extend or interlace fingers to keep fingers above the chest. Straighten arms and position shoulders directly over hands.

Proper hand positioning ensures that the force of compressions is on the sternum, thereby reducing the risk of rib fracture, lung puncture, or liver laceration.

6. Push hard and fast. Chest compressions should depress the sternum 2 inches. Push straight down on the patient's sternum. Perform 30 chest compressions at a rate of 100 per minute, counting "one, two, etc." up to 30, keeping elbows locked, arms straight, and shoulders directly over the hands. Allow full chest recoil (re-expand) after each compression. Chest compression and chest recoil/relaxation times should be approximately equal.

Direct cardiac compression and manipulation of intrathoracic pressure supply blood flow during CPR. Compressing the chest 2 inches ensures that compressions are not too shallow and provides adequate blood flow. Full chest recoil allows adequate venous return to the heart.

7. Give two breaths (as described below) after each set of 30 compressions. Do five complete cycles of 30 compressions and two ventilations.

Breathing and compressions simulate lung and heart function, providing oxygen and circulation.

8. Use the head tilt–chin lift maneuver to open the airway. Place one hand on the patient's forehead and apply

The head tilt–chin lift maneuver lifts the tongue, relieving airway obstruction by the tongue in an unresponsive person.

ACTION	RATIONALE
firm, backward pressure with the palm to tilt the head back. Place the fingers of the other hand under the bony part of the lower jaw near the chin and lift the jaw upward to bring the chin forward and the teeth almost to occlusion.	
9. If trauma to the head or neck is present or suspected, use the jaw-thrust maneuver to open the airway. Place one hand on each side of the patient's head. Rest elbows on the flat surface under the patient, grasp the angle of the patient's lower jaw, and lift with both hands.	The jaw-thrust maneuver may reduce neck and spine movement.
10. Seal the patient's mouth and nose with the face shield, one-way valve mask, or Ambu-bag (handheld resuscitation bag), if available. If not available, seal the patient's mouth with your mouth.	Sealing the patient's mouth and nose prevents air from escaping. Devices such as masks reduce the risk for transmission of infections.
11. Instill two breaths, each lasting 1 second, making the chest rise.	Breathing into the patient provides oxygen to the patient's lungs. Hyperventilation results in increased positive chest pressure and decreased venous return. Blood flow to the lungs during CPR is only about 25% to 33% normal; patient requires less ventilation to provide oxygen and remove carbon dioxide. Longer breaths reduce the amount of blood that refills the heart, reducing blood flow generated by compressions. Delivery of large, forceful breaths may cause gastric inflation and distension.

ACTION	RATIONALE
12. If you are unable to ventilate or the chest does not rise during ventilation, reposition the patient's head and reattempt to ventilate. If still unable to ventilate, resume CPR. Each subsequent time the airway is opened to administer breaths, look for an object. If an object is visible in the mouth, remove it. If no object is visible, continue with CPR.	Inability to ventilate indicates that the airway may be obstructed. Repositioning maneuvers may be sufficient to open the airway and promote spontaneous respirations. It is critical to minimize interruptions in chest compressions, to maintain circulatory perfusion.
13. After 5 complete cycles of CPR, check the carotid pulse, simultaneously evaluating for breathing, coughing, or movement. This assessment should take at least 5 seconds and no more than 10 seconds.	Pulse assessment evaluates cardiac function.
14. If the patient has a pulse, but remains without spontaneous breathing, continue with rescue breathing, without chest compressions. Administer rescue breathing at a rate of one breath every 5 to 6 seconds, for a rate of 10 to 12 breaths per minute.	Rescue breathing maintains adequate oxygenation.
15. If spontaneous breathing resumes, place the patient in the recovery position.	Prevents obstruction of airway.
16. Otherwise, continue CPR until advanced care providers take over, the patient starts to move, you are too exhausted to continue, or a physician discontinues CPR.	Once started, CPR must continue until one of these conditions is met. In a hospital setting, help should arrive within a few minutes.
17. Remove gloves, if used. Perform hand hygiene.	Removing PPE properly reduces the risk for infection transmission and contamination of other items. Hand hygiene prevents transmission of microorganisms.

EVALUATION
- CPR is performed effectively without adverse effect to the patient.
- Patient regains a pulse and respirations.
- Patient's heart and lungs maintain adequate function to sustain life.
- Advanced cardiac life support is initiated.
- Patient does not experience serious injury.

DOCUMENTATION
- Document the time you discovered the patient unresponsive and started CPR. Continued intervention, such as by the code team, is typically documented on a code form, which identifies the actions and drugs provided during the code. Provide a summary of these events in the patient's medical record.

SKILL 28   ASSISTING WITH CAST APPLICATION

A cast is a rigid external immobilizing device that encases a body part. Casts are used to immobilize a body part in a specific position and to apply uniform pressure on the encased soft tissue. They may be used to treat injuries, correct a deformity, stabilize weakened joints, or promote healing after surgery. Casts generally allow the patient mobility while restricting movement of the affected body part. Casts may be made of plaster or synthetic materials, such as fiberglass. Each material has advantages and disadvantages. Nonplaster casts set in 15 minutes and can sustain weight bearing or pressure in 15 to 30 minutes. Plaster casts can take 24 to 72 hours to dry, and weight bearing or pressure is contraindicated during this period. Patient safety is of utmost importance during the application of a cast. Typically, a physician or other advanced practice professional applies the cast. Nursing responsibilities include preparing the patient and equipment and assisting during the application. The nurse provides skin care to the affected area before, during, and after the cast is applied. In some settings, nurses with special preparation may apply or change casts.

DELEGATION CONSIDERATIONS

Assisting with the application of a cast may not be delegated to nursing assistive personnel (NAP) or to unlicensed assistive personnel (UAP). Depending on the state's nurse practice act and the organization's policies and procedures, assisting with the application of a cast may be delegated to licensed practical/vocational nurses (LPN/LVNs). The decision to delegate must be based on careful analysis of the patient's needs and circumstances, as well as the qualifications of the person to whom the task is being delegated. Refer to the Delegation Guidelines in Appendix A.

EQUIPMENT

- Casting materials, such as plaster rolls or fiberglass, depending on the type of cast being applied
- Padding material, such as stockinette, sheet wadding, or Webril, depending on the type of cast being applied
- Plastic bucket or basin filled with warm water
- Disposable, nonsterile gloves and aprons
- Scissors
- Waterproof, disposable pads
- PPE, as indicated

ASSESSMENT

- Assess the skin condition in the affected area, noting redness, contusions, or open wounds.
- Assess the neurovascular status of the affected extremity, including distal pulses, color, temperature, presence of edema, capillary refill to fingers or toes, weakness, sensation, and motion.
- Perform a pain assessment. If the patient reports pain, administer the prescribed analgesic in sufficient time to allow for the full effect of the medication. Assess for muscle spasms and administer the prescribed muscle relaxant in sufficient time to allow for the full effect of the medication.
- Assess for the presence of disease processes that may contraindicate the use of a cast or interfere with wound healing, including skin diseases, peripheral vascular disease, diabetes mellitus, and open or draining wounds.

NURSING DIAGNOSIS

- Risk for Impaired Skin Integrity
- Impaired Physical Mobility
- Risk for Peripheral Neurovascular Dysfunction
- Ineffective Peripheral Tissue Perfusion

OUTCOME IDENTIFICATION AND PLANNING

- Cast is applied without interfering with neurovascular function and that healing occurs.
- Patient is free from complications.
- Patient has knowledge of the treatment regimen.
- Patient experiences increased comfort.

IMPLEMENTATION

ACTION	RATIONALE
1. Review the medical record and medical orders to determine the need for the cast.	Reviewing the medical record and order validates the correct patient and correct procedure.

ACTION	RATIONALE
2. Perform hand hygiene. Put on gloves and/or other PPE, as indicated.	Hand hygiene and PPE prevent the spread of microorganisms. PPE is required based on transmission precautions.
3. Identify the patient. Explain the procedure to the patient and verify area to be casted.	Patient identification validates the correct patient and correct procedure. Discussion and explanation help allay anxiety and prepare the patient for what to expect.
4. Perform a pain assessment and assess for muscle spasm. Administer prescribed medications in sufficient time to allow for the full effect of the analgesic and/or muscle relaxant.	Assessment of pain and analgesic administration ensure patient comfort and enhance cooperation.
5. Close the curtains around the bed and close the door to the room, if possible. Place the bed at an appropriate and comfortable working height, usually elbow height of the caregiver (VISN 8 Patient Safety Center, 2009).	Closing the door or curtains provides privacy. Proper bed height helps reduce back strain while you are performing the procedure.
6. Position the patient, as needed, depending on the type of cast being applied and the location of the injury. Support the extremity or body part to be casted.	Proper positioning minimizes movement, maintains alignment, and increases patient comfort.
7. Drape the patient with the waterproof pads.	Draping provides warmth and privacy and helps protect other body parts from contact with casting materials.
8. Cleanse and dry the affected body part.	Skin care before cast application helps prevent skin breakdown.
9. Position and maintain the affected body part in the position indicated by the physician or advanced practice professional as the stockinette, sheet wadding, and padding are applied	Stockinette and other materials protect the skin from casting materials and create a smooth, padded edge, protecting the skin from abrasion. Padding protects the skin, tissues, and nerves from the pressure of the cast.

ACTION	RATIONALE

(Figure 1). The stockinette should extend beyond the ends of the cast. As the wadding is applied, check for wrinkles.

FIGURE 1 Stockinette in place.

10. Continue to position and maintain the affected body part in the position indicated by the physician or advanced practice professional as the casting material is applied. Assist with finishing by folding the stockinette or other padding down over the outer edge of the cast.

Smooth edges lessen the risk for skin irritation and abrasion.

11. **Support the cast during hardening.** Handle hardening plaster casts with the palms of hands, not fingers (Figure 2). Support the cast on a firm, smooth surface.

Proper handling avoids denting of the cast and development of pressure areas.

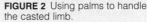

FIGURE 2 Using palms to handle the casted limb.

ACTION	RATIONALE
Do not rest it on a hard surface or sharp edges. Avoid placing pressure on the cast.	
12. **Elevate the injured limb at heart level with pillow or bath blankets, as ordered, making sure pressure is evenly distributed under the cast.**	Elevation promotes venous return. Evenly distributed pressure prevents molding and denting of the cast and development of pressure areas.
13. Place the bed in the lowest position, with the side rails up. Make sure the call bell and other essential items are within easy reach.	Having the bed at proper height and leaving the call bell and other items within reach ensure patient safety.
14. Remove gloves and any other PPE, if used. Perform hand hygiene.	Removing PPE properly reduces the risk for infection transmission and contamination of other items. Hand hygiene prevents the spread of microorganisms.
15. Obtain x-rays, as ordered.	X-rays identify that the affected area is positioned properly.
16. Instruct the patient to report pain, odor, drainage, changes in sensation, abnormal sensation, or the inability to move fingers or toes of the affected extremity.	Pressure within a cast may increase with edema and lead to compartment syndrome. Patient complaints allow for early detection of, and prompt intervention for, complications such as skin irritation or impaired tissue perfusion.
17. Leave the cast uncovered and exposed to the air. Reposition the patient every 2 hours. Depending on facility policy, a fan may be used to dry the cast.	Keeping the cast uncovered promotes drying. Repositioning prevents development of pressure areas. Using a fan helps increase airflow and speeds drying.

EVALUATION
- Neurovascular function is maintained and healing occurs.
- Patient is free from complications.
- Patient has knowledge of the treatment regimen.
- Patient experiences increased comfort.

DOCUMENTATION
- Document the time, date, and site that the cast was applied. Include the skin assessment and care provided before application. Document the patient's response to the cast and the neurovascular status of the extremity.

SKILL 29 CARING FOR A CAST

A cast is a rigid external immobilizing device that encases a body part. Casts, made of plaster or synthetic materials, such as fiberglass, are used to immobilize a body part in a specific position and to apply uniform pressure on the encased soft tissue. They may be used to treat injuries, correct a deformity, stabilize weakened joints, or promote healing after surgery. Casts generally allow the patient mobility while restricting movement of the affected body part. Nursing responsibilities after the cast is in place include maintaining the cast, preventing complications, and providing patient teaching related to cast care.

DELEGATION CONSIDERATIONS

Care of a cast may not be delegated to nursing assistive personnel (NAP) or to unlicensed assistive personnel (UAP). Depending on the state's nurse practice act and the organization's policies and procedures, care of a cast may be delegated to licensed practical/vocational nurses (LPN/LVNs). The decision to delegate must be based on careful analysis of the patient's needs and circumstances, as well as the qualifications of the person to whom the task is being delegated. Refer to the Delegation Guidelines in Appendix A.

EQUIPMENT

- Washcloth
- Towel
- Skin cleanser
- Basin of warm water
- Waterproof pads
- Tape
- Pillows
- PPE, as indicated

ASSESSMENT

- Review the patient's medical record and nursing plan of care to determine the need for cast care and care of the affected area.
- Perform a pain assessment and administer the prescribed medication in sufficient time to allow for the full effect of the analgesic before starting care.
- Assess the neurovascular status of the affected extremity, including distal pulses, color, temperature, presence of edema, capillary refill to fingers or toes, and sensation and motion. Assess the skin distal to

the cast. Note any indications of infection, including any foul odor from the cast, pain, fever, edema, and extreme warmth over an area of the cast.
- Assess for complications of immobility, including alterations in skin integrity, reduced joint movement, decreased peristalsis, constipation, alterations in respiratory function, and signs of thrombophlebitis.
- Inspect the condition of the cast. Be alert for cracks, dents, or the presence of drainage from the cast.
- Assess the patient's knowledge of cast care.

NURSING DIAGNOSIS
- Risk for Peripheral Neurovascular Dysfunction
- Self-Care Deficit (bathing, feeding, dressing, or toileting)
- Risk for Impaired Skin Integrity

OUTCOME IDENTIFICATION AND PLANNING
- Cast remains intact.
- Patient does not experience neurovascular compromise.
- Patient is free from infection.
- Patient experiences only mild pain and slight edema or soreness.
- Patient experiences only slight limitations of range of joint motion.
- Skin around the cast edges remains intact.
- Patient participates in ADLs.
- Patient demonstrates appropriate cast-care techniques.

IMPLEMENTATION

ACTION	RATIONALE
1. Review the medical record and the nursing plan of care to determine the need for cast care and care for the affected body part.	Reviewing the medical record and plan of care validates the correct patient and correct procedure.
2. Perform hand hygiene. Put on PPE, as indicated.	Hand hygiene and PPE prevent the spread of microorganisms. PPE is required based on transmission precautions.
3. Identify the patient. Explain the procedure to the patient.	Patient identification validates the correct patient and correct procedure. Discussion and explanation help allay anxiety and prepare the patient for what to expect.

ACTION	RATIONALE
4. Close the curtains around the bed and close the door to the room, if possible. Place the bed at an appropriate and comfortable working height, usually elbow height of the caregiver (VISN 8 Patient Safety Center, 2009).	Closing the door or curtains provides privacy. Proper bed height helps reduce back strain while you are performing the procedure.
5. If a plaster cast was applied, handle the casted extremity or body area with the palms of your hands for the first 24 to 36 hours, until the cast is fully dry.	Proper handling of a plaster cast prevents dents in the cast, which may create pressure areas on the inside of the cast.
6. If the cast is on an extremity, elevate the affected area on pillows covered with waterproof pads. **Maintain the normal curvatures and angles of the cast.**	Elevation helps reduce edema and enhances venous return. Use of a waterproof pad prevents soiling of linen. Maintaining curvatures and angles maintains proper joint alignment, helps prevent flattened areas on the cast as it dries, and prevents pressure areas.
7. Keep cast (plaster) uncovered until fully dry.	Keeping the cast uncovered allows heat and moisture to dissipate and air to circulate to speed drying.
8. Assess the condition of the cast. Be alert for cracks, dents, or the presence of drainage from the cast. Perform skin and neurovascular assessments according to facility policy, as often as every 1 to 2 hours. **Check for pain, edema, inability to move body parts distal to the cast, pallor, pulses, and abnormal sensations. If the cast is on an extremity, compare it with the noncasted extremity.**	Assessment helps detect abnormal neurovascular function or infection and allows for prompt intervention. Assessing the neurovascular status determines the circulation and oxygenation of tissues. Pressure within a cast may increase with edema and lead to compartment syndrome.
9. If breakthrough bleeding or drainage is noted on the cast, mark the area on the	Marking the area provides a baseline for monitoring the amount of bleeding or drainage.

ACTION	RATIONALE
cast, according to facility policy. Indicate the date and time next to the area. Follow medical orders or facility policy regarding the amount of drainage that needs to be reported to the primary care provider.	
10. Assess for signs of infection. Monitor the patient's temperature. Assess for a foul odor from the cast, increased pain, or extreme warmth over an area of the cast.	Infection deters healing. Assessment allows for early detection and prompt intervention.
11. Reposition the patient every 2 hours. Provide back and skin care frequently. Encourage ROM exercises for unaffected joints. Encourage the patient to cough and breathe deeply.	Repositioning promotes even drying of the cast and reduces the risk for the development of pressure areas under the cast. Frequent skin and back care prevents patient discomfort and skin breakdown. ROM exercises maintain joint function of unaffected areas. Coughing and deep breathing reduce the risk for respiratory complications associated with immobility.
12. Instruct the patient to report pain, odor, drainage, changes in sensation, abnormal sensation, or the inability to move fingers or toes of the affected extremity.	Pressure within a cast may increase with edema and lead to compartment syndrome. The patient's understanding of signs and symptoms allows for early detection and prompt intervention.
13. Place the bed in the lowest position, with the side rails up. Make sure the call bell and other essential items are within easy reach.	Having the bed at proper height and leaving the call bell and other items within reach ensures patient safety.
14. Remove PPE, if used. Perform hand hygiene.	Removing PPE properly reduces the risk for infection transmission and contamination of other items. Hand hygiene prevents the spread of microorganisms.

EVALUATION

- Patient exhibits a cast that is intact without evidence of neurovascular compromise to the affected body part.
- Patient remains free from infection.
- Patient verbalizes only mild pain and slight edema or soreness.
- Patient maintains range of joint motion.
- Patient demonstrates intact skin at cast edges.
- Patient is able to perform ADLs.
- Patient demonstrates appropriate cast-care techniques.

DOCUMENTATION

- Document all assessments and care provided. Document the patient's response to the cast, repositioning, and any teaching.

SKILL 30 | PERFORMING INTERMITTENT CLOSED CATHETER IRRIGATION

Bladder irrigation is not recommended unless obstruction is anticipated, as might occur with bleeding after prostate or bladder surgery (SUNA, 2010, p. 9). Catheter irrigation should be avoided unless necessary to relieve or prevent obstruction (Herter & Wallace Kazer, 2010). If obstruction is anticipated, continuous irrigation is suggested to prevent obstruction (SUNA) (See Skill 15). However, intermittent irrigation is sometimes prescribed to restore or maintain the patency of the drainage system. Sediment or debris, as well as blood clots, might block the catheter, preventing the flow of urine out of the catheter. Irrigations might also be used to instill medications that will act directly on the bladder wall. Irrigating a catheter through a closed system is preferred to opening the catheter because opening the catheter could lead to contamination and infection.

DELEGATION CONSIDERATIONS

Intermittent closed catheter irrigation is not delegated to nursing assistive personnel (NAP) or unlicensed assistive personnel (UAP). Depending on the state's nurse practice act and the organization's policies and procedures, intermittent closed catheter irrigation may be delegated to licensed practical/vocational nurses (LPN/LVNs). The decision to delegate must be based on careful analysis of the patient's needs and circumstances, as well as the qualifications of the person to whom the task is being delegated. Refer to the Delegation Guidelines in Appendix A.

EQUIPMENT

- Sterile basin or container
- Sterile irrigating solution (at room temperature or warmed to body temperature)
- 30- to 60-mL syringe (with 18- or 19-gauge blunt-end needle, if catheter access port is not a needleless system)

- Clamp for drainage tubing
- Bath blanket
- Disposable gloves
- Additional PPE, as indicated
- Waterproof pad
- Alcohol or other disinfectant swab

ASSESSMENT

- Check the medical record for an order to irrigate the catheter, including the type and amount of solution to use for the irrigation.
- Before performing the procedure, assess catheter drainage and amount of urine in drainage bag.
- Assess for bladder fullness, either by palpation or with a handheld bladder ultrasound device.
- Assess for signs of adverse effects, which may include pain, bladder spasm, bladder distension/fullness, or lack of drainage from catheter.

NURSING DIAGNOSIS

- Impaired Urinary Elimination
- Risk for Infection

OUTCOME IDENTIFICATION AND PLANNING

- Patient exhibits the free flow of urine through the catheter.
- Patient's bladder is not distended.
- Patient remains free from pain and free of any signs and symptoms of infection.

IMPLEMENTATION

ACTION	RATIONALE
1. Confirm the order for catheter irrigation in the medical record.	Verifying the medical order ensures that the correct intervention is administered to the right patient.
2. Gather equipment.	Assembling equipment provides for an organized approach to task.
3. Perform hand hygiene and put on PPE, if indicated.	Hand hygiene and PPE prevent the spread of microorganisms. PPE is required based on transmission precautions.
4. Identify the patient.	Identifying the patient ensures the right patient receives the intervention and helps prevent errors.

ACTION	RATIONALE
5. Close curtains around bed and close the door to the room, if possible. Discuss the procedure with patient.	This ensures the patient's privacy. This discussion promotes reassurance and provides knowledge about the procedure. Dialogue encourages patient participation and allows for individualized nursing care.
6. Assemble equipment on overbed table within reach.	Arranging items nearby is convenient, saves time, and avoids unnecessary stretching and twisting of muscles on the part of the nurse.
7. Adjust bed to comfortable working height, usually elbow height of the caregiver (VISN 8 Patient Safety Center, 2009).	Having the bed at the proper height prevents back and muscle strain.
8. Put on gloves. Empty the catheter drainage bag and measure the amount of urine, noting the amount and characteristics of the urine. Remove gloves.	Gloves prevent contact with blood and body fluids. Emptying the drainage bag allows for accurate assessment of drainage after the irrigation solution is instilled. Assessment of urine provides a baseline for future comparison. Proper removal of PPE prevents transmission of microorganisms.
9. Assist patient to comfortable position and expose access port on catheter setup. Place waterproof pad under catheter and aspiration port. Remove catheter from device or tape anchoring catheter to the patient.	This provides adequate visualization. Waterproof pad protects patient and bed from leakage. Removing the catheter from the anchoring device or tape allows for manipulation of the catheter.
10. Open supplies, using aseptic technique. Pour sterile solution into sterile basin. Aspirate the prescribed amount of irrigant (usually 30 to 60 mL) into sterile syringe. Put on gloves.	Use of aseptic technique ensures sterility of irrigating fluid and prevents spread of microorganisms. Gloves prevent contact with blood and body fluids.
11. **Cleanse the access port on catheter with antimicrobial swab.**	Cleaning the port reduces the risk of introducing organisms into the closed urinary system.

ACTION	RATIONALE
12. Clamp or fold catheter tubing below the access port.	This directs the irrigating solution into the bladder, preventing flow into the drainage bag.
13. Attach the syringe to the access port on the catheter using a twisting motion (Figure 1). **Gently instill solution into catheter.**	Gentle irrigation prevents damage to bladder lining. Instillation of fluid dislodges material blocking the catheter.

FIGURE 1 Attaching syringe to access port with twisting motion.

ACTION	RATIONALE
14. Remove syringe from access port. **Unclamp or unfold tubing and allow irrigant and urine to flow into the drainage bag.** Repeat procedure, as necessary.	Gravity aids drainage of urine and irrigant from the bladder.
15. Remove gloves. Secure catheter tubing to the patient's inner thigh or lower abdomen (if a male patient) with anchoring device or tape. Leave some slack in the catheter for leg movement.	Proper attachment prevents trauma to the urethra and meatus from tension on the tubing. Whether to take the drainage tubing over or under the leg depends on gravity flow and patient's mobility and comfort.
16. Assist the patient to a comfortable position. Cover the patient with bed linens. Place the bed in the lowest position.	Positioning and covering provide warmth and promote comfort. Lowering bed contributes to patient safety.
17. Secure drainage bag below the level of the bladder. Check that drainage tubing is not kinked and that movement of side rails does not interfere with catheter or drainage bag.	This facilitates drainage of urine and prevents the backflow of urine.

ACTION	RATIONALE
18. Remove equipment and discard syringe in appropriate receptacle. Remove gloves and additional PPE, if used. Perform hand hygiene.	Proper disposal of equipment prevents transmission of microorganisms. Removing PPE properly reduces the risk for infection transmission and contamination of other items. Hand hygiene prevents the spread of microorganisms.
19. Assess patient's response to the procedure and the quality and amount of drainage after the irrigation.	This provides accurate assessment of the patient's response to the procedure.

EVALUATION

- Patient exhibits the free flow of urine through the catheter.
- The irrigant and urine are returned into the drainage bag.
- Patient's bladder is not distended.
- Patient remains free from pain and free of any signs and symptoms of infection.

DOCUMENTATION

- Document baseline assessment of patient. Document the amount and type of irrigation solution used and the amount and characteristics of drainage returned after the procedure. Document the ease of irrigation and the patient's tolerance of the procedure. Record urine amount emptied from the drainage bag before the procedure and the amount of irrigant used on intake and output record. Subtract irrigant amount from the urine output when totaling output to provide accurate recording of urine output.

SKILL 31   ACCESSING AN IMPLANTED PORT

An implanted port consists of a subcutaneous injection port attached to a catheter. The distal catheter tip dwells in the lower one third of the superior vena cava to the junction of the superior vena cava and the right atrium, and the proximal end or port is usually implanted in a subcutaneous pocket of the upper chest wall. Implanted ports placed in the antecubital area of the arm are referred to as peripheral access system ports. When not in use, no external parts of the system are visible. When venous access is desired, the location of the injection port must be palpated. A special angled, noncoring needle is inserted through the skin and septum and into the port reservoir to access the system. Once accessed, patency is maintained by periodic flushing. The length and gauge of the needle used to access the port should be selected based on the patient's anatomy, amount of subcutaneous tissue at the site, and anticipated infusion requirements. In general, a 0.75-inch 20-gauge needle is frequently used. If the patient has a significant amount of subcutaneous tissue, a longer length (1 or 1.5 inch) may be selected. Site dressings are maintained and changed as outlined in Skill 32.

DELEGATION CONSIDERATIONS

Accessing an implanted port is not delegated to nursing assistive personnel (NAP), to unlicensed assistive personnel (UAP), or to licensed practical/vocational nurses (LPN/LVNs).

EQUIPMENT

- Sterile tape or Steri-Strips
- Sterile semipermeable transparent dressing
- Several 2 × 2 gauzes
- Sterile towel or drape
- Cleansing swabs (>0.5% chlorhexidine preparation with alcohol)
- NSS vial and 10-mL syringe or prefilled 10-mL NSS syringe
- Heparin 100 U/mL in 10-mL syringe
- Noncoring needle (Huber needle) of appropriate length and gauge
- Masks (2), depending on facility policy
- Clean gloves
- Sterile gloves
- Additional PPE, as indicated
- Skin protectant wipe (e.g., SkinPrep)
- Alcohol or other disinfectant wipes
- Positive pressure end cap
- IV securement/stabilization device, as appropriate
- Bath blanket

ASSESSMENT

- Inspect the skin over the port, looking for any swelling, redness, drainage, and pain or tenderness.
- Review the patient's history for the length of time the port has been in place. If the port has been placed recently, assess surgical incision. Note presence of Steri-Strips, approximation, ecchymosis, redness, edema, and/or drainage.

NURSING DIAGNOSIS

- Risk for Infection
- Deficient Knowledge
- Risk for Impaired Skin Integrity

OUTCOME IDENTIFICATION AND PLANNING

- Port is accessed with minimal to no discomfort to the patient.
- Patient experiences no trauma to the site or infection.
- Patient verbalized an understanding of care associated with the port.

IMPLEMENTATION

ACTION	RATIONALE
1. Verify medical order and/or facility policy and procedure. Often, the procedure for accessing an implanted port and dressing changes will be a standing protocol. Gather equipment.	Checking the order and/or policy ensures that the proper procedure is initiated. Preparation promotes efficient time management and an organized approach to the task.
2. Perform hand hygiene and put on PPE, if indicated.	Hand hygiene and PPE prevent the spread of microorganisms. Unclean hands and improper technique are potential sources for infecting a CVAD. PPE is required based on transmission precautions.
3. Identify the patient.	Identifying the patient ensures the right patient receives the intervention and helps prevent errors.
4. Close the curtains around the bed and close the door to the room, if possible. Explain what you are going to do, and why you are going to do it to the patient. Ask the patient about allergies to tape and skin antiseptics.	This ensures the patient's privacy. Explanation relieves anxiety and facilitates cooperation. Possible allergies may exist related to tape or antiseptics.
5. Place a waste receptacle or bag at a convenient location for use during the procedure.	Having a waste container handy means the soiled dressing can be discarded easily, without the spread of microorganisms.
6. Adjust the bed to a comfortable working height, usually elbow height of the caregiver (VISN 8 Patient Safety Center, 2009).	Having the bed at the proper height prevents back and muscle strain.
7. Assist the patient to a comfortable position that provides easy access to the port site. Use the bath blanket to cover any exposed area other than the site.	Patient positioning and use of a bath blanket provide for comfort and warmth.

ACTION	RATIONALE
8. Apply a mask, depending on facility policy. Ask the patient to turn his or her head away from the access site. Alternately, have the patient put on a mask, depending on facility policy. Move the overbed table to a convenient location within easy reach. Set up a sterile field on the table. Open dressing supplies and add to the sterile field. If IV solution is infusing via CVAD, interrupt and place on hold during dressing change. Apply slide clamp on each lumen of the CVAD.	Masks are recommended to help to deter the spread of microorganisms (INS, 2011, p. S64). Patient should wear mask if unable to turn the head away from the site or if based on facility policy. Many facilities have all sterile dressing supplies gathered in a single package. Stopping infusion and clamping each lumen prevents air from entering the CVAD.
9. Put on clean gloves. Palpate the location of the port. Assess site. Note the status of any surgical incisions that may be present. Remove gloves and discard.	Knowledge of location and boundaries of port are necessary to access the site safely.
10. Put on sterile gloves. Connect the end cap to the extension tubing on the noncoring needle. Clean end cap with alcohol wipe. Insert syringe with normal saline into end cap. Fill extension tubing with normal saline and apply clamp. Place on sterile field.	Priming extension tubing removes air from tubing and prevents administration of air when connected to the port.
11. Using the chlorhexidine swab, cleanse the port site. Press the applicator against the skin. **Apply chlorhexidine using a gentle back and forth motion.** Moving outward from the site, use a circular, scrubbing motion to continue to clean, covering at least a 2- to 3-inch area. **Do not wipe or blot. Allow to dry completely.**	Site care and replacement of dressing are accomplished using sterile technique. Organisms on the skin can be introduced into the tissues or the bloodstream with the needle. Chlorhexidine is the preferred antiseptic solution, but iodine, povidone-iodine, and 70% alcohol are considered acceptable alternatives in patients who are allergic to chlorhexidine (INS, 2011). Scrubbing motion

ACTION	RATIONALE
	creates friction and lets the solution more effectively penetrate the epidermal layers (Hadaway, 2006).
12. Using the nondominant hand, locate the port. Hold the port stable, keeping the skin taut.	The edges of the port must be palpated so that the needle can be inserted into the center of the port. Hold the port with your nondominant hand so that the needle is inserted into the port with the dominant hand.
13. Visualize the center of the port. Pick up the needle. Coil extension tubing into the palm of your hand. Holding needle at a 90-degree angle to the skin, insert **through the skin into the port septum until the needle hits the back of the port.**	To function properly, the needle must be located in the middle of the port and inserted to the back of the port.
14. Cleanse the end cap on the extension tubing with an antimicrobial swab and insert the syringe with normal saline. **Open the clamp on extension tubing and flush with 3 to 5 mL of saline, while observing the site for fluid leak or infiltration. It should flush easily, without resistance.**	If needle is not inserted correctly, fluid will leak into tissue, causing the tissue to swell and producing signs of infiltration. Flushing without resistance is also a sign that the needle is inserted correctly.
15. Pull back on the syringe plunger to aspirate for blood return. Do not allow blood to enter the syringe. If positive, instill the solution over 1 minute or flush the line according to facility policy. Remove syringe. Insert heparin syringe and instill the solution over 1 minute or according to facility policy. Remove syringe and clamp the extension tubing. Alternately, if IV fluid infusion	Positive blood return indicates the port is patent. Positive blood return confirms patency before administration of medications and solutions (INS, 2011, p. S60). Not allowing blood to enter the syringe ensures that the needle will be flushed with pure saline. Flushing maintains patency of the IV line. **Amount and number of saline and heparin flushes varies depending on specific CVAD and facility policy.** Action of positive pressure end

ACTION	RATIONALE
is to be started, do not flush with heparin.	cap is maintained with removal of syringe before clamp is engaged. Clamping prevents air from entering the CVAD. CVADs should be 'locked' with a heparin solution (10 U/mL) after each intermittent use to prevent clotting.
16. If using a "Gripper®" needle, remove the gripper portion from the needle by squeezing the sides together and lifting off the needle while holding the needle securely to the port with the other hand.	Gripper facilitates needle insertion and needs to be removed before application of dressing.
17. Apply the skin protectant to the site, avoiding direct application to needle insertion site. Allow to dry.	Skin protectant improves adhesion of dressing and protects skin from damage and irritation when dressing is removed.
18. Apply tape or Steri-Strips in a star-like pattern over the needle to secure it.	Secures needle to help prevent the needle from accidentally pulling out.
19. Apply transparent site dressing or securement/stabilization device, centering over insertion site.	Dressing prevents contamination of the IV catheter and protects the insertion site. Stabilization/securing devices preserve the integrity of the access device, minimize catheter movement at the hub, and prevent catheter dislodgement and loss of access (INS, 2011, p. S46).
20. Label dressing with date, time of change, and initials. If IV fluid infusion is ordered, attach administration set to extension tubing and begin administration. Refer to Skill 129.	Other personnel working with the infusion will know what type of device is being used, the site, and when it was inserted. Replace TSM dressings on CVADs every 5 to 7 days and every 2 days for CVAD sites with gauze dressings (INS, 2011; O'Grady et al., 2011).
21. Apply an IV securement/ stabilization device if not already in place as part of dressing, as indicated, based	These systems are recommended for use on all venous access sites, and particularly central venous access sites, to preserve

ACTION	RATIONALE
on facility policy. Explain to the patient the purpose of the device and the importance of safeguarding the site when using the extremity.	the integrity of the access device, minimize catheter movement at the hub, and prevent catheter dislodgement and loss of access (INS, 2011, p. S46). Some devices act as a site dressing also and may already have been applied.
22. Remove equipment. Ensure patient's comfort. Lower bed, if not in lowest position.	Promotes patient comfort and safety.
23. Remove additional PPE, if used. Perform hand hygiene.	Removing PPE properly reduces the risk for infection transmission and contamination of other items. Hand hygiene prevents transmission of microorganisms.

EVALUATION

- Port is accessed without difficulty or pain.
- Patient remains free of signs and symptoms of infection or trauma.
- Patient verbalizes an understanding of care related to the port.

DOCUMENTATION

- Document the location of the port and the size of needle used to access the port. Document the presence of a blood return and the ease of ability to flush the port. Record the patient's reaction to the procedure and if the patient is experiencing any pain or discomfort related to the port. Document the assessment of the site. Record any appropriate patient teaching.

SKILL 32 — CHANGING THE DRESSING AND FLUSHING CENTRAL VENOUS ACCESS DEVICES

Central venous access devices (CVADs) are venous access devices where the tip of the catheter terminates in the central venous circulation, usually in the superior vena cava near its junction with the right atrium (INS, 2011). Types of CVAD include peripherally inserted central catheters (PICC), nontunneled percutaneous central venous catheters, tunneled percutaneous central venous catheters, and implanted ports.

They provide access for a variety of IV fluids, medications, blood products, and TPN solutions and provide a means for hemodynamic monitoring and blood sampling. The patient's diagnosis, the type of care that is required, and other factors (e.g., limited venous access, irritating drugs, patient request, or the need for long-term intermittent infusions) determine the type of CVAD used.

Dressings are placed at the insertion site to occlude the site and prevent the introduction of microorganisms into the bloodstream. Scrupulous care of the site is required to control contamination. Facility policy generally determines the type of dressing used and the intervals for dressing change. TSM dressings (e.g., Tegaderm or OpSite IV) allow easy inspection of the IV site and permits evaporation of moisture that accumulates under the dressing. Sterile gauze may also be used to cover the catheter site. A gauze dressing is recommended if the patient is diaphoretic or if the site is bleeding or oozing, but this should be replaced with a TSM dressing once this is resolved (O'Grady et al., 2011). Perform site care and replace TSM dressings on CVADs every 5 to 7 days and every 2 days for CVAD sites with gauze dressings (INS, 2011; O'Grady et al., 2011). Change any dressing that is damp, loosened, or soiled immediately. Whenever these dressings need to be changed, it is important to observe meticulous aseptic technique to minimize the possibility of contamination.

DELEGATION CONSIDERATIONS

The changing of a CVAD dressing is not delegated to nursing assistive personnel (NAP) or to unlicensed assistive personnel (UAP). Depending on the state's nurse practice act and the organization's policies and procedures, the changing of a CVAD dressing may be delegated to licensed practical/vocational nurses (LPN/LVNs). The decision to delegate must be based on careful analysis of the patient's needs and circumstances, as well as the qualifications of the person to whom the task is being delegated. Refer to the Delegation Guidelines in Appendix A.

EQUIPMENT

- Sterile tape or Steri-Strips
- Sterile semipermeable transparent dressing
- Several 2 × 2 gauzes
- Sterile towel or drape
- Cleansing swabs (>0.5% chlorhexidine preparation with alcohol)
- NSS vial and 10-mL syringe or prefilled 10-mL NSS syringe; one for each lumen of the CVAD
- Heparin 10 U/mL in 10-mL syringe; one for each lumen of the CVAD
- Masks (2), depending on facility policy
- Clean gloves
- Sterile gloves
- Additional PPE, as indicated
- Skin protectant wipe (e.g., SkinPrep)
- Alcohol or other disinfectant wipes
- Positive pressure end caps; one for each lumen of the CVAD
- IV securement/stabilization device, as appropriate
- Measuring tape
- Bath blanket

ASSESSMENT

- Assess the IV site. The dressing should be intact, adhering to the skin on all edges. Check for any leaks or fluid under or around the dressing, or other indications that the dressing needs to be changed. Inspect the tissue around the IV entry site for swelling, coolness, or pallor. These are signs of fluid infiltration into the tissue around the IV catheter. Also inspect the site for redness, swelling, and warmth. These signs might indicate the development of phlebitis or an inflammation of the blood vessel at the site.
- Ask the patient if he or she is experiencing any pain or discomfort related to the venous access device. Pain or discomfort can be a sign of infiltration, extravasation, phlebitis, thrombophlebitis, and infection related to IV therapy.
- Note the insertion date/access date and date of last dressing change.
- Assess the catheter condition.

NURSING DIAGNOSIS

- Risk for Infection
- Deficient Knowledge
- Risk for Impaired Skin Integrity

OUTCOME IDENTIFICATION AND PLANNING

- Patient will remain free of any signs and symptoms of infection.
- Site will be clean and dry, with an intact dressing, and will show no signs or symptoms of IV complications, such as redness, drainage, swelling, or pain.
- CVAD will remain patent.

IMPLEMENTATION

ACTION	RATIONALE
1. Verify the medical order and/or facility policy and procedure. Determine the need for a dressing change. Often, the procedure for CVAD flushing and dressing changes will be a standing protocol. Gather equipment.	Ensures correct intervention for correct patient. Preparation promotes efficient time management and an organized approach to the task.
2. Perform hand hygiene and put on PPE, if indicated.	Hand hygiene and PPE prevent the spread of microorganisms. Unclean hands and improper technique are potential sources for infecting a CVAD. PPE is required based on transmission precautions.

ACTION	RATIONALE
3. Identify the patient.	Identifying the patient ensures the right patient receives the intervention and helps prevent errors.
4. Close the curtains around the bed and close the door to the room, if possible. Explain what you are going to do and why you are going to do it to the patient. Ask the patient about allergies to tape and skin antiseptics.	This ensures the patient's privacy. Explanation relieves anxiety and facilitates cooperation. Possible allergies may exist related to tape or antiseptics.
5. Place a waste receptacle or bag at a convenient location for use during the procedure.	Having a waste container handy means the soiled dressing can be discarded easily, without the spread of microorganisms.
6. Adjust the bed to a comfortable working height, usually elbow height of the caregiver (VISN 8 Patient Safety Center, 2009).	Having the bed at the proper height prevents back and muscle strain.
7. Assist the patient to a comfortable position that provides easy access to the CVAD insertion site and dressing. If the patient has a PICC, position the patient with the arm extended from the body below heart level. Use the bath blanket to cover any exposed area other than the site.	Patient positioning and use of a bath blanket provide for comfort and warmth. This position is recommended to reduce the risk of air embolism.
8. Apply a mask, depending on facility policy. Ask the patient to turn his or her head away from the access site. Alternately, have the patient put on a mask, depending on facility policy. Move the overbed table to a convenient location within easy reach. Set up a sterile field on the table. Open dressing supplies and add to sterile field. If	Masks are recommended to help to deter the spread of microorganisms (INS, 2011, p. S64). Patient should wear a mask if unable to turn the head away from the site or if based on facility policy. Many facilities have all sterile dressing supplies gathered in a single package. Stopping infusion and clamping each lumen prevents air from entering the CVAD.

ACTION	RATIONALE
IV solution is infusing via CVAD, interrupt and place on hold during dressing change. Apply slide clamp on each lumen of the CVAD.	
9. Put on clean gloves. Assess CVAD insertion site through old dressing. (Refer to Assessment discussion above.) Note the status of any sutures that may be present. Palpate the site, noting pain, tenderness, or discomfort. Remove old dressing by lifting it distally and then working proximally, making sure to stabilize the catheter. Discard dressing in trash receptacle. Remove gloves and discard.	Some CVADs may be sutured in place. Note how the CVAD is secured. Care should be taken to avoid dislodgment when changing dressings. Pain, tenderness, or discomfort on palpation may be a sign of infection. Proper disposal of dressing prevents transmission of microorganisms. Removing gloves properly reduces the risk for infection transmission and contamination of other items.
10. Put on sterile gloves. Starting at the insertion site and continuing in a circle, wipe off any old blood or drainage with a sterile antimicrobial wipe. Using the chlorhexidine swab, cleanse the site. Cleanse directly over the insertion site by pressing the applicator against the skin. **Apply chlorhexidine using a gentle back and forth motion.** Moving outward from the site, use a scrubbing motion to continue to clean, covering at least a 2- to 3-inch area. **Do not wipe or blot. Allow to dry completely.** Apply the skin protectant to the same area, avoiding direct application to the insertion site, and allow to dry.	Site care and replacement of dressing are accomplished using sterile technique. Cleansing is necessary because organisms on the skin can be introduced into the tissues or the bloodstream with venous access. Chlorhexidine is recommended for CVAD site care. Chlorhexidine is the preferred antiseptic solution, but iodine, povidone-iodine, and 70% alcohol are considered acceptable alternatives in patients who are allergic to chlorhexidine (INS, 2011).Scrubbing motion creates friction and lets the solution more effectively penetrate the epidermal layers (Hadaway, 2006). Skin protectant improves adhesion of dressing and protects the skin from damage and irritation when the dressing is removed.
11. Stabilize catheter hub by holding it in place with nondominant hand. Use an alcohol wipe to clean each	Cleansing is necessary because organisms on the skin can be introduced into the tissues or the bloodstream with the device.

ACTION	RATIONALE
lumen of the catheter, starting at the insertion site and moving outward.	
12. Apply transparent site dressing or securement/ stabilization device, centering over insertion site. Measure the length of the catheter that extends out from the insertion site.	Dressing prevents contamination of the IV catheter and protects the insertion site. Stabilization/securing devices preserve the integrity of the access device, minimize catheter movement at the hub, and prevent catheter dislodgement and loss of access (INS, 2011, p. S46). Measurement of the extending catheter can be compared with the documented length at time of insertion to assess if the catheter has migrated inward or moved outward.
13. Working with one lumen at a time, remove end cap. Cleanse the end of the lumen with an alcohol swab and apply new end cap. Repeat for each lumen. Secure catheter lumens and/or tubing that extend outside dressing with tape.	The catheter ends should be cleansed and injection caps changed to prevent infection. Weight of tubing and/or tugging on tubing could cause catheter dislodgment.
14. If required, flush each lumen of the CVAD. Amount of saline and heparin flushes varies depending on specific CVAD and facility policy.	Flushing lumen maintains patency.
15. Cleanse end cap with an antimicrobial swab. Insert the saline flush syringe into the cap on the extension tubing. Pull back on the syringe to aspirate the catheter for positive blood return. If positive, instill the solution over 1 minute or flush the line according to facility policy. Remove syringe. Insert heparin syringe and instill the volume of solution	Cleaning the cap reduces the risk for contamination. Positive blood return confirms patency before administration of medications and solutions (INS, 2011, p. S60). Flushing maintains patency of the IV line. Action of positive pressure end cap is maintained with removal of syringe before clamp is engaged. Clamping prevents air from entering the CVAD. CVADs should be 'locked' with a heparin solution (10 U/mL) after each intermittent use to

ACTION	RATIONALE
designated by facility policy over 1 minute or according to facility policy. Remove syringe and reclamp the lumen. Remove gloves.	prevent clotting (INS, 2011). Removing gloves properly reduces the risk for infection transmission and contamination of other items.
16. Label dressing with date, time of change, and initials. Resume fluid infusion, if indicated. Check that IV flow is accurate and system is patent. (Refer to Skill 129.)	Other personnel working with the infusion will know what type of device is being used, the site, and when it was inserted. Replace TSM dressings on CVADs every 5 to 7 days and every 2 days for CVAD sites with gauze dressings (INS, 2011; O'Grady et al., 2011).
17. Apply an IV securement/ stabilization device if not already in place as part of the dressing, as indicated, based on facility policy. Explain to patient the purpose of the device and the importance of safeguarding the site when using the extremity.	These systems are recommended for use on all venous access sites, and particularly central venous access sites, to preserve the integrity of the access device, minimize catheter movement at the hub, and prevent catheter dislodgement and loss of access (INS, 2011, p. S46). Some devices act as a site dressing also and may already have been applied.
18. Remove equipment. Ensure patient's comfort. Lower bed, if not in lowest position.	Promotes patient comfort and safety.
19. Remove additional PPE, if used. Perform hand hygiene.	Removing PPE properly reduces the risk for infection transmission and contamination of other items. Hand hygiene prevents transmission of microorganisms.

EVALUATION

• Dressing is changed without any complications, including dislodgement of the CVAD.
• Patient exhibits an insertion site that is clean and dry without redness or swelling.
• Site dressing is clean, dry, and intact.
• CVAD remains patent.

DOCUMENTATION

- Document the location, appearance and condition of the CVAD site. Include the presence or absence of signs of erythema, redness, swelling, or drainage. Record if the patient is experiencing any pain or discomfort related to the CVAD. Document the clinical criteria for site complications. Record the subjective comments of the patient regarding the absence or presence of pain at the site. Record the patient's reaction to the procedure and pertinent patient teaching, such as alerting the nurse if the patient experiences any pain from the IV or notices any swelling at the site. The CVAD lumens should flush without difficulty. Report any abnormal findings, such as dislodgement of the CVAD, abnormal insertion assessment findings, or inability to flush the CVAD, to the primary care provider.

SKILL 33 DEACCESSING AN IMPLANTED PORT

When an implanted port will not be used for a period of time, such as when a patient is being discharged, the port is deaccessed. Deaccessing a port involves flushing the port and removing the needle from the port.

DELEGATION CONSIDERATIONS

Deaccessing an implanted port is not delegated to nursing assistive personnel (NAP), to unlicensed assistive personnel (UAP), or to licensed practical/vocational nurses (LPN/LVNs).

EQUIPMENT

- Clean gloves
- Additional PPE, as indicated
- Syringe filled with 10 mL saline
- Syringe filled with 5 mL heparin (100 U/mL or facility's recommendations)
- Sterile gauze sponge
- Alcohol or other disinfectant wipes
- Band-Aid

ASSESSMENT

- Inspect the insertion site, looking for any swelling, redness, drainage, and pain or tenderness.
- Review the patient's history for the length of time the port and needle have been in place.

NURSING DIAGNOSIS

- Risk for Infection
- Deficient Knowledge
- Risk for Injury

OUTCOME IDENTIFICATION AND PLANNING

- Access needle is removed with minimal to no discomfort to the patient.
- Patient experiences no trauma or infection.
- Patient verbalizes an understanding of port care.

IMPLEMENTATION

ACTION	RATIONALE
1. Verify medical order and/or facility policy and procedure. Often, the procedure for deaccessing an implanted port will be a standing protocol. Gather equipment.	Checking the order and/or policy ensures that the proper procedure is initiated. Preparation promotes efficient time management and an organized approach to the task.
2. Perform hand hygiene and put on PPE, if indicated.	Hand hygiene and PPE prevent the spread of microorganisms. Unclean hands and improper technique are potential sources for infecting a CVAD. PPE is required based on transmission precautions.
3. Identify the patient.	Identifying the patient ensures the right patient receives the intervention and helps prevent errors.
4. Close the curtains around the bed and close the door to the room, if possible. Explain what you are going to do and why you are going to do it to the patient.	This ensures the patient's privacy. Explanation relieves anxiety and facilitates cooperation.
5. Adjust bed to a comfortable working height, usually elbow height of the caregiver (VISN 8 Patient Safety Center, 2009).	Having the bed at the proper height prevents back and muscle strain.
6. Assist the patient to a comfortable position that provides easy access to the port site. Use the bath blanket to cover any exposed area other than the site.	Patient positioning and use of a bath blanket provide for comfort and warmth.

ACTION	RATIONALE
7. Put on gloves. Stabilize port needle with nondominant hand. Remove any IV securement/stabilization device that may be in place. Gently pull back transparent dressing, beginning with edges and proceeding around the edge of the dressing. Carefully remove all the tape that is securing the needle in place.	Gloves prevent contact with blood and body fluids. Removal of stabilization device and dressing is necessary to remove access needle. Gently pulling the edges of the dressing is less traumatic to the patient.
8. Clean the end cap on the extension tubing and insert the saline-filled syringe. Unclamp the extension tubing and flush with a minimum of 10 mL of normal saline.	It is important to flush all substances out of the well of the implanted port, because it may be inactive for an extended period of time. **Amount and number of saline and heparin flushes varies depending on specific CVAD and facility policy.**
9. Remove the syringe and insert the heparin-filled syringe, flushing with 5 mL heparin (100 U/mL or per facility policy). Remove syringe and clamp the extension tubing.	**Amount of saline and heparin flushes varies depending on specific CVAD and facility policy.** Action of positive pressure end cap is maintained with removal of syringe before clamp is engaged. Clamping prevents air from entering the CVAD. Implanted ports should be 'locked' with a heparin solution (100 U/mL) before removal on an access needle and/or for periodic access and flushing to prevent clotting (INS, 2011, p. S61).
10. Secure the port on either side with the fingers of your nondominant hand. Grasp the needle/wings with the fingers of dominant hand. Firmly and smoothly, pull the needle straight up at a 90-degree angle from the skin to remove it from the port septum. Engage needle guard, if not automatic on removal.	The port is held in place while the needle is removed.

ACTION	RATIONALE
11. Apply gentle pressure with the gauze to the insertion site. Apply a Band-Aid over the port if any oozing occurs. Otherwise, a dressing is not necessary. Remove gloves.	A small amount of blood may form from the needlestick. Intact skin provides a barrier to infection.
12. Ensure patient's comfort. Lower bed, if not in lowest position. Put on one glove to handle needle. Dispose of needle with extension tubing in sharps container.	Promotes patient comfort and safety. Proper disposal of needle prevents accidental injury.
13. Remove gloves and additional PPE, if used. Perform hand hygiene.	Removing PPE properly reduces the risk for infection transmission and contamination of other items. Hand hygiene prevents transmission of microorganisms.

EVALUATION

- Port flushes easily.
- Access needle is removed without difficulty.
- Site is clean, dry, without evidence of redness, irritation, or warmth.
- Patient verbalizes an understanding of port care.

DOCUMENTATION

- Document the location of the port and the ease or difficulty of flushing the port. Record the locking of the port with heparin (100 U/mL). This may be done on the CMAR/MAR. Document removal of the access needle. Record the appearance of the site, including if there is any drainage, swelling, or redness. Record any appropriate patient teaching.

SKILL 34 | REMOVING A PERIPHERALLY INSERTED CENTRAL CATHETER (PICC)

When PICC is no longer required or when the patient has developed complications, it will be discontinued. Nurses or specialized IV team nurses may be responsible for removing a PICC line. Specific protocols must be followed to prevent breakage or fracture of the catheter.

DELEGATION CONSIDERATIONS

The removal of a PICC is not delegated to nursing assistive personnel (NAP), to unlicensed assistive personnel (UAP), or to licensed practical/vocational nurses (LPN/LVNs).

EQUIPMENT

- Clean gloves
- Additional PPE, as indicated
- Sterile gauze sponges
- Tape
- Disposable measuring tape

ASSESSMENT

- Inspect the insertion site, looking for any swelling, redness, or drainage.
- Check pertinent laboratory values, particularly coagulation times and platelet counts. Patients with alterations in coagulation require that pressure be applied for a longer period of time after catheter removal.
- Measure the length of the PICC after removal.

NURSING DIAGNOSIS

- Risk for Infection
- Risk for Injury
- Deficient Knowledge

OUTCOME IDENTIFICATION AND PLANNING

- PICC is removed with minimal to no discomfort to the patient.
- Patient experiences no trauma or infection.

IMPLEMENTATION

ACTION	RATIONALE
1. Verify medical order for PICC removal and facility policy and procedure. Gather equipment.	Checking the order and/or policy ensures that the proper procedure is initiated. Preparation promotes efficient time management and an organized approach to the task.

ACTION	RATIONALE
2. Perform hand hygiene and put on PPE, if indicated.	Hand hygiene and PPE prevent the spread of microorganisms. Unclean hands and improper technique are potential sources for infecting a CVAD. PPE is required based on transmission precautions.
3. Identify the patient.	Identifying the patient ensures the right patient receives the intervention and helps prevent errors.
4. Close the curtains around the bed and close the door to the room, if possible. Explain what you are going to do and why you are going to do it to the patient.	This ensures the patient's privacy. Explanation relieves anxiety and facilitates cooperation.
5. Adjust the bed to a comfortable working height, usually elbow height of the caregiver (VISN 8 Patient Safety Center, 2009).	Having the bed at the proper height prevents back and muscle strain.
6. Assist the patient to a supine position with the arm straight and the catheter insertion site at or below heart level. Use the bath blanket to cover any exposed area other than the site.	This position is recommended to reduce the risk of air embolism. Use of a bath blanket provides for comfort and warmth.
7. Put on gloves. Stabilize catheter hub with your nondominant hand. Gently pull back transparent dressing, beginning with edges and proceeding around the edge of the dressing. Carefully remove all the tape that is securing the catheter in place.	Gloves prevent contact with blood and body fluids. Gently pulling the edges of the dressing is less traumatic to the patient.
8. Instruct the patient to hold his or her breath, and perform a Valsalva maneuver as the last portion of the catheter is removed; if unable to do	Use of Valsalva maneuver or removal during expiration reduces risk for air embolism (Feil, 2012).

ACTION	RATIONALE
so, time the removal during patient expiration.	
9. Using dominant hand, remove the catheter slowly. Grasp the catheter close to the insertion site and slowly ease it out, keeping it parallel to the skin. Continue removing in small increments, using a smooth and constant motion.	Gentle pressure reduces risk of breakage. Catheter should come out easily.
10. After removal, apply pressure to the site with sterile gauze until hemostasis is achieved (minimum 1 minute). Then apply petroleum-based ointment and a sterile dressing to the access site.	Adequate pressure prevents hematoma formation. Use of a petroleum-based ointment and a sterile dressing at the access site seals the skin-to-vein tract and decreases the risk of air embolus (INS, 2011).
11. Measure the catheter and compare it with the length listed in the chart when it was inserted. Inspect the catheter for patency. Dispose of PICC according to facility policy.	Measurement and inspection ensures entire catheter was removed. Proper disposal reduces transmission of microorganisms and prevents contact with blood and body fluids.
12. Remove gloves. Ensure patient's comfort. Lower bed, if not in lowest position.	Promotes patient comfort and safety.
13. Remove additional PPE, if used. Perform hand hygiene.	Removing PPE properly reduces the risk for infection transmission and contamination of other items. Hand hygiene prevents transmission of microorganisms.

EVALUATION

- PICC is removed with minimal to no discomfort to the patient.
- Patient experiences no trauma or infection.

DOCUMENTATION

- Document the location of the PICC and its removal. Record the catheter length and patency. Record the appearance of the site, including if there is any drainage, swelling, or redness. Record any appropriate patient teaching.

SKILL 35 | APPLYING A TWO-PIECE CERVICAL COLLAR

Patients suspected of having injuries to the cervical spine must be immobilized with a cervical collar to stabilize the neck and prevent further damage to the spinal cord. A cervical collar maintains the neck in a straight line, with the chin slightly elevated and tucked inward. Care must be taken when applying the collar not to hyperflex or hyperextend the patient's neck.

DELEGATION CONSIDERATIONS

Application of a cervical collar is not delegated to nursing assistive personnel (NAP) or to unlicensed assistive personnel (UAP). Depending on the state's nurse practice act and the organization's policies and procedures, application of a cervical collar may be delegated to licensed practical/vocational nurses (LPN/LVNs).The decision to delegate must be based on careful analysis of the patient's needs and circumstances, as well as the qualifications of the person to whom the task is being delegated. Refer to the Delegation Guidelines in Appendix A.

EQUIPMENT

- Nonsterile gloves
- Additional PPE, as indicated
- Tape measure
- Cervical collar of appropriate size
- Washcloth
- Skin cleanser and water
- Towel

ASSESSMENT

- Assess for a patent airway. If airway is occluded, try repositioning using the jaw– thrust–chin lift method, which helps open the airway without moving the patient's neck.
- Inspect and palpate the cervical spine area for tenderness, swelling, deformities, or crepitus. Do not ask the patient to move the neck if a cervical spinal cord injury is suspected.
- Perform a neurologic assessment.
- Assess the patient's level of consciousness and ability to follow commands to determine any neurologic dysfunction. If the patient is able to follow commands, instruct him or her not to move the head or neck.
- Have a second person stabilize the cervical spine by holding the patient's head firmly on either side directly above the ears.

NURSING DIAGNOSIS

- Risk for Injury
- Acute Pain

OUTCOME IDENTIFICATION AND PLANNING

- Patient's cervical spine is immobilized, preventing further injury to the spinal cord.
- Patient maintains head and neck without movement.
- Patient experiences minimal to no pain.
- Patient demonstrates an understanding about the need for immobilization.

IMPLEMENTATION

ACTION	RATIONALE
1. Review the medical record and nursing plan of care to determine the need for placement of a cervical collar. Identify any movement limitations. Gather the necessary supplies.	Reviewing the record and care plan validates the correct patient and correct procedure. Identification of limitations prevents injury. Assembling equipment provides for an organized approach to the task.
2. Perform hand hygiene and put on PPE, if indicated.	Hand hygiene and PPE prevent the spread of microorganisms. PPE is required based on transmission precautions.
3. Identify the patient.	Identifying the patient ensures the right patient receives the intervention and helps prevent errors.
4. Close curtains around the bed and close the door to the room, if possible. Explain what you are going to do and why you are going to do it to the patient.	This ensures the patient's privacy. Explanation relieves anxiety and facilitates cooperation.
5. Assemble equipment on overbed table within reach.	Arranging items nearby is convenient, saves time, and avoids unnecessary stretching and twisting of muscles on the part of the nurse.
6. Assess the patient for any changes in neurologic status.	Patients with cervical spine injuries are at risk for problems with the neurologic system.
7. Place the bed at an appropriate and comfortable working height, usually elbow height of the caregiver (VISN 8	Having the bed at the proper height and lowering the rails prevent back and muscle strain.

ACTION	RATIONALE

Patient Safety Center, 2009). Lower the side rails as necessary.

8. Gently clean the patient's face and neck with a skin cleanser and water. If the patient has experienced trauma, inspect the area for broken glass or other material that could cut the patient or the nurse. Pat the area dry.

Blood, glass, leaves, and twigs may be present on the patient's neck. The area should be clean before applying the cervical collar to prevent skin breakdown.

9. Have a second caregiver in position to hold the patient's head firmly on either side above the ears. Measure from the bottom of the chin to the top of the sternum, and measure around the neck. Match these height and circumference measurements to the manufacturer's recommended size chart.

This action stabilizes the cervical spine by holding the head firmly on either side above the ears. To immobilize the cervical spine and to prevent skin breakdown under the collar, the correct collar size must be used (Apold & Rydrych, 2012).

10. Slide the flattened back portion of the collar under the patient's head. **The center of the collar should line up with the center of the patient's neck. Do not allow the patient's head to move when passing the collar under the head.**

Stabilizing the cervical spine is crucial to prevent the head from moving, which could cause further damage to the cervical spine. Placing the collar in the center ensures that the neck is aligned properly.

11. Place the front of the collar centered over the chin, while ensuring that the chin area fits snugly in the recess. Be sure that the front half of the collar overlaps the back half. Secure Velcro straps on both sides. Check to see that at least one finger can be inserted between collar and patient's neck.

The collar should fit snugly to prevent the patient from moving the neck and causing further damage to the cervical spine. Velcro will help hold the collar securely in place. Collar should not be too tight to cause discomfort.

12. Raise the side rails. Place the bed in lowest position. Make sure the call bell is in reach.

Bed in lowest position and access to call bell contribute to patient safety.

ACTION	RATIONALE
13. Reassess the patient's neurologic status and comfort level.	Reassessment helps to evaluate the effects of movement on the patient.
14. Remove PPE, if used. Perform hand hygiene.	Removing PPE properly reduces the risk for infection transmission and contamination of other items. Hand hygiene prevents transmission of microorganisms.
15. **Check the skin under the cervical collar at least every 4 hours for any signs of skin breakdown. Remove the collar every 8 to 12 hours and inspect and cleanse the skin under the collar. When the collar is removed, have a second person immobilize the cervical spine.**	Skin breakdown may occur under the cervical collar if the skin is not inspected and cleansed (Apold & Rydrych, 2012).

EVALUATION

- Cervical collar is placed without adverse effect.
- Patient's cervical spine is immobilized without further injury.
- Patient verbalizes minimal to no pain.
- Patient demonstrates an understanding of the rationale for cervical spine immobilization.

DOCUMENTATION

- Document the application of the collar, including size and any skin care necessary before the application, condition of skin under the cervical collar, and patient's pain level, and neurologic and any other assessment findings.

SKILL 36   PROVIDING CARE OF A CHEST DRAINAGE SYSTEM

Chest tubes may be inserted to drain fluid (pleural effusion), blood (hemothorax), or air (pneumothorax) from the pleural space. A chest tube is a firm plastic tube with drainage holes in the proximal end that is inserted in the pleural space. Once inserted, the tube is secured with a suture and tape, covered with an airtight dressing, and attached to a drainage system that may or may not be attached to suction. Other components of the system may include a closed water-seal drainage system that prevents air from reentering the chest once it has escaped and a suction control chamber that prevents excess suction pressure from being applied to the pleural cavity. The suction chamber may be a water-filled or a dry chamber. A water-filled suction chamber is regulated by the amount of water in the chamber, whereas dry suction is automatically regulated to changes in the patient's pleural pressure. Many health care agencies use a molded plastic, three-compartment disposable chest drainage unit for management of chest tubes. There are also portable drainage systems that use gravity for drainage. The following procedure is based on the use of a traditional water seal, three-compartment chest drainage system. The Skill Variation following the procedure describes a technique for caring for a chest drainage system using dry seal or suction.

DELEGATION CONSIDERATIONS

Care of a chest tube is not delegated to nursing assistive personnel (NAP) or to unlicensed assistive personnel (UAP). Depending on the state's nurse practice act and the organization's policies and procedures, care of a chest tube may be delegated to licensed practical/vocational nurses (LPN/LVNs). The decision to delegate must be based on careful analysis of the patient's needs and circumstances, as well as the qualifications of the person to whom the task is being delegated. Refer to the Delegation Guidelines in Appendix A.

EQUIPMENT

- Bottle of sterile normal saline or water
- Two pairs of padded or rubber-tipped Kelly clamps
- Pair of clean scissors
- Disposable gloves
- Additional PPE, as indicated
- Foam tape
- Prescribed drainage system, if changing is required

ASSESSMENT

- Assess the patient's vital signs. Significant changes from baseline may indicate complications.
- Assess for restlessness and shortness of breath. Assess the patient's respiratory status, including oxygen saturation level. If the chest tube is not functioning appropriately, the patient may become tachypneic and hypoxic.

- Assess the patient's lung sounds. The lung sounds over the chest tube site may be diminished due to the presence of fluid, blood, or air.
- Assess the patient for pain. Sudden pressure or increased pain indicates potential complications. In addition, many patients report pain at the chest tube insertion site and request medication for the pain.
- Assess the patient's knowledge of the chest tube to ensure that he or she understands the rationale for the chest tube.

NURSING DIAGNOSIS

- Impaired Gas Exchange
- Deficient Knowledge
- Acute Pain

OUTCOME IDENTIFICATION AND PLANNING

- Patient will not experience any complications related to the chest drainage system or respiratory distress.
- Patient understands the need for the chest tube.
- Patient will have adequate pain control at the chest tube insertion site.
- Patient's lung sounds will be clear and equal bilaterally.
- Patient will be able to increase activity tolerance gradually.

IMPLEMENTATION

ACTION	RATIONALE
1. Bring necessary equipment to the bedside stand or over-bed table.	Bringing everything to the bedside conserves time and energy. Arranging items nearby is convenient, saves time, and avoids unnecessary stretching and twisting of muscles on the part of the nurse.
2. Perform hand hygiene and put on PPE, if indicated.	Hand hygiene and PPE prevent the spread of microorganisms. PPE is required based on transmission precautions.
3. Identify the patient.	Identifying the patient ensures the right patient receives the intervention and helps prevent errors.
4. Close the curtains around the bed and close the door to the room, if possible.	This ensures the patient's privacy.

ACTION	RATIONALE
5. Explain what you are going to do and the reason for doing it to the patient.	Explanation relieves anxiety and facilitates cooperation.
6. **Assess the patient's level of pain. Administer prescribed medication, as needed.**	Regular pain assessments are required to maintain adequate analgesic relief from the discomfort and pain caused by chest drains (Crawford, 2011; Sullivan, 2008).
7. Put on clean gloves.	Gloves prevent contact with contaminants and body fluids.

Assessing the Drainage System

ACTION	RATIONALE
8. Move the patient's gown to expose the chest tube insertion site. Keep the patient covered as much as possible, using a bath blanket to drape the patient, if necessary. Observe the dressing around the chest tube insertion site and ensure that it is dry, intact, and occlusive.	Keeping the patient as covered as possible maintains the patient's privacy and limits unnecessary exposure of the patient. If the dressing is not intact and occlusive, air can leak into the space, causing displacement of the lung tissue, and the site could be contaminated. Some patients experience significant drainage or bleeding at the insertion site. If this occurs, the dressing needs to be replaced to maintain occlusion of the site.
9. Check that all connections are securely taped. Gently palpate around the insertion site, feeling for crepitus, a result of air or gas collecting under the skin (subcutaneous emphysema). This may feel crunchy or spongy, or like "popping" under your fingers.	The body will absorb small amounts of subcutaneous emphysema after the chest tube is removed. If larger amounts or increasing amounts are present, it could indicate improper placement of the tube or an air leak and can cause discomfort to the patient.
10. Check drainage tubing to ensure that there are no dependent loops or kinks. Position the drainage collection device below the tube insertion site.	Dependent loops or kinks in the tubing can prevent the tube from draining appropriately (Bauman & Handley, 2011; Sullivan, 2008). The drainage collection device must be positioned below the tube insertion site so that

ACTION	RATIONALE
	drainage can move out of the tubing and into the collection device.
11. If the chest tube is ordered to be connected to suction, note the fluid level in the suction chamber and check it with the amount of ordered suction. Look for bubbling in the suction chamber. Temporarily disconnect the suction to check the level of water in the chamber. Add sterile water or saline, if necessary, to maintain correct amount of suction.	Some fluid is lost due to evaporation. If suction is set too low, the amount needs to be increased to ensure that enough negative pressure is placed in the pleural space to drain the pleural space sufficiently. If suction is set too high, the amount needs to be decreased to prevent any damage to the fragile lung tissue. Gentle bubbling in the suction chamber indicates that suction is being applied to assist drainage.
12. Observe the water-seal chamber for fluctuations of the water level with the patient's inspiration and expiration (tidaling). If suction is used, temporarily disconnect the suction to observe for fluctuation. Assess for the presence of bubbling in the water-seal chamber. Add water, if necessary, to maintain the level at the 2-cm mark, or the mark recommended by the manufacturer.	Fluctuation of the water level in the water-seal chamber with inspiration and expiration is an expected and normal finding. Bubbles in the water-seal chamber after the initial insertion of the tube or when air is being removed are a normal finding. Constant bubbles in the water-seal chamber after initial insertion period indicate an air leak in the system. Leaks can occur within the drainage unit, or at the insertion site.
13. Assess the amount and type of fluid drainage. Measure drainage output at the end of each shift by marking the level on the container or placing a small piece of tape at the drainage level to indicate date and time. The amount should be a running total, because the drainage system is never emptied. If the drainage system fills, remove and replace it (See Guidelines below).	Measurement allows for accurate intake and output measurement and assessment of the effectiveness of therapy, and it contributes to the decision to remove the tube. The drainage system would lose its negative pressure if it were opened.

ACTION	RATIONALE
14. Remove gloves. Assist the patient to a comfortable position. Raise the bed rail and place the bed in the lowest position, as necessary.	Removing PPE properly reduces the risk for infection transmission and contamination of other items. Placing the patient in a comfortable position ensures patient comfort. Proper positioning with raised side rails and proper bed height provide for patient comfort and safety.
15. Remove additional PPE, if used. Perform hand hygiene.	Removing PPE properly reduces the risk for infection transmission and contamination of other items. Hand hygiene prevents the spread of microorganisms.

Changing the Drainage System

16. Obtain two padded Kelly clamps, a new drainage system, and a bottle of sterile water. Add water to the water-seal chamber in the new system until it reaches the 2-cm mark or the mark recommended by the manufacturer. Follow manufacturer's directions to add water to the suction system if suction is ordered.	Gathering equipment provides for an organized approach. Appropriate level of water in the water-seal chamber is necessary to prevent air from entering the chest. Appropriate level of water in the suction chamber provides the ordered suction.
17. Put on clean gloves and additional PPE, as indicated.	Gloves prevent contact with contaminants and body fluids.
18. **Apply Kelly clamps 1.5 to 2.5 inches from insertion site and 1 inch apart, going in opposite directions (Figure 1).**	Clamps provide a more complete seal and prevent air from entering the pleural space through the chest tube.

FIGURE 1 Using padded clamps on chest tube.

ACTION	RATIONALE
19. Remove the suction from the current drainage system. Unroll or use scissors to carefully cut away any foam tape on the connection of the chest tube and drainage system. Using a slight twisting motion, remove the drainage system. **Do not pull on the chest tube.**	Removing suction permits application of new system. In many institutions, bands or foam tape are placed where the chest tube meets the drainage system to ensure that the chest tube and the drainage system remain connected. Due to the negative pressure, a slight twisting motion may be needed to separate the tubes. The chest tube is sutured in place; do not tug on the chest tube and dislodge it.
20. Keeping the end of the chest tube sterile, insert the end of the new drainage system into the chest tube. **Remove Kelly clamps.** Reconnect suction, if ordered. Apply foam tape to chest tube/drainage system connection site.	Chest tube is sterile. Tube must be reconnected to suction to form a negative pressure and allow for re-expansion of lung or drainage of fluid. Prolonged clamping can result in a pneumothorax. Bands or foam tape help prevent the separation of the chest tube from the drainage system.
21. Assess the patient and the drainage system as outlined (Steps 5–15).	Assess for changes related to the manipulation of the system and placement of a new drainage system.
22. Remove additional PPE, if used. Perform hand hygiene.	Removing PPE properly reduces the risk for infection transmission and contamination of other items. Hand hygiene prevents the spread of microorganisms.

EVALUATION

- The chest drainage system is patent and functioning.
- Patient remains free of signs and symptoms of respiratory distress and complications related to the chest drainage system.
- Patient verbalizes adequate pain relief.
- Patient gradually increases activity tolerance.
- Patient demonstrates an understanding of the need for the chest tube.

DOCUMENTATION

- Document the site of the chest tube, amount and type of drainage, amount of suction applied, and presence of any bubbling, tidaling, or subcutaneous emphysema noted. Document the type of dressing in place and the patient's pain level, as well as any measures performed to relieve the patient's pain.

SKILL VARIATION | Caring for a Chest Drainage System Using Dry Seal or Suction

1. Bring necessary equipment to the bedside stand or overbed table.
2. Perform hand hygiene and put on PPE, if indicated.
3. Identify the patient.
4. Close the curtains around the bed and close the door to the room, if possible.
5. Explain what you are going to do and the reason for doing it to the patient.
6. **Assess the patient's level of pain. Administer prescribed medication, as needed.**
7. Put on clean gloves. Move the patient's gown to expose the chest-tube insertion site. Keep the patient covered as much as possible, using a bath blanket to drape the patient, if necessary. Observe the dressing around the chest tube insertion site and ensure that it is dry, intact, and occlusive.
8. Check that all connections are taped securely. Gently palpate around the insertion site, feeling for subcutaneous emphysema, a collec-

tion of air or gas under the skin. This may feel crunchy or spongy, or like "popping" under your fingers.
9. Check drainage tubing to ensure that there are no dependent loops or kinks. The drainage collection device must be positioned below the tube insertion site.
10. If the chest tube is ordered to be to be suctioned, assess the amount of suction set on the chest tube against the amount of suction ordered. Assess for the presence of the suction control indicator, which is a bellows or float device, when adjusting the regulator to the desired level of suction, if prescribed.
11. Assess for fluctuations in the diagnostic indicator with the patient's inspiration and expiration.
12. Check the air-leak indicator for leaks in dry systems with a one-way valve.
13. Assess the amount and type of fluid drainage. Measure drainage output at the end of each shift by marking the level on the container or placing a small piece of tape at the drainage level to indicate date and time. The amount should be a running total, because the drainage

Caring for a Chest Drainage System Using Dry Seal or Suction   *continued*

system is never emptied. If the drainage system fills, it is removed and replaced.

14. Some portable chest drainage systems require manual emptying of the collection chamber. Follow the manufacturer's recommendations for timing of emptying. Typically, the unit should not be allowed to fill completely because drainage could spill out. Wear gloves, clean the syringe

port with an alcohol wipe, use a 60-mL Luer-Lok syringe, screw the syringe into the port, and aspirate to withdraw fluid. Repeat, as necessary, to empty the chamber. Dispose of the fluid according to facility policy.

15. Remove gloves, and additional PPE, if used. Perform hand hygiene.

SKILL 37   ASSISTING WITH REMOVAL OF A CHEST TUBE

Chest tubes are removed after the lung is re-expanded and drainage is minimal. An advanced-practice professional usually performs chest tube removal. The practitioner will determine when the chest tube is ready for removal by evaluating the chest x-ray and assessing the patient and the amount of drainage from the tube.

DELEGATION CONSIDERATIONS

Assisting with the removal of a chest tube is not delegated to nursing assistive personnel (NAP) or to unlicensed assistive personnel (UAP). Depending on the state's nurse practice act and the organization's policies and procedures, assisting with the removal of a chest tube may be delegated to licensed practical/vocational nurses (LPN/LVNs). The decision to delegate must be based on careful analysis of the patient's needs and circumstances, as well as the qualifications of the person to whom the task is being delegated. Refer to the Delegation Guidelines in Appendix A.

EQUIPMENT

- Disposable gloves
- Additional PPE, as indicated
- Suture removal kit (tweezers and scissors)
- Sterile Vaseline-impregnated gauze and 4 × 4 gauze

dressings or other occlusive dressings, based on facility policy
- Occlusive tape, such as foam tape

ASSESSMENT

- Assess the patient's respiratory status, including respiratory rate and oxygen saturation level. This provides a baseline for comparison after the tube is removed. If the patient begins to have respiratory distress, he or she will usually become tachypneic and hypoxic.
- Assess the patient's lung sounds. The lung sounds over the chest tube site may be diminished due to the tube.
- Assess the patient for pain. Many patients report pain at the chest tube insertion site and request medication for the pain. If the patient has not recently received pain medication, give it before the chest tube removal to decrease the pain felt with the procedure and ease anxiety (Bauman & Handley, 2011).

NURSING DIAGNOSIS

- Deficient Knowledge
- Acute Pain
- Risk for Injury

OUTCOME IDENTIFICATION AND PLANNING

- Patient will remain free of respiratory distress.
- Insertion site will remain clean and dry without evidence of infection.
- Patient will experience adequate pain control during the chest tube removal.
- Patient's lung sounds will be clear and equal bilaterally.
- Patient will be able to increase activity tolerance gradually.

IMPLEMENTATION

ACTION	RATIONALE
1. Gather necessary equipment.	Assembling equipment provides for an organized approach to the task.
2. Perform hand hygiene and put on PPE, if indicated.	Hand hygiene and PPE prevent the spread of microorganisms. PPE is required based on transmission precautions.
3. Identify the patient.	Identifying the patient ensures the right patient receives the intervention and helps prevent errors.

ACTION	RATIONALE
4. Administer pain medication, as prescribed. **Premedicate patient before the chest tube removal, at a sufficient interval to allow for the medication to take effect, based on the medication prescribed.**	Most patients report discomfort during chest tube removal.
5. Close the curtains around the bed and close the door to the room, if possible.	This ensures the patient's privacy.
6. Explain what you are going to do and the reason for doing it to the patient. Explain any nonpharmacologic pain interventions the patient may use to decrease discomfort during tube removal.	Explanation relieves anxiety and facilitates cooperation. Nonpharmacologic pain management interventions, such as relaxation exercises, have been shown to help decrease pain during chest tube removal (Ertuğ & Ülker, 2011; Friesner et al., 2006).
7. Teach the patient how to do the Valsalva maneuver. Instruct the patient to take a deep breath, keep the mouth closed, and attempt to exhale forcibly while keeping the mouth and nose closed. Bearing down with abdominal muscles can assist with the process.	The chest tube must be removed during breath holding or expiration to prevent air from reentering the pleural space (Bauman & Handley, 2011; Crawford, 2011). The Valsalva maneuver may be contraindicated in people with cardiovascular problems and other illnesses.
8. Put on clean gloves.	Gloves prevent contact with contaminants and body fluids.
9. Provide reassurance to the patient while the practitioner removes the dressing and then the tube.	The removal of the dressing and the tube can increase the patient's anxiety level. Offering reassurance will help the patient feel more secure and help decrease anxiety.
10. **After the practitioner has removed the chest tube and secured the occlusive dressing, assess patient's lung sounds, vital signs, oxygen saturation, and pain level.**	In most facilities, advanced practice professionals remove chest tubes, but some facilities train nurses to remove them. Once the tube is removed, the patient's respiratory status will need to be assessed to ensure that no distress is present.

ACTION	RATIONALE
11. Anticipate an order for a chest x-ray.	A chest x-ray is performed to evaluate the status of the lungs after chest tube removal, to ensure that the lung is still fully inflated.
12. Dispose of equipment appropriately.	This reduces the risk for transmission of microorganisms and contamination of other items.
13. Remove gloves and additional PPE, if used. Perform hand hygiene.	Removing PPE properly reduces the risk for infection transmission and contamination of other items. Hand hygiene prevents the spread of microorganisms.
14. Continue to monitor the patient's cardiopulmonary status and comfort level. Monitor the site for drainage.	Continued monitoring allows for assessment of possible respiratory distress if lung does not remain inflated. Checking dressing ensures the assessment of changes in patient condition and enables timely intervention to prevent complications.

EVALUATION
- Patient exhibits no signs and symptoms of respiratory distress after the chest tube is removed.
- Patient verbalizes adequate pain control.
- Patient's lung sounds are clear and equal.
- Patient's activity level gradually increases.

DOCUMENTATION
- Document the patient's respiratory rate, oxygen saturation, lung sounds, total chest tube output, and status of the insertion site and dressing.

SKILL 38 APPLYING COLD THERAPY

Cold constricts the peripheral blood vessels, reducing blood flow to the tissues and decreasing the local release of pain-producing substances. Cold reduces the formation of edema and inflammation, reduces muscle spasm, and promotes comfort by slowing the transmission of pain stimuli. The application of cold therapy reduces bleeding and hematoma formation. The application of cold, using ice, is appropriate after direct trauma, for dental pain, for muscle spasms, after muscle sprains, and for the treatment of chronic pain. Ice can be used to apply cold therapy, usually in the form of an ice bag or ice collar, or in a glove. Commercially prepared cold packs are also available. For electronically controlled cooling devices, see the accompanying Skill Variation.

DELEGATION CONSIDERATIONS

The application of cold therapy may be delegated to nursing assistive personnel (NAP) or to unlicensed assistive personnel (UAP), as well as to licensed practical/vocational nurses (LPN/LVNs). The decision to delegate must be based on careful analysis of the patient's needs and circumstances, as well as the qualifications of the person to whom the task is being delegated. Refer to the Delegation Guidelines in Appendix A.

EQUIPMENT

- Ice
- Ice bag, ice collar, glove
- Commercially prepared cold packs
- Small towel or washcloth
- PPE, as indicated
- Disposable waterproof pad
- Gauze wrap or tape
- Bath blanket

ASSESSMENT

- Assess the situation to determine the appropriateness for the application of cold therapy.
- Assess the patient's physical and mental status and the condition of the body area to be treated with the cold therapy.
- Confirm the medical order, including frequency, type of therapy, body area to be treated, and length of time for the application.
- Assess the equipment to be used to make sure it will function properly.

NURSING DIAGNOSIS

- Acute Pain
- Delayed Surgical Recovery
- Chronic Pain

OUTCOME IDENTIFICATION AND PLANNING

- Patient experiences increased comfort.
- Patient experiences decreased muscle spasms.

- Patient experiences decreased inflammation.
- Patient does not show signs of bleeding or hematoma at the treatment site.

IMPLEMENTATION

ACTION	RATIONALE
1. Review the medical order or nursing plan of care for the application of cold therapy, including frequency, type of therapy, body area to be treated, and length of time for the application. Gather necessary supplies.	Reviewing the order validates the correct patient and correct procedure. Preparation promotes efficient time management and an organized approach to the task.
2. Perform hand hygiene and put on PPE, if indicated.	Hand hygiene and PPE prevent the spread of microorganisms. PPE is required based on transmission precautions.
3. Identify the patient. Determine if the patient has had any previous adverse reaction to hypothermia therapy.	Identifying the patient ensures the right patient receives the intervention and helps prevent errors. Individual differences exist in tolerating specific therapies.
4. Assemble equipment on overbed table within reach.	Organization facilitates performance of task.
5. Close the curtains around the bed and close the door to the room, if possible. Explain what you are going to do and why you are going to do it to the patient.	This ensures the patient's privacy. Explanation relieves anxiety and facilitates cooperation.
6. Assess the condition of the skin where the cold is to be applied.	Assessment supplies baseline data for posttreatment comparison and identifies any conditions that may contraindicate the application.
7. Assist the patient to a comfortable position that provides easy access to the area to be treated. Expose the area and drape the patient with a bath blanket if needed. Put the waterproof pad under the wound area, if necessary.	Patient positioning and use of a bath blanket provide for comfort and warmth. Waterproof pad protects the patient and the bed linens.

ACTION	RATIONALE
8. Prepare device:	
Fill the bag, collar, or glove about three-fourths full with ice. **Remove any excess air from the device.** Securely fasten the end of the bag or collar; tie the glove closed, checking for holes and leakage of water. Prepare commercially prepared ice pack, according to manufacturer's directions, if appropriate.	Ice provides a cold surface. Excess air interferes with cold conduction. Fastening the end prevents leaks.
9. **Cover the device with a towel or washcloth; commercially prepared devices may come with a cover.** (If the device has a cloth exterior, this is not necessary.)	The cover protects the skin and absorbs condensation.
10. Position cooling device on top of designated area and lightly secure in place as needed.	Proper positioning ensures the cold therapy to the specified body area.
11. **Remove the ice and assess the site for redness after 30 seconds. Ask the patient about the presence of burning sensations.**	These actions prevent tissue injury.
12. Replace the device snugly against the site if no problems are evident. Secure it in place with gauze wrap, ties, or tape.	Wrapping or taping stabilizes the device in the proper location.
13. Reassess the treatment area every 5 minutes or according to facility policy.	Assessment of the patient's skin is necessary for early detection of adverse effects, thereby allowing prompt intervention to avoid complications.
14. **After 20 minutes or the prescribed amount of time, remove the ice and dry the skin.**	Limiting the time of application prevents injury due to overexposure to cold. Prolonged application of cold may result in decreased blood flow with resulting tissue ischemia. A compensatory vasodilation or rebound phenomenon may occur as a means to provide warmth to the area.

ACTION	RATIONALE
15. Remove PPE, if used. Perform hand hygiene.	Removing PPE properly reduces the risk for infection transmission and contamination of other items. Hand hygiene prevents the spread of microorganisms.

EVALUATION

• Patient reports relief of pain and increased comfort.
• Patient verbalizes a decrease in muscle spasms.
• Patient exhibits a reduction in inflammation.
• Patient remains free of any injury, including signs of bleeding or hematoma at the treatment site.

DOCUMENTATION

• Document the location of the application, time of placement, and time of removal. Record the assessment of the area where the cold therapy was applied, including the patient's mobility, sensation, color, temperature, and any presence of numbness, tingling, or pain. Document the patient's response, such as any decrease in pain or change in sensation. Include any pertinent patient and family education.

SKILL VARIATION | **Applying an Electronically Controlled Cooling Device**

Electronically controlled cooling devices are used in situations to deliver a constant cooling effect. After ortho-pedic surgery, those patients as well as other patients with acute musculoskeletal injuries may benefit from this therapy. A medical order is required for use of this device. Initial assessment of the extremity is involved, as well as ongoing assessment throughout the period of use. As with applica-tion of any electronic device, ongoing monitoring for proper

functioning and temperature regulation is necessary.

1. Gather equipment and verify the medical order.
2. Perform hand hygiene. Put on PPE, as indicated.

3. Identify the patient and explain the proce-dure.

4. Assess the involved extremity or body part.

Applying an Electronically Controlled Cooling Device *continued*

5. Set the correct temperature on the device.
6. Wrap the cooling water-flow pad around the involved body part.
7. Wrap an Ace bandage or gauze pads around the water-flow pads.
8. Assess to ensure that the cooling pads are functioning properly.

9. Remove PPE, if used. Perform hand hygiene.

10. Recheck frequently to ensure proper functioning of equipment.
11. Unwrap at intervals to assess skin integrity of the body part.

SKILL 39   IRRIGATING A COLOSTOMY

Colostomy irrigation is a way of achieving fecal continence and control (Perston, 2010). Irrigations are used to promote regular evacuation of some colostomies. Colostomy irrigation may be indicated in patients who have a left-sided end colostomy in the descending or sigmoid colon, are mentally alert, have adequate vision, and have adequate manual dexterity needed to perform the procedure. Contraindications to colostomy irrigation include irritable bowel syndrome, peristomal hernia, postradiation damage to the bowel, diverticulitis, and Crohn's disease (Carlsson, et al., 2010). Ileostomies are not irrigated because the fecal content of the ileum is liquid and cannot be controlled.

Once the patient has established a routine and bowel continence has been established, a small appliance can be worn over the stoma. These "stoma caps" are small capacity appliances with a pad to soak up discharge and a flatus filter (Perston, 2010). If a colostomy irrigation is to be implemented, the nurse should consult facility policy regarding the accepted procedure and, ideally, consult with a wound, ostomy, and continence nurse for patient education and support.

DELEGATION CONSIDERATIONS

Colostomy irrigation is not delegated to nursing assistive personnel (NAP) or to unlicensed assistive personnel (UAP). Depending on the state's nurse practice act and the organization's policies and procedures, the administration of a small-volume cleansing enema may be delegated to licensed practical/vocational nurses (LPN/LVNs). The decision to delegate must be based on careful analysis of the patient's needs and circumstances, as well as the qualifications of the person to whom the task is being delegated. Refer to the Delegation Guidelines in Appendix A.

EQUIPMENT

- Disposable irrigation system and irrigation sleeve
- Waterproof pad
- Bedpan or toilet
- Water-soluble lubricant
- IV pole
- Disposable gloves
- Additional PPE, as indicated
- Solution at a temperature of 98.6°F (37°C) (normally tap water)
- Washcloth, skin cleanser, and towels
- Paper towel
- New ostomy appliance, if needed, or stoma cover

ASSESSMENT

- Ask patient if he or she has been experiencing any abdominal discomfort.
- Ask patient about date of last irrigation and whether there have been any changes in stool pattern or consistency. If the patient irrigates his or her colostomy at home, ask if he or she has any special routines during irrigation, such as reading the newspaper or listening to music. Determine how much solution the patient typically uses for irrigation. The normal amount of irrigation fluid varies, but is usually around 500 mL to 1,000 mL for an adult. If this is a first irrigation, the normal irrigation volume is around 500 mL.
- Assess the ostomy, ensuring that the diversion is a colostomy. Note placement of colostomy on abdomen, color and size of ostomy, color and condition of stoma, and amount and consistency of stool.

NURSING DIAGNOSIS

- Deficient Knowledge
- Anxiety
- Disturbed Body Image

OUTCOME IDENTIFICATION AND PLANNING

- The expected outcome to be met when irrigating a colostomy is that the patient expels soft, formed stool.
- Patient remains free of any evidence of trauma to the stoma and intestinal mucosa.
- Patient demonstrates the ability to participate in care.
- Patient voices increased confidence with ostomy care.
- Patient demonstrates positive coping mechanisms.

IMPLEMENTATION

ACTION	RATIONALE
1. Verify the order for the irrigation. Gather equipment.	Verifying the medical order is crucial to ensuring that the proper treatment is administered to the right patient. Assembling

ACTION	RATIONALE
	equipment provides for an organized approach to the task.
2. Perform hand hygiene and put on PPE, if indicated.	Hand hygiene and PPE prevent the spread of microorganisms. PPE is required based on transmission precautions.
3. Identify the patient.	Identifying the patient ensures the right patient receives the intervention and helps prevent errors.
4. Close the curtains around the bed and close the door to the room, if possible. Explain what you are going to do and why you are going to do it to the patient. Plan where the patient will receive irrigation. Assist the patient onto bedside commode or into nearby bathroom.	This ensures the patient's privacy. Explanation relieves anxiety and facilitates cooperation. Discussion promotes cooperation and helps to minimize anxiety. The patient cannot hold the irrigation solution. A large immediate return of irrigation solution and stool usually occurs.
5. Assemble equipment on overbed table within reach.	Arranging items nearby is convenient, saves time, and avoids unnecessary stretching and twisting of muscles on the part of the nurse.
6. Warm solution in amount ordered and check temperature with a bath thermometer, if available. If bath thermometer is not available, warm to room temperature or slightly higher, and test on inner wrist. If tap water is used, adjust temperature as it flows from faucet.	If the solution is too cool, the patient may experience cramps or nausea. Solution that is too warm or too hot can cause irritation and trauma to intestinal mucosa.
7. Add irrigation solution to container. Release clamp and allow fluid to progress through tube before reclamping.	This causes any air to be expelled from the tubing. Although allowing air to enter the intestine is not harmful, it may further distend the intestine.

ACTION	RATIONALE
8. Hang container on IV pole so that bottom of bag will be at the patient's shoulder level when seated.	Gravity forces the solution to enter the intestine. The amount of pressure determines the rate of flow and pressure exerted on the intestinal wall.
9. Put on gloves.	Gloves prevent contact with blood, body fluids, and micro-organisms.
10. Remove ostomy appliance and attach irrigation sleeve. Place drainage end into toilet bowl or commode.	The irrigation sleeve directs all irrigation fluid and stool into the toilet or bedpan for easy disposal.
11. Lubricate end of cone with water-soluble lubricant.	This facilitates passage of the cone into the stoma opening.
12. Insert the cone through the top of the irrigation sleeve and into the stoma (Figure 1-A). Introduce solution slowly over a period of 5 to 10 minutes. Hold cone and tubing (or if patient is able, allow patient to hold) all the time that solution is being instilled (Figure 1-B). Control rate of flow by closing or opening the clamp.	If the irrigation solution is administered too quickly, the patient may experience nausea and cramps due to rapid distention and increased pressure in the intestine.

FIGURE 1 Colostomy irrigation. (**A**) Inserting irrigation cone. (**B**) Instilling irrigating fluid with sleeve in place.

13. Hold cone in place for an additional 10 seconds after the fluid is infused.	This will allow a small amount of dwell time for the irrigation solution.

ACTION	RATIONALE
14. Remove cone. Patient should remain seated on toilet or bedside commode.	An immediate return of solution and stool will usually occur, followed by a return in spurts for up to 45 more minutes.
15. After majority of solution has returned, allow the patient to clip (close) the bottom of irrigating sleeve and continue with daily activities.	An immediate return of solution and stool will usually occur, followed by a return in spurts for up to 45 more minutes. Leaving the sleeve in place allows the patient to continue with daily activities until return of solution is complete.
16. After solution has stopped flowing from stoma, put on clean gloves. Remove irrigating sleeve and cleanse skin around stoma opening with skin cleanser and water. Gently pat peristomal skin dry.	Gloves prevent contact with blood and body fluids. Peristomal skin must be clean and free of any liquid or stool before application of a new appliance.
17. Attach new appliance to stoma or stoma cover (see Skill 120), as needed.	Some patients will not require an appliance, but may use a stoma cover. Protects stoma.
18. Remove gloves. Return the patient to a comfortable position. Make sure the linens under the patient are dry, if appropriate. Ensure that the patient is covered.	Removing contaminated gloves prevents spread of microorganisms. Promotes patient comfort.
19. Raise side rail. Lower bed height and adjust head of bed to a comfortable position, as necessary.	Promotes patient safety.
20. Remove gloves and additional PPE, if used. Perform hand hygiene.	Removing PPE properly reduces the risk for infection transmission and contamination of other items. Hand hygiene prevents the spread of microorganisms.

EVALUATION

• Irrigation solution flows easily into the stoma opening and the patient expels soft, formed stool.

- Patient remains free of any evidence of trauma to the stoma and intestinal mucosa.
- Patient participates in irrigation with increasing confidence.
- Patient demonstrates positive coping mechanisms.

DOCUMENTATION

- Document the procedure, including the amount of irrigating solution used; color, amount, and consistency of stool returned; condition of stoma; degree of patient participation; and patient's reaction to irrigation.

SKILL 40 | PROMOTING PATIENT COMFORT

The nurse can promote increased comfort and relieve patient discomfort and pain through various pain management therapies. Interventions can include the administration of analgesics, emotional support, comfort measures, and nonpharmacologic interventions. Nonpharmacologic methods of pain management can diminish the emotional components of pain, strengthen coping abilities, give patients a sense of control, contribute to pain relief, decrease fatigue, and promote sleep. The following skill identifies potential interventions related to discomfort and pain. The interventions are listed sequentially for teaching purposes; the order is not sequential and should be adjusted based on patient assessment and nursing judgment. Not every intervention discussed will be appropriate for every patient. Additional interventions for discomfort and pain are discussed in other skills, such as the application of cold or heat therapy (Skills 38 and 81), and the administration of medications for pain relief (Skills 95, 100, 105, 126, 127).

DELEGATION CONSIDERATIONS

The assessment of a patient's pain is not delegated to nursing assistive personnel (NAP) or to unlicensed assistive personnel (UAP). The assessment of a patient's pain may be delegated to licensed practical/vocational nurses (LPN/LVNs). The use of nonpharmacologic interventions related to patient comfort may be delegated to nursing assistive personnel (NAP) or to unlicensed assistive personnel (UAP), as well as to licensed practical/vocational nurses (LPN/LVNs). The decision to delegate must be based on careful analysis of the patient's needs and circumstances, as well as the qualifications of the person to whom the task is being delegated. Refer to the Delegation Guidelines in Appendix A.

EQUIPMENT

- Pain assessment tool and pain scale
- Oral hygiene supplies
- Nonsterile gloves, if necessary
- Additional PPE, as indicated

ASSESSMENT

- Review the patient's medical record and plan of care for information about the patient's status and contraindications to any of the potential interventions.
- Inquire about any allergies.
- Assess the patient's level of discomfort. Assess the patient's pain using an appropriate assessment tool and pain scale. Assess the characteristics of any pain and for other symptoms that often occur with the pain, such as headache or restlessness. Ask the patient what interventions have and have not been successful in the past to promote comfort and relieve pain.
- Assess the patient's vital signs.
- Check the patient's medication administration record for the time an analgesic was last administered.
- Assess cultural beliefs related to pain.
- Assess the patient's response to a particular intervention to evaluate effectiveness and presence of adverse effect.

NURSING DIAGNOSIS

- Acute Pain
- Chronic Pain
- Disturbed Sleep Pattern

OUTCOME IDENTIFICATION AND PLANNING

- Patient experiences relief from discomfort and/or pain without adverse effect.
- Patient experiences decreased anxiety and improved relaxation.
- Patient is able to participate in activities of daily living (ADLs).
- Patient verbalizes an understanding of, and satisfaction with, the pain management plan.

IMPLEMENTATION

ACTION	RATIONALE
1. Perform hand hygiene and put on PPE, if indicated.	Hand hygiene and PPE prevent the spread of microorganisms. PPE is required based on transmission precautions.
2. Identify the patient.	Identifying the patient ensures the right patient receives the intervention and helps prevent errors.

ACTION	RATIONALE
3. Discuss pain with the patient, acknowledging that the patient's pain exists. Explain how pain medications and other pain management therapies work together to provide pain relief. Allow the patient to help choose interventions for pain relief.	Pain discussion and patient involvement strengthen the nurse–patient relationship and promote pain relief (Taylor et al., 2015). Explanation encourages patient understanding and cooperation and reduces apprehension.
4. Assess the patient's pain, using an appropriate assessment tool and measurement scale.	Accurate assessment is necessary to guide treatment/relief interventions and evaluate the effectiveness of pain control measures.
5. Provide pharmacologic interventions, if indicated and ordered.	Analgesics and adjuvant drugs reduce perception of pain and alter responses to discomfort.
6. Adjust the patient's environment to promote comfort.	The environment can improve or detract from the patient's sense of well-being and can be a source of stimulation that aggravates pain and reduces comfort.
a. Adjust and maintain the room temperature per the patient's preference.	A too warm or too cool environment can be a source of stimulation that aggravates pain and reduces comfort.
b. Reduce harsh lighting, but provide adequate lighting per the patient's preference.	Harsh lighting can be a source of stimulation that aggravates pain and reduces comfort.
c. Reduce harsh and unnecessary noise. Avoid having conversations immediately outside the patient's room.	Noise, including talking, can be a source of stimuli that aggravates pain and reduce comfort.
d. Close the room door and/or curtain whenever possible.	Closing the door or curtain provides privacy and reduces noise and other extraneous stimuli that may aggravate pain and reduce comfort.
e. Provide good ventilation in the patient's room. Reduce unpleasant odors by promptly emptying bedpans, urinals, and	Odors can be a source of stimuli that aggravate pain and reduce comfort.

ACTION	RATIONALE

emesis basins after use. Remove trash and laundry promptly.

7. Prevent unnecessary interruptions and coordinate patient activities to group activities together. Allow for and plan rest periods without disturbance.

Frequent interruptions and disturbances for assessment or treatment can be a source of stimuli that aggravate pain and reduce comfort. Fatigue reduces tolerance for pain and can increase the pain experience.

8. Assist the patient to change position frequently. Assist the patient to a comfortable position, maintaining good alignment and supporting extremities as needed. Raise the head of the bed as appropriate.

Positioning in proper alignment with supports ensures that the patient will be able to maintain the desired position and reduces pressure.

9. Provide oral hygiene as often as necessary (e.g., every 1 to 2 hours) to keep the mouth and mucous membranes clean and moist. This is especially important for patients who cannot drink or are not permitted fluids by mouth.

Moisture helps maintain the integrity of mucous membranes. Dry mucous membranes can be a source of stimuli that aggravate pain and reduce comfort.

10. Ensure the availability of appropriate fluids for drinking, unless contraindicated. Make sure the patient's water pitcher is filled and within reach. Have other fluids of the patient's choice available.

Thirst and dry mucous membranes can be sources of stimuli that reduce comfort and aggravate pain.

11. Remove physical situations that might cause discomfort.

a. Change soiled and/or wet dressings; replace soiled and/or wet bed linens.

Moisture can cause discomfort and irritation to skin.

b. Smooth wrinkles in bed linens.

Wrinkled bed linens apply pressure to skin and can cause discomfort and irritation to skin.

c. Ensure patient is not lying or sitting on tubes, tubing, wires, or other equipment.

Tubing and equipment apply pressure to skin and can cause discomfort and irritation to skin.

ACTION	RATIONALE
12. Assist the patient as necessary with ambulation, and active or passive range-of-motion exercises (ROM), as appropriate.	Activity prevents stiffness and loss of mobility, which can reduce comfort and aggravate pain.
13. Assess the patient's spiritual needs related to the pain experience. Ask the patient if he/she would like a spiritual counselor to visit.	Some people's spiritual beliefs facilitate positive coping with the effects of illness, including pain.
14. Consider the use of distraction. Distraction requires the patient to focus on something other than the pain.	Conscious attention often appears to be necessary to experience pain. Preoccupation with other things has been observed to distract the patient from pain. Distraction is thought to raise the threshold of pain and/or increase pain tolerance (Taylor et al., 2015).

a. Have the patient recall a pleasant experience or focus attention on an enjoyable experience.

b. Offer age or developmentally appropriate games, toys, books, audiobooks, access to television, and/or videos, or other items of interest to the patient.

c. Encourage the patient to hold or stroke a loved person, pet, or toy.

d. Offer access to music the patient prefers. Turn on the music when pain begins, or before anticipated painful stimuli. The patient can close his or her eyes and concentrate on listening. Raising or lowering the volume as pain increases or decreases can be helpful.

ACTION	RATIONALE
15. Consider the use of guided imagery.	Guided imagery helps the patient gradually become less aware of the discomfort or pain. Positive emotions evoked by the image help reduce the pain experience.

15. Consider the use of guided imagery.

   a. Help the patient to identify a scene or experience that the patient describes as happy, pleasant, or peaceful.

   b. Encourage the patient to begin with several minutes of focused breathing, relaxation, or meditation. (Refer to specific information in steps 16 and 17.)

   c. Help the patient concentrate on the peaceful, pleasant image.

   d. If indicated, read a description of the identified scene or experience, using a soothing, soft voice.

   e. Encourage the patient to concentrate on the details of the image, such as its sight, sounds, smells, tastes, and touch.

16. Consider the use of relaxation activities, such as deep breathing.

Relaxation techniques reduce skeletal muscle tension and lessen anxiety, both of which can reduce comfort and aggravate pain. Relaxation can also be a distraction, providing help in reducing the pain experience (Kwekkeboom et al., 2008; Taylor et al., 2015).

   a. Have the patient sit or recline comfortably and place hands on stomach. Close the eyes.

   b. Ask the patient to mentally count to maintain a comfortable rate and rhythm. Have the patient

ACTION	RATIONALE

inhale slowly and deeply while letting the abdomen expand as much as possible. Have the patient hold his or her breath for a few seconds.

c. Tell the patient to exhale slowly through the mouth, blowing through puckered lips. Have the patient continue to count to maintain comfortable rate and rhythm, concentrating on the rise and fall of the abdomen.

d. When the patient's abdomen feels empty, have the patient begin again with a deep inhalation.

e. Encourage patient to practice at least twice a day, for 10 minutes, and then use the technique as needed to assist with pain management.

17. Consider the use of relaxation activities, such as progressive muscle relaxation.

Relaxation techniques reduce skeletal muscle tension and lessen anxiety, both of which can reduce comfort and aggravate pain. Relaxation can also be a distraction, providing help in reducing the pain experience (Kwekkeboom et al., 2008; Taylor et al., 2015).

a. Assist the patient to a comfortable position.

b. Direct the patient to focus on a particular muscle group. Start with the muscles of the jaw, then repeat with the muscles of the neck, shoulder, upper and lower arm, hand, abdomen, buttocks, thigh, lower leg, and foot.

ACTION	RATIONALE

c. Ask the patient to tighten the muscle group and note the sensation that the tightened muscles produce. After 5 to 7 seconds, tell the patient to relax the muscles all at once and concentrate on the sensation of the relaxed state, noting the difference in feeling in the muscles when contracted and relaxed.

d. Have the patient continue to tighten–hold–relax each muscle group until the entire body has been covered.

e. Encourage the patient to practice at least twice a day, for 10 minutes, and then use the technique, as needed, to assist with pain management.

18. Consider the use of cutaneous stimulation, such as the intermittent application of heat or cold, or both.

Heat helps relieve pain by stimulating specific nerve fibers, closing the gate that allows the transmission of pain stimuli to centers in the brain. Heat accelerates the inflammatory response to promote healing, and reduces muscle tension to promote relaxation and help to relieve muscle spasms and joint stiffness. Cold reduces blood flow to tissues and decreases the local release of pain-producing substances such as histamine, serotonin, and bradykinin, and reduces the formation of edema and inflammation.

Cold reduces muscle spasm, alters tissue sensitivity (producing numbness), and promotes comfort by slowing the transmission of pain stimuli (Taylor et al., 2015).

ACTION	RATIONALE
19. Consider the use of cutaneous stimulation, such as massage (see Skill 6).	Cutaneous stimulation techniques stimulate the skin's surface, closing the gating mechanism in the spinal cord, decreasing the number of pain impulses that reach the brain for perception.
20. Discuss the potential for use of cutaneous stimulation, such as TENS, with the patient and primary care provider. (See Skill 164.)	Cutaneous stimulation techniques stimulate the skin's surface, closing the gating mechanism in the spinal cord, decreasing the number of pain impulses that reach the brain for perception.
21. Remove equipment and return patient to a position of comfort. Remove gloves, if used. Raise side rail and lower bed.	Equipment removal and repositioning promote patient comfort. Removing gloves properly reduces the risk for infection transmission and contamination of other items. Lowering bed promotes patient safety.
22. Remove additional PPE, if used. Perform hand hygiene.	Removing PPE properly reduces the risk for infection transmission and contamination of other items. Hand hygiene prevents transmission of microorganisms.
23. Evaluate the patient's response to interventions. Reassess level of discomfort or pain using original assessment tools. Reassess and alter plan of care as appropriate.	Evaluation allows for individualization of plan of care and promotes optimal patient comfort.

EVALUATION

- Patient experiences relief from discomfort and/or pain without adverse effect.
- Patient experiences decreased anxiety and improved relaxation.
- Patient is able to participate in ADLs.
- Patient verbalizes an understanding of, and satisfaction with, the pain management plan.

DOCUMENTATION

- Document pain assessment and other significant assessments. Document pain relief therapies used and patient responses. Record alternative treatments to consider, if appropriate. Document reassessment of pain and comfort after interventions, at an appropriate interval, based on specific interventions used.

SKILL 41 ASSISTING WITH THE USE OF A BEDSIDE COMMODE

Patients who experience difficulty getting to the bathroom may benefit from the use of a bedside commode. Bedside commodes are portable toilet substitutes that can be used for voiding and defecation. A bedside commode can be placed close to the bed for easy use. Many have armrests attached to the legs that may interfere with ease of transfer. The legs usually have some type of end cap on the bottom to reduce movement, but care must be taken to prevent the commode from moving during transfer, resulting in patient injury or falls.

DELEGATION CONSIDERATIONS

Assisting a patient with the use of a commode may be delegated to nursing assistive personnel (NAP) or to unlicensed assistive personnel (UAP), as well as to licensed practical/vocational nurses (LPN/LVNs). The decision to delegate must be based on careful analysis of the patient's needs and circumstances, as well as the qualifications of the person to whom the task is being delegated. Refer to the Delegation Guidelines in Appendix A.

EQUIPMENT

- Commode with cover (usually attached)
- Toilet tissue
- Nonsterile gloves
- Additional PPE, as indicated
- Disposable washcloths and skin cleanser
- Moist towelettes, skin cleanser and water, or hand sanitizer

ASSESSMENT

- Assess the patient's normal elimination habits.
- Determine why the patient needs to use a commode, such as weakness or unsteady gait. Assess the patient's degree of limitation and ability to help with the activity.
- Check for the presence of drains, dressings, intravenous fluid infusion sites/equipment, or other devices that could interfere with the patient's ability to help with the procedure or that could become dislodged.
- Assess the characteristics of the urine and the patient's skin.

NURSING DIAGNOSIS

- Risk for Falls
- Impaired Urinary Elimination
- Toileting Self-Care Deficit

OUTCOME IDENTIFICATION AND PLANNING

- Patient is able to void with assistance.
- Patient maintains continence.
- Patient demonstrates how to use the commode.
- Patient maintains skin integrity.
- Patient remains free from injury.

IMPLEMENTATION

ACTION	RATIONALE
1. Review the patient's chart for any limitations in physical activity. Gather equipment.	Physical limitations may require adaptations in performing the skill. Assembling equipment provides for an organized approach to the task.
2. Obtain assistance for patient transfer from another staff member, if necessary.	Assistance from another person may be required to transfer the patient safely to the commode.
3. Perform hand hygiene and put on PPE, if indicated.	Hand hygiene and PPE prevent the spread of microorganisms. PPE is required based on transmission precautions.
4. Identify the patient.	Identifying the patient ensures the right patient receives the intervention and helps prevent errors.
5. Close the curtains around the bed and close the door to the room, if possible. Discuss the procedure with the patient and assess the patient's ability to assist with the procedure, as well as personal hygiene preferences.	This ensures the patient's privacy. Discussion promotes reassurance and provides knowledge about the procedure. Dialogue encourages patient participation and allows for individualized nursing care.
6. Place the commode close to, and parallel with, the bed. Raise or remove the seat cover.	Allows for easy access.

ACTION	RATIONALE

7. Assist the patient to a standing position and then help the patient pivot to the commode. **While bracing one commode leg with your foot, ask the patient to place his or her hands one at a time on the armrests. Assist the patient to lower himself/herself slowly onto the commode seat.**

Standing and then pivoting ensures safe patient transfer. Bracing the commode leg with a foot prevents the commode from shifting while the patient is sitting down.

8. Cover the patient with a blanket. Place call bell and toilet tissue within easy reach. Leave patient if it is safe to do so. Remove PPE, if used, and perform hand hygiene.

Covering the patient promotes warmth. Falls can be prevented if the patient does not have to reach for items he or she needs. Leaving patient alone, if possible, promotes self-esteem and shows respect for privacy. Removing PPE properly reduces the risk for infection transmission and contamination of other items. Hand hygiene prevents the spread of microorganisms.

Assisting Patient Off Commode

9. Perform hand hygiene. Put on gloves and additional PPE, as indicated.

Hand hygiene deters the spread of microorganisms. Gloves prevent exposure to blood and body fluids.

10. Assist the patient to a standing position. If the patient needs assistance with hygiene, wrap toilet tissue around your hand several times, and wipe the patient clean, using one stroke from the pubic area toward the anal area. Discard tissue in an appropriate receptacle, according to facility policy, and continue with additional tissue until patient is dry. Place tissue in receptacle. Use warm, moist disposable washcloth and skin cleanser to clean

Cleaning area from front to back minimizes fecal contamination of the vagina and urinary meatus. Cleaning the patient after he or she has used the commode prevents offensive odors and irritation to the skin.

ACTION	RATIONALE
perineal area as necessary, and as per patient request.	
11. Do not place toilet tissue in the commode if a specimen is required or if output is being recorded. Replace or lower the seat cover.	Mixing toilet tissue with a specimen makes laboratory examination more difficult and interferes with accurate output measurement. Covering the commode helps to prevent the spread of microorganisms.
12. Remove your gloves. Return the patient to the bed or chair. If the patient returns to the bed, raise side rails, as appropriate. Ensure that the patient is covered and call bell is readily within reach.	Removing contaminated gloves prevents spread of microorganisms. Returning the patient to the bed or chair promotes patient comfort. Side rails assist with patient movement in the bed. Having the call bell readily available promotes patient safety.
13. Offer patient supplies to wash and dry his or her hands, assisting as necessary.	Washing hands after using the commode helps prevent the spread of microorganisms.
14. Put on clean gloves. Empty and clean the commode, measuring urine in graduated container, as necessary.	Gloves prevent exposure to blood and body fluids. Accurate measurement of urine is necessary for accurate intake and output records.
15. Remove gloves and additional PPE, if used. Perform hand hygiene.	Removing PPE properly reduces the risk for infection transmission and contamination of other items. Hand hygiene prevents the spread of microorganisms.

EVALUATION

- Patient successfully uses the bedside commode.
- Patient remains dry and does not experience episodes of incontinence.
- Patient demonstrates measures to assist with using the commode.
- Patient does not experience impaired skin integrity or falls.

DOCUMENTATION

Document the patient's tolerance of the activity, including his or her ability to use the commode. Record the amount of urine voided and/or stool passed on the intake and output record, if appropriate. Document any other assessments, such as unusual urine or stool characteristics or alterations in the patient's skin.

Warm, moist compresses are used to help promote circulation, encourage healing, decrease edema, promote consolidation of exudate, and decrease pain and discomfort. Moist heat softens crusted material and is less drying to the skin. Moist heat also penetrates tissues more deeply than dry heat. The heat of a warm compress dissipates quickly, so the compresses must be changed frequently. If a constant warm temperature is required, a heating device such as an Aquathermia pad (refer to Skill 81) is applied over the compress. However, **because moisture conducts heat, a low temperature setting is needed on the heating device.** Many facilities have warming devices to heat the dressing package to an appropriate temperature for the compress. These devices help reduce the risk of burning or skin damage.

DELEGATION CONSIDERATIONS

The application of a warm compress may be delegated to nursing assistive personnel (NAP) or unlicensed assistive personnel (UAP), as well as to licensed practical/vocational nurses (LPN/LVNs). The decision to delegate must be based on careful analysis of the patient's needs and circumstances, as well as the qualifications of the person to whom the task is being delegated. Refer to the Delegation Guidelines in Appendix A.

EQUIPMENT

- Prescribed solution to moisten the compress material, warmed to 105°F to 110°F
- Container for solution
- Gauze dressings or compresses
- Alternately, obtain the appropriate number of commercially packaged prewarmed dressings from the warming device
- Clean, disposable gloves
- Additional PPE, as indicated
- Waterproof pad and bath blanket
- Dry bath towel
- Tape or ties
- Aquathermia or other external heating device, if ordered or required to maintain the temperature of the compress

ASSESSMENT

- Assess for circulatory compromise in the area where the compress will be applied, including skin color, pulses distal to the site, evidence of edema, and the presence of sensation.
- Assess the situation to determine the appropriateness for the application of heat.
- Confirm the medical order for the compresses, including the solution to be used, frequency, body area to be treated, and length of time for the application.
- Assess the equipment to be used, if necessary, including the condition of cords, plugs, and heating elements. Look for fluid leaks.

Once the equipment is turned on, make sure there is a consistent distribution of heat and the temperature is within safe limits.
• Assess the application site frequently during the treatment, as tissue damage can occur.

NURSING DIAGNOSIS
• Impaired Tissue Integrity
• Chronic Pain
• Risk for Impaired Skin Integrity

OUTCOME IDENTIFICATION AND PLANNING
• Patient shows signs such as decreased inflammation, decreased muscle spasms, or decreased pain that indicate problems have been relieved.
• Patient experiences improved healing, and the patient remains free from injury.

IMPLEMENTATION

ACTION	RATIONALE
1. Review the medical order for the application of a moist warm compress, including frequency and length of time for the application. Gather necessary supplies.	Reviewing the order and plan of care validates the correct patient and correct procedure. Preparation promotes efficient time management and an organized approach to the task.
2. Perform hand hygiene and put on PPE, if indicated.	Hand hygiene and PPE prevent the spread of microorganisms. PPE is required based on transmission precautions.
3. Identify the patient.	Identifying the patient ensures the right patient receives the intervention and helps prevent errors.
4. Assemble equipment on overbed table within reach.	Organization facilitates performance of task.
5. Assess the patient for possible need for nonpharmacologic pain-reducing interventions or analgesic medication before beginning the procedure. Administer appropriate analgesic, as ordered, and allow enough time for	Pain is a subjective experience influenced by past experience. Depending on the site of application, manipulation of the area may cause pain for some patients.

ACTION	RATIONALE
the analgesic to achieve its effectiveness before beginning the procedure.	
6. Close the curtains around the bed and close the door to room, if possible. Explain what you are going to do and why you are going to do it to the patient.	This ensures the patient's privacy. Explanation relieves anxiety and facilitates cooperation.
7. If using an electronic heating device, check that the water in the unit is at the appropriate level. Fill the unit two-thirds full with distilled water, or to the fill mark, if necessary. Check the temperature setting on the unit to ensure it is within the safe range. (Refer to Skill 81.)	Sufficient water in the unit is necessary to ensure proper function of the unit. Tap water leaves mineral deposits in the unit. Checking the temperature setting helps to prevent skin or tissue damage.
8. Assist the patient to a comfortable position that provides easy access to the area. Use a bath blanket to cover any exposed area other than the intended site. Place a waterproof pad under the site.	Patient positioning and use of a bath blanket provide for comfort and warmth. Waterproof pad protects underlying surfaces.
9. Place a waste receptacle at a convenient location for use during the procedure.	Having a waste container handy means that the used materials may be discarded easily, without the spread of microorganisms.
10. Pour the warmed solution into the container and drop the gauze for the compress into the solution. Alternately, if commercially packaged, prewarmed gauze is used, open packaging.	Prepares compress for application.
11. Put on clean gloves. Assess the application site for inflammation, skin color, and ecchymosis.	Gloves protect the nurse from potential contact with microorganisms. Assessment provides information about the area, the healing process, and the presence of infection, and allows for

ACTION	RATIONALE

documentation of the condition of the area before the compress is applied.

12. Retrieve the compress from the warmed solution, squeezing out any excess moisture. Alternately, remove pre-warmed gauze from open package. **Apply the compress by gently and carefully molding it to the intended area. Ask the patient if the application feels too hot.**

Excess moisture may contaminate the surrounding area and is uncomfortable for the patient. Molding the compress to the skin promotes retention of warmth around the site.

13. Cover the site with a single layer of gauze and with a clean dry bath towel; secure in place with tape or roller gauze, if necessary.

Towel provides extra insulation.

14. Place the Aquathermia or heating device, if used, over the towel.

Use of heating device maintains the temperature of the compress and extends the therapeutic effect.

15. Remove gloves and discard them appropriately. Perform hand hygiene and remove additional PPE, if used.

Hand hygiene prevents the spread of microorganisms. Removing PPE properly reduces the risk for infection transmission and contamination of other items.

16. **Monitor the time the compress is in place to prevent burns and skin/tissue damage. Monitor the condition of the patient's skin and the patient's response at frequent intervals.**

Extended use of heat results in an increased risk for burns from the heat. Impaired circulation may affect the patient's sensitivity to heat.

17. After the prescribed time for the treatment (up to 30 minutes), remove the external heating device (if used). Put on gloves.

Gloves protect the nurse from potential contact with microorganisms.

18. Carefully remove the compress while assessing the skin condition around the site and observing the patient's

Assessment provides information about the healing process; the presence of irritation or infection should be documented.

ACTION	RATIONALE
response to the heat application. Note any changes in the application area.	
19. Remove gloves. Place the patient in a comfortable position. Lower the bed. Dispose of any other supplies appropriately.	Repositioning promotes patient comfort and safety.
20. Remove additional PPE, if used. Perform hand hygiene.	Removing PPE properly reduces the risk for infection transmission and contamination of other items. Hand hygiene prevents the spread of microorganisms.

EVALUATION
- Patient reports relief of symptoms, such as decreased inflammation, pain, or muscle spasms.
- Patient remains free of signs and symptoms of injury.

DOCUMENTATION
- Document the procedure, the length of time the compress was applied, including any use of an Aquathermia pad. Record the temperature of the Aquathermia pad and length of application time. Include a description of the application area, noting any edema, redness, or ecchymosis. Document the patient's reaction to the procedure including pain assessment. Record any patient and family education provided.

SKILL 43 | APPLYING AN EXTERNAL CONDOM CATHETER

When voluntary control of urination is not possible for male patients, an alternative to an indwelling catheter is the external condom catheter. This soft, pliable sheath made of silicone material is applied externally to the penis. Most devices are self-adhesive. The condom catheter is connected to drainage tubing and a collection bag. The collection bag may be a leg bag. The risk for urinary tract infection (UTI) with a condom catheter is lower than the risk associated with an indwelling urinary catheter. Nursing care of a patient with a condom catheter includes vigilant skin care to prevent excoriation. This includes removing the condom catheter daily, washing the penis with skin cleanser and water and drying carefully, and inspecting the skin for irritation. In hot, humid weather, more frequent changing may be required. Always follow the manufacturer's instructions for applying the condom catheter because there are several variations. In all cases, take care to fasten the condom securely enough to prevent leakage, yet not so tightly as to constrict the blood vessels in the area. In addition, the tip of the tubing should be kept 1 to 2 inches (2.5 to 5 cm) beyond the tip of the penis to prevent irritation to the sensitive glans area.

Maintaining free urinary drainage is another nursing priority. Institute measures to prevent the tubing from becoming kinked and urine from backing up in the tubing. Urine can lead to excoriation of the glans, so position the tubing that collects the urine from the condom so that it draws urine away from the penis.

Always use a measuring or sizing guide supplied by the manufacturer to ensure the correct size of sheath is applied. Apply skin barriers, such as Cavilon or Skin Prep to the penis to protect penile skin from irritation and changes in integrity.

DELEGATION CONSIDERATIONS

The application of an external condom catheter may be delegated to nursing assistive personnel (NAP) or to unlicensed assistive personnel (UAP), as well as to licensed practical/vocational nurses (LPN/LVNs). The decision to delegate must be based on careful analysis of the patient's needs and circumstances, as well as the qualifications of the person to whom the task is being delegated. Refer to the Delegation Guidelines in Appendix A.

EQUIPMENT

- Condom sheath in appropriate size
- Skin protectant, such as Cavilon or Skin Prep
- Velcro leg strap, catheter securing device, or tape
- Bath blanket
- Reusable leg bag with tubing or urinary drainage setup

- Basin of warm water and skin cleanser
- Disposable gloves
- Additional PPE, as indicated
- Washcloth and towel
- Scissors

ASSESSMENT

- Assess the patient's knowledge of the need for catheterization.
- Ask the patient about any allergies, especially to latex or tape.
- Assess the size of the patient's penis to ensure that the appropriate-sized condom catheter is used.
- Inspect the skin in the groin and scrotal area, noting any areas of redness, irritation, or breakdown.

NURSING DIAGNOSIS

• Impaired Urinary Elimination
• Functional Urinary Incontinence
• Risk for Impaired Skin Integrity

OUTCOME IDENTIFICATION AND PLANNING

• Patient's urinary elimination will be maintained, with a urine output of at least 30 mL/hour, and the bladder is not distended.
• Patient's skin remains clean, dry, and intact, without evidence of irritation or breakdown.

IMPLEMENTATION

ACTION	RATIONALE
1. Gather equipment.	Assembling equipment provides for an organized approach to the task.
2. Perform hand hygiene and put on PPE, if indicated.	Hand hygiene and PPE prevent the spread of microorganisms. PPE is required based on transmission precautions.
3. Identify the patient.	Identifying the patient ensures the right patient receives the intervention and helps prevent errors.
4. Close the curtains around the bed and close the door to the room, if possible. Discuss the procedure with the patient. Ask the patient if he has any allergies, especially to latex.	This ensures the patient's privacy. This discussion promotes reassurance and provides knowledge about the procedure. Dialogue encourages patient participation and allows for individualized nursing care. Some condom catheters are made of latex.
5. Assemble equipment on overbed table within reach.	Arranging items nearby is convenient, saves time, and avoids unnecessary stretching and twisting of muscles on the part of the nurse.
6. Adjust the bed to a comfortable working height, usually elbow height of the caregiver (VISN 8 Patient Safety	Having the bed at the proper height prevents back and muscle strain. Positioning on one side allows for ease of use of

ACTION	RATIONALE
Center, 2009). Stand on the patient's right side if you are right-handed, or on patient's left side if you are left-handed.	dominant hand for catheter application.
7. Prepare urinary drainage setup or reusable leg bag for attachment to the condom sheath.	Provides for an organized approach to the task.
8. Position the patient on his back with thighs slightly apart. Drape patient so that only the area around the penis is exposed. Slide waterproof pad under the patient.	Positioning allows access to the site. Draping prevents unnecessary exposure and promotes warmth. The waterproof pad will protect bed linens from moisture.
9. Put on disposable gloves. Trim any long pubic hair that is in contact with the penis.	Gloves prevent contact with blood and body fluids. Trimming pubic hair prevents pulling of hair by adhesive without the risk of infection associated with shaving.
10. Clean the genital area with washcloth, skin cleanser, and warm water. If patient is uncircumcised, retract foreskin and clean glans of penis. Replace foreskin. Clean the tip of the penis first, moving the washcloth in a circular motion from the meatus outward. Wash the shaft of the penis using downward strokes toward the pubic area. Rinse and dry. Remove gloves. Perform hand hygiene again.	Washing removes urine, secretions, and microorganisms. The penis must be clean and dry to minimize skin irritation. If the foreskin is left retracted, it may cause venous congestion in the glans of the penis, leading to edema.
11. Apply skin protectant to penis and allow to dry.	Skin protectant minimizes the risk of skin irritation from adhesive and moisture and increases the adhesive's ability to adhere to skin.
12. Roll condom sheath outward onto itself. Grasp penis firmly with nondominant	Rolling the condom sheath outward allows for easier application. The space prevents irritation

ACTION	RATIONALE

hand. Apply condom sheath by rolling it onto the penis with dominant hand (Figure 1). Leave 1 to 2 inches (2.5 to 5 cm) of space between the tip of the penis and the end of the condom sheath.

to tip of penis and allows free drainage of urine.

FIGURE 1 Unrolling sheath onto penis.

13. **Apply pressure to the sheath at the base of the penis for 10 to 15 seconds.**

Application of pressure ensures good adherence of adhesive with skin.

14. Connect condom sheath to drainage setup. Avoid kinking or twisting drainage tubing.

The collection device keeps the patient dry. Kinked tubing encourages backflow of urine.

15. Remove gloves. Secure drainage tubing to the patient's inner thigh with Velcro leg strap or tape. Leave some slack in tubing for leg movement.

Proper attachment prevents tension on the sheath and potential inadvertent removal.

16. Assist the patient to a comfortable position. Cover the patient with bed linens. Place the bed in the lowest position.

Positioning and covering provide warmth and promote comfort. Bed in the lowest position promotes patient safety.

17. Secure drainage bag below the level of the bladder. Check that drainage tubing is not kinked and that movement of side rails does not interfere with the drainage bag.

Facilitates drainage of urine and prevents the backflow of urine.

ACTION	RATIONALE
18. Remove equipment. Remove gloves and additional PPE, if used. Perform hand hygiene.	Proper disposal of equipment prevents transmission of microorganisms. Removing PPE properly reduces the risk for infection transmission and contamination of other items. Hand hygiene prevents the spread of microorganisms.

EVALUATION

- Condom catheter is applied without adverse effect.
- Patient's urinary elimination is maintained, with a urine output of at least 30 mL/hour.
- Patient's skin remains clean, dry, and intact, without evidence of irritation or breakdown.

DOCUMENTATION

- Document the assessment data supporting the decision to use a condom catheter, the application of the condom catheter, and the condition of the patient's skin. Record urine output on the intake and output record.

SKILL 44   REMOVING CONTACT LENSES

If a patient wears contact lenses but cannot remove them, the nurse is responsible for removing them. Leaving contact lenses in place for long periods could result in permanent eye damage. Before removing lenses, use gentle pressure to center the lens on the cornea. Once removed, be sure to identify the lenses as being for the right or left eye, because the two lenses are not necessarily identical. If an eye injury is present, do not try to remove lenses because of the danger of causing an additional injury.

DELEGATION CONSIDERATIONS

The removal of contact lenses may be delegated to nursing assistive personnel (NAP) or to unlicensed assistive personnel (UAP), as well as to licensed practical/vocational nurses (LPN/LVNs). The decision to delegate must be based on careful analysis of the patient's needs and circumstances, as well as the qualifications of the person to whom the task is being delegated. Refer to the Delegation Guidelines in Appendix A.

EQUIPMENT

- Disposable gloves
- Additional PPE, if indicated
- Container for contact lenses (if unavailable, two small sterile containers marked "L" and "R" will suffice)
- Sterile normal saline solution
- Rubber pincer, if available (for removal of soft lenses)
- Suction-cup remover, if available (for removal of rigid lenses)

ASSESSMENT

- Assess both eyes for contact lenses; some people wear them in only one eye.
- Assess eyes for any redness or drainage.
- Assess for any eye injury. If an injury is present, notify the primary care provider about the presence of a contact lens. Do not try to remove the contact lens in this situation due to the risk for additional eye injury.

NURSING DIAGNOSIS

- Risk for Injury
- Deficient Knowledge

OUTCOME IDENTIFICATION AND PLANNING

- The lenses are removed without trauma to the eye and stored safely.

IMPLEMENTATION

ACTION	RATIONALE
1. Perform hand hygiene and put on PPE, if indicated.	Hand hygiene and PPE prevent the spread of microorganisms. PPE is required based on transmission precautions.
2. Identify the patient. Explain the procedure to the patient.	Patient identification validates the correct patient and correct procedure. Discussion and explanation help allay anxiety and prepare the patient for what to expect.
3. Assemble equipment on overbed table within reach.	Organization facilitates performance of task.
4. Close the curtains around the bed and close the door to the room, if possible.	This ensures the patient's privacy.
5. Assist the patient to a supine position. Raise the bed to a comfortable working	Supine position with the bed raised and the side rail down is the least stressful position for

ACTION	RATIONALE
position, usually elbow height of the caregiver (VISN 8 Patient Safety Center, 2009). Lower side rail closest to you.	removing a contact lens. Proper bed height helps reduce back strain while performing the procedure.
6. If containers are not already labeled, do so now. Place 5 mL of normal saline in each container.	Many patients have different prescription strengths for each eye. The saline will prevent the contact from drying out.
7. Put on gloves. Remove soft contact lens:	Gloves prevent the spread of microorganisms.

7. (continued)

a. Have the patient look forward. Retract the lower lid with one hand. Using the pad of the index finger of the other hand, move the lens down to the sclera (Figure 1).

b. Using the pads of the thumb and index finger, grasp the lens with a gentle pinching motion and remove it (Figure 2).

See the accompanying Skill Variation for other techniques for removing both rigid and soft lenses.

FIGURE 1 Retracting lower lid with one hand and using pad of index finger of other hand to move lens down to sclera.

FIGURE 2 Using pads of thumb and index finger to grasp lens with a gentle pinching motion to remove it.

ACTION	RATIONALE
8. Place the first lens in its designated cup in the storage case before removing the second lens.	Lenses may be different for each eye. Avoids mixing them up.
9. Repeat actions to remove other contact lens.	
10. If patient is awake and has glasses at bedside, offer patient glasses.	Not being able to see clearly creates anxiety.
11. Remove equipment and return the patient to a position of comfort. Remove your gloves. Raise side rail and lower bed.	Promotes patient comfort and safety. Removing gloves properly reduces the risk for infection transmission and contamination of other items.
12. Remove additional PPE, if used. Perform hand hygiene.	Removing PPE properly reduces the risk for infection transmission and contamination of other items. Hand hygiene prevents transmission of microorganisms.

EVALUATION
- Patient remains free of injury as the contact lenses are removed.
- Patient's eye exhibits no signs and symptoms of trauma, irritation, or redness.
- Contact lenses are stored safely.

DOCUMENTATION
- Record your assessment, significant observations, and unusual findings, such as drainage or pain. Document any teaching done. Document the removal of the contact lenses, their storage, and patient response.

SKILL VARIATION | Removing Different Types of Contact Lens

1. Perform hand hygiene and put on PPE, if indicated.

2. Identify the patient.

continued on page 236

3. Explain what you are going to do and the reason for doing it to the patient.

4. Assemble necessary equipment on the bedside stand or overbed table.

5. Close the curtains around the bed and close the door to the room, if possible.

6. Assist the patient to a supine position. Raise bed to a comfortable working position, usually elbow height of the caregiver (VISN 8 Patient Safety Center, 2009). Lower side rail closest to you.

7. If containers are not already labeled, do so now. Place 5 mL of normal saline in each container.

8. Put on clean gloves.

To Remove Hard Contact Lenses—Patient Is Able to Blink:

a. If the lens is not centered over the cornea, apply gentle pressure on the lower eyelid to center the lens.

b. Gently pull the outer corner of the eye toward the ear.

c. Position the other hand below the lens to catch it and ask patient to blink.

To Remove Hard Contact Lenses—Patient Is Unable to Blink:

a. Gently spread the eyelids beyond the top and bottom edges of the lens.

b. Gently press the lower eyelid up against the bottom of the lens.

c. After the lens is tipped slightly, move the eyelids toward one another to cause the lens to slide out between the eyelids.

To Remove Hard Contact Lenses With a Suction Cup—Patient Is Unable to Blink:

a. Ensure that contact lens is centered on the cornea. Place a drop of sterile saline on the suction cup.

b. Place the suction cup in the center of the contact lens and gently pull the contact lens off the eye.

c. To remove the suction cup from the lens, slide the lens off sideways.

To Remove Soft Contact Lenses With a Rubber Pincer:

a. Locate the contact lens and place the rubber pincers in the center of the lens.

b. Gently squeeze the pincers and remove the lens from the eye.

9. Place the first lens in its designated cup in the storage case before removing the second lens.

10. Repeat actions to remove other contact lens. Remove gloves.

11. If patient is awake and has glasses at bedside, offer patient glasses. Lower bed. Assist patient to a comfortable position.

12. Remove additional PPE, if used. Perform hand hygiene.

A continuous passive motion (CPM) device passively moves a joint within a certain ROM (Viswanathan & Kidd, 2010). It is frequently prescribed after total knee arthroplasty as well as after surgery on other joints, such as shoulders. The degree of flexion and extension of the joint and the cycle rate (the number of revolutions per minute) are determined by the prescriber, but nurses place the patient in and out of the device and monitor the patient's response to the therapy.

DELEGATION CONSIDERATIONS

The application and removal of a continuous passive motion (CPM) device is not delegated to nursing assistive personnel (NAP) or to unlicensed assistive personnel (UAP). The application and removal of a continuous passive motion (CPM) device may be delegated to licensed practical/vocational nurses (LPN/LVNs). The decision to delegate must be based on careful analysis of the patient's needs and circumstances, as well as the qualifications of the person to whom the task is being delegated. Refer to the Delegation Guidelines in Appendix A.

EQUIPMENT

- CPM device
- Single patient use soft-goods kit
- Tape measure
- Goniometer
- Nonsterile gloves and/or other PPE, if indicated

ASSESSMENT

- Review the medical record and nursing plan of care for orders for degrees of flexion and extension.
- Assess the neurovascular status of the involved extremity.
- Perform a pain assessment. Administer the prescribed medication in sufficient time to allow for the full effect of the analgesic before starting the device.
- Assess for proper alignment of the joint in the CPM device. Assess the patient's ability to tolerate the prescribed treatment.

NURSING DIAGNOSIS

- Impaired Physical Mobility
- Risk for Peripheral Neurovascular Dysfunction
- Risk for Impaired Skin Integrity
- Risk for Injury

OUTCOME IDENTIFICATION AND PLANNING

- Patient experiences increased joint mobility.
- Patient displays improved or maintained muscle strength and muscle atrophy and contractures are prevented.

- Circulation is promoted in the affected extremity.
- Effects of immobility are decreased and healing is stimulated.

IMPLEMENTATION

ACTION	RATIONALE
1. Review the medical record and nursing plan of care for the appropriate degrees of flexion and extension, the cycle rate, and the length of time the CPM is to be used.	Reviewing the medical record and plan of care validates the correct patient and correct procedure and reduces the risk for injury.
2. Obtain equipment. Apply the soft goods to the CPM device.	Equipment preparation promotes efficient time management and provides an organized approach to the task. The soft goods help to prevent friction to the extremity during motion.
3. Perform hand hygiene. Put on PPE, as indicated.	Hand hygiene and PPE prevent the spread of microorganisms. PPE is required based on transmission precautions.
4. Identify the patient. Explain the procedure to the patient.	Patient identification validates the correct patient and correct procedure. Discussion and explanation help allay anxiety and prepare the patient for what to expect.
5. Close the curtains around the bed and close the door to the room, if possible. Place the bed at an appropriate and comfortable working height, usually elbow height of the caregiver (VISN 8 Patient Safety Center, 2009).	Closing the door or curtains provides privacy. Proper bed height helps reduce back strain.
6. Using the tape measure, determine the distance between the gluteal crease and the popliteal space.	The thigh length on the CPM device is adjusted based on this measurement.
7. Measure the leg from the knee to 14 inches beyond the bottom of the foot.	The position of the footplate is adjusted based on this measurement.

ACTION	RATIONALE
8. Position the patient in the middle of the bed. Make sure the affected extremity is in a slightly abducted position.	Proper positioning promotes correct body alignment and prevents pressure on the unaffected extremity.
9. Support the affected extremity and elevate it, placing it in the padded CPM device.	Support and elevation assist in movement of the affected extremity without injury.
10. Make sure the knee is at the hinged joint of the CPM device.	Proper positioning in the device prevents injury.
11. Adjust the footplate to maintain the patient's foot in a neutral position. Assess the patient's position to make sure the leg is not internally or externally rotated.	Adjustment helps ensure proper positioning and prevent injury.
12. Apply the restraining straps under the CPM device and around the leg. Check that two fingers fit between the strap and the leg (Figure 1).	Restraining straps maintain the leg in position. Leaving a space between the strap and leg prevents injury from excessive pressure from the strap.

FIGURE 1 Using two fingers to check the fit between the straps and the leg.

ACTION	RATIONALE
13. Explain the use of the STOP/ GO button to the patient. Set the controls to the prescribed levels of flexion and extension and cycles per minute. Turn on the power to the CPM.	Explanation decreases anxiety by allowing the patient to participate in care.
14. Set the device to ON and start the therapy by pressing the GO button. Observe the patient and the device during	Observation ensures that the device is working properly, thereby ensuring patient safety. Measuring with a goniometer

ACTION	RATIONALE
the first cycle. Determine the angle of flexion when the device reaches its greatest height using the goniometer (Figure 2). Compare with prescribed degree.	ensures the device is set to the prescribed parameters.

FIGURE 2 Determining the angle of joint flexion, using the goniometer.

ACTION	RATIONALE
15. Check the patient's level of comfort and perform skin and neurovascular assessments at least every 8 hours or per facility policy.	Frequent assessments provide for early detection and prompt intervention should problems arise.
16. Place the bed in the lowest position, with the side rails up. Make sure the call bell and other essential items are within easy reach.	Having the bed at the proper height and having the call bell and other items handy ensure patient safety.
17. Remove PPE, if used. Perform hand hygiene.	Removing PPE properly reduces the risk for infection transmission and contamination of other items. Hand hygiene prevents the spread of microorganisms.

EVALUATION
- Patient demonstrates increased joint mobility.
- Patient exhibits improved muscle strength without evidence of atrophy or contractures.

DOCUMENTATION
- Document the time and date of application of the CPM, the extension and flexion settings, the speed of the device, the patient's response to the therapy, and your assessment of the extremity.

SKILL 46 | TEACHING DEEP BREATHING EXERCISES, COUGHING, AND SPLINTING

During surgery, the cough reflex is suppressed, mucus accumulates in the tracheobronchial passages, and the lungs do not ventilate fully. After surgery, respirations are often less effective as a result of anesthesia, pain medication, and pain from the incision, particularly thoracic and high abdominal incisions. Alveoli do not inflate and may collapse. Along with retained secretions, this increases the risk for atelectasis and respiratory infection.

Deep breathing exercises hyperventilate the alveoli and prevent them from collapsing again, improve lung expansion and volume, help to expel anesthetic gases and mucus, and facilitate tissue oxygenation. Coughing, which helps to remove mucus from the respiratory tract, usually is taught in conjunction with deep breathing. Because coughing is often painful for the patient with a thoracic or abdominal incision, it is important to teach the patient how to splint the incision when coughing. This technique provides support to the incision and helps reduce pain during coughing and movement.

DELEGATION CONSIDERATIONS

Preoperative assessment and teaching is not delegated to nursing assistive personnel (NAP) or to unlicensed assistive personnel (UAP). Depending on the state's nurse practice act and the organization's policies and procedures, preoperative teaching may be delegated to licensed practical/vocational nurses (LPN/LVNs) after an assessment of education needs by the registered nurse. The decision to delegate must be based on careful analysis of the patient's needs and circumstances, as well as the qualifications of the person to whom the task is being delegated. Refer to the Delegation Guidelines in Appendix A.

EQUIPMENT

- Small pillow or folded bath blanket
- PPE, as indicated

ASSESSMENT

- Identify patients who are considered at greater risk for respiratory complications after surgery, such as the very young and very old; obese or malnourished patients; patients with fluid and electrolyte imbalances; patients with chronic disease; patients who have underlying lung or cardiac disease; patients who have decreased mobility; and patients who are at risk for decreased compliance with postoperative activities, such as those with alterations in cognitive function. Depending on the particular at-risk patient, specific assessments and interventions may be warranted.
- Assess the patient's current level of knowledge regarding deep breathing, coughing, and splinting.

NURSING DIAGNOSIS

- Deficient Knowledge
- Risk for Infection
- Impaired Physical Mobility

OUTCOME IDENTIFICATION AND PLANNING

- Patient and/or significant other verbalizes an understanding of the instructions and is able to demonstrate the activities.

IMPLEMENTATION

ACTION	RATIONALE
1. Check the patient's medical record for the type of surgery and review the medical orders. Gather the necessary supplies.	This check ensures that the care will be provided for the right patient and any specific teaching based on the type of surgery will be addressed. Preparation promotes efficient time management and an organized approach to the task.
2. Perform hand hygiene and put on PPE, if indicated.	Hand hygiene and PPE prevent the spread of microorganisms. PPE is required based on transmission precautions.
3. Identify the patient.	Identifying the patient ensures the right patient receives the intervention and helps prevent errors.
4. Close curtains around the bed and close the door to the room, if possible. Explain what you are going to do and why you are going to do it to the patient. Place necessary supplies on the bedside stand or overbed table, within easy reach.	This ensures the patient's privacy. Explanation relieves anxiety and facilitates cooperation. Bringing everything to the bedside conserves time and energy. Arranging items nearby is convenient, saves time, and avoids unnecessary stretching and twisting of muscles on the part of the nurse.
5. Identify the patient's learning needs and the patient's level of knowledge regarding deep breathing exercises, coughing, and splinting of	Identification of baseline knowledge contributes to individualized teaching. Previous surgical experience may impact preoperative/postoperative care positively or

ACTION	RATIONALE

the incision. If the patient has had surgery before, ask about this experience.

negatively, depending on this experience.

6. Explain the rationale for performing deep breathing exercises, coughing, and splinting of the incision.

Explanation facilitates patient cooperation. An understanding of the rationale may contribute to increased compliance.

7. Teach the patient how to perform deep breathing exercises.

Deep breathing exercises improve lung expansion and volume, help expel anesthetic gases and mucus from the airway, and facilitate the oxygenation of body tissues.

a. Assist or ask the patient to sit up (semi- or high-Fowler's position), with the neck and shoulders supported. Ask the patient to place the palms of both hands along the lower anterior rib cage.

The upright position promotes chest expansion and lessens exertion of the abdominal muscles. Positioning the hands on the rib cage allows the patient to feel the chest rise and the lungs expand as the diaphragm descends.

b. Ask the patient to exhale gently and completely.

c. Instruct the patient to breathe in through the nose as deeply as possible and hold breath for 3 to 5 seconds.

Deep inhalation promotes lung expansion.

d. Instruct the patient to exhale through the mouth, pursing the lips like when whistling.

e. Have the patient practice the breathing exercise three times. Instruct the patient that this exercise should be performed every 1 to 2 hours for the first 24 hours after surgery, and as necessary thereafter, depending on risk factors and pulmonary status.

Return demonstration ensures that the patient is able to perform the exercises properly. Practice promotes effectiveness and compliance.

8. Provide teaching regarding coughing and splinting.

Coughing helps remove retained mucus from the respiratory tract. Splinting minimizes pain while coughing or moving.

ACTION	RATIONALE
a. Ask the patient to sit up (semi-Fowler's position), leaning forward. Apply a folded bath blanket or pillow against the part of the body where the incision will be (e.g., abdomen or chest).	These interventions aim to decrease discomfort while coughing.
b. Ask the patient to inhale and exhale deeply and slowly through the nose three times.	
c. Ask the patient to take a deep breath and hold it for 3 seconds and then cough out three short times.	
d. Ask the patient to take a quick breath through the mouth and strongly and deeply cough again one or two times.	
e. Ask the patient to take another deep breath.	
f. Instruct the patient that he or she should perform these actions every 2 hours when awake after surgery.	
9. Validate the patient's understanding of the information. Ask the patient to give a return demonstration. Ask the patient if he or she has any questions. Encourage the patient to practice the activities and ask questions, if necessary.	Validation facilitates patient's understanding of information and performance of activities.
10. Remove PPE, if used. Perform hand hygiene.	Removing PPE properly reduces the risk for infection transmission and contamination of other items. Hand hygiene prevents the spread of microorganisms.

EVALUATION

• The expected outcome is met when the patient and/or significant other verbalizes an understanding of the instructions related to deep breathing, coughing, and splinting, and is able to demonstrate the activities.

DOCUMENTATION

• Document the components of teaching related to deep breathing exercises, coughing, and splinting that were reviewed with the patient and family, if present. Record the patient's ability to demonstrate deep breathing exercises, coughing, and splinting and his or her response to the teaching; note if any follow-up instruction needs to be performed.

SKILL 47 — PERFORMING EMERGENCY AUTOMATED EXTERNAL DEFIBRILLATION

Early defibrillation, as part of cardiopulmonary resuscitation (CPR), is critical to survival from sudden cardiac arrest (Link et al., 2010). The interval from collapse to defibrillation is one of the most important determinants of survival from sudden cardiac arrest with ventricular fibrillation or pulseless ventricular tachycardia (AHA, 2011). The most frequent initial cardiac rhythm in out-of-hospital witnessed sudden cardiac arrest is ventricular fibrillation (Link et al., 2010). Electrical therapy can be administered by defibrillation, cardioversion, or a pacemaker. Early defibrillation is critical to increase patient survival (AHA, 2011; Link et al., 2010).

Defibrillation delivers large amounts of electric current to a patient over brief periods of time. It is the standard treatment for ventricular fibrillation (VF) and is also used to treat pulseless ventricular tachycardia (VT). The goal is to depolarize the irregularly beating heart temporarily and allow more coordinated contractile activity to resume. It does so by completely depolarizing the myocardium, producing a momentary asystole. This provides an opportunity for the natural pacemaker centers of the heart to resume normal activity.

The automated external defibrillator (AED) is a portable external defibrillator that automatically detects and interprets the heart's rhythm and informs the operator if a shock is indicated. AEDs are appropriate for use in situations where the patient is unresponsive, not breathing, and has no pulse (AHA, 2011). The defibrillator responds to the patient information by advising 'shock' or 'no shock.' Fully automatic models automatically perform rhythm analysis and shock, if indicated. These are usually found in out-of-hospital settings. Semiautomatic models require the operator to press an 'Analyze' button to initiate rhythm analysis and then press a

'Shock' button to deliver the shock, if indicated. Semiautomatic models are usually found in the hospital setting. An AED will not deliver a shock unless the electrode pads are correctly attached and a shockable rhythm is detected. Some AEDs have motion-detection devices that ensure the defibrillator will not discharge if there is motion, such as motion from personnel in contact with the patient. The strength of the charge is preset. Once the pads are in place and the device is turned on, follow the prompts given by the device. The following guidelines are based on the American Heart Association (AHA, 2011) guidelines. AHA guidelines state that these recommendations may be modified for the in-hospital setting, where continuous electrocardiographic or hemodynamic monitoring may be in place. CPR should be immediately initiated and the AED/defibrillator should be used as soon as it is available (Link et al., 2010).

Current recommendations call for the application of the AED as soon as it is available, allowing for analysis of cardiac status and delivery of an initial shock, if indicated, for adults and children. After an initial shock, deliver five cycles of chest compressions/ventilations (30/2), and then reanalyze cardiac rhythm. Provide sets of one shock alternating with 2 minutes of CPR until the AED indicates a 'no shock indicated' message or until advanced cardiac life support (ACLS) is available (AHA, 2011).

In the hospital setting, it is imperative that personnel be aware of the patient's stated instructions regarding a wish not to be resuscitated. This should be clearly expressed and documented in the patient's medical record.

DELEGATION CONSIDERATIONS

The initiation and provision of cardiopulmonary resuscitation, including use of an AED, is appropriate for all health care providers.

EQUIPMENT

- Automated external defibrillator (AED) (some models have the pads, cables, and AED pre-connected).
- Self-adhesive, pregelled monitor-defibrillator pads (6)
- Cables to connect the pads and AED
- Razor
- Towel

ASSESSMENT

- Assess the patient for unresponsiveness, effective breathing, and signs of circulation.
- Assess the patient's vital parameters and determine the patient's level of responsiveness.
- Check for partial or complete airway obstruction.
- Assess for the absence or ineffectiveness of respirations.
- Assess for the absence of signs of circulation and pulses.
- AED should be used only when a patient is unresponsive, not breathing, or not breathing normally, and without signs of circulation (pulseless, lack of effective respirations, coughing, movement).

- Determine the age of the patient; some AED systems are designed to deliver both adult and child shock doses. Choose correct electrode pad for size/age of patient. If available, use child pads or a child system for children less than 8 years of age.
- Determine whether special situations exist that require additional actions before the AED is used or that contraindicate its use.

NURSING DIAGNOSIS

- Decreased Cardiac Output
- Impaired Spontaneous Ventilation
- Risk for Ineffective Cerebral Tissue Perfusion

OUTCOME IDENTIFICATION AND PLANNING

- Automatic external defibrillation is performed correctly without adverse effect to the patient.
- Patient regains signs of circulation, with organized electrical rhythm and pulse.
- Patient regains respirations.
- Patient's heart and lungs maintain adequate function to sustain life.
- Patient does not experience serious injury.
- Advanced cardiac life support is initiated.

IMPLEMENTATION

ACTION	RATIONALE
1. Assess responsiveness. Look for breathing. If the patient is not responsive and is not breathing or not breathing normally, call for help, pull call bell, and call the facility emergency response number. Call for the AED. Put on gloves, if available. Begin cardiopulmonary resuscitation (CPR) (see Skill 27).	Assessing responsiveness prevents starting CPR on a conscious patient. Activating the emergency response system initiates a rapid response. Gloves prevent contact with blood and body fluids. Initiating CPR preserves heart and brain function while awaiting defibrillation.
2. **Provide defibrillation at the earliest possible moment, as soon as AED becomes available.**	The interval from collapse to defibrillation is one of the most important determinants of survival from sudden cardiac arrest (AHA, 2011).
3. Prepare the AED. Power on the AED. Push the power button. Some devices will turn on automatically when the lid or case is opened.	Proper setup ensures proper functioning.

ACTION	RATIONALE
4. Attach AED cables to the adhesive electrode pads (may be preconnected).	Proper setup ensures proper functioning.
5. Stop chest compressions. Peel away the covering from the electrode pads to expose the adhesive surface. Attach the electrode pads to the patient's chest. Place one pad on the upper right sternal border, directly below the clavicle. Place the second pad lateral to the left nipple, with the top margin of the pad a few inches below the axilla (anterolateral positioning) (Figure 1). Alternately, if two or more rescuers are present, one rescuer should continue chest compressions while another rescuer attaches the AED pads. Attach the AED connecting cables to the AED box, if not preconnected.	Proper setup ensures proper functioning. AHA (2011) specifies anterolateral placement. See note below in *Special Considerations* for alternate electrode placement. Application by second rescuer minimizes interruptions in chest compressions.

FIGURE 1 AED electrode pad placement.

| 6. Once the pads are in place and the device is turned on, follow the prompts given by the device. Clear the patient | Movement and electrical impulses cause artifact during analysis. Avoidance of artifact ensures accurate rhythm analysis. |

ACTION	RATIONALE
and analyze the rhythm. Ensure no one is touching the patient. Loudly state a "Clear the patient" message. Press 'Analyze' button to initiate analysis, if necessary. Some devices automatically begin analysis when the pads are attached. Avoid all movement affecting the patient during analysis.	Avoidance of contact with the patient avoids accidental shock to personnel.
7. If a shockable rhythm is present, the device will announce that a shock is indicated and begin charging. Once the AED is charged, a message will be delivered to shock the patient.	Shock message is delivered through a written or visual message on the AED screen, an auditory alarm, or a voice-synthesized statement.
8. **Before pressing the 'Shock' button, loudly state a "Clear the patient" message. Visually check that no one is in contact with the patient.** Press the 'Shock' button. If the AED is fully automatic, a shock will be delivered automatically.	Ensuring a clear patient avoids accidental shocking of personnel.
9. Immediately resume CPR, beginning with chest compressions. After five cycles (about 2 minutes), allow the AED to analyze the heart rhythm. If a shock is not advised, resume CPR, beginning with chest compressions. Do not recheck to see if there is a pulse. Follow the AED voice prompts.	Resuming CPR provides optimal treatment. CPR preserves heart and neurologic function (based on AHA 2011 recommended guidelines). Even when a shock eliminates the dysrhythmia, it may take several minutes for a heart rhythm to establish and even longer to achieve perfusion. Chest compressions can provide coronary and cerebral perfusion during this period. Some AEDs in the community for use by lay persons are automatically programmed to cycle through three analysis/shock cycles in one set. This would necessitate turning off the AED after the first shock

ACTION	RATIONALE
	and turning it back on for future analysis and defibrillation. Be familiar with the type of AED available for use.
10. Continue CPR until advanced care providers take over, the patient starts to move, you are too exhausted to continue, or a physician discontinues CPR.	Once started, CPR must continue until one of these conditions is met. In a hospital setting, help should arrive within a few minutes.
11. Remove gloves, if used. Perform hand hygiene.	Removing PPE properly reduces the risk for infection transmission and contamination of other items. Hand hygiene prevents transmission of microorganisms.

EVALUATION

- Automatic external defibrillation is applied correctly without adverse effect to the patient.
- Patient regains signs of circulation.
- Patient regains respirations.
- Patient's heart and lungs maintain adequate function to sustain life.
- Patient does not experience injury.
- Advanced cardiac life support is initiated.

DOCUMENTATION

- Document the time you discovered the patient unresponsive and started CPR. Document the time(s) AED shocks are initiated. Continued intervention, such as by the code team, is typically documented on a code form, which identifies the actions and drugs provided during the code. Provide a summary of these events in the patient's medical record.

Electrical therapy is used to terminate or control potentially lethal dysrhythmias quickly. Electrical therapy can be administered by defibrillation, cardioversion, or a pacemaker. Early defibrillation is critical to increase patient survival (AHA, 2011; Link et al., 2010). Defibrillation delivers large amounts of electric current to a patient over brief periods of time. It is the standard treatment for ventricular fibrillation (VF) and is also used to treat ventricular tachycardia (VT), in which the patient has no pulse. The goal is temporarily to depolarize the irregularly beating heart and allow more coordinated contractile activity to resume. It does so by completely depolarizing the myocardium, producing a momentary asystole. This provides an opportunity for the natural pacemaker centers of the heart to resume normal activity. The electrode paddles delivering the current may be placed on the patient's chest or, during cardiac surgery, directly on the myocardium.

Manual defibrillation is accomplished with an external defibrillator and it depends on the operator for analysis of rhythm, charging, proper application of the paddles to the patient's thorax, and delivery of counter shock. It requires the user to have immediate and accurate dysrhythmia recognition skills. The following guidelines are based on the American Heart Association 2011 guidelines.

In the hospital setting, it is imperative that personnel be aware of the patient's stated instructions regarding a wish not to be resuscitated. This should be clearly expressed and documented in the patient's medical record.

DELEGATION CONSIDERATIONS

The initiation and provision of manual external defibrillation should be performed by health care providers who are certified in Advanced Cardiac Life Support measures.

EQUIPMENT

- Defibrillator (monophasic or biphasic)
- External paddles (or internal paddles sterilized for cardiac surgery)
- Conductive medium pads
- Electrocardiogram (ECG) monitor with recorder (often part of the defibrillator)
- Oxygen therapy equipment
- Handheld resuscitation bag
- Airway equipment
- Emergency pacing equipment
- Emergency cardiac medications

ASSESSMENT

- Assess the patient for unresponsiveness, effective breathing, and signs of circulation.

- Assess the patient's vital parameters and determine the patient's level of responsiveness.
- Check for partial or complete airway obstruction. Assess for the absence or ineffectiveness of respirations.
- Assess for the absence of signs of circulation and pulses.
- Call for help and perform cardiopulmonary resuscitation (CPR) until the defibrillator and other emergency equipment arrive.

NURSING DIAGNOSIS
- Decreased Cardiac Output
- Impaired Spontaneous Ventilation
- Risk for Injury

OUTCOME IDENTIFICATION AND PLANNING
- Defibrillation is performed correctly without adverse effect to the patient, and the patient regains signs of circulation.
- Patient regains respirations.
- Patient's heart and lungs maintain adequate function to sustain life.
- Patient does not experience serious injury.
- Advanced cardiac life support is initiated.

IMPLEMENTATION

ACTION	RATIONALE
1. Assess responsiveness. If the patient is not responsive, call for help, pull call bell, and call the facility emergency response number. Call for the AED. Put on gloves, if available. Begin cardiopulmonary resuscitation (CPR).	Assessing responsiveness prevents starting CPR on a conscious victim. Activating the emergency response system initiates a rapid response. Gloves prevent contact with blood and body fluids. Initiating CPR preserves heart and brain function while awaiting defibrillation.
2. Turn on the defibrillator.	Charging and placement prepare for defibrillation.
3. If the defibrillator has "quick-look" capability, place the paddles on the patient's chest. Otherwise, connect the monitoring leads of the defibrillator to the patient and assess the cardiac rhythm.	Connecting the monitor leads to the patient allows for a quick view of the cardiac rhythm.
4. Expose the patient's chest, and apply conductive pads at the paddle placement positions. For anterolateral placement,	This placement ensures that the electrical stimulus needs to travel only a short distance to the heart.

ACTION	RATIONALE

ACTION

place one pad to the right of the upper sternum, just below the right clavicle, and the other over the fifth or sixth intercostal space at the left anterior axillary line (Figure 1). For anteroposterior placement, place the anterior pad/paddle directly over the heart at the precordium, to the left of the lower sternal border. Place the flat posterior pad/paddle under the patient's body beneath the heart and immediately below the scapulae (but not on the vertebral column) (Figure 2). 'Hands-free' defibrillator pads can be used with the same placement positions, if available.

FIGURE 1 Anterolateral placement of conductive pads and defibrillator paddles.

Posterior   Anterior

FIGURE 2 Anteroposterior placement of conductive pads and defibrillator paddles (From Hinkle, J. L. & Cheever, K. H. (2014). Brunner and Suddarth's textbook of medical-surgical nursing (13th ed.). Philadelphia, PA: Wolters Kluwer Health/Lippincott Williams & Wilkins, with permission, Figure 26-25).

ACTION	RATIONALE
5. Set the energy level for 360 J (joules) for an adult patient when using a monophasic defibrillator. Use clinically appropriate energy levels for biphasic defibrillators, beginning with 120 to 200 J, depending on device (Morton & Fontaine, 2013).	Proper setup ensures proper functioning.
6. Charge the paddles by pressing the charge buttons, which are located either on the machine or on the paddles themselves.	Proper setup ensures proper functioning.
7. **Place the paddles over the conductive pads and press firmly against the patient's chest, using 25 pounds (11 kg) of pressure. If using hands-off pads, do not touch the paddles.**	Proper setup ensures proper functioning. Solid adhesion is necessary for conduction.
8. Reassess the cardiac rhythm.	The rhythm may have changed during preparation.
9. **If the patient remains in VF or pulseless VT, instruct all personnel to stand clear of the patient and the bed, including the operator.**	Standing clear of the bed and patient helps prevent electrical shocks to personnel.
10. Discharge the current by pressing both paddle charge buttons simultaneously. If using remote defibrillator pads, press the discharge or shock button on the machine.	Pressing the charge buttons discharges the electric current for defibrillation.
11. After the shock, immediately resume CPR, beginning with chest compressions. After five cycles (about 2 minutes), reassess the cardiac rhythm. Continue until advanced care providers take over, the patient starts to move, you are too exhausted to continue, or a physician discontinues CPR.	Resuming CPR provides optimal treatment. CPR preserves heart, and neurologic function. Even when a shock eliminates the dysrhythmia, it may take several minutes for a heart rhythm to establish and even longer to achieve perfusion. Chest compressions can provide coronary and cerebral perfusion during this period (Zed et al., 2008).

ACTION	RATIONALE
12. If necessary, prepare to defibrillate a second time.	Additional shocking may be needed to stimulate the heart.
13. Announce that you are preparing to defibrillate and follow the procedure described above.	Additional shocking may be needed to stimulate the heart.
14. If defibrillation restores a normal rhythm:	
a. Check for signs of circulation; check the central and peripheral pulses, and obtain a blood pressure reading, heart rate, and respiratory rate.	The patient will need continuous monitoring to prevent further problems. Continuous monitoring helps provide for early detection and prompt intervention should additional problems arise.
b. If signs of circulation are present, check breathing. If breathing is inadequate, assist breathing. Start rescue breathing (one breath every 5 seconds).	
c. If breathing is adequate, place the patient in the recovery position. Continue to assess the patient.	
d. Assess the patient's level of consciousness, cardiac rhythm, blood pressure, breath sounds, skin color, and temperature.	Reassessment determines the need for continued intervention. Provides optimal treatment.
e. Obtain baseline ABG levels (Skill 24) and a 12-lead ECG (Skill 61), if ordered.	
f. Provide supplemental oxygen, ventilation, and medications, as needed.	
g. Anticipate the possible use of induced therapeutic hypothermia.	Cooling the patient after cardiac arrest protects the brain and may preserve neurologic function by reducing the cerebral metabolic rate of oxygen (Morton & Fontaine, 2013; Bucher et al., 2012).

ACTION	RATIONALE
15. Check the chest for electrical burns and treat them, as ordered, with corticosteroid- or lanolin-based creams. If using 'hands-free' pads, keep pads on in case of recurrent ventricular tachycardia or ventricular fibrillation.	Skin inspection identifies injury. Keeping pads in place provides preparation for future use.
16. Remove gloves, if used. Perform hand hygiene.	Removing PPE properly reduces the risk for infection transmission and contamination of other items. Hand hygiene prevents transmission of microorganisms.
17. Prepare the defibrillator for immediate reuse.	A patient may remain unstable and could require further intervention.

EVALUATION

- Defibrillation is performed correctly without adverse effect to the patient and the patient regains signs of circulation.
- Patient regains respirations.
- Patient's heart and lungs maintain adequate function to sustain life.
- Patient does not experience serious injury.
- Advanced cardiac life support is initiated.

DOCUMENTATION

- Document the time you discovered the patient unresponsive and started CPR. Document the procedure, including the patient's ECG rhythms both before and after defibrillation; the number of times defibrillation was performed; the voltage used during each attempt; whether a pulse returned; the dosage, route, and time of drug administration; whether CPR was used; how the airway was maintained; and the patient's outcome. Continued intervention, such as by the code team, is typically documented on a code form, which identifies the actions and drugs provided during the code. Provide a summary of these events in the patient's medical record.

Plaque, which can accumulate on dentures, can promote oropharyngeal colonization of pathogens. Diligent oral hygiene care can improve oral health and decrease the incidence of aspiration pneumonia, community-acquired pneumonia, ventilator-associated pneumonia, and other systemic diseases. It is important to brush dentures twice a day and to remove and rinse dentures and mouth after meals. Dentures may be cleaned more often, based on need and the patient's personal preference. Dentures are often removed at night. Handle dentures with care to prevent breakage.

DELEGATION CONSIDERATIONS

The implementation of denture care may be delegated to nursing assistive personnel (NAP) or to unlicensed assistive personnel (UAP), as well as to licensed practical/vocational nurses (LPN/LVNs). The decision to delegate must be based on careful analysis of the patient's needs and circumstances, as well as the qualifications of the person to whom the task is being delegated. Refer to the Delegation Guidelines in Appendix A.

EQUIPMENT

- Soft toothbrush or denture brush
- Toothpaste
- Denture cleaner (optional)
- Denture adhesive (optional)
- Glass of cool water
- Emesis basin
- Denture cup (optional)
- Nonsterile gloves
- Additional PPE, as indicated
- Towel
- Mouthwash (optional)
- Washcloth or paper towel
- Lip lubricant (optional)
- Gauze

ASSESSMENT

- Assess the patient's oral hygiene preferences: frequency, time of day, and type of hygiene products.
- Assess for any physical activity limitations, difficulty chewing, pain, tenderness, and discomfort.
- Assess patient's oral cavity.
- Assess patient's ability to perform own care.

NURSING DIAGNOSIS

- Ineffective Health Maintenance
- Impaired Oral Mucous Membrane
- Disturbed Body Image

OUTCOME IDENTIFICATION AND PLANNING

- The patient's mouth and dentures will be clean.
- The patient will exhibit a positive body image.
- The patient will verbalize the importance of oral care.

IMPLEMENTATION

ACTION	RATIONALE
1. Perform hand hygiene and put on PPE, if indicated.	Hand hygiene and PPE prevent the spread of microorganisms. PPE is required based on transmission precautions.
2. Identify patient. Explain procedure to the patient.	Identifying the patient ensures the right patient receives the intervention and helps prevent errors. Explanation facilitates cooperation.
3. Assemble equipment on overbed table within reach.	Organization facilitates performance of task.
4. Provide privacy for the patient.	Cleaning another person's mouth is invasive and may be embarrassing. Patient may be embarrassed by removal of dentures.
5. Lower side rail and assist patient to sitting position, if permitted, or turn patient onto side. Place towel across patient's chest. Raise bed to a comfortable working position, usually elbow height of the caregiver (VISN 8 Patient Safety Center, 2009). Put on gloves.	The sitting or side-lying position prevents aspiration of fluids into the lungs. The towel protects the patient from dampness. Proper bed height helps reduce back strain while performing the procedure. Gloves prevent the spread of microorganisms.
6. Apply gentle pressure with 4 × 4 gauze to grasp upper denture plate and remove it (Figure 1).	Rocking motion breaks suction between denture and gum. Using 4 × 4 gauze prevents slippage

FIGURE 1 Removing dentures with a gauze sponge.

ACTION	RATIONALE
Place it immediately in denture cup. Lift lower dentures with gauze, using slight rocking motion. Remove, and place in denture cup.	and discourages spread of microorganisms.
7. Place paper towels or washcloth in sink while brushing. Using the toothbrush and paste, brush all denture surfaces gently but thoroughly. If patient prefers, add denture cleaner to cup with water and follow directions on preparation.	Putting paper towels or a washcloth in the sink protects against breakage. Dentures collect food and microorganisms and require daily cleaning.
8. Rinse thoroughly with water. Apply denture adhesive, if appropriate.	Water aids in removal of debris and acts as a cleaning agent.
9. Use a toothbrush and paste to gently clean gums, mucous membranes, and tongue. Offer water and/or mouthwash so patient can rinse mouth before replacing dentures.	Cleaning removes food particles and plaque, permitting proper fit and preventing infection. Mouthwash leaves a pleasant taste in the mouth.
10. Insert upper denture in mouth and press firmly. Insert lower denture. Check that the dentures are securely in place and comfortable.	This ensures patient comfort.
11. If the patient desires, dentures can be stored in the denture cup in cold water, instead of returning to the mouth. Label the cup and place it in the patient's bedside table.	Storing in water prevents warping of dentures. Proper storage prevents loss and damage.
12. Remove equipment and return the patient to a position of comfort. Remove your gloves. Raise side rail and lower bed.	Promotes patient comfort and safety. Removing gloves properly reduces the risk for infection transmission and contamination of other items.
13. Remove additional PPE, if used. Perform hand hygiene.	Removing PPE properly reduces the risk for infection transmission and contamination of other items. Hand hygiene prevents transmission of microorganisms.

EVALUATION

- Patient's oral cavity and dentures are clean and free from complications.
- Patient states or demonstrates improved body image.
- Patient verbalizes a basic understanding of the need for oral care.

DOCUMENTATION

- Record oral assessment, significant observations and unusual findings, such as bleeding or inflammation. Document any teaching done. Document procedure and patient response.

SKILL 50   CARING FOR A HEMOVAC DRAIN

A Hemovac drain is placed into a vascular cavity where blood drainage is expected after surgery, such as with abdominal and orthopedic surgery. The drain consists of perforated tubing connected to a portable vacuum unit. Suction is maintained by compressing a spring-like device in the collection unit. After a surgical procedure, the surgeon places one end of the drain in or near the area to be drained. The other end passes through the skin via a separate incision. These drains are usually sutured in place. The site may be treated as an additional surgical wound, but often these sites are left open to air 24 hours after surgery. As the drainage accumulates in the collection unit, it expands and suction is lost, requiring recompression. Typically, the drain is emptied every 4 or 8 hours and when it is half full of drainage or air. However, based on the medical orders and nursing assessment and judgment, it could be emptied and recompressed more frequently.

DELEGATION CONSIDERATIONS

Care for a Hemovac drain insertion site is not delegated to nursing assistive personnel (NAP) or to unlicensed assistive personnel (UAP). Depending on the organization's policies and procedures, the drain may be emptied and reconstituted by nursing assistive personnel (NAP) or unlicensed assistive personnel (UAP). Depending on the state's nurse practice act and the organization's policies and procedures, these procedures may be delegated to licensed practical/vocational nurses (LPN/LVNs). The decision to delegate must be based on careful analysis of the patient's needs and circumstances, as well as the qualifications of the person to whom the task is being delegated. Refer to the Delegation Guidelines in Appendix A.

EQUIPMENT

- Graduated container for measuring drainage
- Clean, disposable gloves
- Additional PPE, as indicated

- Cleansing solution, usually sterile normal saline
- Sterile gauze pads
- Skin-protectant wipes
- Dressing materials for site dressing, if used

ASSESSMENT

- Assess the situation to determine the need for wound cleaning, a dressing change, or emptying of the drain.
- Assess the patient's level of comfort and the need for analgesics before wound care. Assess if the patient experienced any pain related to prior dressing changes and the effectiveness of interventions employed to minimize the patient's pain.
- Assess the current dressing. Assess for the presence of excess drainage or bleeding or saturation of the dressing.
- Assess the patency of the Hemovac drain and the drain site. Note the characteristics of the drainage in the collection bag.
- Inspect the wound and the surrounding tissue. Assess the appearance of the incision for the approximation of wound edges, the color of the wound and surrounding area, and signs of dehiscence. Note the stage of the healing process and characteristics of any drainage. Also assess the surrounding skin for color, temperature, and edema, ecchymosis, or maceration.

NURSING DIAGNOSIS

- Risk for Infection
- Disturbed Body Image
- Impaired Skin Integrity
- Deficient Knowledge

OUTCOME IDENTIFICATION AND PLANNING

- Drain is patent and intact.
- Drain care is accomplished without contaminating the wound area and/or without causing trauma to the wound.
- Patient does not experience pain or discomfort.
- Wound continues to show signs of progression of healing.
- Drainage amounts are measured accurately at the frequency required by facility policy and recorded as part of the intake and output record.
- Patient demonstrates understanding of drain care.

IMPLEMENTATION

ACTION	RATIONALE
1. Review the medical orders for wound care or the nursing plan of care related to	Reviewing the order and plan of care validates the correct patient and correct procedure. Preparation

ACTION	RATIONALE
wound/drain care. Gather necessary supplies.	promotes efficient time management and an organized approach to the task.
2. Perform hand hygiene and put on PPE, if indicated.	Hand hygiene and PPE prevent the spread of microorganisms. PPE is required based on transmission precautions.
3. Identify the patient.	Identifying the patient ensures the right patient receives the intervention and helps prevent errors.
4. Assemble equipment on overbed table within reach.	Organization facilitates performance of the task.
5. Close the curtains around the bed and close the door to the room, if possible. Explain what you are going to do and why you are going to do it to the patient.	This ensures the patient's privacy. Explanation relieves anxiety and facilitates cooperation.
6. Assess the patient for possible need for nonpharmacologic pain-reducing interventions or analgesic medication before wound care dressing change. Administer appropriate prescribed analgesic. Allow enough time for analgesic to achieve its effectiveness before beginning the procedure.	Pain is a subjective experience influenced by past experience. Wound care and dressing changes may cause pain for some patients.
7. Place a waste receptacle at a convenient location for use during the procedure.	Having a waste container handy means that the soiled dressing may be discarded easily, without the spread of microorganisms.
8. Adjust bed to comfortable working height, usually elbow height of the caregiver (VISN 8, 2009).	Having the bed at the proper height prevents back and muscle strain.
9. Assist the patient to a comfortable position that provides easy access to the drain and/or wound area. Use a bath	Patient positioning and use of a bath blanket provide for comfort and warmth. Waterproof pad protects underlying surfaces.

ACTION	**RATIONALE**

blanket to cover any exposed area other than the wound. Place a waterproof pad under the wound site.

10. Put on clean gloves; put on mask or face shield, as indicated.

Gloves prevent the spread of microorganisms; mask reduces the risk of transmission should splashing occur.

11. Place the graduated collection container under the drain outlet. **Without contaminating the outlet, pull off the cap. The chamber will expand completely as it draws in air. Empty the chamber's contents completely into the container. Use the gauze pad to clean the outlet. Fully compress the chamber by pushing the top and bottom together with your hands. Keep the device tightly compressed while you apply the cap (Figure 1).**

Emptying the drainage allows for accurate measurement. Cleaning the outlet reduces the risk of contamination and helps prevent the spread of microorganisms. Compressing the chamber reestablishes the suction.

FIGURE 1 Compressing Hemovac and securing cap.

12. Check the patency of the equipment. **Make sure the tubing is free from twists and kinks.**

Patent, untwisted, or unkinked tubing promotes appropriate drainage from wound.

13. Secure the Hemovac drain to the patient's gown below the wound with a safety pin, **making sure that there is no tension on the tubing.**

Securing the drain prevents injury to the patient and accidental removal of the drain.

ACTION	RATIONALE
14. Carefully measure and record the character, color, and amount of the drainage. Discard the drainage according to facility policy.	Documentation promotes continuity of care and communication. Appropriate disposal of biohazard material reduces the risk for microorganism transmission. Proper disposal of gloves deters transmission of microorganisms.
15. Put on clean gloves. If the drain site has a dressing, re-dress the site as outlined in Skill 55. Include cleaning of the sutures with the gauze pad moistened with normal saline. Dry sutures with gauze before applying new dressing.	Dressing protects the site. Cleaning and drying sutures deters growth of microorganisms.
16. If the drain site is open to air, observe the sutures that secure the drain to the skin. Look for signs of pulling, tearing, swelling, or infection of the surrounding skin. Gently clean the sutures with the gauze pad moistened with normal saline. Dry with a new gauze pad. Apply skin protectant to the surrounding skin, if needed.	Early detection of problems leads to prompt intervention and prevents complications. Gentle cleaning and drying prevent the growth of microorganisms. Skin protectant prevents skin irritation and breakdown.
17. Remove and discard gloves. Remove all remaining equipment; place the patient in a comfortable position, with side rails up and bed in the lowest position.	Proper removal and disposal of gloves prevents spread of microorganisms. Proper patient and bed positioning promotes safety and comfort.
18. Remove additional PPE, if used. Perform hand hygiene.	Removing PPE properly reduces the risk for infection transmission and contamination of other items. Hand hygiene prevents the spread of microorganisms.
19. Check drain status at least every 4 hours. Check all wound dressings every shift. More frequent checks may be needed if the wound is more complex or dressings become saturated quickly.	Checking drain ensures proper functioning and early detection of problems. Checking dressings ensures the assessment of changes in patient condition and timely intervention to prevent complications.

EVALUATION

- Patient exhibits a patent and intact Hemovac drain with a wound area that is free of contamination and trauma.
- Patient verbalizes minimal to no pain or discomfort.
- Patient exhibits signs and symptoms of progressive wound healing.
- Drainage measured accurately at the frequency required by facility policy, and amounts recorded as part of the intake and output record.
- Patient verbalizes an understanding of the rationale for and/or the technique for drain care.

DOCUMENTATION

- Document the location of the wound and drain, the assessment of the wound and drain site, and patency of the drain. Note if sutures are intact. Document the presence and characteristics of drainage on the old dressing upon removal. Include the appearance of the surrounding skin. Document cleansing of the drain site. Record any skin care and any dressing applied. Note that the drain was emptied and recompressed. Note pertinent patient and family education and any patient reaction to this procedure, including patient's pain level and effectiveness of nonpharmacologic interventions or analgesia if administered. Document the amount and characteristics of drainage obtained on the appropriate intake and output record.

SKILL 51 CARING FOR A JACKSON-PRATT DRAIN

A Jackson-Pratt (J-P) or grenade drain collects wound drainage in a bulblike device that is compressed to create gentle suction. It consists of perforated tubing connected to a portable vacuum unit. After a surgical procedure, the surgeon places one end of the drain in or near the area to be drained. The other end passes through the skin via a separate incision. These drains are usually sutured in place. The site may be treated as an additional surgical wound, but often these sites are left open to air 24 hours after surgery. They are typically used with breast and abdominal surgery. As the drainage accumulates in the bulb, the bulb expands and suction is lost, requiring recompression. Typically, these drains are emptied every 4 to 8 hours, and when they are half full of drainage or air. However, based on nursing assessment and judgment, the drain could be emptied and recompressed more frequently.

DELEGATION CONSIDERATIONS

Care for a Jackson-Pratt drain insertion site is not delegated to nursing assistive personnel (NAP) or to unlicensed assistive personnel (UAP). Depending on the organization's policies and procedures, the drain may be emptied and reconstituted by nursing assistive personnel (NAP) or unlicensed assistive personnel (UAP). Depending on the state's nurse practice act and the organization's policies and procedures, these procedures may be delegated to licensed practical/vocational nurses (LPN/LVNs). The decision to delegate must be based on careful analysis of the patient's needs and circumstances, as well as the qualifications of the person to whom the task is being delegated. Refer to the Delegation Guidelines in Appendix A.

EQUIPMENT

- Graduated container for measuring drainage
- Clean, disposable gloves
- Additional PPE, as indicated
- Cleansing solution, usually sterile normal saline
- Sterile gauze pads
- Skin-protectant wipes
- Dressing materials for site dressing, if used

ASSESSMENT

- Assess the situation to determine the need for wound cleaning, a dressing change, or emptying of the drain.
- Assess the patient's level of comfort and the need for analgesics before wound care. Assess if the patient experienced any pain related to prior dressing changes and the effectiveness of interventions employed to minimize the patient's pain.
- Assess the current dressing. Assess for the presence of excess drainage or bleeding or saturation of the dressing.
- Assess the patency of the Jackson-Pratt drain and the drain site. Note the characteristics of the drainage in the collection bag.
- Inspect the wound and the surrounding tissue. Assess the appearance of the incision for the approximation of wound edges, the color of the wound and surrounding area, and signs of dehiscence. Note the stage of the healing process and characteristics of any drainage. Also assess the surrounding skin for color, temperature, and edema, ecchymosis, or maceration.

NURSING DIAGNOSIS

- Risk for Infection
- Impaired Skin Integrity
- Disturbed Body Image
- Deficient Knowledge

OUTCOME IDENTIFICATION AND PLANNING

- Drain is patent and intact.
- Drain care is accomplished without contaminating the wound area and/or without causing trauma to the wound.
- Patient does not experience pain or discomfort.
- Wound continues to show signs of progression of healing.

- Drainage amounts are measured accurately at the frequency required by facility policy and recorded as part of the intake and output record.
- Patient demonstrates an understanding of drain care.

IMPLEMENTATION

ACTION	RATIONALE
1. Review the medical orders for wound care or the nursing plan of care related to wound/drain care. Gather necessary supplies.	Reviewing the order and plan of care validates the correct patient and correct procedure. Preparation promotes efficient time management and organized approach to the task.
2. Perform hand hygiene and put on PPE, if indicated.	Hand hygiene and PPE prevent the spread of microorganisms. PPE is required based on transmission precautions.
3. Identify the patient.	Identifying the patient ensures the right patient receives the intervention and helps prevent errors.
4. Assemble equipment on overbed table within reach.	Organization facilitates performance of the task.
5. Close the curtains around the bed and close the door to the room, if possible. Explain what you are going to do and why you are going to do it to the patient.	This ensures the patient's privacy. Explanation relieves anxiety and facilitates cooperation.
6. Assess the patient for possible need for nonpharmacologic pain-reducing interventions or analgesic medication before wound care dressing change. Administer appropriate prescribed analgesic. Allow enough time for the analgesic to achieve its effectiveness before beginning the procedure.	Pain is a subjective experience influenced by past experience. Wound care and dressing changes may cause pain for some patients.
7. Place a waste receptacle at a convenient location for use during the procedure.	Having a waste container handy means that the soiled dressing may be discarded easily, without the spread of microorganisms.

ACTION	RATIONALE
8. Adjust bed to comfortable working height, usually elbow height of the caregiver (VISN 8, 2009).	Having the bed at the proper height prevents back and muscle strain.
9. Assist the patient to a comfortable position that provides easy access to the drain and/or wound area. Use a bath blanket to cover any exposed area other than the wound. Place a waterproof pad under the wound site.	Patient positioning and use of a bath blanket provide for comfort and warmth. Waterproof pad protects underlying surfaces.
10. Put on clean gloves; put on mask or face shield, as indicated.	Gloves prevent the spread of microorganisms; mask reduces the risk of transmission should splashing occur.
11. Place the graduated collection container under the drain outlet. Without contaminating the outlet valve, pull off the cap. The chamber will expand completely as it draws in air. **Empty the chamber's contents completely into the container. Use the gauze pad to clean the outlet. Fully compress the chamber with one hand and replace the cap with your other hand (Figure 1).**	Emptying the drainage allows for accurate measurement. Cleaning the outlet reduces the risk of contamination and helps prevent the spread of microorganisms. Compressing the chamber reestablishes the suction.

FIGURE 1 Compressing Jackson-Pratt drain and replacing cap.

ACTION	RATIONALE
12. Check the patency of the equipment. **Make sure the tubing is free from twists and kinks.**	Patent, untwisted, or unkinked tubing promotes appropriate wound drainage.
13. Secure the Jackson-Pratt drain to the patient's gown below the wound with a safety pin, **making sure that there is no tension on the tubing.**	Securing the drain prevents injury to the patient and accidental removal of the drain.
14. Carefully measure and record the character, color, and amount of the drainage. Discard the drainage according to facility policy. Remove gloves.	Documentation promotes continuity of care and communication. Appropriate disposal of biohazard material reduces the risk for microorganism transmission.
15. Put on clean gloves. If the drain site has a dressing, re-dress the site as outlined in Skill 55. Include cleaning of the sutures with the gauze pad moistened with normal saline. Dry sutures with gauze before applying new dressing.	Dressing protects the site. Cleaning and drying sutures deters growth of microorganisms.
16. If the drain site is open to air, observe the sutures that secure the drain to the skin. Look for signs of pulling, tearing, swelling, or infection of the surrounding skin. Gently clean the sutures with the gauze pad moistened with normal saline. Dry with a new gauze pad. Apply skin protectant to the surrounding skin, if needed.	Early detection of problems leads to prompt intervention and prevents complications. Gentle cleaning and drying prevent the growth of microorganisms. Skin protectant prevents skin irritation and breakdown.
17. Remove and discard gloves. Remove all remaining equipment; place the patient in a comfortable position, with side rails up and bed in the lowest position.	Proper removal of gloves prevents spread of microorganisms. Proper patient and bed positioning promotes safety and comfort.

ACTION	RATIONALE
18. Remove additional PPE, if used. Perform hand hygiene.	Removing PPE properly reduces the risk for infection transmission and contamination of other items. Hand hygiene prevents the spread of microorganisms.
19. Check drain status at least every 4 hours. Check all wound dressings every shift. Perform more frequent checks if the wound is more complex or dressings become saturated quickly.	Checking drain ensures proper functioning and early detection of problems. Checking dressings ensures the assessment of changes in patient condition and timely intervention to prevent complications.

EVALUATION

- Patient exhibits a patent and intact Jackson-Pratt drain with a wound area that is free of contamination and trauma.
- Patient verbalizes minimal to no pain or discomfort.
- Patient exhibits signs and symptoms of progressive wound healing, with drainage being measured accurately at the frequency required by facility policy, and amounts recorded as part of the intake and output record.
- Patient verbalizes an understanding of the rationale for and/or the technique for drain care.

DOCUMENTATION

- Document the location of the wound and drain, the assessment of the wound and drain site, and patency of the drain. Note if sutures are intact. Document the presence and characteristics of drainage on the old dressing upon removal. Include the appearance of the surrounding skin. Document cleansing the drain site. Record any skin care and the dressing applied. Note that the drain was emptied and recompressed. Note pertinent patient and family education and any patient reaction to this procedure, including patient's pain level and effectiveness of nonpharmacologic interventions or analgesia, if administered. Document the amount and characteristics of drainage obtained on the appropriate intake and output record.

SKILL 52 — CARING FOR A PENROSE DRAIN

Drains are inserted into or near a wound when it is anticipated that a collection of fluid in a closed area would delay healing. A Penrose drain is a hollow, open-ended rubber tube. It allows fluid to drain via capillary action into absorbent dressings. Penrose drains are commonly used after a surgical procedure or for drainage of an abscess. After a surgical procedure, the surgeon places one end of the drain in or near the area to be drained. The other end passes through the skin, directly through the incision or through a separate opening referred to as a stab wound. A Penrose drain is not sutured. A large safety pin is usually placed in the part outside the wound to prevent the drain from slipping back into the incised area. This type of drain can be advanced or shortened to drain different areas. The patency and placement of the drain are included in the wound assessment.

DELEGATION CONSIDERATIONS

Care for a Penrose drain insertion site and wound care is not delegated to nursing assistive personnel (NAP) or to unlicensed assistive personnel (UAP). Depending on the state's nurse practice act and the organization's policies and procedures, these procedures may be delegated to licensed practical/vocational nurses (LPN/LVNs). The decision to delegate must be based on careful analysis of the patient's needs and circumstances, as well as the qualifications of the person to whom the task is being delegated. Refer to the Delegation Guidelines in Appendix A.

EQUIPMENT

- Sterile gloves
- Gauze dressings
- Sterile cotton-tipped applicators, if appropriate
- Sterile drain sponges
- Surgical or abdominal pads
- Sterile dressing set or suture set (for the sterile scissors and forceps)
- Sterile cleaning solution as ordered (commonly 0.9% normal saline solution)
- Sterile container to hold cleaning solution
- Clean safety pin
- Clean, disposable gloves
- Plastic bag or other appropriate waste container for soiled dressings
- Waterproof pad and bath blanket
- Tape or ties
- Skin-protectant wipes, if needed
- Additional dressings and supplies needed or as required for ordered wound care

ASSESSMENT

- Assess the situation to determine the necessity for wound cleaning and a dressing change.

- Confirm any medical orders relevant to drain care and any drain care included in the nursing plan of care.
- Assess the patient's level of comfort and the need for analgesics before wound care. Assess if the patient experienced any pain related to prior dressing changes and the effectiveness of interventions employed to minimize the patient's pain.
- Assess the current dressing to determine if it is intact, and assess for the presence of excess drainage, bleeding, or saturation of the dressing.
- Assess the patency of the Penrose drain.
- Inspect the wound and the surrounding tissue. Assess the appearance of the wound for the approximation of wound edges, the color of the wound and surrounding area, and signs of dehiscence. Note the stage of the healing process and the characteristics of any drainage. Assess the surrounding skin for color, temperature, and the presence of edema, ecchymosis, or maceration.

NURSING DIAGNOSIS

- Risk for Infection
- Disturbed Body Image
- Deficient Knowledge

OUTCOME IDENTIFICATION AND PLANNING

- Drain remains patent and intact.
- Drain care is accomplished without contaminating the wound area, or causing trauma to the wound, and without causing the patient to experience pain or discomfort.
- Wound shows signs of progressive healing without evidence of complications.
- Patient demonstrates an understanding of drain care.

IMPLEMENTATION

ACTION	RATIONALE
1. Review the medical orders for wound care or the nursing plan of care related to wound/drain care. Gather necessary supplies.	Reviewing the order and plan of care validates the correct patient and correct procedure. Preparation promotes efficient time management and an organized approach to the task.
2. Perform hand hygiene and put on PPE, if indicated.	Hand hygiene and PPE prevent the spread of microorganisms. PPE is required based on transmission precautions.

ACTION	RATIONALE
3. Identify the patient.	Identifying the patient ensures the right patient receives the intervention and helps prevent errors.
4. Assemble equipment on overbed table within reach.	Organization facilitates performance of the task.
5. Close the curtains around the bed and close the door to the room, if possible. Explain what you are going to do and why you are going to do it to the patient.	This ensures the patient's privacy. Explanation relieves anxiety and facilitates cooperation.
6. Assess the patient for possible need for nonpharmacologic pain-reducing interventions or analgesic medication before wound care dressing change. Administer appropriate prescribed analgesic. Allow enough time for the analgesic to achieve its effectiveness before beginning procedure.	Pain is a subjective experience influenced by past experience. Wound care and dressing changes may cause pain for some patients.
7. Place a waste receptacle at a convenient location for use during the procedure.	Having a waste container handy means that the soiled dressing may be discarded easily, without the spread of microorganisms.
8. Adjust bed to comfortable working height, usually elbow height of the caregiver (VISN 8, 2009).	Having the bed at the proper height prevents back and muscle strain.
9. Assist the patient to a comfortable position that provides easy access to the drain and/or wound area. Use a bath blanket to cover any exposed area other than the wound. Place a waterproof pad under the wound site.	Patient positioning and use of a bath blanket provide for comfort and warmth. Waterproof pad protects underlying surfaces.
10. Put on clean gloves. Check the position of the drain or drains before removing the dressing. Carefully and	Gloves protect the nurse from handling contaminated dressings. Checking the position ensures that a drain is not removed

ACTION	RATIONALE
gently remove the soiled dressings. If there is resistance, use a silicone-based adhesive remover to help remove the tape. If any part of the dressing sticks to the underlying skin, use small amounts of sterile saline to help loosen and remove it.	accidentally if one is present. Cautious removal of the dressing is more comfortable for the patient and ensures that any drain present is not removed. A silicone-based adhesive remover allows for the easy, rapid, and painless removal without the associated problems of skin stripping (Denyer, 2011; Benbow, 2011). Sterile saline moistens the dressing for easier removal and minimizes damage and pain.
11. After removing the dressing, note the presence, amount, type, color, and odor of any drainage on the dressings. Place soiled dressings in the appropriate waste receptacle.	The presence of drainage should be documented. Discarding dressings appropriately prevents the spread of microorganisms.
12. Inspect the drain site for appearance and drainage. Assess if any pain is present.	The wound healing process and/or the presence of irritation or infection must be documented.
13. Using sterile technique, prepare a sterile work area and open the needed supplies.	Supplies are within easy reach and sterility is maintained.
14. Open the sterile cleaning solution. Pour it into the basin. Add the gauze sponges.	Sterility of dressings and solution is maintained.
15. Put on sterile gloves.	Sterile gloves help to maintain surgical asepsis and sterile technique and prevent the spread of microorganisms.
16. Cleanse the drain site with the cleaning solution. Use the forceps and the moistened gauze or cotton-tipped applicators. **Start at the drain insertion site, moving in a circular motion toward the periphery. Use each gauze sponge or applicator only once.** Discard and use new gauze if additional cleansing is needed.	Using a circular motion ensures that cleaning occurs from the least to most contaminated area and a previously cleaned area is not contaminated again.

ACTION	RATIONALE
17. Dry the skin with a new gauze pad in the same manner. Apply skin protectant to the skin around the drain; extend out to include the area of skin that will be taped. Place a pre-split drain sponge under and around the drain (Figure 1). Closely observe the safety pin in the drain. If the pin or drain is crusted, replace the pin with a new sterile pin. **Take care not to dislodge the drain.**	Drying prevents skin irritation. Skin protectant prevents skin irritation and breakdown. The gauze absorbs drainage and prevents the drainage from accumulating on the patient's skin. Microorganisms grow more easily in a soiled environment. The safety pin ensures proper placement because the drain is not sutured in place.

FIGURE 1 Pre-split dressing around Penrose drain.

ACTION	RATIONALE
18. Apply gauze pads over the drain. Apply ABD pads over the gauze.	The gauze absorbs drainage. Pads provide both extra absorption for excess drainage and a moisture barrier.
19. Remove and discard gloves. Apply tape, Montgomery straps, or roller gauze to secure the dressings.	Proper disposal of gloves prevents the spread of microorganisms. Tape or other securing products are easier to apply after gloves have been removed.
20. After securing the dressing, label dressing with date and time. Remove all remaining equipment; place the patient in a comfortable position, with side rails up and bed in the lowest position.	Recording date and time provides communication and demonstrates adherence to plan of care. Proper patient and bed positioning promotes safety and comfort.
21. Remove additional PPE, if used. Perform hand hygiene.	Removing PPE properly reduces the risk for infection transmission and contamination of other items. Hand hygiene prevents the spread of microorganisms.

ACTION	RATIONALE
22. Check all wound dressings every shift. More frequent checks may be needed if the wound is more complex or dressings become saturated quickly.	Checking dressings ensures the assessment of changes in patient condition and timely intervention to prevent complications.

EVALUATION

- Patient exhibits a wound that is clean, dry, and intact, with a patent, intact Penrose drain.
- Patient remains free of wound contamination and trauma.
- Patient reports minimal to no pain or discomfort.
- Patient exhibits signs and symptoms of progressive wound healing.
- Patient verbalizes an understanding of the rationale for and/or the technique for drain care.

DOCUMENTATION

- Document the location of the wound and drain, the assessment of the wound and drain site, and intactness of the Penrose drain. Document the presence of drainage and characteristics on the old dressing upon removal. Include the appearance of the surrounding skin. Document cleansing of the drain site. Record any skin care and the dressing applied. Note pertinent patient and family education and any patient reaction to this procedure, including patient's pain level and effectiveness of nonpharmacologic interventions or analgesia if administered.

SKILL 53 CARING FOR A T-TUBE DRAIN

A biliary drain, or T-tube, is sometimes placed in the common bile duct after removal of the gallbladder (cholecystectomy) or a portion of the bile duct (choledochostomy). The tube drains bile while the surgical site is healing. A portion of the tube is inserted into the common bile duct and the remaining portion is anchored to the abdominal wall, passed through the skin, and connected to a closed drainage system. Often, a three-way valve is inserted between the drain tube and the drainage system to allow for clamping and flushing of the tube, if necessary. The drainage amount is measured every shift, recorded, and included in output totals.

DELEGATION CONSIDERATIONS

Care for a T-tube drain insertion site is not delegated to nursing assistive personnel (NAP) or to unlicensed assistive personnel (UAP). Depending on the organization's policies and procedures, the drain may be emptied and reconstituted by nursing assistive personnel (NAP) or unlicensed assistive personnel (UAP). Depending on the state's nurse practice act and the organization's policies and procedures, these procedures may be delegated to licensed practical/vocational nurses (LPN/LVNs). The decision to delegate must be based on careful analysis of the patient's needs and circumstances, as well as the qualifications of the person to whom the task is being delegated. Refer to the Delegation Guidelines in Appendix A.

EQUIPMENT

- Sterile gloves
- Clean, disposable gloves
- Additional PPE, as indicated
- Sterile gauze pads
- Sterile drain sponges
- Cleansing solution, usually sterile normal saline
- Sterile cotton-tipped applicators (if appropriate)
- Transparent dressing
- Graduated collection container
- Waste receptacle
- Sterile basin
- Sterile forceps
- Tape
- Skin-protectant wipes
- Waterproof pad and bath blanket, if needed

ASSESSMENT

- Assess the situation to determine the need for wound cleaning, a dressing change, or emptying of the drain. Confirm any medical orders relevant to drain care and any drain care included in the nursing plan of care.
- Assess the patient's level of comfort and the need for analgesics before wound care. Assess if the patient experienced any pain related to prior dressing changes and the effectiveness of interventions employed to minimize the patient's pain.
- Assess the current dressing to determine if it is intact, and assess for evidence of excessive drainage or bleeding or saturation of the dressing.
- Assess the patency of the T-tube and the drain site. Note the characteristics of the drainage in the collection bag.
- Inspect the wound and the surrounding tissue. Assess the appearance of the incision for the approximation of wound edges, the color of the wound and surrounding area, and signs of dehiscence. Note the stage of the healing process and characteristics of any drainage. Assess the surrounding skin for color, temperature, and edema, ecchymosis, or maceration.

NURSING DIAGNOSIS

- Risk for Infection
- Deficient Knowledge

- Disturbed Body Image
- Impaired Skin Integrity

OUTCOME IDENTIFICATION AND PLANNING

- Drain remains patent and intact.
- Drain care is accomplished without contaminating the wound area and/or without causing trauma to the wound.
- Patient does not experience pain or discomfort.
- Wound continues to show signs of progression of healing.
- Drainage amounts are measured accurately at the frequency required by facility policy and recorded as part of the intake and output record.
- Patient demonstrates an understanding of drain care.

IMPLEMENTATION

ACTION	RATIONALE
1. Review the medical orders for wound care or the nursing plan of care related to wound/drain care. Gather necessary supplies.	Reviewing the order and plan of care validates the correct patient and correct procedure. Preparation promotes efficient time management and an organized approach to the task.
2. Perform hand hygiene and put on PPE, if indicated.	Hand hygiene and PPE prevent the spread of microorganisms. PPE is required based on transmission precautions.
3. Identify the patient.	Identifying the patient ensures the right patient receives the intervention and helps prevent errors.
4. Assemble equipment on overbed table within reach.	Organization facilitates performance of the task.
5. Close the curtains around the bed and close the door to the room, if possible. Explain what you are going to do and why you are going to do it to the patient.	This ensures the patient's privacy. Explanation relieves anxiety and facilitates cooperation.
6. Assess the patient for possible need for nonpharmacologic pain-reducing interventions or analgesic	Pain is a subjective experience influenced by past experience. Wound care and dressing changes may cause pain for some patients.

ACTION	RATIONALE
medication before wound care dressing change. Administer appropriate prescribed analgesic. Allow enough time for the analgesic to achieve its effectiveness before beginning the procedure.	
7. Place a waste receptacle at a convenient location for use during the procedure.	Having a waste container handy means that the soiled dressing may be discarded easily, without the spread of microorganisms.
8. Adjust bed to comfortable working height, usually elbow height of the caregiver (VISN 8, 2009).	Having the bed at the proper height prevents back and muscle strain.
9. Assist the patient to a comfortable position that provides easy access to the drain and/or wound area. Use a bath blanket to cover any exposed area other than the wound. Place a waterproof pad under the wound site.	Patient positioning and use of a bath blanket provide for comfort and warmth. Waterproof pad protects underlying surfaces.

Emptying Drainage

ACTION	RATIONALE
10. Put on clean gloves; put on mask or face shield, as indicated.	Gloves prevent the spread of microorganisms; mask reduces the risk of transmission should splashing occur.
11. Using sterile technique, open a gauze pad, making a sterile field with the outer wrapper.	Using sterile technique deters the spread of microorganisms.
12. Place the graduated collection container under the outlet valve of the drainage bag. **Without touching the outlet, pull off the cap and empty the bag's contents completely into the container. Use the gauze to wipe the outlet, and replace the cap.**	Draining contents into a container allows for accurate measurement of the drainage. Touching the outlet with gloves or other surface contaminates the valve, potentially introducing pathogens. Wiping the outlet with gauze prevents contamination of the valve. Recapping prevents the spread of microorganisms.

ACTION	RATIONALE
13. Carefully measure and note the characteristics of the drainage. Discard the drainage according to facility policy.	Documentation promotes continuity of care and communication. Appropriate disposal of biohazard material reduces the risk for microorganism transmission.
14. Remove gloves and perform hand hygiene.	Proper glove removal and performing hand hygiene prevent spread of microorganisms.

Cleaning the Drain Site

ACTION	RATIONALE
15. Put on clean gloves. Check the position of the drain or drains before removing the dressing. Carefully and gently remove the soiled dressings. If there is resistance, use a silicone-based adhesive remover to help remove the tape. If any part of the dressing sticks to the underlying skin, use small amounts of sterile saline to help loosen and remove it. Do not reach over the drain site.	Gloves protect the nurse from handling contaminated dressings. Checking the position ensures that a drain is not removed accidentally if one is present. Cautious removal of the dressing is more comfortable for the patient and ensures that any drain present is not removed. A silicone-based adhesive remover allows for the easy, rapid, and painless removal without the associated problems of skin stripping (Denyer, 2011; Benbow, 2011). Sterile saline moistens the dressing for easier removal and minimizes damage and pain.
16. After removing the dressing, note the presence, amount, type, color, and odor of any drainage on the dressings. Place soiled dressings in the appropriate waste receptacle. Remove gloves and dispose of them in appropriate waste receptacle.	The presence of drainage should be documented. Proper disposal of gloves prevents spread of microorganisms.
17. Inspect the drain site for appearance and drainage. Assess if any pain is present.	Wound healing process and/or the presence of irritation or infection should be documented.
18. Using sterile technique, prepare a sterile work area and open the needed supplies.	Preparing a sterile work area ensures that supplies are within easy reach and sterility is maintained.

ACTION	RATIONALE
19. Open the sterile cleaning solution. Pour it into the basin. Add the gauze sponges.	Sterility of dressings and solution is maintained.
20. Put on sterile gloves.	Use of sterile gloves maintains surgical asepsis and sterile technique and reduces the risk of microorganism transmission.
21. Cleanse the drain site with the cleaning solution. Use the forceps and the moistened gauze or cotton-tipped applicators. **Start at the drain insertion site, moving in a circular motion toward the periphery. Use each gauze sponge only once.** Discard and use new gauze if additional cleansing is needed.	Cleaning is done from the least to most contaminated area so that a previously cleaned area is not contaminated again.
22. Dry with new sterile gauze in the same manner. Apply skin protectant to the skin around the drain; extend out to include the area of skin that will be taped.	Drying prevents skin irritation. Skin protectant prevents skin irritation and breakdown.
23. Place a pre-split drain sponge under the drain. Apply gauze pads over the drain. Remove and discard gloves.	The gauze absorbs drainage and prevents the drainage from accumulating on the patient's skin. Proper disposal of gloves prevents spread of microorganisms.
24. Secure the dressings with tape, as needed. Alternatively, before removing gloves, place a transparent dressing over the tube and insertion site. **Be careful not to kink the tubing.**	Kinked tubing could block drainage. Type of dressing used is often determined by facility policy.
25. After securing the dressing, label it with date and time. Remove all remaining equipment; place the patient in a comfortable position, with side rails up and bed in the lowest position.	Recording date and time provides communication and demonstrates adherence to plan of care. Proper patient and bed positioning promotes safety and comfort.

ACTION	RATIONALE
26. Remove additional PPE, if used. Perform hand hygiene.	Removing PPE properly reduces the risk for infection transmission and contamination of other items. Hand hygiene prevents the spread of microorganisms.
27. Check drain status at least every 4 hours. Check all wound dressings every shift. Perform more frequent checks if the wound is more complex or dressings become saturated quickly.	Checking drain ensures proper functioning and early detection of problems. Checking dressings ensures the assessment of changes in patient condition and timely intervention to prevent complications.

EVALUATION

- Patient exhibits a patent and intact T-tube drain with a wound area that is free of contamination and trauma.
- Patient verbalizes minimal to no pain or discomfort.
- Patient exhibits signs and symptoms of progressive wound healing.
- Drainage is measured accurately at the frequency required by facility policy, and amounts recorded as part of the intake and output record.
- Patient verbalizes an understanding of the rationale for and/or the technique for drain care.

DOCUMENTATION

- Document the location of the wound and drain, the assessment of the wound and drain site, and patency of the drain. Note if sutures are intact. Document the presence and characteristics of drainage on the old dressing upon removal. Include the appearance of the surrounding skin. Document cleansing of the drain site. Record any skin care and the dressing applied. Note pertinent patient and family education and any patient reaction to this procedure, including patient's pain level and effectiveness of nonpharmacologic interventions or analgesia, if administered. Document the amount of bile drainage obtained from the drainage bag on the appropriate intake and output record.

SKILL 54 | CHANGING A PERIPHERAL VENOUS ACCESS DRESSING

The IV site is a potential entry point for microorganisms into the bloodstream. To prevent this, sealed IV dressings are used to occlude the site and prevent complications. Transparent semipermeable membrane (TSM) dressings are used most commonly to protect the insertion site. TSM dressings (e.g., Tegaderm or OpSite IV) allow easy inspection of the IV site and permit evaporation of moisture that accumulates under the dressing. Sterile gauze may also be used to cover the catheter site. A gauze dressing is recommended if the patient is diaphoretic or if the site is bleeding or oozing. However, the gauze dressing should be replaced with a TSM once this is resolved (O'Grady et al., 2011). The particular facility's policies determine the type of dressing used and when these dressings are changed. Routine site care and dressing changes are not performed on peripheral catheters unless the dressing is soiled or no longer intact (INS, 2011). However, dressing changes might be required more often, based on nursing assessment and judgment. Any access site dressing that is damp, loosened, or soiled should be changed immediately. Whenever these dressings need to be changed, it is important to observe meticulous aseptic technique to minimize the possibility of contamination.

DELEGATION CONSIDERATIONS

The changing of a peripheral venous access dressing is not delegated to nursing assistive personnel (NAP) or to unlicensed assistive personnel (UAP). Depending on the state's nurse practice act and the organization's policies and procedures, the changing of a peripheral venous access dressing may be delegated to licensed practical/vocational nurses (LPN/LVNs). The decision to delegate must be based on careful analysis of the patient's needs and circumstances, as well as the qualifications of the person to whom the task is being delegated. Refer to the Delegation Guidelines in Appendix A.

EQUIPMENT

- Transparent occlusive dressing
- Cleansing swabs (chlorhexidine preferred; 70% alcohol, iodine, or povidone-iodine are also acceptable)
- Adhesive remover (optional)
- Alcohol or other disinfectant wipes
- Skin protectant wipe (e.g., SkinPrep)
- IV securement/stabilization device, as appropriate
- Tape
- Clean gloves
- Towel or disposable pad
- Additional PPE, as indicated

ASSESSMENT

- Assess the IV site. The dressing should be intact, adhering to the skin on all edges. Check for any leaks or fluid under or around

283

the dressing, or other indications that the dressing needs to be changed.

- Inspect the tissue around the IV entry site for swelling, coolness, or pallor. These are signs of fluid infiltration into the tissue around the IV catheter.
- Inspect the site for redness, swelling, and warmth. These signs might indicate the development of phlebitis or an inflammation of the blood vessel at the site.
- Ask the patient if he/she is experiencing any pain or discomfort related to the IV line. Pain or discomfort can be a sign of infiltration, extravasation, phlebitis, thrombophlebitis, and infection related to IV therapy.
- Note the insertion date and date of last dressing change, if different from insertion date.
- Assess the patient's need to maintain venous access. If patient does not need the access, discuss the possibility of discontinuation with the primary care provider.
- Ask the patient about any allergies.

NURSING DIAGNOSIS

- Risk for Infection
- Risk for Injury
- Risk for Impaired Skin Integrity

OUTCOME IDENTIFICATION AND PLANNING

- Patient will exhibit an access site that is clean, dry, and without evidence of any signs and symptoms of infection, infiltration, or phlebitis.
- Dressing will be clean, dry, and intact.
- Patient will not experience injury.

IMPLEMENTATION

ACTION	RATIONALE
1. Determine the need for a dressing change. Check facility policy. Gather equipment.	The particular facility's policies determine the type of dressing used and when these dressings are changed. Dressing changes might be required more often, based on nursing assessment and judgment. Immediately change any access site dressing that is damp, loosened, or soiled. Preparation promotes efficient time management and an organized approach to the task.

ACTION	RATIONALE
2. Perform hand hygiene and put on PPE, if indicated.	Hand hygiene and PPE prevent the spread of microorganisms. PPE is required based on transmission precautions.
3. Identify the patient.	Identifying the patient ensures the right patient receives the intervention and helps prevent errors.
4. Close the curtains around the bed and close the door to the room, if possible. Explain what you are going to do and why you are going to do it to the patient. Ask the patient about allergies to tape and skin antiseptics.	This ensures the patient's privacy. Explanation relieves anxiety and facilitates cooperation. Possible allergies may exist related to tape or antiseptics.
5. Put on gloves. Place towel or disposable pad under the arm with the venous access. If solution is currently infusing, temporarily stop the infusion. Hold the catheter in place with your nondominant hand and **carefully remove old dressing and/or stabilization/securing device.** Use adhesive remover as necessary. Discard dressing.	Gloves prevent contact with blood and body fluids. Pad protects underlying surface. Proper disposal of dressing prevents transmission of microorganisms.
6. **Inspect IV site for presence of phlebitis (inflammation), infection, or infiltration.** Discontinue and relocate IV, if noted.	Inflammation (phlebitis), infection, or infiltration causes trauma to tissues and necessitates removal of the venous access device.
7. **Cleanse the site with an antiseptic solution, such as chlorhexidine, or according to facility policy. Press applicator against the skin and apply chlorhexidine using a gentle back and forth motion. Do not wipe or blot. Allow to dry completely.**	Cleansing the skin is necessary because organisms on the skin can be introduced into the tissues or the bloodstream with the venous access. Chlorhexidine is the preferred antiseptic solution, but iodine, povidone-iodine, and 70% alcohol are considered acceptable alternatives (INS, 2011). A

ACTION	RATIONALE
	scrubbing motion creates friction and lets the solution more effectively penetrate the epidermal layers (Hadaway, 2006).
8. Open the skin protectant wipe. Apply it to the site, making sure to cover at minimum the area to be covered with the dressing. Allow to dry. Place sterile transparent dressing or catheter securing/stabilization device over the venipuncture site.	Skin protectant aids in adhesion of the dressing and decreases the risk for skin trauma when the dressing is removed. Transparent dressing allows easy visualization and protects the site. Stabilization/securing devices preserve the integrity of the access device, minimize catheter movement at the hub, and prevent catheter dislodgement and loss of access (INS, 2011, p. S46). Some stabilization devices act as a site dressing also.
9. Label dressing with date, time of change, and initials. Loop the tubing near the entry site, and anchor with tape (nonallergenic) close to site. Resume fluid infusion, if indicated. Check that IV flow is accurate and system is patent.	Other personnel working with the infusion will know what type of device is being used, the site, and when it was inserted. Peripheral venous catheter IV insertion sites are changed every 72 to 96 hours for an adult (O'Grady et al., 2011).
10. Apply an IV securement/stabilization device if not already in place as part of the dressing, as indicated, based on facility policy. Explain to patient the purpose of the device and the importance of safeguarding the site when using the extremity.	These systems are recommended for use on all venous access sites, and particularly central venous access sites, to preserve the integrity of the access device, minimize catheter movement at the hub, and prevent catheter dislodgement and loss of access (INS, 2011, p. S46). Some devices also act as a site dressing and may already have been applied.
11. Remove equipment. Ensure patient's comfort. Remove gloves. Lower bed, if not in lowest position.	Promotes patient comfort and safety. Removing gloves properly reduces the risk for infection transmission and contamination of other items.

ACTION	RATIONALE
12. Remove additional PPE, if used. Perform hand hygiene.	Removing PPE properly reduces the risk for infection transmission and contamination of other items. Hand hygiene prevents transmission of microorganisms.

EVALUATION

- Patient remains free of any signs and symptoms of infection, phlebitis, or infiltration at the venous access site.
- Access site dressing is clean, dry, and intact.
- Patient has not experienced injury.

DOCUMENTATION

- Document the location of the venous access as well as the condition of the site. Include the presence or absence of signs of erythema, redness, swelling, or drainage. Document the clinical criteria for site complications. Record the subjective comments of the patient regarding the absence or presence of pain at the site. Record the patient's reaction to the procedure and pertinent patient teaching, such as alerting the nurse if the patient experiences any pain from the IV or notices any swelling at the site.

SKILL 55 CLEANING A WOUND AND APPLYING A DRY, STERILE DRESSING

The goal of wound care is to promote tissue repair and regeneration to restore skin integrity. Often, wound care includes cleaning of the wound and the use of a dressing as a protective covering over the wound. Wound cleansing is performed to remove debris, contaminants, and excess exudate. Sterile normal saline or a commercially prepared cleanser is the preferred cleansing solution. There is no standard frequency for how often dressings should be changed. It depends on the amount of drainage, the primary practitioner's preference, the nature of the wound, and the particular wound care product being used. It is customary for the surgeon or other advanced practice professional to perform the first dressing change on a surgical wound, usually within 24 to 48 hours after surgery.

DELEGATION CONSIDERATIONS

Wound care and procedures requiring the use of a sterile field and other sterile items are not delegated to nursing assistive personnel (NAP) or unlicensed assistive personnel (UAP). Depending on the state's nurse practice act and the organization's policies and procedures, these procedures may be delegated to licensed practical/vocational nurses (LPN/LVNs). The decision to delegate must be based on careful analysis of the patient's needs and circumstances, as well as the qualifications of the person to whom the task is being delegated. Refer to the Delegation Guidelines in Appendix A.

EQUIPMENT

- Sterile gloves
- Clean, disposable gloves
- Additional PPE, as indicated
- Gauze dressings
- Surgical or abdominal pads
- Sterile dressing set or suture set (for the sterile scissors and forceps)
- Sterile cleaning solution as ordered (commonly 0.9% normal saline solution, or a commercially prepared wound cleanser)
- Sterile basin (may be optional)
- Sterile drape (may be optional)
- Plastic bag or other appropriate waste container for soiled dressings
- Waterproof pad and bath blanket
- Tape or ties
- Bath blanket or other linens for draping patient
- Additional dressings and supplies needed or required by the primary care provider's order

ASSESSMENT

- Assess the situation to determine the need for wound cleaning and a dressing change. Confirm any medical orders relevant to wound care and any wound care included in the nursing plan of care.
- Assess the patient's level of comfort and the need for analgesics before wound care. Assess if the patient experienced any pain related to prior dressing changes and the effectiveness of interventions employed to minimize the patient's pain.
- Assess the current dressing to determine if it is intact. Assess for excess drainage, bleeding, or saturation of the dressing.
- Inspect the wound and the surrounding tissue. Assess the appearance of the wound for the approximation of wound edges, the color of the wound and surrounding area, and signs of dehiscence. Assess for the presence of sutures, staples, or adhesive closure strips. Note the stage of the healing process and characteristics of any drainage. Also assess the surrounding skin for color, temperature, and edema, ecchymosis, or maceration.

NURSING DIAGNOSIS

- Risk for Infection
- Disturbed Body Image
- Acute Pain
- Impaired Skin Integrity
- Delayed Surgical Recovery

OUTCOME IDENTIFICATION AND PLANNING

- Wound is cleaned and protected with a dressing without contaminating the wound area, causing trauma to the wound, and/or causing the patient to experience pain or discomfort.
- Wound continues to show signs of progression of healing.
- Patient demonstrates an understanding of the need for wound care and dressing change.

IMPLEMENTATION

ACTION	RATIONALE
1. Review the medical order for wound care or the nursing plan of care related to wound care. Gather necessary supplies.	Reviewing the order and plan of care validates the correct patient and correct procedure. Preparation promotes efficient time management and an organized approach to the task.
2. Perform hand hygiene and put on PPE, if indicated.	Hand hygiene and PPE prevent the spread of microorganisms. PPE is required based on transmission precautions.
3. Identify the patient.	Identifying the patient ensures the right patient receives the intervention and helps prevent errors.
4. Assemble equipment on overbed table within reach.	Organization facilitates performance of the task.
5. Close the curtains around the bed and close the door to the room if possible. Explain to the patient what you are going to do and why you are going to do it.	This ensures the patient's privacy. Explanation relieves anxiety and facilitates cooperation.
6. Assess the patient for the possible need for nonpharmacologic pain-reducing interventions or analgesic medication before wound care dressing change. Administer appropriate prescribed analgesic. Allow enough time for the analgesic to achieve its effectiveness.	Pain is a subjective experience influenced by past experience. Wound care and dressing changes may cause pain for some patients.

ACTION	RATIONALE
7. Place a waste receptacle or bag at a convenient location for use during the procedure.	Having a waste container handy means the soiled dressing may be discarded easily, without the spread of microorganisms.
8. Adjust the bed to a comfortable working height, usually elbow height of the caregiver (VISN 8, 2009).	Having the bed at the proper height prevents back and muscle strain.
9. Assist the patient to a comfortable position that provides easy access to the wound area. Use the bath blanket to cover any exposed area other than the wound. Place a waterproof pad under the wound site.	Patient positioning and use of a bath blanket provide for comfort and warmth. Waterproof pad protects underlying surfaces.
10. Check the position of drains, tubes, or other adjuncts before removing the dressing. Put on clean, disposable gloves and loosen tape on the old dressings. If necessary, use an adhesive remover to help get the tape off.	Checking ensures that a drain is not removed accidentally if one is present. Gloves protect the nurse from contaminated dressings and prevent the spread of microorganisms. Adhesive-tape remover helps reduce patient discomfort during dressing removal.
11. Carefully remove the soiled dressings. If there is resistance, use a silicone-based adhesive remover to help remove the tape. If any part of the dressing sticks to the underlying skin, use small amounts of sterile saline to help loosen and remove it.	Cautious removal of the dressing is more comfortable for the patient and ensures that any drain present is not removed. A silicone-based adhesive remover allows for the easy, rapid, and painless removal without the associated problems of skin stripping (Denyer, 2011; Benbow, 2011). Sterile saline moistens the dressing for easier removal and minimizes damage and pain.
12. After removing the dressing, note the presence, amount, type, color, and odor of any drainage on the dressings. Place soiled dressings in the appropriate waste receptacle. Remove your gloves and dispose of them in an appropriate waste receptacle.	The presence of drainage should be documented. Proper disposal of soiled dressings and used gloves prevents the spread of microorganisms.

ACTION	RATIONALE

13. Inspect the wound site for size, appearance, and drainage. Assess if any pain is present. Check the status of sutures, adhesive closure strips, staples, and drains or tubes, if present. Note any problems to include in your documentation.

Wound healing or the presence of irritation or infection should be documented.

14. **Using sterile technique, prepare a sterile work area and open the needed supplies.**

Supplies are within easy reach and sterility is maintained.

15. Open the sterile cleaning solution. Depending on the amount of cleaning needed, the solution might be poured directly over gauze sponges over a container for small cleaning jobs, or into a basin for more complex or larger cleaning.

Sterility of dressings and solution is maintained.

16. Put on sterile gloves. Alternately, clean gloves (clean technique) may be used when cleaning a chronic wound or pressure ulcer.

Use of sterile gloves maintains surgical asepsis and sterile technique and reduces the risk for spreading microorganisms. Clean technique is appropriate for cleaning chronic wounds or pressure ulcers.

17. Clean the wound. **Clean the wound from top to bottom and from the center to the outside.** Following this pattern, use new gauze for each wipe, placing the used gauze in the waste receptacle. Alternately, spray the wound from top to bottom with a commercially prepared wound cleanser.

Cleaning from top to bottom and center to outside ensures that cleaning occurs from the least to most contaminated area and a previously cleaned area is not contaminated again. Using a single gauze for each wipe ensures that the previously cleaned area is not contaminated again.

18. Once the wound is cleaned, dry the area using a gauze sponge in the same manner. Apply ointment or perform other treatments, as ordered.

Moisture provides a medium for growth of microorganisms. The growth of microorganisms may be inhibited and the healing process improved with the use

ACTION	RATIONALE
	of ordered ointments or other applications.
19. If a drain is in use at the wound location, clean around the drain. Refer to Skills 50, 51, 52, and 53.	Cleaning the insertion site helps prevent infection.
20. Apply a layer of dry, sterile dressing over the wound. Forceps may be used to apply the dressing.	Primary dressing serves as a wick for drainage. Use of forceps helps ensure that sterile technique is maintained.
21. Place a second layer of gauze over the wound site, as necessary.	A second layer provides for increased absorption of drainage.
22. Apply a surgical or abdominal pad (ABD) over the gauze at the site as the outermost layer of the dressing, as necessary.	The dressing acts as additional protection for the wound against microorganisms in the environment and increased absorption of drainage.
23. Remove and discard gloves. Apply tape, Montgomery straps, or roller gauze to secure the dressings. Alternately, many commercial wound products are self-adhesive and do not require additional tape.	Proper disposal of gloves prevents the spread of microorganisms. Tape or other securing products are easier to apply after gloves have been removed.
24. After securing the dressing, label it with date and time. Remove all remaining equipment; place the patient in a comfortable position, with side rails up and bed in the lowest position.	Recording date and time provides communication and demonstrates adherence to plan of care. Proper patient and bed positioning promotes safety and comfort.
25. Remove PPE, if used. Perform hand hygiene.	Removing PPE properly reduces the risk for infection transmission and contamination of other items. Hand hygiene prevents the spread of microorganisms.
26. Check all wound dressings every shift. More frequent checks may be needed if the wound is more complex or dressings become saturated quickly.	Checking dressings ensures the assessment of changes in patient condition and timely intervention to prevent complications.

EVALUATION
- Patient exhibits a clean, intact wound with a clean dressing in place.
- Wound is free of contamination and trauma.
- Patient reports little to no pain or discomfort during care.
- Patient demonstrates signs and symptoms of progressive wound healing.

DOCUMENTATION
- Document the location of the wound and that the dressing was removed. Record your assessment of the wound, including approximation of wound edges; presence of sutures, staples, or adhesive closure strips; and the condition of the surrounding skin. Note if redness, edema, or drainage is observed. Document cleansing of the incision with normal saline and any application of antibiotic ointment as ordered. Record the type of dressing that was reapplied. Note pertinent patient and family education and any patient reaction to this procedure, including patient's pain level and effectiveness of nonpharmacologic interventions or analgesia if administered.

SKILL 56 | APPLYING A HYDROCOLLOID DRESSING

Hydrocolloid dressings are wafer-shaped dressings that come in many shapes, sizes, and thicknesses. An adhesive backing provides adherence to the wound and surrounding skin. They absorb drainage, maintain a moist wound surface, and decrease the risk for infection by covering the wound surface. Many commercially prepared dressing and wound care products are applied in a similar manner. It is very important for the nurse to be aware of the products available in a particular facility and be familiar with the indications for, and correct use of, each type of dressing and wound care product.

DELEGATION CONSIDERATIONS

Wound care and procedures requiring the use of a sterile field and other sterile items are not delegated to nursing assistive personnel (NAP) or unlicensed assistive personnel (UAP). In some settings, such as long-term care, the application of a wound dressing using clean technique for a chronic wound may be delegated to NAPs/UAPs. However, the assessment of the wound is performed by the RN. Depending on the state's nurse practice act and the organization's policies and procedures, these procedures may be delegated to licensed practical/vocational nurses (LPN/LVNs). The decision to delegate must be based on careful analysis of the patient's needs and circumstances, as well as the qualifications of the person to whom the task is being delegated. Refer to the Delegation Guidelines in Appendix A.

EQUIPMENT

- Hydrocolloid dressing
- Clean, disposable gloves
- Sterile gloves, if indicated
- Additional PPE, as indicated
- Sterile dressing instrument set or suture set (for the scissors and forceps)
- Sterile cleaning solution as ordered (commonly 0.9% normal saline solution)
- Skin-protectant wipes
- Additional supplies needed for wound cleansing
- Sterile cotton-tipped applicators
- Waterproof pad
- Bath blanket
- Measuring tape or other supplies, such as sterile flexible applicator, for assessing wound measurements, as indicated

ASSESSMENT

- Assess the situation to determine the need for a dressing change. Check the date when the current dressing (if present) was placed.
- Confirm any medical orders relevant to wound care and any wound care included in the nursing plan of care.
- Assess the patient's level of comfort and the need for analgesics before wound care. Assess if the patient experienced any pain related to prior dressing changes and the effectiveness of interventions employed to minimize the patient's pain.
- Assess the current dressing to determine if it is intact. Assess for excess drainage or bleeding or saturation of the dressing. Inspect the wound and the surrounding tissue.
- Assess the location, appearance of the wound, stage (if appropriate), drainage, and types of tissue present in the wound. Measure the wound. Note the stage of the healing process and characteristics of any drainage. Also assess the surrounding skin for color, temperature, and edema, ecchymosis, or maceration.

NURSING DIAGNOSIS

- Impaired Skin Integrity
- Chronic Pain
- Impaired Tissue Integrity

OUTCOME IDENTIFICATION AND PLANNING

- Procedure is accomplished without contaminating the wound area, causing trauma to the wound, and/or causing the patient to experience pain or discomfort.
- Sterile technique is maintained (if appropriate) and wound healing is promoted.
- Surrounding skin is without signs of irritation, infection, and maceration; and wound continues to show signs of progression of healing.

IMPLEMENTATION

ACTION	RATIONALE
1. Review the medical orders for wound care or the nursing plan of care related to wound care. Gather necessary supplies.	Reviewing the order and plan of care validates the correct patient and correct procedure. Preparation promotes efficient time management and an organized approach to the task.
2. Perform hand hygiene and put on PPE, if indicated.	Hand hygiene and PPE prevent the spread of microorganisms. PPE is required based on transmission precautions.
3. Identify the patient.	Identifying the patient ensures the right patient receives the intervention and helps prevent errors.
4. Assemble equipment on overbed table within reach.	Organization facilitates performance of the task.
5. Close the curtains around the bed and close the door to the room if possible. Explain what you are going to do and why you are going to do it to the patient.	This ensures the patient's privacy. Explanation relieves anxiety and facilitates cooperation.
6. Assess the patient for possible need for nonpharmacologic pain-reducing interventions or analgesic medication before wound care dressing change. Administer appropriate prescribed analgesic. Allow enough time for the analgesic to achieve its effectiveness before beginning the procedure.	Pain is a subjective experience influenced by past experience. Wound care and dressing changes may cause pain for some patients.
7. Place a waste receptacle or bag at a convenient location for use during the procedure.	Having a waste container handy means the soiled dressing may be discarded easily, without the spread of microorganisms.
8. Adjust the bed to a comfortable working height, usually elbow height of the caregiver (VISN 8, 2009).	Having the bed at the proper height prevents back and muscle strain.

ACTION	RATIONALE
9. Assist the patient to a comfortable position that provides easy access to the wound area. Position the patient so the wound cleanser or irrigation solution will flow from the clean end of the wound toward the dirtier end, if being used (see Skill 55 for wound cleansing and Skill 185 for irrigation techniques). Use the bath blanket to cover any exposed area other than the wound. Place a waterproof pad under the wound site.	Patient positioning and use of a bath blanket provide for comfort and warmth. Gravity directs the flow of liquid from the least contaminated to the most contaminated area. Waterproof pad protects underlying surfaces.
10. Put on clean gloves. Carefully and gently remove the soiled dressings. If there is resistance, use a silicone-based adhesive remover to help remove the tape. If any part of the dressing sticks to the underlying skin, use small amounts of sterile saline to help loosen and remove it.	Gloves protect the nurse from handling contaminated dressings. Cautious removal of the dressing is more comfortable for the patient and ensures that any drain present is not removed. A silicone-based adhesive remover allows for the easy, rapid, and painless removal without the associated problems of skin stripping (Denyer, 2011; Benbow, 2011). Sterile saline moistens the dressing for easier removal and minimizes damage and pain.
11. After removing the dressing, note the presence, amount, type, color, and odor of any drainage on the dressings. Place soiled dressings in the appropriate waste receptacle.	The presence of drainage should be documented. Discarding dressings appropriately prevents the spread of microorganisms.
12. Assess the wound for appearance, stage, presence of eschar, granulation tissue, epithelialization, undermining, tunneling, necrosis, sinus tract, and drainage. Assess the appearance of the surrounding tissue. Measure the wound.	This information provides evidence about the wound healing process and/or the presence of infection.

ACTION	RATIONALE
13. Remove your gloves and put them in the receptacle.	Discarding gloves prevents the spread of microorganisms.
14. Set up a sterile field, if indicated, and wound cleaning supplies. Put on sterile gloves. Alternately, clean gloves (clean technique) may be used when cleaning a chronic wound or pressure ulcer.	Sterile gloves maintain surgical asepsis. Clean technique is appropriate for cleaning chronic wounds or pressure ulcers.
15. Clean the wound. Refer to Skill 55. Alternately, irrigate the wound, as ordered or required (see Skill 185).	Cleaning the wound removes previous drainage and wound debris.
16. Dry the surrounding skin with gauze dressings.	Moisture provides a medium for growth of microorganisms. Excess moisture can contribute to skin irritation and breakdown.
17. Apply a skin protectant to the surrounding skin.	A skin protectant prevents skin irritation and breakdown.
18. Cut the dressing to size, if indicated, using sterile scissors. Size the dressing generously, allowing at least a 1-inch margin of healthy skin around the wound to be covered with the dressing.	These actions ensure proper adherence, coverage of the wound, and wear of the dressing.
19. Remove the release paper from the adherent side of the dressing. Apply the dressing to the wound without stretching the dressing. Smooth wrinkles as the dressing is applied (Figure 1).	Proper application prevents shearing force on the wound and minimizes irritation.

FIGURE 1 Hydrocolloid dressing in place.

ACTION	RATIONALE
20. If necessary, secure the dressing edges with tape. Apply additional skin barrier to the areas to be covered with tape, if necessary. Dressings that are near the anus need to have the edges taped. Apply additional skin barrier to the areas to be covered with tape, if necessary.	Taping helps keep the dressing intact. Skin protectant prevents surrounding skin irritation and breakdown. Taping the edges of dressings near the anus prevents wound contamination from fecal material.
21. After securing the dressing, label it with date and time. Remove all remaining equipment; place the patient in a comfortable position, with side rails up and bed in the lowest position.	Recording date and time provides communication and demonstrates adherence to plan of care. Proper patient and bed positioning promotes safety and comfort.
22. Remove PPE, if used. Perform hand hygiene.	Removing PPE properly reduces the risk for infection transmission and contamination of other items. Hand hygiene prevents the spread of microorganisms.
23. Check all wound dressings every shift. More frequent checks may be needed if the wound is more complex or dressings become saturated quickly.	Checking dressings ensures the assessment of changes in patient condition and timely intervention to prevent complications.

EVALUATION

- Procedure is accomplished without contaminating the wound area, causing trauma to the wound, and/or causing the patient to experience pain or discomfort.
- Sterile technique is maintained (if appropriate).
- Wound healing is promoted.
- Surrounding skin is without signs of irritation, infection, and maceration; and the wound continues to show signs of progression of healing.

DOCUMENTATION

- Document the location of the wound and that the dressing was removed. Record your assessment of the wound, including evidence of granulation tissue, presence of necrotic tissue, stage (if appropriate), and characteristics of drainage. Include the appearance of the surrounding skin. Document the cleansing or irrigation of the wound and solution used. Record the type of hydrocolloid dressing that was applied. Note pertinent patient and family education and any patient reaction to this procedure, including the patient's pain level and effectiveness of nonpharmacologic interventions or analgesia if administered.

SKILL 57 APPLYING A SALINE-MOISTENED DRESSING

Gauze or other dressing materials can be moistened with saline to keep the surface of open wounds moist. A saline-moistened dressing promotes moist wound healing and protects the wound from contamination and trauma. A moist wound surface enhances the cellular migration necessary for tissue repair and healing. It is important that the dressing material be moist, not wet, when placed in open wounds. Dressing materials are soaked in normal saline solution and squeezed to remove excess saline so that the dressing is only slightly moist. The dressing can be loosely packed in the wound bed, if appropriate, and then covered with a secondary dressing to absorb drainage. In addition, many commercially prepared wound care products are also available to maintain a moist wound environment. These dressing and wound care products are applied in a similar manner. It is very important for the nurse to be aware of the products available in a particular facility and to be familiar with the indications for, and correct use of, each type of dressing and wound care product.

DELEGATION CONSIDERATIONS

Wound care and procedures requiring the use of a sterile field and other sterile items are not delegated to nursing assistive personnel (NAP) or to unlicensed assistive personnel (UAP). Depending on the state's nurse practice act and the organization's policies and procedures, these procedures may be delegated to licensed practical/vocational nurses (LPN/LVNs). The decision to delegate must be based on careful analysis of the patient's needs and circumstances, as well as the qualifications of the person to whom the task is being delegated. Refer to the Delegation Guidelines in Appendix A.

EQUIPMENT

- Clean, disposable gloves
- Sterile gloves, if indicated
- Additional PPE, as indicated
- Sterile dressing set or suture set (for the sterile scissors and forceps)
- Sterile thin-mesh gauze dressing for packing, if ordered
- Sterile gauze dressings
- Surgical or abdominal pads
- Skin-protectant wipes
- Sterile basin
- Sterile cleaning solution as ordered (commonly 0.9% normal saline solution)
- Sterile saline

- Tape or ties
- Plastic bag or other appropriate waste container for soiled dressings
- Sterile cotton-tipped applicators
- Supplies for wound cleansing or irrigation, as necessary
- Waterproof pad and bath blanket

ASSESSMENT

- Assess the situation to determine the need for a dressing change. Confirm any medical orders relevant to wound care and any wound care included in the nursing plan of care.
- Assess the patient's level of comfort and the need for analgesics before wound care. Assess if the patient experienced any pain related to previous dressing changes and the effectiveness of interventions employed to minimize the patient's pain.
- Assess the current dressing to determine if it is intact. Assess for excess drainage or bleeding or saturation of the dressing. Inspect the wound and the surrounding tissue.
- Assess the location, appearance of the wound, wound stage (if appropriate), drainage, and types of tissue present in the wound. Measure the wound. Note the stage of the healing process and characteristics of any drainage. Also assess the surrounding skin for color, temperature, and edema, ecchymosis, or maceration.

NURSING DIAGNOSIS

- Disturbed Body Image
- Impaired Skin Integrity
- Acute Pain
- Impaired Tissue Integrity

OUTCOME IDENTIFICATION AND PLANNING

- Procedure is accomplished without contaminating the wound area, causing trauma to the wound, and/or causing the patient to experience pain or discomfort.
- Wound healing is promoted.
- Surrounding skin is without signs of irritation, infection, and maceration.
- Wound continues to show signs of progression of healing.

IMPLEMENTATION

ACTION	RATIONALE
1. Review the medical orders for wound care or the nursing plan of care related to wound care. Gather necessary supplies.	Reviewing the order and plan of care validates the correct patient and correct procedure. Preparation promotes efficient time management and an organized approach to the task.

ACTION	RATIONALE
2. Perform hand hygiene and put on PPE, if indicated.	Hand hygiene and PPE prevent the spread of microorganisms. PPE is required based on transmission precautions.
3. Identify the patient.	Identifying the patient ensures the right patient receives the intervention and helps prevent errors.
4. Assemble equipment on overbed table within reach.	Organization facilitates performance of the task.
5. Close the curtains around the bed and close the door to the room if possible. Explain what you are going to do and why you are going to do it to the patient.	This ensures the patient's privacy. Explanation relieves anxiety and facilitates cooperation.
6. Assess the patient for possible need for nonpharmacologic pain-reducing interventions or analgesic medication before wound care dressing change. Administer appropriate prescribed analgesic. Allow enough time for the analgesic to achieve its effectiveness.	Pain is a subjective experience influenced by past experience. Wound care and dressing changes may cause pain for some patients.
7. Place a waste receptacle or bag at a convenient location for use during the procedure.	Having a waste container handy means the soiled dressing may be discarded easily, without the spread of microorganisms.
8. Adjust the bed to a comfortable working height, usually elbow height of the caregiver (VISN 8, 2009).	Having the bed at the proper height prevents back and muscle strain.
9. Assist the patient to a comfortable position that provides easy access to the wound area. Position the patient so the wound cleanser or irrigation solution will flow from the clean end of the wound toward the dirtier end, if being	Patient positioning and use of a bath blanket provide for comfort and warmth. Gravity directs the flow of liquid from the least contaminated to the most contaminated area. Waterproof pad protects underlying surfaces.

ACTION	RATIONALE

used (see Skill 55 for wound cleansing and Skill 185 for irrigation techniques). Use the bath blanket to cover any exposed area other than the wound. Place a waterproof pad under the wound site.

10. Put on clean gloves. Carefully and gently remove the soiled dressings. If there is resistance, use a silicone-based adhesive remover to help remove the tape. If any part of the dressing sticks to the underlying skin, use small amounts of sterile saline to help loosen and remove it.

Gloves protect the nurse from handling contaminated dressings. Cautious removal of the dressing is more comfortable for the patient and ensures that any drain present is not removed. A silicone-based adhesive remover allows for the easy, rapid, and painless removal without the associated problems of skin stripping (Denyer, 2011; Benbow, 2011). Sterile saline moistens the dressing for easier removal and minimizes damage and pain.

11. After removing the dressing, note the presence, amount, type, color, and odor of any drainage on the dressings. Place soiled dressings in the appropriate waste receptacle.

The presence of drainage should be documented. Discarding dressings appropriately prevents the spread of microorganisms.

12. Assess the wound for appearance, stage, the presence of eschar, granulation tissue, epithelialization, undermining, tunneling, necrosis, sinus tract, and drainage. Assess the appearance of the surrounding tissue. Measure the wound.

This information provides evidence about the wound healing process and/or the presence of infection.

13. Remove your gloves and put them in the receptacle.

Discarding gloves prevents the spread of microorganisms.

14. Using sterile technique, open the supplies and dressings. Place the fine-mesh gauze into the basin and pour the ordered solution over the mesh to saturate it.

Gauze touching the wound surface must be moistened to increase the absorptive ability and promote healing.

ACTION	RATIONALE
15. Put on sterile gloves. Alternately, clean gloves (clean technique) may be used to clean a chronic wound or pressure ulcer.	Sterile gloves maintain surgical asepsis. Clean technique is appropriate when cleaning chronic wounds and pressure ulcers.
16. Clean the wound. Refer to Skill 55. Alternately, irrigate the wound, as ordered or required (see Skill 185).	Cleaning the wound removes previous drainage and wound debris.
17. Dry the surrounding skin with sterile gauze dressings.	Moisture provides a medium for growth of microorganisms.
18. Apply a skin protectant to the surrounding skin, if needed.	A skin protectant prevents skin irritation and breakdown.
19. If not already on, put on sterile gloves. Squeeze excess fluid from the gauze dressing. Unfold and fluff the dressing.	Sterile gloves prevent contamination of the dressing material. The gauze provides a thin, moist layer to contact all the wound surfaces.
20. Gently press to loosely pack the moistened gauze into the wound. If necessary, use the forceps or cotton-tipped applicator to press the gauze into all wound surfaces.	The dressing provides a moist environment for all wound surfaces. Avoid overpacking the gauze; loosely pack to prevent too much pressure in the wound bed, which could impede wound healing.
21. Apply several dry, sterile gauze pads over the wet gauze.	Dry gauze absorbs excess moisture and drainage.
22. Place the ABD pad over the gauze.	The ABD pad prevents contamination.
23. Remove and discard gloves. Apply tape, Montgomery straps, or roller gauze to secure the dressings. Alternately, many commercial wound products are self-adhesive and do not require additional tape.	Proper disposal of gloves prevents the spread of microorganisms. Tape or other securing products are easier to apply after gloves have been removed.
24. After securing the dressing, label dressing with date and time. Remove all remaining equipment; place the patient	Recording date and time provides communication and demonstrates adherence to plan of care. Proper patient and bed

ACTION	RATIONALE
in a comfortable position, with side rails up and bed in the lowest position.	positioning promotes safety and comfort.
25. Remove PPE, if used. Perform hand hygiene.	Removing PPE properly reduces the risk for infection transmission and contamination of other items. Hand hygiene prevents the spread of microorganisms.
26. Check all wound dressings every shift. More frequent checks may be needed if the wound is more complex or dressings become saturated quickly.	Checking dressings ensures the assessment of changes in patient condition and timely intervention to prevent complications.

EVALUATION

- The expected outcome when applying a saline-moistened dressing is met when the procedure is accomplished without contaminating the wound area, causing trauma to the wound, and/or causing the patient to experience pain or discomfort. Other outcomes are met when sterile technique is maintained (if appropriate); wound healing is promoted; the surrounding skin is without signs of irritation, infection, and maceration; and the wound continues to show signs of progression of healing.

DOCUMENTATION

- Document the location of the wound and that the dressing was removed. Record your assessment of the wound, including evidence of granulation tissue, presence of necrotic tissue, stage (if appropriate), and characteristics of drainage. Include the appearance of the surrounding skin. Document the cleansing or irrigation of the wound and solution used. Record the type of dressing that was reapplied. Note pertinent patient and family education and any patient reaction to this procedure, including patient's pain level and effectiveness of nonpharmacologic interventions or analgesia if administered.

SKILL 58 INSTILLING EAR DROPS

Drugs are instilled into the auditory canal for their local effect. They are used to soften wax, relieve pain, apply local anesthesia, and treat infections. The tympanic membrane separates the external ear from the middle ear. Normally, it is intact and closes the entrance to the middle ear completely. If it is ruptured or has been opened by surgical intervention, the middle ear and the inner ear have a direct passage to the external ear. When this occurs, perform instillations with the greatest of care to prevent forcing materials from the outer ear into the middle ear and the inner ear. Use sterile technique to prevent infection.

DELEGATION CONSIDERATIONS

The administration of medication via drops in the ear is not delegated to nursing assistive personnel (NAP) or to unlicensed assistive personnel (UAP). Depending on the state's nurse practice act and the organization's policies and procedures, the administration of ear drops may be delegated to licensed practical/vocational nurses (LPN/LVNs). The decision to delegate must be based on careful analysis of the patient's needs and circumstances, as well as the qualifications of the person to whom the task is being delegated. Refer to the Delegation Guidelines in Appendix A.

EQUIPMENT

- Medication (warmed to 37°C [98.6°F])
- Dropper
- Tissue
- Cotton balls (optional)
- Gloves
- Additional PPE, as indicated
- Washcloth (optional)
- Normal saline solution
- Computer-generated Medication Administration Record (CMAR) or Medication Administration Record (MAR)

ASSESSMENT

- Assess the affected ear for redness, erythema, edema, drainage, or tenderness.
- Assess the patient for allergies.
- Verify patient name, dose, route, and time of administration.
- Assess the patient's knowledge of medication and procedure. If the patient has a knowledge deficit about the medication, this may be an appropriate time to begin education about the medication.
- Assess the patient's ability to cooperate with the procedure.

NURSING DIAGNOSIS

- Anxiety
- Risk for Injury
- Acute Pain

OUTCOME IDENTIFICATION AND PLANNING

- Drops are administered successfully into the ear.
- Patient understands the rationale for the ear drop instillation and has decreased anxiety.
- Patient remains free from pain.
- Patient experiences no allergy response or injury.

IMPLEMENTATION

ACTION	RATIONALE
1. Gather equipment. Check medication order against the original order in the medical record, according to facility policy. Clarify any inconsistencies. Check the patient's chart for allergies.	This comparison helps to identify errors that may have occurred when orders were transcribed. The primary care provider's order is the legal record of medication orders for each facility.
2. Know the actions, special nursing considerations, safe dose ranges, purpose of administration, and adverse effects of the medication to be administered. Consider the appropriateness of the medication for this patient.	This knowledge aids the nurse in evaluating the therapeutic effect of the medication in relation to the patient's disorder and can also be used to educate the patient about the medication.
3. Perform hand hygiene.	Hand hygiene prevents the spread of microorganisms.
4. Move the medication cart to the outside of the patient's room or prepare for administration in the medication area.	Organization facilitates error-free administration and saves time.
5. Unlock the medication cart or drawer. Enter pass code and scan employee identification, if required.	Locking the cart or drawer safeguards each patient's medication supply. Hospital accrediting organizations require medication carts to be locked when not in use. Entering pass code and scanning ID allows only authorized users into the system and identifies the user for documentation by the computer.

ACTION	RATIONALE
6. **Prepare medications for one patient at a time.**	This prevents errors in medication administration.
7. Read the CMAR/MAR and select the proper medication from the patient's medication drawer or unit stock.	This is the *first* check of the label.
8. Compare the label with the CMAR/MAR. Check expiration dates and perform calculations, if necessary. Scan the bar code on the package, if required.	This is the *second* check of the label. Verify calculations with another nurse to ensure safety, if necessary.
9. **Depending on facility policy, the third check of the label may occur at this point. If so, when all medications for one patient have been prepared, recheck the labels with the CMAR/MAR before taking the medications to the patient.**	This *third* check ensures accuracy and helps to prevent errors. *Note:* Many facilities require the *third* check to occur at the bedside, after identifying the patient and before administration.
10. Lock the medication cart before leaving it.	Locking the cart or drawer safeguards the patient's medication supply. Hospital accrediting organizations require medication carts to be locked when not in use.
11. Transport medications to the patient's bedside carefully, and keep the medications in sight at all times.	Careful handling and close observation prevent accidental or deliberate disarrangement of medications.
12. **Ensure that the patient receives the medications at the correct time.**	Check agency policy, which may allow for administration within a period of 30 minutes before or 30 minutes after the designated time.
13. Perform hand hygiene and put on PPE, if indicated.	Hand hygiene and PPE prevent the spread of microorganisms. PPE is required based on transmission precautions.

ACTION	RATIONALE

14. **Identify the patient.** 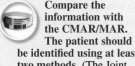 **Compare the information with the CMAR/MAR. The patient should be identified using at least two methods.** (The Joint Commission, 2013):

Identifying the patient ensures the right patient receives the medications and helps prevent errors. The patient's room number or physical location is not used as an identifier (The Joint Commission, 2013). Replace the identification band if it is missing or inaccurate in any way.

   a. Check the name on the patient's identification band.
   b. Check the identification number on the patient's identification band.
   c. Check the birth date on the patient's identification band.
   d. Ask the patient to state his or her name and birth date, based on facility policy.

This requires a response from the patient, but illness and strange surroundings often cause patients to be confused.

15. **Complete necessary assessments before administering medications. Check the patient's allergy bracelet or ask the patient about allergies. Explain the purpose and action of each medication to the patient.**

Assessment is a prerequisite to administration of medications.

16. Scan the patient's bar code on the identification band, if required.

Provides an additional check to ensure that the medication is given to the right patient.

17. **Based on facility policy, the third check of the label may occur at this point. If so, recheck the labels with the CMAR/MAR before administering the medications to the patient.**

Many facilities require the *third* check to occur at the bedside, after identifying the patient and before administration. If facility policy directs the *third* check at this time, this *third* check ensures accuracy and helps to prevent errors.

18. Put on gloves.

Gloves protect the nurse from potential contact with mucous membranes and body fluids.

ACTION	RATIONALE
19. Cleanse external ear of any drainage with cotton ball or washcloth moistened with normal saline.	Debris and drainage may prevent some of the medication from entering the ear canal.
20. Place patient on his or her unaffected side in bed, or, if ambulatory, have patient sit with head well tilted to the side so that the affected ear is uppermost.	This positioning prevents the drops from escaping from the ear.
21. Draw up the amount of solution needed in the dropper. Do not return excess medication to stock bottle. A pre-packaged, monodrip plastic container may also be used.	Risk for contamination is increased when medication is returned to the stock bottle.
22. Straighten auditory canal by pulling cartilaginous portion of pinna up and back for an adult.	Pulling on the pinna as described helps to straighten the canal properly for ear drop instillation.
23. Hold dropper in the ear with its tip above the auditory canal. Do not touch the dropper to the ear. For an infant or an irrational or confused patient, protect the dropper with a piece of soft tubing to help prevent injury to the ear.	By holding the dropper in the ear, most of the medication will enter the ear canal. Touching the dropper to the ear contaminates the dropper and medication. The hard tip of the dropper can damage the tympanic membrane if it is jabbed into the ear.
24. **Allow drops to fall on the side of the canal. Avoid instilling in the middle of the canal, to avoid instilling directly onto the tympanic membrane.**	It is uncomfortable for the patient if the drops fall directly onto the tympanic membrane.
25. Release pinna after instilling drops, and have patient maintain the head position to prevent escape of medication.	Medication should remain in ear canal for at least 5 minutes.
26. Gently press on the tragus a few times.	Pressing on the tragus causes medication from the canal to move toward the tympanic membrane.

ACTION	RATIONALE
27. If ordered, loosely insert a cotton ball into the ear canal.	A cotton ball can help prevent medication from leaking out of the ear canal.
28. Remove gloves. Assist the patient to a comfortable position.	This ensures patient comfort.
29. Remove additional PPE, if used. Perform hand hygiene.	Removing PPE properly reduces the risk for infection transmission and contamination of other items. Hand hygiene prevents the spread of microorganisms.
30. Document the administration of the medication immediately after administration.	Timely documentation helps to ensure patient safety.
31. Evaluate the patient's response to medication within an appropriate time frame.	The patient needs to be evaluated for therapeutic and adverse effects from the medication.

EVALUATION

- Patient receives the ear drops successfully.
- Patient verbalizes an understanding of the rationale for ear drop instillation.
- Patient exhibits no or decreased anxiety.
- Patient experiences no or minimal pain.
- Patient experiences no allergy response or injury.

DOCUMENTATION

- Document the administration of the medication immediately after administration, including date, time, dose, route of administration, and site of administration, specifically right, left, or both ears, on the CMAR/MAR or record using the required format. If using a bar-code system, medication administration is automatically recorded when the bar code is scanned. PRN medications require documentation of the reason for administration. Prompt recording avoids the possibility of accidentally repeating the administration of the drug. Document pre- and post-administration assessments, characteristics of any drainage, and the patient's response to the treatment, if appropriate. If the drug was refused or omitted, record this in the appropriate area on the medication record and notify the primary care provider. This verifies the reason medication was omitted and ensures that the primary care provider is aware of the patient's condition.

SKILL 59 | ADMINISTERING AN EAR IRRIGATION

Irrigations of the external auditory canal are ordinarily performed for cleaning purposes or for applying heat to the area. Typically, a normal saline solution is used, although an antiseptic solution may be indicated for local action. To prevent pain, make sure the irrigation solution is at least room temperature. Usually, an irrigation syringe is used. However, an irrigating container with tubing and an ear tip may also be used, especially if the purpose of the irrigation is to apply heat to the area.

DELEGATION CONSIDERATIONS

The administration of an irrigation of the ear is not delegated to nursing assistive personnel (NAP) or to unlicensed assistive personnel (UAP). Depending on the state's nurse practice act and the organization's policies and procedures, the irrigation of the ear may be delegated to licensed practical/vocational nurses (LPN/LVNs). The decision to delegate must be based on careful analysis of the patient's needs and circumstances, as well as the qualifications of the person to whom the task is being delegated. Refer to the Delegation Guidelines in Appendix A.

EQUIPMENT

- Prescribed irrigating solution (warmed to 37°C [98.6°F])
- Irrigation set (container and irrigating or bulb syringe)
- Waterproof pad
- Emesis basin
- Cotton-tipped applicators
- Gloves
- Additional PPE, as indicated
- Cotton balls
- Computer-generated Medication Administration Record (CMAR) or Medication Administration Record (MAR)

ASSESSMENT

- Assess the affected ear for redness, erythema, edema, drainage, or tenderness.
- Assess the patient's ability to hear.
- Assess the patient for allergies.
- Verify patient name, dose, route, and time of administration.
- Assess the patient's knowledge of medication and procedure. If the patient has a knowledge deficit about the medication, this may be an appropriate time to begin education about the medication.
- Assess the patient's ability to cooperate with the procedure.

NURSING DIAGNOSIS

- Acute Pain
- Risk for Injury
- Deficient Knowledge

OUTCOME IDENTIFICATION AND PLANNING

- Irrigation is administered successfully.
- Patient remains free from pain and injury.
- Patient experiences improved hearing.
- Patient understands the rationale for the procedure.

IMPLEMENTATION

ACTION	RATIONALE
1. Gather equipment. Check medication order against the original order in the medical record, according to facility policy. Clarify any inconsistencies. Check the patient's chart for allergies.	This comparison helps to identify errors that may have occurred when orders were transcribed. The primary care provider's order is the legal record of medication orders for each facility.
2. Know the actions, special nursing considerations, safe dose ranges, purpose of administration, and adverse effects of the medication to be administered. Consider the appropriateness of the medication for this patient.	This knowledge aids the nurse in evaluating the therapeutic effect of the medication in relation to the patient's disorder and can also be used to educate the patient about the medication.
3. Perform hand hygiene.	Hand hygiene prevents the spread of microorganisms.
4. Move the medication cart to the outside of the patient's room or prepare for administration in the medication area.	Organization facilitates error-free administration and saves time.
5. Unlock the medication cart or drawer. Enter pass code and scan employee identification, if required.	Locking the cart or drawer safeguards each patient's medication supply. Hospital accrediting organizations require medication carts to be locked when not in use. Entering pass code and scanning ID allows only authorized users into the computer system and identifies the user for documentation by the computer.

ACTION	RATIONALE
6. **Prepare medications for one patient at a time.**	This prevents errors in medication administration.
7. Read the CMAR/MAR and select the proper medication from unit stock or the patient's medication drawer.	This is the *first* check of the label.
8. Compare the label with the CMAR/MAR. Check expiration dates and perform calculations, if necessary. Scan the bar code on the package, if required.	This is the *second* check of the label. Verify calculations with another nurse to ensure safety, if necessary.
9. **Depending on facility policy, the third check of the label may occur at this point. If so, when all medications for one patient have been prepared, recheck the labels with the CMAR/MAR before taking the medications to the patient.**	This *third* check ensures accuracy and helps to prevent errors. *Note:* Many facilities require the *third* check to occur at the bedside, after identifying the patient and before administration.
10. Lock the medication cart before leaving it.	Locking the cart or drawer safeguards the patient's medication supply. Hospital accrediting organizations require medication carts to be locked when not in use.
11. Transport medications to the patient's bedside carefully, and keep the medications in sight at all times.	Careful handling and close observation prevent accidental or deliberate disarrangement of medications.
12. **Ensure that the patient receives the medications at the correct time.**	Check agency policy, which may allow for administration within a period of 30 minutes before or 30 minutes after the designated time.
13. Perform hand hygiene and put on PPE, if indicated.	Hand hygiene and PPE prevent the spread of microorganisms. PPE is required based on transmission precautions.

ACTION	RATIONALE

14. **Identify the patient.** 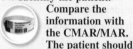 **Compare the information with the CMAR/MAR. The patient should be identified using at least two methods** (The Joint Commission, 2013):

Identifying the patient ensures the right patient receives the medications and helps prevent errors. The patient's room number or physical location is not used as an identifier (The Joint Commission, 2013). Replace the identification band if it is missing or inaccurate in any way.

   a. Check the name on the patient's identification band.

   b. Check the identification number on the patient's identification band.

   c. Check the birth date on the patient's identification band.

   d. Ask the patient to state his or her name and birth date, based on facility policy.

This requires a response from the patient, but illness and strange surroundings often cause patients to be confused.

15. Explain the procedure to the patient.

Explanation facilitates cooperation and reassures the patient.

16. Scan the patient's bar code on the identification band, if required.

Provides an additional check to ensure that the medication is given to the right patient.

17. Assemble equipment at patient's bedside.

This provides for an organized approach to the task.

18. Put on gloves.

Gloves protect the nurse from potential contact with contaminants and body fluids.

19. Have the patient sit up or lie with head tilted toward side of the affected ear. Protect the patient and bed with a waterproof pad. Have the patient support the basin under the ear to receive the irrigating solution.

Gravity causes the irrigating solution to flow from the ear to the basin.

20. Clean pinna and meatus of auditory canal, as necessary, with moistened cotton-tipped applicators dipped in warm tap water or the irrigating solution.

Materials lodged on the pinna and at the meatus may be washed into the ear.

ACTION	RATIONALE
21. Fill bulb syringe with warm solution. If an irrigating container is used, prime the tubing.	Priming the tubing allows air to escape from the tubing. Air forced into the ear canal is noisy and therefore unpleasant for the patient.
22. Straighten the auditory canal by pulling the cartilaginous portion of pinna up and back for an adult.	Straightening the ear canal allows solution to reach all areas of the canal easily.
23. **Direct a steady, slow stream of solution against the roof of the auditory canal, using only enough force to remove secretions. Do not occlude the auditory canal with the irrigating nozzle. Allow solution to flow out unimpeded.**	Directing the solution at the roof of the canal helps prevent injury to the tympanic membrane. Continuous in-and-out flow of the irrigating solution helps to prevent pressure in the canal.
24. When irrigation is complete, place a cotton ball loosely in the auditory meatus and have the patient lie on side of affected ear on a towel or absorbent pad.	The cotton ball absorbs excess fluid, and gravity allows the remaining solution in the canal to escape from the ear.
25. Remove gloves. Assist the patient to a comfortable position.	This ensures patient comfort.
26. Remove additional PPE, if used. Perform hand hygiene.	Removing PPE properly reduces the risk for infection transmission and contamination of other items. Hand hygiene prevents the spread of microorganisms.
27. Document the administration of the medication immediately after administration.	Timely documentation helps to ensure patient safety.
28. Evaluate the patient's response to the procedure. Return in 10 to 15 minutes and remove cotton ball and assess drainage. Evaluate the patient's response to the medication within an appropriate time frame.	The patient needs to be evaluated for any adverse effects from the procedure. Drainage or pain may indicate injury to the tympanic membrane. The patient needs to be evaluated for therapeutic and adverse effects from the medication.

EVALUATION

- Ear canal is irrigated successfully.
- Patient experiences no or minimal pain or discomfort.
- Patient's hearing is improved.
- Patient understands the rationale for the ear irrigation procedure.

DOCUMENTATION

- Document the procedure, site, the type of solution and volume used, length of time irrigation performed, pre- and postprocedure assessments, characteristics of any drainage, and the patient's response to the treatment.

SKILL 60   ASSISTING A PATIENT WITH EATING

The primary care provider will order a diet for the patient, based on the patient's condition. Many patients can independently meet their nutritional needs by feeding themselves. Other patients, especially the very young and some older adult patients, such as people with arthritis of the hands, may have some difficulty opening juice containers, and so on. Patients with paralysis of the hands or advanced dementia may be unable to feed themselves. For these patients, the nurse should provide assistance, as needed. This skill is frequently delegated to nursing assistants. However, the nurse is responsible for the initial and ongoing assessment of the patient for potential complications related to feeding. Before this skill can be delegated, it is paramount for the nurse to make sure that the nursing assistant has been educated to observe for any swallowing difficulties and has knowledge of aspiration precautions

DELEGATION CONSIDERATIONS

Assisting patients to eat may be delegated to nursing assistive personnel (NAP) or to unlicensed assistive personnel (UAP), as well as to licensed practical/vocational nurses (LPN/LVNs). See previous discussion. The decision to delegate must be based on careful analysis of the patient's needs and circumstances, as well as the qualifications of the person to whom the task is being delegated. Refer to the Delegation Guidelines in Appendix A.

EQUIPMENT

- Patient tray of food, based on prescribed diet
- Wet wipes for hand hygiene
- Mouth care materials
- Patient's dentures, eyeglasses, hearing aid, if needed
- Special adaptive utensils, as needed
- Napkins, protective covering or towel
- PPE, as indicated

ASSESSMENT

- Confirm the type of diet that has been ordered for the patient.
- Assess for any food allergies and religious or cultural preferences, as appropriate.
- Check to make sure the patient does not have any scheduled laboratory or diagnostic studies that may impact whether he/she is able to eat a meal.
- Assess for any swallowing difficulties.
- Assess the patient's abdomen.

NURSING DIAGNOSIS

- Feeding Self-Care Deficit
- Risk for Aspiration
- Impaired Swallowing

OUTCOME IDENTIFICATION AND PLANNING

- Patient consumes 50% to 60% of the contents of the meal tray.
- Patient does not aspirate during or after the meal.
- Patient expresses contentment related to eating, as appropriate.

IMPLEMENTATION

ACTION	RATIONALE
1. Check the medical order for the type of diet prescribed for the patient.	Ensures the correct diet for the patient.
2. Perform hand hygiene and put on PPE, if indicated.	Hand hygiene and PPE prevent the spread of microorganisms. PPE is required based on transmission precautions.
3. Identify the patient.	Identifying the patient ensures the right patient receives the intervention and helps prevent errors.
4. Explain the procedure to the patient.	Explanations provide reassurance and facilitate cooperation of the patient.
5. **Assess level of consciousness, for any physical limitations, decreased hearing or visual acuity. If patient uses a hearing aid or wears**	Alertness is necessary for the patient to swallow and consume food. Using a hearing aid, glasses, and dentures for chewing facilitates the intake of food.

ACTION	RATIONALE
glasses or dentures, provide, as needed. Ask if the patient has any cultural or religious preferences and food likes and dislikes, if possible.	Patient preferences should be considered in food selection as much as possible to increase the intake of food and maximize the benefit of the meal.
6. Pull the patient's bedside curtain. Assess the abdomen. Ask the patient if he/she has any nausea. Ask the patient if he/she has any difficulty swallowing. Assess the patient for nausea or pain and administer an antiemetic or analgesic, as needed.	Provides for privacy. A functioning GI tract is essential for digestion. The presence of pain or nausea will diminish appetite. If the patient is medicated, wait for the appropriate time for absorption of the medication before beginning the feeding.
7. Offer to assist the patient with any elimination needs.	Promotes comfort and may avoid interruptions for toileting during meals.
8. Provide hand hygiene and mouth care as needed.	May improve appetite and promote comfort.
9. Remove any bedpans or undesirable equipment and odors, if possible, from the vicinity where the meal will be eaten. Perform hand hygiene.	Unpleasant odors and equipment may decrease the patient's appetite. Hand hygiene prevents the spread of microorganisms.
10. Open the patient's bedside curtain. Assist to, or position the patient in, a high Fowler's or sitting position in the bed or chair. Position the bed in the low position if the patient remains in bed.	Proper positioning improves swallowing ability and reduces the risk of aspiration.
11. Place protective covering or towel over the patient if desired.	Prevents soiling of the patient's gown.
12. Check tray to make sure that it is the correct tray before serving. Place tray on the overbed table so the patient can see food if able. Ensure that hot foods are hot and cold foods are cold. Use caution with hot beverages, allowing sufficient time for	Ensures that the correct tray is given to the patient. Encouraging the patient choice promotes patient dignity and respect. Close observation is necessary to assess for signs of aspiration or difficulty with meal.

ACTION	RATIONALE
cooling, if needed. Ask the patient for his/her preference related to what foods are desired first. Cut food into small pieces, as needed. Observe swallowing ability throughout the meal.	
13. If possible, sit facing the patient while feeding is taking place. If the patient is able, encourage him/her to hold finger foods and feed self as much as possible. Converse with patient during the meal, as appropriate. If, however, the patient has dysphagia, limit questioning or conversation that would require patient response during eating. Play relaxation music if patient desires.	In general, optimal meal time involves social interaction and conversation. Talking during eating is contraindicated for patients with dysphagia, because of increased risk for aspiration.
14. Allow enough time for the patient to chew and swallow the food adequately. The patient may need to rest for short periods during eating.	Eating requires energy and many medical conditions can weaken patients. Rest can restore energy for eating.
15. When the meal is completed or the patient is unable to eat any more, remove the tray from the room. **Note the amount and types of food consumed. Note the volume of liquid consumed.**	Nutrition plays an important role in healing and overall health. If the patient is not eating enough to meet nutritional requirements, alternative methods need to be considered.
16. Reposition the overbed table, remove the protective covering, offer hand hygiene, as needed, and offer the bedpan. Assist the patient to a position of comfort and relaxation.	Promotes the comfort of the patient, meets possible elimination needs, and facilitates digestion.
17. Remove PPE, if used. Perform hand hygiene.	Removing PPE properly reduces the risk for infection transmission and contamination of other items. Hand hygiene prevents the spread of microorganisms.

EVALUATION

- Patient consumes an adequate amount of nutrients.
- Patient expresses an appetite for the food, relating likes and dislikes.
- Patient experiences no nausea, vomiting, or aspiration episodes.

DOCUMENTATION

- Document the condition of the abdomen. Record that head of bed was elevated to at least 30 to 45 degrees. Note any swallowing difficulties and the patient's response to the meal. Document the percentage of the intake from the meal. If the patient had a poor intake, document the need for further consultation with the primary care provider and dietitian, as needed. Record any pertinent teaching that was conducted. Record liquids consumed on intake and output record, as appropriate.

SKILL 61 | OBTAINING AN ELECTROCARDIOGRAM (ECG)

Electrocardiography (ECG [also abbreviated as EKG in some references]) is one of the most valuable and frequently used diagnostic tools. ECG measures the heart's electrical activity. Impulses moving through the heart's conduction system create electric currents that can be monitored on the body's surface. Electrodes attached to the skin can detect these electric currents and transmit them to an instrument that produces a record, the electrocardiogram, of cardiac activity. The data are graphed as waveforms. ECG can be used to identify myocardial ischemia and infarction, rhythm and conduction disturbances, chamber enlargement, electrolyte imbalances, and drug toxicity.

The standard 12-lead ECG uses a series of electrodes placed on the extremities and the chest wall to assess the heart from 12 different viewpoints (leads) by attaching ten cables with electrodes to the patient's limbs and chest: four limb electrodes and six chest electrodes (Figure 1). Each lead provides an electrographic snapshot of electrochemical activity of the myocardial cell membrane. The ECG device measures and averages the differences between the electrical potential of the electrode sites for each lead and graphs them over time, creating the standard ECG complex, called PQRST. These electrodes provide views of the heart from the frontal plane as well as the horizontal plane. It is essential that connection or placement of the ECG electrodes/leads is accurate to prevent misdiagnosis. The ECG tracing needs to be clear to enable accurate and reliable interpretation (Jevon, 2010).

An ECG is typically accomplished using a multichannel method. All electrodes are attached to the patient at once and the machine prints a simultaneous view of all leads. It is important to reassure the patient that the leads just sense and record and do not transmit any electricity. The patient

FIGURE 1 12-lead ECG lead placement. (From Morton, P.G., & Fontaine, D.K. (2013). *Essentials of critical care nursing. A holistic approach.* Philadelphia: Wolters Kluwer Health/Lippincott Williams & Wilkins, with permission.)

must be able to lie still and refrain from speaking to prevent body movement from creating artifact in the ECG. Variations of standard ECG include exercise ECG (stress ECG) and ambulatory ECG (Holter monitoring).

Interpreting the ECG requires the following actions:
• Determine the rhythm.
• Determine the rate.
• Evaluate the P wave.
• Determine the duration of the PR interval.
• Determine the duration of the QRS complex.
• Evaluate the T waves.
• Determine the duration of the QT interval.
• Evaluate any other components.

DELEGATION CONSIDERATIONS

Obtaining an electrocardiogram is not delegated to nursing assistive personnel (NAP) or to unlicensed assistive personnel (UAP). Depending on the state's nurse practice act and the organization's policies and procedures, this procedure may be delegated to licensed practical/vocational nurses (LPN/LVNs). The decision to delegate must be based on careful analysis of the patient's needs and circumstances, as well as the qualifications of the person to whom the task is being delegated. Refer to the Delegation Guidelines in Appendix A.

EQUIPMENT

- ECG machine
- Recording paper
- Disposable pregelled electrodes
- Adhesive remover swabs
- 4 × 4 gauze pads
- Skin cleanser and water, if necessary
- Additional PPE, as indicated
- Bath blanket

ASSESSMENT

- Review the patient's medical record and plan of care for information about the patient's need for an ECG.
- Assess the patient's cardiac status, including heart rate, blood pressure, and auscultation of heart sounds.
- If the patient is already connected to a cardiac monitor, remove the electrodes to accommodate the precordial leads and minimize electrical interference on the ECG tracing.
- Keep the patient away from objects that might cause electrical interference, such as equipment, fixtures, and power cords.
- Inspect the patient's chest for areas of irritation, breakdown, or excessive hair that might interfere with electrode placement.

NURSING DIAGNOSIS

- Decreased Cardiac Output
- Acute Pain
- Activity Intolerance

OUTCOME IDENTIFICATION AND PLANNING

- Cardiac electrical tracing is obtained without any complications.
- Patient displays an increased understanding about the ECG.
- Patient has reduced anxiety about the procedure.

IMPLEMENTATION

ACTION	RATIONALE
1. Verify the order for an ECG in the patient's medical record.	This ensures that the correct intervention is performed on the correct patient.

ACTION	RATIONALE
2. Gather all equipment.	Assembling equipment provides for an organized approach to the task.
3. Perform hand hygiene and put on PPE, if indicated.	Hand hygiene and PPE prevent the spread of microorganisms. PPE is required based on transmission precautions.
4. Identify the patient.	Identifying the patient ensures the right patient receives the intervention and helps prevent errors.
5. Close curtains around the bed and close the door to the room, if possible. As you set up the machine to record a 12-lead ECG, explain the procedure to the patient. Tell the patient that the test records the heart's electrical activity, and it may be repeated at certain intervals. Emphasize that no electrical current will enter his/her body. Tell the patient the test typically takes about 5 minutes. Ask the patient about allergies to adhesive, as appropriate.	This ensures the patient's privacy. Explanation relieves anxiety and facilitates cooperation. Possible allergies may exist related to adhesive on ECG leads.
6. Place the ECG machine close to the patient's bed, and plug the power cord into the wall outlet.	Having equipment available saves time and facilitates accomplishment of the task.
7. If the bed is adjustable, raise it to a comfortable working height, usually elbow height of the caregiver (VISN 8 Patient Safety Center, 2009).	Having the bed at the proper height prevents back and muscle strain.
8. Have the patient lie supine in the center of the bed with the arms at the sides. Raise the head of the bed if necessary to promote comfort.	Proper positioning helps increase patient comfort and will produce a better tracing. Proper positioning and relaxation of the arms and legs minimizes muscle

ACTION	RATIONALE

Expose the patient's arms and legs, and drape appropriately. Encourage the patient to relax the arms and legs. Ensure the wrists do not touch the waist. Make sure the feet do not touch the bed's footboard.

tension and trembling and electrical interference.

9. If necessary, prepare the skin for electrode placement. If an area is excessively hairy, clip the hair. **Do not shave hair.** Clean excess oil or other substances from the skin with skin cleanser and water and dry it completely. If wet gel electrodes are used, shaving and abrading skin is not necessary. If solid gel electrodes are used, clean, degrease, and debrade the skin (gently rub with gauze pad) and clip hair, if necessary.

Shaving causes microabrasions on the chest skin. Oils and excess hair interfere with electrode contact and function. Alcohol, benzoin, and antiperspirant are not recommended to prepare skin.

10. Apply the limb electrodes, then connect the limb lead wires to the electrodes. The tip of each lead wire is lettered and color coded for easy identification. The white or RA lead goes to the right arm, just above the wrist bone; the green or RL lead to the right leg, just above the ankle bone; the red or LL lead to the left leg, just above the ankle bone; the black or LA lead to the left arm, just above the wrist bone. Peel the contact paper off the self-sticking disposable electrode and apply directly to the prepared site, as recommended by the manufacturer. Refer to Figure 1 for electrode placement.

Use of recommended standard sites for limb electrodes is essential to obtain accurate recording (Crawford & Doherty, 2010; SCST, 2010).

ACTION	RATIONALE
11. Expose the patient's chest. Apply the chest electrodes, and then connect the chest lead wires to the electrodes. The tip of each lead wire is lettered and color coded for easy identification. The V_1 to V_6 leads are applied to the chest. Peel the contact paper off the self-sticking, disposable electrode and apply directly to the prepared site, as recommended by the manufacturer. Position chest electrodes as follows (refer to Figure 1): • V_1: (Red) Fourth intercostal space at right sternal border • V_2: (Yellow) Fourth intercostal space at left sternal border • V_3: (Green) Exactly midway between V_2 and V_4 • V_4: (Blue) Fifth intercostal space at the left midclavicular line • V_5: (Orange) Left anterior axillary line, same horizontal plane as V_4 and V_6 • V_6: (Purple) Left midaxillary line, same horizontal plane as V_4 and V_5	Proper lead placement is necessary for accurate test results (SCST, 2010; Kligfield et al., 2007).
12. After the application of all the leads, ensure that the cables are not pulling on the electrodes or lying over each other. Make sure the paper-speed selector is set to the standard 25 m/second and that the machine is set to full voltage.	Minimizes electrical artifact and improves quality and accuracy of the ECG (Roberts, 2002, in Jevon, 2010). The machine will record a normal standardization mark—a square that is the height of 2 large squares or 10 small squares on the recording paper.
13. If necessary, enter the appropriate patient identification data into the machine.	This allows for proper identification of the ECG strip.

ACTION	RATIONALE
14. Ask the patient to relax and breathe normally. **Instruct the patient to lie still and not to talk while you record the ECG.**	Lying still and not talking produces a better tracing.
15. Press the AUTO button. Observe the tracing quality. The machine will record all 12 leads automatically, recording 3 consecutive leads simultaneously. Some machines have a display screen so you can preview waveforms before the machine records them on paper. Adjust waveform, if necessary. If any part of the waveform extends beyond the paper when you record the ECG, adjust the normal standardization to half-standardization and repeat. Note this adjustment on the ECG strip, because this will need to be considered in interpreting the results.	Observation of tracing quality allows for adjustments to be made, if necessary. Notation of adjustments ensures accurate interpretation of results.
16. When the machine finishes recording the 12-lead ECG, remove the electrodes and clean the patient's skin, if necessary, with adhesive remover for sticky residue.	Removal and cleaning promote patient comfort.
17. After disconnecting the lead wires from the electrodes, dispose of the electrodes. Return the patient to a comfortable position. Lower bed height and adjust the head of bed to a comfortable position.	Proper disposal deters the spread of microorganisms. Positioning with head adjustment promotes patient comfort. Lowering the bed height promotes patient safety.
18. Clean the ECG machine per facility policy. If not done electronically from data entered into the machine, label the ECG with the patient's name, date of birth, location, date and time of	Cleaning equipment between patient uses decreases the risk for transmission of microorganisms. Accurate labeling ensures the ECG is recorded for the correct patient and accurate and reliable interpretation.

ACTION	RATIONALE
recording, and other relevant information, such as symptoms that occurred during the recording (Jevon, 2010). Note any deviations to the standard approach to the recording, such as alternative placement of leads.	
19. Remove additional PPE, if used. Perform hand hygiene.	Removing PPE properly reduces the risk for infection transmission and contamination of other items. Hand hygiene prevents transmission of microorganisms.

EVALUATION

- ECG reading is obtained without any undue patient anxiety or complications or injury.
- Patient verbalizes an understanding of the reason for the ECG.

DOCUMENTATION

- Document significant assessment findings, the date and time that the ECG was obtained, and the patient's response to the procedure. Label the ECG recording with the patient's name, room number, and facility identification number, if this was not done by the machine. Also record the date and time as well as any appropriate clinical information on the ECG, such as blood pressure measurement, if the patient was experiencing chest pain. Record any deviations to the standard approach to the recording, such as alternative placement of leads.

SKILL 62   SECURING AN ENDOTRACHEAL TUBE

Endotracheal tubes provide an airway for patients who cannot maintain a sufficient airway on their own. A tube is passed through the mouth or nose into the trachea. Patients who have an endotracheal tube have a high risk for skin breakdown related to the securing of the endotracheal tube, compounded by the risk of increased secretions. The endotracheal tube should be retaped every 24 hours to prevent skin breakdown and to ensure that the tube is secured properly. Retaping an endotracheal tube requires two people. There are other ways of securing an endotracheal tube besides using tape. To secure with another device, follow the manufacturer's recommendations. However, the literature suggests using tape to secure an endotracheal tube may be the best method (Shimizu et al., 2011; Carlson et al., 2007). One example of taping an endotracheal tube is provided below, but this skill might be performed differently in your facility. Always refer to specific agency policy.

DELEGATION CONSIDERATIONS

Securing an endotracheal tube is not delegated to nursing assistive personnel (NAP) or to unlicensed assistive personnel (UAP). Depending on the state's nurse practice act and the organization's policies and procedures, securing of an endotracheal tube in a stable situation, such as long-term care and other community-based care settings, may be delegated to licensed practical/vocational nurses (LPN/LVNs). The decision to delegate must be based on careful analysis of the patient's needs and circumstances, as well as the qualifications of the person to whom the task is being delegated. Refer to the Delegation Guidelines in Appendix A.

EQUIPMENT

- Assistant (nurse or respiratory therapist)
- Portable or wall suction unit with tubing
- Sterile suction catheter with Y-port
- 1-inch tape (adhesive or water-proof tape)
- Disposable gloves
- Mask and goggles or face shield
- Additional PPE, as indicated
- Sterile suctioning kit

- Oral suction catheter
- Two 3-mL syringes or tongue blade
- Scissors
- Washcloth and cleaning agent
- Skin barrier (e.g., 3M or Skin-Prep)
- Adhesive remover swab
- Towel
- Razor (optional)
- Shaving cream (optional)
- Sterile saline or water
- Handheld pressure gauge

ASSESSMENT

- Assess for the need for retaping, which may include loose or soiled tape, pressure on mucous membranes, or repositioning of tube.
- Assess endotracheal tube length. The tube has markings on the side to ensure it is not moved during the retaping. Note the centimeter (cm) marking at the patient's lip or naris.
- Assess lung sounds to obtain a baseline. Ensure that the lung sounds are still heard throughout the lobes. Assess oxygen saturation level. If the tube is dislodged, the oxygen saturation level may change. Assess the chest for symmetric rise and fall during respiration. If the tube is dislodged, the rise and fall of the chest will change.
- Assess the patient's need for pain medication or sedation. Assess pain. The patient should be calm, free of pain, and relaxed during the retaping so as not to move and cause an accidental extubation.

• Inspect the area on the posterior portion of the neck for any skin breakdown that may result from irritation or pressure from tape or endotracheal tube holder.

NURSING DIAGNOSIS

• Risk for Impaired Skin Integrity
• Impaired Oral Mucous Membrane
• Risk for Infection
• Risk for Injury

OUTCOME IDENTIFICATION AND PLANNING

• Endotracheal tube remains in place.
• Patient maintains bilaterally equal and clear lung sounds.
• Patient demonstrates understanding about the reason for the endotracheal tube.
• Patient's skin remains intact.
• Patient's oxygen saturation remains within acceptable parameters, or greater than 95%.
• Patient's chest rises symmetrically and airway remains clear.

IMPLEMENTATION

ACTION	RATIONALE
1. Bring necessary equipment to the bedside stand or overbed table.	Bringing everything to the bedside conserves time and energy. Arranging items nearby is convenient, saves time, and avoids unnecessary stretching and twisting of muscles on the part of the nurse.
2. Perform hand hygiene and put on PPE, if indicated.	Hand hygiene and PPE prevent the spread of microorganisms. PPE is required based on transmission precautions.
3. Identify the patient.	Identifying the patient ensures the right patient receives the intervention and helps prevent errors.
4. Close the curtains around the bed and close the door to the room, if possible.	This ensures the patient's privacy.
5. Assess the need for endotracheal tube retaping. **Administer pain medication or**	Retaping the endotracheal tube can stimulate coughing, which may be painful for patients, particularly

ACTION	RATIONALE
sedation, as prescribed, before attempting to retape endotracheal tube. Explain what you are going to do and the reason for doing it to the patient, even if the patient does not appear to be alert.	those with surgical incisions. Explanation alleviates fears, facilitates cooperation, and provides reassurance for the patient. Any procedure that may compromise respiration is frightening for the patient. Even if the patient appears unconscious, the nurse should explain what is happening.
6. Obtain the assistance of a second individual to hold the endotracheal tube in place while the old tape is removed and the new tape is placed.	This prevents accidental extubation.
7. Adjust the bed to a comfortable working position, usually elbow height of the caregiver (VISN 8 Patient Safety Center, 2009). Lower side rail closest to you. **If conscious, place the patient in a semi-Fowler's position. If unconscious, place the patient in the lateral position, facing you.** Move the overbed table close to your work area and raise to waist height. Place a trash receptacle within easy reach of the work area.	Having the bed at the proper height prevents back and muscle strain. A sitting position helps the patient to cough and makes breathing easier. Gravity also facilitates catheter insertion. The lateral position prevents the airway from becoming obstructed and promotes drainage of secretions. The overbed table provides work surface and maintains sterility of objects on the work surface. Placing the trash receptacle within reach allows for an organized approach to care.
8. Put on face shield or goggles and mask. Suction patient as described in Skill 63 or 64.	Personal protective equipment prevents exposure to contaminants. Suctioning decreases the likelihood of the patient coughing during the retaping of the endotracheal tube. If the patient coughs, the tube may become dislodged.
9. Measure a piece of tape for the length needed to reach around the patient's neck to the mouth plus 8 inches. Cut tape. Lay it adhesive-side up on the table.	Extra length is needed so that tape can be wrapped around the endotracheal tube.
10. Cut another piece of tape long enough to reach from one jaw around the back of	This prevents the tape from sticking to the patient's hair and the back of the neck.

ACTION	RATIONALE

the neck to the other jaw. Lay this piece on the center of the longer piece on the table, matching the tapes' adhesive sides together.

11. Take one 3-mL syringe or tongue blade and wrap the sticky tape around the syringe until the nonsticky area is reached. Do this for the other side as well.

This helps the nurse or respiratory therapist to manage the tape without it sticking to the sheets or the patient's hair.

12. Take one of the 3-mL syringes or tongue blades and pass it under the patient's neck so that there is a 3-mL syringe on either side of the patient's head.

This makes the tape easy to access when retaping the tube.

13. Put on disposable gloves. Have the assistant put on gloves as well.

Gloves protect hands from exposure to contaminants.

14. Provide oral care, including suctioning the oral cavity.

This helps to decrease secretions in the oral cavity and pharynx region.

15. Take note of the 'cm' position markings on the tube. Begin to unwrap old tape from around the endotracheal tube. After one side is unwrapped, have assistant hold the endotracheal tube as close to the lips or nares as possible to offer stabilization.

Assistant should hold the tube to prevent accidental extubation. Holding the tube as close to lips or nares as possible prevents accidental dislodgement of tube.

16. Carefully remove the remaining tape from the endotracheal tube. **After tape is removed, have assistant gently and slowly move endotracheal tube (if orally intubated) to the other side of the mouth. Assess mouth for any skin breakdown. Before applying new tape, make sure that markings on endotracheal tube are at same spot as when retaping began.**

The endotracheal tube may cause pressure ulcers if left in the same place over time. By moving the tube, the risk for pressure ulcers is reduced.

ACTION	RATIONALE
17. Remove old tape from cheeks and side of face. Use adhesive remover to remove excess adhesive from tape. Clean the face and neck with washcloth and cleanser. If patient has facial hair, consider shaving cheeks. Pat cheeks dry with the towel.	To prevent skin breakdown, remove old adhesive. Shaving helps to decrease pain when tape is removed. Cheeks must be dry before new tape is applied to ensure that it sticks.
18. Apply the skin barrier to the patient's face (under nose, on cheeks, and lower lip) where the tape will sit. Unroll one side of the tape. Ensure that nonstick part of tape remains behind the patient's neck while pulling firmly on the tape. Place adhesive portion of tape snugly against the patient's cheek. Keep track of the pilot balloon from the endotracheal tube, to avoid taping it to the patient's face. Split the tape in half from the end to the corner of the mouth.	Skin barrier protects the skin from injury with subsequent tape removal and helps the tape adhere better to the skin. The tape should be snug to the side of the patient's face to prevent accidental extubation.
19. Place the top-half piece of tape under the patient's nose (Figure 1). Wrap the lower half around the tube in one direction, such as over and around the tube. Fold over tab on end of tape.	By placing one piece of tape on the lip and the other piece of tape on the tube, the tube remains secure. Tab makes tape removal easier.

FIGURE 1 Putting new tape in place.

| 20. Unwrap second side of tape. Split to corner of the mouth. | Alternating the placement of the top and bottom pieces of tape |

ACTION	RATIONALE

Place the bottom-half piece of tape along the patient's lower lip. Wrap the top half around the tube in the opposite direction, such as below and around the tube. Fold over tab on end of tape. Ensure tape is secure (Figure 2). Remove gloves.

provides more anchorage for the tube. Wrapping the tape in an alternating manner ensures that the tape will not accidentally be unwound.

FIGURE 2 Ensuring tape is securely stabilizing the tube.

21. **Auscultate lung sounds. Assess for cyanosis, oxygen saturation, chest symmetry, and endotracheal tube stability. Again check to ensure that the tube is at the correct depth.**

If the tube has been moved from original place, the lung sounds may change, as well as oxygen saturation and chest symmetry. The tube should be stable and should not move with each respiration cycle.

22. **If the endotracheal tube is cuffed, check pressure of the balloon by attaching a handheld pressure gauge to the pilot balloon of the endotracheal tube.**

It is thought cuff pressure should be maintained at less than 25 cm H_2O to prevent excessive pressure on tracheal mucosal wall and surrounding structures (Sultan et al., 2011). Maximal cuff pressures should not exceed 24 to 30 cm H_2O to prevent tracheal ischemia and necrosis.

23. Assist the patient to a comfortable position. Raise the bed rail and place the bed in the lowest position.

Ensures patient comfort. Proper positioning with raised side rails and proper bed height provide for patient comfort and safety.

24. Remove face shield or goggles and mask. Remove additional PPE, if used. Perform hand hygiene.

Removing PPE properly reduces the risk for infection transmission and contamination of other items. Hand hygiene prevents the spread of microorganisms.

EVALUATION

- Endotracheal tube tape is changed without dislodgement or a depth change of the tube.
- Patient's lung sounds remain equal.
- No pressure ulcers are noted.
- Patient's airway remains clear.
- Patient's oxygen saturation remains within acceptable parameters, or greater than 95%, chest rises symmetrically, and skin remains acyanotic.
- Endotracheal tube cuff pressure is maintained at 20 to 25 cm H_2O.

DOCUMENTATION

- Document the procedure, including the depth of the endotracheal tube from teeth or lips; the amount, consistency, and color of secretions suctioned; presence of any skin or mucous membrane changes or pressure ulcers; and your before and after assessments, including lung sounds, oxygen saturation, skin color, cuff pressure, and chest symmetry.

SKILL 63 | SUCTIONING AN ENDOTRACHEAL TUBE: CLOSED SYSTEM

The purpose of suctioning is to maintain a patent airway and remove pulmonary secretions, blood, vomitus, or foreign material from the airway. When suctioning via an endotracheal tube, the goal is to remove secretions that are not accessible to cilia bypassed by the tube itself. Tracheal suctioning can lead to hypoxemia, cardiac dysrhythmias, trauma, atelectasis, infection, bleeding, and pain. It is imperative to be diligent in maintaining aseptic technique and following facility guidelines and procedures to prevent potential hazards. Suctioning frequency is based on clinical assessment to determine the need for suctioning.

Suctioning removes secretions not accessible to bypassed cilia, so recommendation is to insert the catheter only as far as the end of the endotracheal tube. Catheter contact and suction cause tracheal mucosal damage, loss of cilia, edema, and fibrosis, and increase the risk of infection and bleeding for the patient. Insertion of the suction catheter to a predetermined distance, no more than 1 cm past the length of the endotracheal tube, avoids contact with the trachea and carina, reducing the effects of tracheal mucosal damage (Hahn, 2010; Ireton, 2007; Pate, 2004; Pate & Zapata, 2002).

Closed system suction may be used routinely or when a patient must be suctioned frequently and quickly due to an excess of secretions, depending on the policies of the facility. One drawback of closed suctioning is thought to be the hindrance of the sheath when rotating the suction catheter upon removal.

DELEGATION CONSIDERATIONS

Suctioning an endotracheal tube is not delegated to nursing assistive personnel (NAP) or to unlicensed assistive personnel (UAP). Depending on the state's nurse practice act and the organization's policies and procedures, suctioning of an endotracheal tube in a stable situation, such as long-term care and other community-based care settings, may be delegated to licensed practical/vocational nurses (LPN/LVNs). The decision to delegate must be based on careful analysis of the patient's needs and circumstances, as well as the qualifications of the person to whom the task is being delegated. Refer to the Delegation Guidelines in Appendix A.

EQUIPMENT

- Portable or wall suction unit with tubing
- Closed suction device of appropriate size for patient
- 3 mL or 5 mL normal saline solution in dosette or syringe
- Sterile gloves
- Additional PPE, as indicated

ASSESSMENT

- Assess lung sounds. Patients who need to be suctioned may have wheezes, crackles, or gurgling present.
- Assess oxygen saturation level. Oxygen saturation usually decreases when a patient needs to be suctioned.
- Assess respiratory status, including respiratory rate and depth. Patients may become tachypneic when they need to be suctioned. Assess patient for signs of respiratory distress, such as nasal flaring, retractions, or grunting.
- Additional indications for suctioning via an endotracheal tube include secretions in the tube, acute respiratory distress, and frequent or sustained coughing.
- Assess for pain and the potential to cause pain during the intervention. Perform individualized pain management in response to the patient's needs (Arroyo-Novoa et al., 2008). Administer pain medication, as prescribed, before suctioning.
- Assess appropriate suction catheter depth.
- Assess the characteristics and amount of secretions while suctioning.

NURSING DIAGNOSIS

- Ineffective Airway Clearance
- Risk for Aspiration
- Risk for Infection
- Impaired Gas Exchange

OUTCOME IDENTIFICATION AND PLANNING

- Patient will exhibit improved breath sounds and a clear, patent airway.
- Patient will exhibit an oxygen saturation level within acceptable parameters.

- Patient will demonstrate a respiratory rate and depth within age-acceptable parameters.
- Patient will remain free of any signs of respiratory distress.

IMPLEMENTATION

ACTION	RATIONALE
1. Bring necessary equipment to the bedside stand or overbed table.	Bringing everything to the bedside conserves time and energy. Arranging items nearby is convenient, saves time, and avoids unnecessary stretching and twisting of muscles on the part of the nurse.
2. Perform hand hygiene and put on PPE, if indicated.	Hand hygiene and PPE prevent the spread of microorganisms. PPE is required based on transmission precautions.
3. Identify the patient.	Identifying the patient ensures the right patient receives the intervention and helps prevent errors.
4. Close the curtains around the bed and close the door to the room, if possible.	This ensures the patient's privacy.
5. Determine the need for suctioning. Verify the suction order in the patient's medical record. **Assess for pain or the potential to cause pain. Administer pain medication, as prescribed, before suctioning.**	To minimize trauma to airway mucosa, suctioning should be done only when secretions have accumulated or adventitious breath sounds are audible. Suctioning can cause moderate to severe pain for patients. Individualized pain management is imperative (Arroyo-Novoa et al., 2008). Suctioning stimulates coughing, which is painful for patients with surgical incisions.
6. Explain what you are going to do and the reason for doing it to the patient, even if the patient does not appear to be alert. Reassure the patient you will interrupt the procedure if he/she indicates respiratory difficulty.	Explanation alleviates fears. Even if the patient appears unconscious, the nurse should explain what is happening. Any procedure that compromises respiration is frightening for the patient.

ACTION	RATIONALE
7. Adjust the bed to a comfortable working position, usually elbow height of the caregiver (VISN 8 Patient Safety Center, 2009). Lower side rail closest to you. **If conscious, place the patient in a semi-Fowler's position. If unconscious, place the patient in the lateral position, facing you.** Move the overbed table close to your work area and raise to waist height.	Having the bed at the proper height prevents back and muscle strain. A sitting position helps the patient to cough and makes breathing easier. Gravity also facilitates catheter insertion. The lateral position prevents the airway from becoming obstructed and promotes drainage of secretions. The overbed table provides work surface and maintains sterility of objects on work surface.
8. Turn suction to appropriate pressure: • For a wall unit for an adult: 100–150 mm Hg; neonates: 60–80 mm Hg; infants: 80–125 mm Hg; children: 80–125 mm Hg; adolescents: 80–150 mm Hg (Hess et al., 2012). • For a portable unit for an adult: 10–15 cm Hg; neonates: 6–8 cm Hg; infants: 8–10 cm Hg; children: 8–10 cm Hg; adolescents: 8–15 cm Hg.	Higher pressures can cause excessive trauma, hypoxemia, and atelectasis.
9. Open the package of the closed suction device using aseptic technique. Make sure that the device remains sterile.	The device must remain sterile to prevent a nosocomial infection.
10. Put on sterile gloves.	Gloves deter the spread of microorganisms.
11. Using nondominant hand, disconnect ventilator from endotracheal tube. Place ventilator tubing in a convenient location so that the inside of the tubing remains sterile or continue to hold the tubing in your nondominant hand.	This provides access to the endotracheal tube while keeping one hand sterile. The inside of the ventilator tubing should remain sterile to prevent a nosocomial infection.

ACTION	RATIONALE
12. **Using dominant hand and keeping device sterile, connect the closed suctioning device so that the suctioning catheter is in line with the endotracheal tube.**	Keeping the device sterile decreases the risk for a nosocomial infection.
13. **Keeping the inside of the ventilator tubing sterile, attach ventilator tubing to port perpendicular to the endotracheal tube.** Attach suction tubing to suction catheter.	The inside of the ventilator tubing must remain sterile to prevent a nosocomial infection. By connecting the ventilator tubing to the port, the patient does not need to be disconnected from the ventilator to be suctioned.
14. Pop top off sterile normal saline dosette. Open plug to port by suction catheter and insert saline dosette or syringe.	The saline will help to clean the catheter between suctioning.
15. Hyperventilate the patient by using the sigh button on the ventilator before suctioning. Turn safety cap on suction button of catheter so that button is depressed easily.	Hyperoxygenating and hyperventilating before suctioning helps to decrease the effects of oxygen removal during suctioning. The safety button keeps the patient from accidentally depressing the button and decreasing the oxygen saturation.
16. Grasp suction catheter through protective sheath, about 6 inches (15 cm) from the endotracheal tube. Gently insert the catheter into the endotracheal tube (Figure 1). Release the catheter while holding on to the protective sheath. Move hand farther	The sheath keeps the suction catheter sterile. Catheter contact and suction cause tracheal mucosal damage, loss of cilia, edema, and fibrosis, and increase the risk of infection and bleeding for the patient. Insertion of the suction catheter to a predetermined distance, no more than

FIGURE 1 Inserting catheter through sheath and into endotracheal tube.

ACTION	RATIONALE

back on catheter. **Grasp catheter through sheath and repeat movement, advancing the catheter to the predetermined length. Do not occlude Y-port when inserting the catheter.**

1 cm past the length of the endotracheal tube, avoids contact with the trachea and carina, reducing the effects of tracheal mucosal damage (Hahn, 2011; Ireton, 2007; Pate, 2004; Pate & Zapata, 2002). If resistance is met, the carina or tracheal mucosa has been hit. Withdraw the catheter at least 0.5 inch before applying suction. Suctioning when inserting the catheter increases the risk for trauma to airway mucosa and increases the risk of hypoxemia.

17. Apply intermittent suction by depressing the suction button with thumb of nondominant hand. Gently rotate the catheter with thumb and index finger of dominant hand as catheter is being withdrawn. **Do not suction for more than 10 to 15 seconds at a time.** Hyperoxygenate or hyperventilate with sigh button on ventilator, as ordered.

Turning the catheter while withdrawing it helps clean surfaces of the respiratory tract and prevents injury to tracheal mucosa. Suctioning for longer than 10 to 15 seconds robs the respiratory tract of oxygen, which may result in hypoxemia. Suctioning too quickly may be ineffective at clearing all secretions. Hyperoxygenation and hyperventilation reoxygenate the lungs.

18. Once the catheter is withdrawn back into the sheath (Figure 2), depress the suction button while gently squeezing the normal saline dosette until the catheter is clean. **Allow at least a 30-second to 1-minute interval if additional suctioning is needed.**

Flushing cleans and clears the catheter and lubricates it for next insertion. Allowing time interval and replacing oxygen delivery setup help compensate for hypoxia induced by the suctioning. Excessive suction passes contribute to complications.

FIGURE 2 Removing suction catheter by pulling back into sheath.

ACTION	RATIONALE
No more than three suction passes should be made per suctioning episode.	
19. When the procedure is completed, **ensure that the catheter is withdrawn into the sheath,** and turn the safety button. Remove normal saline dosette and apply cap to port.	By turning the safety button, the suction is blocked at the catheter so the suction cannot remove oxygen from the endotracheal tube.
20. Suction the oral cavity with a separate single-use, disposable catheter and perform oral hygiene. Remove gloves. Turn off suction.	Suctioning of the oral cavity removes secretions that may be stagnant in the mouth and pharynx, reducing the risk for infection. Oral hygiene offers comfort to the patient. Removing PPE properly reduces the risk for infection transmission and contamination of other items.
21. Assist the patient to a comfortable position. Raise the bed rail and place the bed in the lowest position.	Ensures patient comfort. Proper positioning with raised side rails and proper bed height provide for patient comfort and safety.
22. Reassess the patient's respiratory status, including respiratory rate, effort, oxygen saturation, and lung sounds.	These assess effectiveness of suctioning and the presence of complications.
23. Remove additional PPE, if used. Perform hand hygiene.	Removing PPE properly reduces the risk for infection transmission and contamination of other items. Hand hygiene prevents the spread of microorganisms.

EVALUATION
- Patient exhibits improved breath sounds and a clear and patent airway.
- Patient's oxygen saturation level is within acceptable parameters.
- Patient does not exhibit signs or symptoms of respiratory distress or complications.

DOCUMENTATION
- Document the time of suctioning, your assessments before and after intervention, reason for suctioning, oxygen saturation levels, and the characteristics and amount of secretions.

SKILL 64 SUCTIONING AN ENDOTRACHEAL TUBE: OPEN SYSTEM

The purpose of suctioning is to maintain a patent airway and remove pulmonary secretions, blood, vomitus, or foreign material from the airway. When suctioning via an endotracheal tube, the goal is to remove secretions that are not accessible to cilia bypassed by the tube itself. Remember, tracheal suctioning can lead to hypoxemia, cardiac dysrhythmias, trauma, atelectasis, infection, bleeding, and pain. Therefore, it is imperative to be diligent in maintaining aseptic technique and in following facility guidelines and procedures to prevent potential hazards. Frequency of suctioning is based on clinical assessment.

Because suctioning removes secretions not accessible to bypassed cilia, the recommendation is to insert the catheter only as far as the end of the endotracheal tube. Catheter contact and suction can cause tracheal mucosal damage, loss of cilia, edema, and fibrosis, and increase the risk of infection and bleeding for the patient. Insertion of the suction catheter to a predetermined distance, no more than 1 cm past the length of the endotracheal tube, avoids contact with the trachea and carina, reducing the effects of tracheal mucosal damage (Hahn, 2010; Ireton, 2007; Pate, 2004; Pate & Zapata, 2002).

Some consider open system suctioning to be the most efficient way to suction the endotracheal tube, arguing that there are no limitations to the movement of the suction catheter while suctioning. However, the nurse may unknowingly contaminate an open system during the procedure. In addition, with the open system, the patient must be removed from the ventilator during suctioning.

DELEGATION CONSIDERATIONS

Suctioning an endotracheal tube is not delegated to nursing assistive personnel (NAP) or to unlicensed assistive personnel (UAP). Depending on the state's nurse practice act and the organization's policies and procedures, suctioning of an endotracheal tube in a stable situation, such as long-term care and other community-based care settings, may be delegated to licensed practical/vocational nurses (LPN/LVNs). The decision to delegate must be based on careful analysis of the patient's needs and circumstances, as well as the qualifications of the person to whom the task is being delegated. Refer to the Delegation Guidelines in Appendix A.

EQUIPMENT

- Portable or wall suction unit with tubing
- A commercially prepared suction kit with an appropriate size catheter (see General Considerations) or
- Sterile suction catheter with Y-port in the appropriate size
- Sterile, disposable container
- Sterile gloves
- Towel or waterproof pad

- Goggles and mask or face shield
- Additional PPE, as indicated
- Disposable, clean gloves
- Resuscitation bag connected to 100% oxygen
- Assistant (optional)

ASSESSMENT

- Assess lung sounds. Patients who need to be suctioned may have wheezes, crackles, or gurgling present.
- Assess oxygen saturation level. Oxygen saturation usually decreases when a patient needs to be suctioned.
- Assess respiratory status, including respiratory rate and depth. Patients may become tachypneic when they need to be suctioned. Assess patient for signs of respiratory distress, such as nasal flaring, retractions, or grunting.
- Additional indications for suctioning via an endotracheal tube include secretions in the tube, acute respiratory distress, and frequent or sustained coughing.
- Assess for pain and the potential to cause pain during the intervention. Perform individualized pain management in response to the patient's needs (Arroyo-Novoa et al., 2008). Administer pain medication, as prescribed, before suctioning.
- Assess appropriate suction catheter depth. Assess the characteristics and amount of secretions while suctioning.

NURSING DIAGNOSIS

- Ineffective Airway Clearance
- Risk for Aspiration
- Risk for Infection
- Impaired Gas Exchange

OUTCOME IDENTIFICATION AND PLANNING

- Patient will exhibit improved breath sounds and a clear, patent airway.
- Patient will exhibit an oxygen saturation level within acceptable parameters.
- Patient will demonstrate a respiratory rate and depth within age-acceptable parameters.
- Patient will remain free of any signs of respiratory distress.

IMPLEMENTATION

ACTION	RATIONALE
1. Bring necessary equipment to the bedside stand or over-bed table.	Bringing everything to the bedside conserves time and energy. Arranging items nearby is convenient, saves time, and avoids unnecessary stretching

ACTION	RATIONALE
	and twisting of muscles on the part of the nurse.
2. Perform hand hygiene and put on PPE, if indicated.	Hand hygiene and PPE prevent the spread of microorganisms. PPE is required based on transmission precautions.
3. Identify the patient.	Identifying the patient ensures the right patient receives the intervention and helps prevent errors.
4. Close the curtains around the bed and close the door to the room, if possible.	This ensures the patient's privacy.
5. Determine the need for suctioning. Verify the suction order in the patient's medical record. **Assess for pain or the potential to cause pain. Administer pain medication, as prescribed, before suctioning.**	To minimize trauma to airway mucosa, suctioning should be done only when secretions have accumulated or adventitious breath sounds are audible. Suctioning can cause moderate to severe pain for patients. Individualized pain management is imperative (Arroyo-Novoa et al., 2008). Suctioning stimulates coughing, which is painful for patients with surgical incisions.
6. Explain what you are going to do and the reason for doing it to the patient, even if the patient does not appear to be alert. Reassure the patient you will interrupt the procedure if he/she indicates respiratory difficulty.	Explanation alleviates fears. Even if the patient appears unconscious, the nurse should explain what is happening. Any procedure that compromises respiration is frightening for the patient.
7. Adjust the bed to a comfortable working position, usually elbow height of the caregiver (VISN 8 Patient Safety Center, 2009). Lower side rail closest to you. **If conscious, place the patient in a semi-Fowler's position. If unconscious,**	Having the bed at the proper height prevents back and muscle strain. A sitting position helps the patient to cough and makes breathing easier. Gravity also facilitates catheter insertion. The lateral position prevents the airway from becoming obstructed and

ACTION	RATIONALE
place the patient in the lateral position, facing you. Move the overbed table close to your work area and raise it to waist height.	promotes drainage of secretions. The overbed table provides a work surface and maintains sterility of objects on work surface.
8. Place towel or waterproof pad across the patient's chest.	This protects bed linens and the patient.
9. Turn suction to appropriate pressure: • For a wall unit for an adult: 100–150 mm Hg; neonates: 60–80 mm Hg; infants: 80–125 mm Hg; children: 80–125 mm Hg; adolescents: 80–150 mm Hg (Hess et al., 2012). • For a portable unit for an adult: 10–15 cm Hg; neonates: 6–8 cm Hg; infants: 8–10 cm Hg; children: 8–10 cm Hg; adolescents: 8–15 cm Hg.	Higher pressures can cause excessive trauma, hypoxemia, and atelectasis.
10. Put on a disposable, clean glove and occlude the end of the connecting tubing to check suction pressure. Place the connecting tubing in a convenient location. Place the resuscitation bag connected to oxygen within convenient reach, if using.	Glove prevents contact with blood and body fluids. Checking pressure ensures equipment is working properly. Allows for an organized approach to the procedure.
11. Open sterile suction package using aseptic technique. The open wrapper becomes a sterile field to hold other supplies. Carefully remove the sterile container, touching only the outside surface. Set it up on the work surface and pour sterile saline into it.	Sterile normal saline or water is used to lubricate the outside of the catheter, minimizing irritation of mucosa during introduction. It is also used to clear the catheter between suction attempts.
12. Put on face shield or goggles and mask. Put on sterile gloves. **The dominant**	Handling the sterile catheter using a sterile glove helps prevent introducing organisms

ACTION	RATIONALE

hand will manipulate the catheter and must remain sterile. The nondominant hand is considered clean rather than sterile and will control the suction valve (Y-port) on the catheter.

into the respiratory tract; the clean glove protects the nurse from microorganisms.

13. With dominant gloved hand, pick up sterile catheter. Pick up the connecting tubing with the nondominant hand and connect the tubing and suction catheter.

Sterility of the suction catheter is maintained.

14. Moisten the catheter by dipping it into the container of sterile saline, unless it is a silicone catheter. Occlude Y-tube to check suction.

Lubricating the inside of the catheter with saline helps move secretions in the catheter. Silicone catheters do not require lubrication. Checking suction ensures equipment is working properly.

15. Hyperventilate the patient using your nondominant hand and a manual resuscitation bag and delivering three to six breaths or use the sigh mechanism on a mechanical ventilator.

Hyperventilation and hyperoxygenation aids in preventing hypoxemia during suctioning.

16. Open the adapter on the mechanical ventilator tubing or remove the manual resuscitation bag with your nondominant hand.

This exposes the endotracheal tube without contaminating sterile gloved hand.

17. Using your dominant hand, gently and quickly insert the catheter into the trachea (Figure 1). **Advance the**

Catheter contact and suction cause tracheal mucosal damage, loss of cilia, edema, and fibrosis, and increase the risk of

FIGURE 1 Inserting suction catheter into endotracheal tube.

ACTION	RATIONALE

catheter to the predetermined length. Do not occlude Y-port when inserting the catheter.

infection and bleeding for the patient. Insertion of the suction catheter to a predetermined distance, no more than 1 cm past the length of the endotracheal tube, avoids contact with the trachea and carina, reducing the effects of tracheal mucosal damage (Hahn, 2010; Ireton, 2007; Pate, 2004; Pate & Zapata, 2002). If resistance is met, the carina or tracheal mucosa has been hit. Withdraw the catheter at least 0.5 inch before applying suction. Occluding the Y-port (i.e., suctioning) when inserting the catheter increases the risk for trauma to the airway mucosa and increases the risk of hypoxemia.

18. Apply suction by intermittently occluding the Y-port on the catheter with the thumb of your nondominant hand, and gently rotate the catheter as it is being withdrawn (Figure 2). Do not suction for more than 10 to 15 seconds at a time.

Turning the catheter as it is withdrawn minimizes trauma to the mucosa. Suctioning for longer than 10 to 15 seconds robs the respiratory tract of oxygen, which may result in hypoxemia. Suctioning too quickly may be ineffective at clearing all secretions.

FIGURE 2 Withdrawing suction catheter and intermittently occluding Y-port with thumb to apply suction.

19. Hyperventilate the patient using your nondominant hand and a manual resuscitation bag and delivering three to six breaths. Replace the oxygen delivery device, if applicable, using your

Suctioning removes air from the patient's airway and can cause hypoxemia. Hyperventilation and hyperoxygenation can help prevent suction-induced hypoxemia.

ACTION	RATIONALE
nondominant hand and have the patient take several deep breaths. If the patient is mechanically ventilated, close the adapter on the mechanical ventilator tubing or replace the ventilator tubing and use the sigh mechanism on a mechanical ventilator.	
20. Flush catheter with saline. Assess the effectiveness of suctioning and repeat, as needed, and according to patient's tolerance.	Flushing clears the catheter and lubricates it for next insertion. Reassessment determines need for additional suctioning.
Wrap the suction catheter around your dominant hand between attempts.	Wrapping the catheter prevents inadvertent contamination of the catheter.
21. **Allow at least a 30-second to 1-minute interval if additional suctioning is needed. Do not make more than three suction passes per suctioning episode.** Suction the oropharynx after suctioning the trachea. Do not reinsert in the endotracheal tube after suctioning the mouth.	The interval allows for reventilation and reoxygenation of airways. Excessive suction passes contribute to complications. Suctioning the oropharynx clears the mouth of secretions. More microorganisms are usually present in the mouth, so it is suctioned last to prevent transmission of contaminants.
22. When suctioning is completed, remove gloves from dominant hand over the coiled catheter, pulling off inside-out. Remove glove from nondominant hand and dispose of gloves, catheter, and container with solution in the appropriate receptacle. Assist patient to a comfortable position. Raise bed rail and place bed in the lowest position.	This technique of glove removal and disposal of equipment reduces transmission of microorganisms. Proper positioning with raised side rails and proper bed height provide for patient comfort and safety.
23. Turn off suction. Remove face shield or goggles and mask. Perform hand hygiene.	Removing face shield or goggles and mask properly reduces the risk for infection transmission and contamination of other items. Hand hygiene prevents transmission of microorganisms.

ACTION	RATIONALE
24. Perform oral hygiene after suctioning.	Respiratory secretions that are allowed to accumulate in the mouth are irritating to mucous membranes and unpleasant for the patient.
25. Reassess the patient's respiratory status, including respiratory rate, effort, oxygen saturation, and lung sounds.	These assess effectiveness of suctioning and the presence of complications.
26. Remove additional PPE, if used. Perform hand hygiene.	Removing PPE properly reduces the risk for infection transmission and contamination of other items. Hand hygiene prevents the spread of microorganisms.

EVALUATION

- Patient exhibits improved breath sounds and a clear and patent airway.
- Patient's oxygen saturation level is within acceptable parameters.
- Patient does not exhibit signs or symptoms of respiratory distress or complications.

DOCUMENTATION

- Document the time of suctioning, your assessments before and after interventions, reason for suctioning, oxygen saturation levels, and the characteristics and amount of secretions.

SKILL 65 ADMINISTERING A LARGE-VOLUME CLEANSING ENEMA

Cleansing enemas are given to remove feces from the colon. Some of the reasons for administering a cleansing enema include relieving constipation or fecal impaction, preventing involuntary escape of fecal material during surgical procedures, promoting visualization of the intestinal tract by radiographic or instrument examination, and helping to establish regular bowel function during a bowel training program. Cleansing enemas are classified as either large-volume or small-volume. This skill addresses administering a large-volume enema. (Small-volume enemas are addressed in Skill 67.) Large-volume enemas are known as hypotonic or isotonic, depending on the solution used. Hypotonic (tap water) and isotonic (normal saline solution) enemas are large-volume enemas that result in rapid colonic emptying. However, using large volumes of solution (adults: 500 to 1,000 mL; infants: 150 to 250 mL) may be dangerous for patients with weakened intestinal walls, such as those with bowel inflammation or bowel infection. Large-volume enema solutions often require special preparation and equipment.

DELEGATION CONSIDERATIONS

The administration of some types of enemas may be delegated to nursing assistive personnel (NAP) or to unlicensed assistive personnel (UAP) who have received appropriate training. The administration of a large-volume cleansing enema may be delegated to licensed practical/vocational nurses (LPN/LVNs). The decision to delegate must be based on careful analysis of the patient's needs and circumstances, as well as the qualifications of the person to whom the task is being delegated. Refer to the Delegation Guidelines in Appendix A.

EQUIPMENT

- Enema solution as ordered at a temperature of 105°F to 110°F (40°C to 43°C) for adults in the prescribed amount. (Amount will vary depending on type of solution, patient's age, and patient's ability to retain the solution. Average cleansing enema for an adult may range from 750 to 1,000 mL.)
- Disposable enema set, which includes a solution container and tubing
- Water-soluble lubricant
- IV pole
- Necessary additives, as ordered
- Waterproof pad
- Bath thermometer (if available)
- Bath blanket
- Bedpan and toilet tissue
- Disposable gloves
- Additional PPE, as indicated
- Paper towel
- Washcloth, skin cleanser, and towel

ASSESSMENT

- Ask the patient when he/she had the last bowel movement.
- Assess the patient's abdomen, including auscultating for bowel sounds, and palpating for tenderness and/or firmness. Because the goal of a cleansing enema is to increase peristalsis, which should increase bowel sounds, assess the abdomen before and after the enema.
- Assess the rectal area for any fissures, hemorrhoids, sores, or rectal tears. If any of these are present, take added care while inserting the tube.
- Assess the results of the patient's laboratory work, specifically the platelet count and white blood cell (WBC) count. An enema is contraindicated for patients with a low platelet count or low WBC

count. An enema may irritate or traumatize the GI mucosa, causing bleeding, bowel perforation, or infection in these patients. Any unnecessary procedures that would place the patient with a low platelet count or low WBC count at risk for bleeding or infection should not be performed.

- Assess for dizziness, light-headedness, diaphoresis, and clammy skin. The enema may stimulate a vagal response, which increases parasympathetic stimulation, causing a decrease in heart rate.
- Do not administer enemas to patients who have severe abdominal pain, bowel obstruction, bowel inflammation or bowel infection, or after rectal, prostate, or colon surgery.

NURSING DIAGNOSIS

- Acute Pain
- Constipation
- Risk for Constipation

OUTCOME IDENTIFICATION AND PLANNING

- Patient expels feces.
- Patient verbalizes decreased discomfort.
- Abdominal distention is absent.
- Patient remains free of any evidence of trauma to the rectal mucosa or other adverse effects.

IMPLEMENTATION

ACTION	RATIONALE
1. Verify the order for the enema. Gather equipment.	Verifying the medical order is crucial to ensuring that the proper enema is administered to the right patient. Assembling equipment provides for an organized approach to the task.
2. Perform hand hygiene and put on PPE, if indicated.	Hand hygiene and PPE prevent the spread of microorganisms. PPE is required based on transmission precautions.
3. Identify the patient. 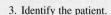	Identifying the patient ensures the right patient receives the intervention and helps prevent errors.
4. Explain the procedure to the patient and provide the	Explanation facilitates patient cooperation and reduces anxiety.

ACTION	RATIONALE

rationale why the tube is needed. Discuss the associated discomforts that may be experienced and possible interventions that may allay this discomfort. Answer any questions, as needed.

5. Assemble equipment on overbed table within reach.

Arranging items nearby is convenient, saves time, and avoids unnecessary stretching and twisting of muscles on the part of the nurse.

6. Close the curtains around the bed and close the door to the room, if possible. Discuss where the patient will defecate. Have a bedpan, commode, or nearby bathroom ready for use.

This ensures the patient's privacy. Explanation relieves anxiety and facilitates cooperation. The patient is better able to relax and cooperate if he or she is familiar with the procedure and knows everything is in readiness when the urge to defecate is felt. Defecation usually occurs within 5 to 15 minutes.

7. Warm the enema solution in amount ordered, and check temperature with a bath thermometer, if available. If bath thermometer is not available, warm to room temperature or slightly higher, and test on inner wrist. If tap water is used, adjust temperature as it flows from the faucet.

Warming the solution prevents chilling the patient, adding to the discomfort of the procedure. Cold solution could cause cramping; a too-warm solution could cause trauma to intestinal mucosa.

8. Add enema solution to container. Release clamp and allow fluid to progress through tube before reclamping.

This causes any air to be expelled from the tubing. Although allowing air to enter the intestine is not harmful, it may further distend the intestine.

9. Adjust the bed to a comfortable working height, usually elbow height of the caregiver (VISN 8 Patient Safety Center, 2009). Position the patient on the left side (Sims' position), as dictated by

Having the bed at the proper height prevents back and muscle strain. Sims' position facilitates flow of solution via gravity into the rectum and colon, optimizing solution retention. Folding back the linen in this manner minimizes

ACTION	RATIONALE
patient comfort and condition. Fold top linen back just enough to allow access to the patient's rectal area. Drape the patient with the bath blanket, as necessary, to maintain privacy and warmth. Place a waterproof pad under the patient's hip.	unnecessary exposure and promotes the patient's comfort and warmth. The waterproof pad will protect the bed.
10. Put on gloves.	Gloves prevent contact with contaminants and body fluids.
11. Elevate solution so that it is no higher than 18 inches (45 cm) above level of anus. Plan to give the solution slowly over a period of 5 to 10 minutes. Hang the container on an IV pole or hold it at the proper height.	Gravity forces the solution to enter the intestine. The amount of pressure determines the rate of flow and pressure exerted on the intestinal wall. Giving the solution too quickly causes rapid distention and pressure, poor defecation, or damage to the mucous membrane.
12. Generously lubricate end of rectal tube 2 to 3 inches (5 to 7 cm). A disposable enema set may have a prelubricated rectal tube.	Lubrication facilitates passage of the rectal tube through the anal sphincter and prevents injury to the mucosa.
13. Lift buttock to expose anus. Ask patient to take several deep breaths. Slowly and gently insert the enema tube 3 to 4 inches (7 to 10 cm) for an adult. Direct it at an angle pointing toward the umbilicus, not the bladder.	Good visualization of the anus helps prevent injury to tissues. Deep breathing helps relax the anal sphincters. The anal canal is about 1 to 2 inches (2.5 to 5 cm) long. Insertion 3 to 4 inches ensures the tube is inserted past the external and internal anal sphincters; further insertion may damage intestinal mucous membrane. The suggested angle follows the normal intestinal contour and thus will help to prevent perforation of the bowel. Slow insertion of the tube minimizes spasms of the intestinal wall and sphincters.
14. If resistance is met while inserting the tube, permit a	Resistance may be due to spasms of the intestine or failure of the

ACTION	RATIONALE
small amount of solution to enter, withdraw tube slightly, and then continue to insert it. **Do not force entry of the tube.** Ask the patient to take several deep breaths.	internal sphincter to open. The solution may help to reduce spasms and relax the sphincter, thus making continued insertion of the tube safe. Forcing a tube may injure the intestinal mucosa wall. Taking deep breaths helps relax the anal sphincter.
15. Introduce solution slowly over a period of 5 to 10 minutes. Hold tubing all the time that solution is being instilled. Assess for dizziness, light-headedness, nausea, diaphoresis, and clammy skin during administration. **If the patient experiences any of these symptoms, stop the procedure immediately, monitor the patient's heart rate and blood pressure, and notify the primary care provider.**	Introducing the solution slowly helps prevent rapid distention of the intestine and a desire to defecate. Assessment allows for detection of a vagal response. The enema may stimulate a vagal response, which increases parasympathetic stimulation, causing a decrease in heart rate.
16. Clamp tubing or lower container if patient desires to defecate or cramping occurs. Instruct the patient to take small, fast breaths or to pant.	These techniques help relax muscles and prevent premature expulsion of the solution.
17. After the solution has been given, clamp tubing and remove tube. Have paper towel ready to receive tube as it is withdrawn.	Wrapping tube in paper towel prevents dripping of solution.
18. Return the patient to a comfortable position. Encourage the patient to hold the solution until the urge to defecate is strong, usually in about 5 to 15 minutes. Make sure the linens under the patient are dry. Remove your gloves and ensure that the patient is covered.	This amount of time usually allows muscle contractions to become sufficient to produce good results. Promotes patient comfort. Removing contaminated gloves prevents spread of microorganisms.

ACTION	RATIONALE
19. Raise side rail. Lower bed height and adjust head of bed to a comfortable position.	Promotes patient safety.
20. Remove additional PPE, if used. Perform hand hygiene.	Removing PPE properly reduces the risk for infection transmission and contamination of other items. Hand hygiene prevents the spread of microorganisms.
21. When patient has a strong urge to defecate, place him/her in a sitting position on a bedpan or assist to commode or bathroom. Offer toilet tissues, if not in the patient's reach. Stay with the patient or have call bell readily accessible.	The sitting position is most natural and facilitates defecation. Fall prevention is a high priority due to the urgency of reaching the commode.
22. Remind patient not to flush the commode before you inspect results of enema.	The results need to be observed and recorded. Additional enemas may be necessary if the physician has ordered enemas "until clear."
23. Put on gloves and assist patient, if necessary, with cleaning anal area. Offer washcloths, skin cleanser, and water for handwashing. Remove gloves.	Cleaning the anal area and proper hygiene deter the spread of microorganisms. Gloves prevent contact with contaminants and body fluids.
24. Leave the patient clean and comfortable. Care for equipment properly.	Bacteria that grow in the intestine can be spread to others if equipment is not properly cleaned.
25. Perform hand hygiene.	Hand hygiene deters the spread of microorganisms.

EVALUATION
- Patient expels feces.
- Patient verbalizes decreased discomfort.
- Abdominal distention is absent.
- Patient remains free of any evidence of trauma to the rectal mucosa or other adverse effect.

DOCUMENTATION

- Document the amount and type of enema solution used; amount, consistency, and color of stool; pain assessment rating; assessment of perineal area for any irritation, tears, or bleeding; and the patient's reaction to the procedure.

SKILL 66 ADMINISTERING A RETENTION ENEMA

Retention enemas are ordered for various reasons. *Oil-retention* enemas help to lubricate the stool and intestinal mucosa, making defecation easier. *Carminative* enemas help to expel flatus from the rectum and relieve distention secondary to flatus. *Medicated* enemas are used to administer a medication rectally. *Anthelmintic* enemas are administered to destroy intestinal parasites.

DELEGATION CONSIDERATIONS

The administration of some types of enemas may be delegated to nursing assistive personnel (NAP) or to unlicensed assistive personnel (UAP) who have received appropriate training. The administration of a retention enema may be delegated to licensed practical/vocational nurses (LPN/LVNs). The decision to delegate must be based on careful analysis of the patient's needs and circumstances, as well as the qualifications of the person to whom the task is being delegated. Refer to the Delegation Guidelines in Appendix A.

EQUIPMENT

- Enema solution (varies depending on reason for enema), often prepackaged, commercially prepared solutions
- Nonsterile gloves
- Additional PPE, as indicated
- Waterproof pad
- Bath blanket
- Washcloth, skin cleanser, and towel
- Bedpan or commode
- Toilet tissue
- Water-soluble lubricant

ASSESSMENT

- Ask the patient when he or she had the last bowel movement.
- Assess the patient's abdomen, including auscultating for bowel sounds, and palpating. Because the goal of a cleansing enema is to increase peristalsis, which should increase bowel sounds, assess the abdomen before and after the enema.
- Assess the rectal area for any fissures, hemorrhoids, sores, or rectal tears. If present, added care should be taken while inserting the tube.

- Assess the results of the patient's laboratory work, specifically the platelet count and white blood cell (WBC) count. An enema is contraindicated for patients with a low platelet count or low WBC count. An enema may irritate or traumatize the GI mucosa, causing bleeding, bowel perforation, or infection in these patients. Any unnecessary procedures that would place the patient with a low platelet count or low WBC count at risk for bleeding or infection should not be performed.
- Assess for dizziness, light-headedness, diaphoresis, nausea, and clammy skin. The enema may stimulate a vagal response, which increases parasympathetic stimulation, causing a decrease in heart rate.
- Do not administer enemas to patients who have severe abdominal pain, bowel obstruction, bowel inflammation or bowel infection, or after rectal, prostate, and colon surgery.

NURSING DIAGNOSIS
- Constipation
- Acute Pain
- Risk for Injury

OUTCOME IDENTIFICATION AND PLANNING
- Patient retains the solution for the prescribed, appropriate length of time and experiences the expected therapeutic effect of the solution.
- Patient verbalizes decreased discomfort.
- Abdominal distention is absent.
- Patient demonstrates signs and symptoms indicative of a resolving infection.
- Patient remains free of any evidence of trauma to the rectal mucosa or other adverse effect.

IMPLEMENTATION

ACTION	RATIONALE
1. Verify the order for the enema. Gather equipment.	Verifying the medical order is crucial to ensuring that the proper enema is administered to the right patient. Assembling equipment provides for an organized approach to the task.
2. Perform hand hygiene and put on PPE, if indicated.	Hand hygiene and PPE prevent the spread of microorganisms. PPE is required based on transmission precautions.

ACTION	RATIONALE
3. Identify the patient.	Identifying the patient ensures the right patient receives the intervention and helps prevent errors.
4. Explain the procedure to the patient and provide the rationale why the tube is needed. Discuss the associated discomforts that may be experienced and possible interventions that may allay this discomfort. Answer any questions, as needed.	Explanation facilitates patient cooperation and reduces anxiety.
5. Assemble equipment on overbed table within reach. Warm the enema solution to body temperature by placing the container in a bowl of warm water.	Arranging items nearby is convenient, saves time, and avoids unnecessary stretching and twisting of muscles on the part of the nurse. A cold solution can cause intestinal cramping.
6. Close the curtains around the bed and close the door to the room, if possible. Discuss where the patient will defecate. Have a bedpan, commode, or nearby bathroom ready for use.	This ensures the patient's privacy. Explanation relieves anxiety and facilitates cooperation. The patient is better able to relax and cooperate if he or she is familiar with the procedure and knows everything is in readiness if the urge to dispel the enema is felt.
7. Adjust the bed to a comfortable working height, usually elbow height of the caregiver (VISN 8 Patient Safety Center, 2009). Position the patient on the left side (Sims' position), as dictated by patient comfort and condition. Fold top linen back just enough to allow access to the patient's rectal area. Drape the patient with the bath blanket, as necessary, to maintain privacy and provide warmth. Place a waterproof pad under the patient's hip.	Having the bed at the proper height prevents back and muscle strain. Sims' position facilitates flow of solution via gravity into the rectum and colon, optimizing retention of the solution. Folding back the linen in this manner minimizes unnecessary exposure and promotes the patient's comfort and warmth. The waterproof pad will protect the bed.

ACTION	RATIONALE
8. Put on gloves.	Gloves prevent contact with blood and body fluids.
9. Remove cap of prepackaged enema solution. Apply a generous amount of lubricant to the tube.	Lubrication is necessary to minimize trauma on insertion.
10. Lift buttock to expose anus. Ask the patient to take several deep breaths. Slowly and gently insert the rectal tube 3 to 4 inches (7 to 10 cm) for an adult. Direct it at an angle pointing toward the umbilicus.	Good visualization of the anus helps prevent injury to tissues. Deep breathing helps relax the anal sphincters. The anal canal is about 1 to 2 inches (2.5 to 5 cm) long. Inserting 3 to 4 inches ensures the tube is inserted past the external and internal anal sphincters; further insertion may damage intestinal mucous membrane. The suggested angle follows the normal intestinal contour and thus will help to prevent perforation of the bowel. Slow insertion of the tube minimizes spasms of the intestinal wall and sphincters. Deep breathing helps relax the anal sphincters.
11. Compress the container with your hands. Roll the end up on itself, toward the rectal tip. Administer all the solution in the container. Assess for dizziness, lightheadedness, nausea, diaphoresis, and clammy skin during administration. **If the patient experiences any of these symptoms, stop the procedure immediately, monitor the patient's heart rate and blood pressure, and notify the primary care provider.**	Rolling the container aids administration of all of the contents of the container. Assessment allows for detection of a vagal response. The enema may stimulate a vagal response, which increases parasympathetic stimulation, causing a decrease in heart rate.
12. **Remove the container while keeping it compressed.** Have paper towel ready to receive tube as it is withdrawn.	If container is released, a vacuum will form, allowing some of the enema solution to re-enter the container.

ACTION	RATIONALE
13. **Instruct the patient to retain the enema solution for at least 30 minutes or as indicated, per manufacturer's direction.**	Solution needs to dwell for at least 30 minutes, or per manufacturer's direction, to allow for its optimal action.
14. Remove your gloves. Return the patient to a comfortable position. Make sure the linens under the patient are dry and ensure that the patient is covered.	Removing contaminated gloves prevents spread of microorganisms. Promotes patient comfort.
15. Raise side rail. Lower bed height and adjust head of bed to a comfortable position.	Promotes patient safety.
16. Remove additional PPE, if used. Perform hand hygiene.	Removing PPE properly reduces the risk for infection transmission and contamination of other items. Hand hygiene prevents the spread of microorganisms.
17. When the patient has a strong urge to dispel the solution, place him or her in a sitting position on bedpan or assist to commode or bathroom. Stay with the patient or have call bell readily accessible.	The sitting position is most natural and facilitates defecation. Fall prevention is a high priority due to the urgency of reaching the commode.
18. Remind the patient not to flush the commode before you inspect the results of enema, if used for bowel evacuation. Record character of stool, as appropriate, and the patient's reaction to the enema.	The results need to be observed and recorded.
19. Put on gloves and assist patient, if necessary, with cleaning of anal area. Offer washcloths, skin cleanser, and water for handwashing. Remove gloves.	Cleaning the anal area and proper hygiene deter the spread of microorganisms. Removing PPE properly reduces the risk for infection transmission and contamination of other items.
20. Leave patient clean and comfortable. Care for equipment properly.	Bacteria that grow in the intestine can be spread to others if equipment is not properly cleaned.

ACTION	RATIONALE
21. Perform hand hygiene.	Hand hygiene deters the spread of microorganisms.

EVALUATION

- Patient expels feces without evidence of trauma to the rectal mucosa.
- Depending on the reason for the retention enema, other outcomes met may include the patient verbalizes a decrease in pain after the enema; and the patient demonstrates signs and symptoms indicative of a resolving infection.

DOCUMENTATION

- Document the amount and type of enema solution used; length of time retained by the patient; amount, consistency, and color of stool, as appropriate; pain assessment rating; assessment of perineal area for any irritation, tears, or bleeding; and the patient's reaction to procedure.

SKILL 67   ADMINISTERING A SMALL-VOLUME CLEANSING ENEMA

Cleansing enemas are given to remove feces from the colon. Some of the reasons for administering a cleansing enema include relieving constipation or fecal impaction, preventing involuntary escape of fecal material during surgical procedures, promoting visualization of the intestinal tract by radiographic or instrument examination, and helping to establish regular bowel function during a bowel training program. Cleansing enemas are classified as either large-volume or small-volume. This skill addresses administering a small-volume enema. (Large-volume enemas are addressed in Skill 65.) Small-volume enemas (adult: 70 to 130 mL) are also known as hypertonic enemas. These hypertonic solutions work by drawing water into the colon, which stimulates the defecation reflex. They may be contraindicated in patients for whom sodium retention is a problem. They are also contraindicated for patients with renal impairment or reduced renal clearance, because these patients have compromised ability to excrete phosphate adequately, with resulting hyperphosphatemia (Jacobson et al., 2010).

DELEGATION CONSIDERATIONS

The administration of some types of enemas may be delegated to nursing assistive personnel (NAP) or to unlicensed assistive personnel (UAP) who have received appropriate training. The administration of a small-volume cleansing enema may be delegated to licensed practical/vocational nurses (LPN/LVNs). The decision to delegate must be based on careful analysis of the patient's needs and circumstances, as well as the qualifications of the person to whom the task is being delegated. Refer to the Delegation Guidelines in Appendix A.

EQUIPMENT

- Commercially prepared enema with rectal tip
- Water-soluble lubricant
- Waterproof pad
- Bath blanket
- Bedpan and toilet tissue
- Disposable gloves
- Additional PPE, as indicated
- Paper towel
- Washcloth, skin cleanser, and towel

ASSESSMENT

- Assess the patient's abdomen, including auscultating for bowel sounds, and palpating the abdomen.
- Assess the abdomen before and after the enema. The goal of a cleansing enema is to increase peristalsis, which should increase bowel sounds.
- Inspect the rectal area for any fissures, hemorrhoids, sores, or rectal tears. If any of these are noted, take added care while administering the enema.
- Check the results of the patient's laboratory work, specifically the platelet count and white blood cell (WBC) count. A normal platelet count ranges from 150,000 to 400,000/mm^3. A platelet count of less than 20,000 may seriously compromise the patient's ability to clot blood. Therefore, do not perform any unnecessary procedures that would place the patient at risk for bleeding or infection. A low WBC count places the patient at risk for infection.
- Assess for dizziness, light-headedness, diaphoresis, nausea, and clammy skin. The enema may stimulate a vagal response, which increases parasympathetic stimulation, causing a decrease in heart rate.
- Do not administer enemas to patients who have severe abdominal pain, bowel obstruction, bowel inflammation or bowel infection, or after rectal, prostate, and colon surgery.

NURSING DIAGNOSIS

- Acute Pain
- Constipation
- Risk for Constipation

OUTCOME IDENTIFICATION AND PLANNING

- Patient expels feces and reports a decrease in pain and discomfort.
- Patient remains free of any evidence of trauma to the rectal mucosa.

IMPLEMENTATION

ACTION	RATIONALE
1. Verify the order for the enema. Gather equipment.	Verifying the medical order is crucial to ensuring that the proper enema is administered to the right patient. Assembling equipment provides for an organized approach to the task.
2. Perform hand hygiene and put on PPE, if indicated.	Hand hygiene and PPE prevent the spread of microorganisms. PPE is required based on transmission precautions.
3. Identify the patient.	Identifying the patient ensures the right patient receives the intervention and helps prevent errors.
4. Explain the procedure to the patient and provide the rationale why the tube is needed. Discuss the associated discomforts that may be experienced and possible interventions that may allay this discomfort. Answer any questions, as needed.	Explanation facilitates patient cooperation and reduces anxiety.
5. Assemble equipment on overbed table within reach. Warm the enema solution to body temperature by placing the container in a bowl of warm water.	Arranging items nearby is convenient, saves time, and avoids unnecessary stretching and twisting of muscles on the part of the nurse. A cold solution can cause intestinal cramping.
6. Close the curtains around the bed and close the door to the room, if possible. Discuss where the patient will defecate. Have a bedpan, commode, or nearby bathroom ready for use.	This ensures the patient's privacy. Explanation relieves anxiety and facilitates cooperation. The patient is better able to relax and cooperate if he or she is familiar with the procedure and knows everything is in readiness

ACTION	RATIONALE
	when the urge to defecate is felt. Defecation usually occurs within 5 to 15 minutes.
7. Adjust the bed to a comfortable working height, usually elbow height of the caregiver (VISN 8 Patient Safety Center, 2009). Position the patient on the left side (Sims' position), as dictated by patient comfort and condition. Fold top linen back just enough to allow access to the patient's rectal area. Drape the patient with the bath blanket, as necessary, to maintain privacy and provide warmth. Place a waterproof pad under the patient's hip.	Having the bed at the proper height prevents back and muscle strain. Sims' position facilitates flow of solution via gravity into the rectum and colon, optimizing retention of solution. Folding back the linen in this manner minimizes unnecessary exposure and promotes the patient's comfort and warmth. The waterproof pad will protect the bed.
8. Put on gloves.	Gloves prevent contact with contaminants and body fluids.
9. Remove the cap and generously lubricate end of rectal tube 2 to 3 inches (5 to 7 cm).	Lubrication facilitates passage of the rectal tube through the anal sphincter and prevents injury to the mucosa.
10. Lift buttock to expose anus. Ask the patient to take several deep breaths. Slowly and gently insert the rectal tube 3 to 4 inches (7 to 10 cm) for an adult. Direct it at an angle pointing toward the umbilicus, not bladder. **Do not force entry of the tube.**	Good visualization of the anus helps prevent injury to tissues. Deep breathing helps relax the anal sphincters. The anal canal is about 1 to 2 inches (2.5 to 5 cm) long. Insertion 3 to 4 inches ensures the tube is inserted past the external and internal anal sphincters; further insertion may damage intestinal mucous membrane. The suggested angle follows the normal intestinal contour, helping prevent perforation of the bowel. Forcing a tube may injure the intestinal mucosa wall.
11. Compress the container with your hands. Roll the end up on itself, toward the rectal tip. Administer all the	Rolling the container aids administration of all of its contents. Assessment allows for detection of a vagal response. The enema

ACTION	RATIONALE
solution in the container. Assess for dizziness, light-headedness, nausea, dia-phoresis, and clammy skin during administration. **If the patient experiences any of these symptoms, stop the procedure immediately, monitor the patient's heart rate and blood pressure, and notify the primary care provider.**	may stimulate a vagal response, which increases parasympathetic stimulation, causing a decrease in heart rate.
12. After the solution has been given, remove the tube, **keeping the container com-pressed.** Have paper towel ready to receive tube as it is withdrawn. Encourage the patient to hold the solution until the urge to defecate is strong, usually in about 5 to 15 minutes.	If the container is released, a vacuum will form, allowing some of the enema solution to re-enter the container. This amount of time usually allows muscle contractions to become sufficient to produce good results.
13. Remove gloves. Return the patient to a comfortable posi-tion. Make sure the linens under the patient are dry. Ensure that the patient is covered.	Promotes patient comfort. Removing contaminated gloves prevents spread of microorgan-isms.
14. Raise side rail. Lower bed height and adjust head of bed to a comfortable position.	Promotes patient safety.
15. Remove additional PPE, if used. Perform hand hygiene.	Removing PPE properly reduces the risk for infection transmission and contamination of other items. Hand hygiene prevents the spread of microorganisms.
16. When patient has a strong urge to defecate, place him/her in a sitting position on a bedpan or assist to com-mode or bathroom. Stay with patient or have call bell readily accessible.	The sitting position is most natu-ral and facilitates defecation. Fall prevention is a high priority due to the urgency of reaching the commode.

ACTION	RATIONALE
17. Remind the patient not to flush the toilet or empty the commode before you inspect the results of the enema.	The results need to be observed and recorded. Additional enemas may be necessary if the physician has ordered enemas "until clear."
18. Put on gloves and assist patient, if necessary, with cleaning of anal area. Offer washcloths, skin cleanser, and water for handwashing. Remove gloves.	Cleaning the anal area and proper hygiene deter the spread of microorganisms.
19. Leave the patient clean and comfortable. Care for equipment properly.	Bacteria that grow in the intestine can be spread to others if equipment is not properly cleaned.
20. Perform hand hygiene.	Hand hygiene deters the spread of microorganisms.

EVALUATION

- Patient expels feces.
- Patient verbalizes decreased discomfort.
- Abdominal distention is absent.
- Patient remains free of any evidence of trauma to the rectal mucosa or other adverse effect.

DOCUMENTATION

- Document the amount and type of enema solution used; amount, consistency, and color of stool; pain assessment rating; assessment of perineal area for any irritation, tears, or bleeding; and patient's reaction to the procedure.

SKILL 68   CARING FOR A PATIENT RECEIVING EPIDURAL ANALGESIA

Epidural analgesia is being used more commonly to provide pain relief during the immediate postoperative phase (particularly after thoracic, abdominal, orthopedic, and vascular surgery), procedural pain, trauma pain, and for chronic pain situations (Sawhney, 2012). Epidural pain management is also being used with infants and children (Kyle & Carman, 2013). The anesthesiologist or radiologist usually inserts the catheter in the mid-lumbar region into the epidural space that exists between the walls of the vertebral canal and the dura mater or outermost connective tissue membrane surrounding the spinal cord. For temporary therapy, the catheter exits directly over the spine, and the tubing is positioned over the patient's shoulder with the end of the catheter taped to the chest. For long-term therapy, the catheter is usually tunneled subcutaneously and exits on the side of the body or on the abdomen.

The epidural analgesia can be administered as a bolus dose (either one time or intermittently), via a continuous infusion pump, or by a patient-controlled epidural analgesia (PCEA) pump (Taylor et al., 2015). Additional information specific to PCA administration is discussed in Skill 127. Epidural catheters used for the management of acute pain are typically removed 36 to 72 hours after surgery, when oral medication can be substituted for pain relief.

DELEGATION CONSIDERATIONS

The care related to epidural analgesia is not delegated to nursing assistive personnel (NAP) or to unlicensed assistive personnel (UAP). Depending on the state's nurse practice act and the organization's policies and procedures, specific aspects of the care related to epidural analgesia, such as monitoring the infusion and assessment of patient response, may be delegated to licensed practical/vocational nurses (LPN/LVNs). The decision to delegate must be based on careful analysis of the patient's needs and circumstances, as well as the qualifications of the person to whom the task is being delegated. Refer to the Delegation Guidelines in Appendix A.

EQUIPMENT

- Volume infusion device
- Epidural infusion tubing
- Prescribed epidural analgesic solutions
- Computerized medication administration record (CMAR) or medication administration record (MAR)
- Pain assessment tool and/or measurement scale
- Transparent dressing or gauze pads

- Labels for epidural infusion line
- Tape
- Emergency drugs and equipment, such as naloxone, oxygen, endotracheal intubation set, handheld resuscitation bag, per facility policy
- Gloves
- Additional PPE, as indicated

ASSESSMENT

- Review the patient's medical record and plan of care for specific instructions related to epidural analgesia therapy, including the medical order for the drug and conditions indicating the need for therapy.
- Review the patient's history for conditions that might contraindicate therapy, such as local or systemic infections, increased intracranial

pressure, neurologic disease, coagulopathy or use of anticoagulant therapy, spinal arthritis or spinal deformity, hypotension, marked hypertension, allergy to the prescribed medication, or psychiatric disorder.
- Check to ensure proper functioning of the unit.
- Assess the patient's level of consciousness and understanding of epidural analgesia therapy and the rationale for its use.
- Assess the patient's level of discomfort and pain using an appropriate assessment tool. Assess the characteristics of any pain. Assess for other symptoms that often occur with the pain, such as headache or restlessness. Ask the patient what interventions have and have not been successful in the past to promote comfort and relieve pain.
- Assess the patient's vital signs and respiratory status, including rate, depth, and rhythm, oxygen saturation level using pulse oximetry, and level of carbon dioxide concentration using capnography.
- Assess the patient's sedation score.
- Assess the patient's response to the intervention to evaluate effectiveness and for the presence of adverse effects.

NURSING DIAGNOSIS
- Acute Pain
- Chronic Pain
- Risk for Infection
- Deficient Knowledge

OUTCOME IDENTIFICATION AND PLANNING
- Patient reports increased comfort and/or decreased pain, without adverse effects, oversedation, and respiratory depression.
- Patient displays decreased anxiety.
- Patient displays improved coping skills.
- Patient remains free from infection.
- Patient verbalizes an understanding of the therapy and the reason for its use.

IMPLEMENTATION

ACTION	RATIONALE
1. Gather equipment. Check the medication order against the original order in the medical record, according to facility policy. Clarify any inconsistencies. Check the patient's medical record for allergies.	This comparison helps to identify errors that may have occurred when orders were transcribed. The medical order is the legal record-of-medication order for each agency.

ACTION	RATIONALE
2. Know the actions, special nursing considerations, safe dose ranges, purpose of administration, and adverse effects of the medications to be administered. Consider the appropriateness of the medication for this patient.	This knowledge aids the nurse in evaluating the therapeutic effect of the medication in relation to the patient's disorder and can also be used to educate the patient about the medication.
3. Prepare the medication syringe or other container for administration, based on facility policy.	Proper preparation and administration prevent errors.
4. Perform hand hygiene and put on PPE, if indicated.	Hand hygiene and PPE prevent the spread of microorganisms. PPE is required based on transmission precautions.
5. Identify the patient.	Identifying the patient ensures that the right patient receives the intervention and helps prevent errors.
6. Show the patient the device, and explain the function of the device and the reason for it use. Explain the purpose and action of the medication to the patient.	Explanation encourages patient understanding and cooperation and reduces apprehension.
7. Close the door to the room or pull the bedside curtain.	Closing the door or curtain provides patient privacy.
8. Complete necessary assessments before administering the medication. Check allergy bracelet or ask the patient about allergies. Assess the patient's pain, using an appropriate assessment tool and measurement scale. Put on gloves.	Assessment is a prerequisite to administration of medications. Accurate assessment is necessary to guide treatment and relief interventions and to evaluate the effectiveness of pain control measures. Gloves are indicated for potential contact with blood or body fluids.
9. **Have an ampule of 0.4 mg naloxone (Narcan) and a syringe at the bedside.**	Naloxone reverses the respiratory depressant effect of opioids.

ACTION	RATIONALE
10. After the catheter has been inserted and the infusion initiated by the anesthesiologist or radiologist, **check the label on the medication container and rate of infusion with the medication record and patient identification.** Obtain verification of information from a second nurse, according to facility policy. If using a barcode administration system, scan the barcode on the medication label, if required.	This action verifies that the correct drug and dosage will be administered to the correct patient. Confirmation of information by a second nurse helps prevent errors. Scanning the barcode provides an additional check to ensure that the medication is given to the right patient.
11. Tape all connection sites. Label the bag, tubing, and pump apparatus "For Epidural Infusion Only." **Do not administer any other narcotics or adjuvant drugs without the approval of the clinician responsible for the epidural injection.**	Taping prevents accidental dislodgement. Labeling prevents inadvertent administration of other IV medications through this setup. Additional medication may potentiate the action of the opioid, increasing the risk for respiratory depression.
12. Assess the catheter exit site and apply a transparent dressing over the catheter insertion site, if not already in place. Remove gloves and additional PPE, if used. Perform hand hygiene.	The transparent dressing protects the site while still allowing assessment. Removing PPE properly reduces the risk for infection transmission and contamination of other items. Hand hygiene reduces transmission of microorganisms.
13. Monitor the infusion rate according to facility policy. Assess and record sedation level and respiratory status, including the patient's oxygen saturation, continuously for the first 20 minutes after initiation, then at least every hour for the first 12 hours, every 2 hours up to 24 hours, then at 4-hour intervals (or according to facility policy) (Sawhney, 2012). **Notify the**	Monitoring the infusion rate prevents incorrect administration of the medication. Opioids can depress the respiratory center in the medulla. A change in the level of consciousness is usually the first sign of altered respiratory function.

ACTION	RATIONALE
physician if the sedation rating is 3 or 4, the respiratory depth decreases, or the respiratory rate falls below 10 breaths per minute. Also monitor end-tidal carbon dioxide level (capnography) for patients at high risk of respiratory depression (Sawhney, 2012).	
14. Keep the head of bed elevated 30 degrees unless contraindicated.	Elevation of the patient's head minimizes upward migration of the opioid in the spinal cord, thus decreasing the risk for respiratory depression.
15. Assess the patient's level of pain and the effectiveness of pain relief.	This information helps in determining the need for subsequent *breakthrough* pain medication.
16. Monitor the patient's blood pressure and pulse.	Hypotension can result from the use of epidural analgesia.
17. Monitor urinary output and assess for bladder distention.	Opioids can cause urinary retention.
18. Assess motor strength and sensation every 4 hours.	The catheter may migrate into the intrathecal space and allow opioids to block the transmission of nerve impulses completely through the spinal cord to the brain.
19. Monitor for adverse effects (pruritus, nausea, and vomiting).	Opioids may spread into the trigeminal nerve, causing itching, or resulting in nausea and vomiting owing to slowed gastrointestinal function or stimulation of a chemoreceptor trigger zone in the brain. Medications are available to treat these adverse effects.
20. Assess for signs of infection at the insertion site.	Inflammation or local infection can develop at the catheter insertion site.
21. Assess the catheter-site dressing for drainage, based on facility policy. Notify the anesthesia provider or pain management team	Catheter-site dressing should remain clean, dry and intact. Abnormalities in the dressing may indicate leakage of cerebrospinal fluid or catheter

ACTION	RATIONALE
immediately of any abnormalities. Change the dressing over the catheter exit site per facility policy using aseptic technique. Change the infusion tubing every 48 hours or as specified by facility policy.	dislodgement. Dressing and tubing changes using aseptic technique reduce the risk for infection.

EVALUATION

- Patient verbalizes pain relief.
- Patient exhibits a dry, intact dressing, and the catheter exit site is free of signs and symptoms of complications, injury, or infection.
- Patient reports a decrease in anxiety and increased ability to cope with pain.
- Patient verbalizes information related to the functioning of the epidural catheter and the reasons for its use.

DOCUMENTATION

- Document catheter patency; the condition of the insertion site and dressing; sedation score, oxygen saturation, vital signs, and assessment information; any change in infusion rate, solution, or tubing; analgesics administered; and the patient's response.

SKILL 69   CARING FOR A PATIENT WITH AN EXTERNAL FIXATION DEVICE

External fixation devices are used to manage open fractures with soft-tissue damage. They consist of one of a variety of frames to hold pins that are drilled into or through bones. External fixators provide stable support for severely crushed or splintered fractures and access to and treatment for soft-tissue injuries. The use of these devices allows treatment of the fracture and damaged soft tissues while promoting patient comfort, early mobility, and active exercise of adjacent uninvolved joints. Complications related to disuse and immobility are minimized. Nursing responsibilities include reassuring the patient, maintaining the device, monitoring neurovascular status, promoting exercise, preventing complications from the therapy, preventing infection by providing pin-site care, and providing teaching to ensure compliance and self-care. A growing evidence base supports effective management of pin sites, but no clear consensus (Walker, 2012; Lagerquist et al., 2012). Pin-site care often varies based on primary care provider and facility policy. Dressings are often applied for the first 48 to 72 hours, and then sites may be left open to air. Pin-site care may be performed frequently in the first 48 to 72 hours after application, when drainage may be heavy; other evidence suggests pin care should begin after the first 48 to 72 hours. Pin-site care may be done daily or weekly (Timms & Pugh, 2012; Lagerquist et al., 2012). Refer to specific patient medical orders and facility guidelines.

Nurses play a major role in preparing the patient psychologically for the application of an external fixator. The devices appear clumsy and large. In addition, the nurse needs to clarify misconceptions regarding pain and discomfort associated with the device.

DELEGATION CONSIDERATIONS

The care of a patient with an external fixator device may not be delegated to nursing assistive personnel (NAP) or to unlicensed assistive personnel (UAP). Depending on the state's nurse practice act and the organization's policies and procedures, care for these patients may be delegated to licensed practical/vocational nurses (LPN/LVNs). The decision to delegate must be based on careful analysis of the patient's needs and circumstances, as well as the qualifications of the person to whom the task is being delegated. Refer to the Delegation Guidelines in Appendix A.

EQUIPMENT

Equipment varies with the type of fixator and the type and location of the fracture but may include:
- Sterile applicators
- Cleansing solution, usually sterile normal saline or chlorhexidine, per primary care provider order or facility policy
- Ice bag

- Antimicrobial ointment, per primary care provider order or facility policy
- Sterile gauze or dressing, per primary care provider order or facility policy
- Analgesic, as ordered
- Sterile gloves for performing pin care, depending on facility policy
- Additional PPE, as indicated

ASSESSMENT

- Review the patient's medical record and the nursing plan of care to determine the type of device being used and prescribed care.
- Assess the patient's pain and need for analgesia before providing care.
- Assess the external fixator to ensure proper function and position.
- Perform skin and neurovascular assessments.
- Inspect the pin insertion sites for signs of inflammation and infection, including swelling, cloudy or offensive drainage, pain, or redness.
- Assess the patient's knowledge regarding the device and self-care activities and responsibilities.

NURSING DIAGNOSIS

- Risk for Infection
- Anxiety
- Acute Pain
- Self-Care Deficit (toileting, bathing, or dressing)

OUTCOME IDENTIFICATION AND PLANNING

- Patient shows no evidence of complication, such as infection, contractures, venous stasis, thrombus formation, or skin breakdown.
- Patient shows signs of healing.
- Patient experiences relief from pain.
- Patient is free from injury.

IMPLEMENTATION

ACTION	RATIONALE
1. Review the medical record and the nursing plan of care to determine the type of device being used and prescribed care.	Reviewing the medical record and plan of care validates the correct patient and correct procedure.
2. Perform hand hygiene. Put on PPE, as indicated.	Hand hygiene and PPE prevent the spread of microorganisms. PPE is required based on transmission precautions.
3. Identify the patient. Explain the procedure to the patient. Assure the patient that there will be little pain after the fixation device is in place. Reinforce that the patient will be able to adjust to the device and will be able to move about with the device, allowing him or her to resume normal activities more quickly.	Patient identification validates the correct patient and correct procedure. Discussion and explanation allay anxiety and prepare the patient psychologically for the application of the device.
4. **After the fixation device is in place, apply ice to the surgical site, as ordered or per facility policy. Elevate the affected body part, if appropriate.**	Ice and elevation help reduce swelling, relieve pain, and reduce bleeding.

ACTION	RATIONALE
5. Perform a pain assessment and assess for muscle spasm. Administer prescribed medications in sufficient time to allow for the full effect of the analgesic and/or muscle relaxant.	Pain assessment and analgesic administration help promote patient comfort.
6. Administer analgesics, as ordered, before exercising or mobilizing the affected body part.	Administration of analgesics promotes patient comfort and facilitates movement.
7. Perform neurovascular assessments, per facility policy or medical order, usually every 2 to 4 hours for 24 hours, then every 4 to 8 hours. Assess the affected body part for color, motion, sensation, edema, capillary refill, and pulses. If appropriate, compare with the unaffected side. Assess for pain not relieved by analgesics, and for burning, tingling, and numbness.	Assessment promotes early detection and prompt intervention for abnormal neurovascular function, nerve damage, or circulatory impairment. Assessment of neurovascular status determines the circulation and oxygenation of tissues.
8. Close the curtains around the bed and close the door to the room, if possible. Place the bed at an appropriate and comfortable working height, usually elbow height of the caregiver (VISN 8 Patient Safety Center, 2009).	Closing the door or curtains provides for privacy. Proper bed height prevents back and muscle strain.
9. Assess the pin site for redness, tenting of the skin, prolonged or purulent drainage, swelling, and bowing, bending, or loosening of the pins. Monitor body temperature.	Assessing pin sites aids in early detection of infection and stress on the skin and allows for appropriate intervention.
10. Perform pin-site care.	Performing pin-site care prevents crusting at the site that could lead to fluid buildup, infection, and osteomyelitis.

ACTION	RATIONALE
a. Using sterile technique, open the applicator package and pour the cleansing agent into the sterile container.	Using sterile technique reduces the risk for transmission of microorganisms.
b. Put on the sterile gloves.	Gloves prevent contact with blood and/or body fluids.
c. Place the applicators into the solution.	
d. **Clean the pin site starting at the insertion area and working outward, away from the pin site (Figure 1).**	Cleaning from the center outward promotes movement from the least to most contaminated area.

FIGURE 1 Cleaning around pin sites with normal saline on an applicator.

ACTION	RATIONALE
e. **Use each applicator once. Use a new applicator for each pin site.**	Using each applicator only once prevents transfer of microorganisms.
11. Depending on medical order and facility policy, apply the antimicrobial ointment to pin sites and apply a dressing. Remove gloves and dispose of them appropriately.	Antimicrobial ointment helps reduce the risk of infection. A dressing aids in protecting the pin sites from contamination and containing any drainage. Disposing of gloves reduces the risk of microorganism transmission.
12. Perform range-of-motion exercises on all joint areas, unless contraindicated. Encourage the patient to cough and deep breathe every 2 hours.	Range-of-motion exercises promote joint mobility. Coughing and deep breathing reduce the risk of respiratory complications related to immobility.
13. Place the bed in the lowest position that still allows the weight to hang freely, with	Proper bed positioning ensures effective application of traction without patient injury. Leaving the

ACTION	RATIONALE
the side rails up. Make sure the call bell and other essential items are within easy reach.	call bell and other items within reach ensures patient safety.
14. Remove PPE, if used. Perform hand hygiene.	Removing PPE properly reduces the risk for infection transmission and contamination of other items. Hand hygiene prevents the spread of microorganisms.

EVALUATION

- Patient exhibits an external fixation device in place with pin sites that are clean, dry, and intact, without evidence of infection.
- Patient remains free of complications, such as contractures, venous stasis, thrombus formation, or skin breakdown.
- Patient verbalizes pain relief.
- Patient remains free of injury.
- Patient demonstrates knowledge of pin-site care.

DOCUMENTATION

- Document the time, date, and type of device in place. Include the skin assessment, pin site assessment, and pin-site care. Document the patient's response to the device and the neurovascular status of the affected area.

SKILL 70 INSTILLING EYE DROPS

Eye drops are instilled for their local effects, such as for pupil dilation or constriction when examining the eye, for infection treatment, or for controlling intraocular pressure (for patients with glaucoma). The type and amount of solution administered depends on the purpose of the instillation.

The eye is a delicate organ, highly susceptible to infection and injury. Although the eye is never free of microorganisms, the secretions of the conjunctiva protect against many pathogens. For maximal safety for the patient, the equipment, solutions, and ointments introduced into the conjunctival sac should be sterile. If this is not possible, follow careful guidelines for medical asepsis.

DELEGATION CONSIDERATIONS

The administration of medication via drops in the eye is not delegated to nursing assistive personnel (NAP) or to unlicensed assistive personnel (UAP). Depending on the state's nurse practice act and the organization's policies and procedures, the administration of eye drops may be delegated to licensed practical/vocational nurses (LPN/LVNs). The decision to delegate must be based on careful analysis of the patient's needs and circumstances, as well as the qualifications of the person to whom the task is being delegated. Refer to the Delegation Guidelines in Appendix A.

EQUIPMENT

- Gloves
- Additional PPE, as indicated
- Medication
- Tissues
- Normal saline solution
- Washcloth, cotton balls, or gauze squares
- Computer-generated Medication Administration Record (CMAR) or Medication Administration Record (MAR)

ASSESSMENT

- Assess the patient for any allergies.
- Check the expiration date before administering the medication.
- Assess the appropriateness of the drug for the patient.
- Review assessment and laboratory data that may influence drug administration.
- Verify patient name, dose, route, and time of administration.
- Assess the affected eye for any drainage, erythema, or swelling.
- Assess the patient's knowledge of the medication. If the patient has a knowledge deficit about the medication, this may be the appropriate time to begin education about the medication.
- If the medication may affect the patient's vital signs, assess them before administration.

NURSING DIAGNOSIS

- Risk for Allergy Response
- Deficient Knowledge
- Risk for Injury

OUTCOME IDENTIFICATION AND PLANNING

- Medication is delivered successfully into the eye.
- Patient experiences no allergy response.
- Patient does not exhibit systemic effects of the medication.
- Patient's eye remains free from injury.
- Patient understands the rationale for medication administration.

IMPLEMENTATION

ACTION	RATIONALE
1. Gather equipment. Check medication order against the original order in the medical record, according to facility policy. Clarify any inconsistencies. Check the patient's chart for allergies.	This comparison helps to identify errors that may have occurred when orders were transcribed. The primary care provider's order is the legal record of medication orders for each facility.
2. Know the actions, special nursing considerations, safe dose ranges, purpose of administration, and adverse effects of the medications to be administered. Consider the appropriateness of the medication for this patient.	This knowledge aids the nurse in evaluating the therapeutic effect of the medication in relation to the patient's disorder and can also be used to educate the patient about the medication.
3. Perform hand hygiene.	Hand hygiene prevents the spread of microorganisms.
4. Move the medication cart to the outside of the patient's room or prepare for administration in the medication area.	Organization facilitates error-free administration and saves time.
5. Unlock the medication cart or drawer. Enter pass code and scan employee identification, if required.	Locking the cart or drawer safeguards each patient's medication supply. Hospital accrediting organizations require medication carts to be locked when not in use. Entering pass code and scanning ID allows only authorized users into the system and identifies the user for documentation by the computer.
6. **Prepare medications for one patient at a time.**	This prevents errors in medication administration.
7. Read the CMAR/MAR and select the proper medication from the patient's medication drawer or unit stock.	This is the *first* check of the label.
8. Compare the label with the CMAR/MAR. Check	This is the *second* check of the label. Verify calculations with

ACTION	RATIONALE
expiration dates and perform calculations, if necessary. Scan the bar code on the package, if required.	another nurse to ensure safety, if necessary.
9. **Depending on facility policy, the third check of the label may occur at this point. If so, when all medications for one patient have been prepared, recheck the labels with the CMAR/MAR before taking the medications to the patient.**	This *third* check ensures accuracy and helps to prevent errors. *Note:* Many facilities require the *third* check to occur at the bedside, after identifying the patient and before administration.
10. Lock the medication cart before leaving it.	Locking the cart or drawer safeguards the patient's medication supply. Hospital accrediting organizations require medication carts to be locked when not in use.
11. Transport medications to the patient's bedside carefully, and keep the medications in sight at all times.	Careful handling and close observation prevent accidental or deliberate disarrangement of medications.
12. **Ensure that the patient receives the medications at the correct time.**	Check agency policy, which may allow for administration within a period of 30 minutes before or 30 minutes after the designated time.
13. Perform hand hygiene and 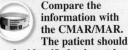 put on PPE, if indicated.	Hand hygiene and PPE prevent the spread of microorganisms. PPE is required based on transmission precautions.
14. **Identify the patient. Compare the information with the CMAR/MAR. The patient should be identified using at least two methods** (The Joint Commission, 2013):	Identifying the patient ensures the right patient receives the medications and helps prevent errors. The patient's room number or physical location is not used as an identifier (The Joint Commission, 2013). Replace the identification band if it is missing or inaccurate in any way.
a. Check the name on the patient's identification band.	

ACTION	RATIONALE

b. Check the identification number on the patient's identification band.

c. Check the birth date on the patient's identification band.

d. Ask the patient to state his or her name and birth date, based on facility policy.

This requires a response from the patient, but illness and strange surroundings often cause patients to be confused.

15. **Complete necessary assessments before administering medications. Check the patient's allergy bracelet or ask the patient about allergies. Explain the purpose and action of each medication to the patient.**

Assessment is a prerequisite to administration of medications.

16. Scan the patient's bar code on the identification band, if required.

Provides an additional check to ensure that the medication is given to the right patient.

17. **Based on facility policy, the third check of the label may occur at this point. If so, recheck the labels with the CMAR/MAR before administering the medications to the patient.**

Many facilities require the *third* check to occur at the bedside, after identifying the patient and before administration. If facility policy directs the *third* check at this time, this *third* check ensures accuracy and helps to prevent errors.

18. Put on gloves.

Gloves protect the nurse from potential contact with mucous membranes and body fluids.

19. Offer tissue to patient.

Solution and tears may spill from the eye during the procedure.

20. Cleanse the eyelids and eyelashes of any drainage with a washcloth, cotton balls, or gauze squares moistened with normal saline solution. Use each area of the cleaning surface once, moving from the inner toward the outer canthus.

Debris can be carried into the eye when the conjunctival sac is exposed. Using each area of the gauze once and moving from the inner canthus to the outer canthus prevents carrying debris to the lacrimal ducts.

ACTION	RATIONALE
21. Tilt the patient's head back slightly if sitting, or place the patient's head over a pillow if lying down. **Tilting the patient's head should be avoided if the patient has a cervical spine injury.** The head may be turned slightly to the affected side to prevent solution or tears from flowing toward the opposite eye.	Tilting the patient's head back slightly makes it easier to reach the conjunctival sac. Turning the head to the affected side helps to prevent solution or tears from flowing toward the opposite eye.
22. Remove the cap from the medication bottle, being careful not to touch the inner side of the cap.	Touching the inner side of the cap may contaminate the bottle of medication.
23. Invert the monodrip plastic container that is commonly used to instill eye drops. Have the patient look up and focus on something on the ceiling.	By having the patient look up and focus on something else, the procedure is less traumatic and keeps the eye still.
24. Place thumb or two fingers near margin of lower eyelid immediately below eye-lashes, and exert pressure downward over bony cheek prominence. The lower con-junctival sac is exposed as the lower lid is pulled down.	The eye drop should be placed in the conjunctival sac, not directly on the eyeball.
25. **Hold the dropper close to the eye, but avoid touching eyelids or lashes.** Squeeze container and allow prescribed number of drops to fall in lower conjunctival sac.	Touching the eye, eyelids, or lashes can contaminate the medication in the bottle; startle the patient, causing blinking; or injure the eye. Do not allow medication to fall onto the cornea. This may injure the cornea or cause the patient to have an unpleasant sensation.
26. Release lower lid after eye drops are instilled. Ask patient to close eyes gently.	This allows the medication to be distributed over the entire eye.
27. Apply gentle pressure over inner canthus to prevent eye drops from flowing into tear duct.	This minimizes the risk of systemic effects from the medication.

ACTION	RATIONALE
28. Instruct patient not to rub affected eye.	This prevents injury and irritation to the eye.
29. Remove gloves. Assist the patient to a comfortable position.	This ensures patient comfort.
30. Remove additional PPE, if used. Perform hand hygiene.	Removing PPE properly reduces the risk for infection transmission and contamination of other items. Hand hygiene prevents the spread of microorganisms.
31. Document the administration of the medication immediately after administration. See Documentation section below.	Timely documentation helps to ensure patient safety.
32. Evaluate the patient's response to the medication within an appropriate time frame.	The patient needs to be evaluated for therapeutic and adverse effects from the medication.

EVALUATION

- Patient receives the eye drops.
- Patient experiences no adverse effects, including allergy response, systemic effects, or injury.
- Patient verbalizes an understanding of the rationale for the medication administration.

DOCUMENTATION

- Document the administration of the medication immediately after administration, including date, time, dose, route of administration, and site of administration, specifically right, left, or both eyes, on the CMAR/MAR or record using the required format. If using a bar-code system, medication administration is automatically recorded when the bar code is scanned. PRN medications require documentation of the reason for administration. Prompt recording avoids the possibility of accidentally repeating the administration of the drug. If the drug was refused or omitted, record this in the appropriate area on the medication record and notify the primary care provider. This verifies the reason medication was omitted and ensures that the primary care provider is aware of the patient's condition.

SKILL 71 | ADMINISTERING AN EYE IRRIGATION

Eye irrigation is performed to remove secretions or foreign bodies or to cleanse and soothe the eye. When irrigating one eye, take care that the overflowing irrigation fluid does not contaminate the other eye.

DELEGATION CONSIDERATIONS

The administration of an eye irrigation is not delegated to nursing assistive personnel (NAP) or to unlicensed assistive personnel (UAP). Depending on the state's nurse practice act and the organization's policies and procedures, the administration of an eye irrigation may be delegated to licensed practical/vocational nurses (LPN/LVNs). The decision to delegate must be based on careful analysis of the patient's needs and circumstances, as well as the qualifications of the person to whom the task is being delegated. Refer to the Delegation Guidelines in Appendix A.

EQUIPMENT

- Sterile irrigation solution (warmed to 37°C [98.6°F])
- Sterile irrigation set (sterile container and irrigating or bulb syringe)
- Emesis basin or irrigation basin
- Washcloth
- Waterproof pad
- Towel
- Gloves
- Additional PPE, as indicated

ASSESSMENT

- Assess the patient's eyes for redness, erythema, edema, drainage, or tenderness.
- Assess the patient for allergies.
- Verify patient name, dose, route, and time of administration.
- Assess the patient's knowledge of the procedure. If the patient has a knowledge deficit about the procedure, this may be an appropriate time to begin patient education.
- Assess the patient's ability to cooperate with the procedure.

NURSING DIAGNOSIS

- Deficient Knowledge
- Risk for Injury
- Acute Pain

OUTCOME IDENTIFICATION AND PLANNING

- Patient's eye is cleansed successfully.
- Patient understands the rationale for the procedure and is able to participate.
- Patient's eye remains free from injury.
- Patient remains free from pain.

IMPLEMENTATION

ACTION	RATIONALE
1. Gather equipment. Check the original order in the medical record for the irrigation, according to facility policy. Clarify any inconsistencies. Check the patient's chart for allergies.	This comparison helps to identify errors that may have occurred when orders were transcribed. The primary care provider's order is the legal record of medication orders for each facility.
2. Perform hand hygiene and put on PPE, if indicated.	Hand hygiene and PPE prevent the spread of microorganisms. PPE is required based on transmission precautions.
3. **Identify the patient. Compare the information with the CMAR/MAR. The patient should be identified using at least two methods** (The Joint Commission, 2013):	Identifying the patient ensures the right patient receives the medication and helps prevent errors. The patient's room number or physical location is not used as an identifier (The Joint Commission, 2013). Replace the identification band if it is missing or inaccurate in any way.
a. Check the name on the patient's identification.	
b. Check the identification number on the patient's identification band.	
c. Check the birth date on the patient's identification band.	
d. Ask the patient to state his or her name and birth date, based on facility policy.	This requires a response from the patient, but illness and strange surroundings often cause patients to be confused.
4. Explain the procedure to the patient.	Explanation facilitates cooperation and reassures the patient.
5. Scan the patient's bar code on the identification band, if required.	Provides an additional check to ensure that the medication is given to the right patient.
6. Assemble equipment at the patient's bedside.	This provides for an organized approach to the task.

ACTION	RATIONALE
7. Have the patient sit or lie with head tilted toward side of affected eye. Protect the patient and bed with a waterproof pad.	Gravity aids flow of the solution away from the unaffected eye and from the inner canthus of the affected eye toward the outer canthus.
8. Put on gloves. Clean lids and lashes with washcloth moistened with normal saline or the solution ordered for the irrigation. Wipe from inner canthus to outer canthus. Use a different corner of washcloth with each wipe.	Gloves protect the nurse from contact with mucous membranes, body fluids, and contaminants. Materials lodged on lids or in lashes may be washed into the eye. Wiping from the inner to outer canthus protects the nasolacrimal duct and the other eye. Use of a different part of the washcloth prevents transmission of bacteria.
9. Place curved basin at cheek on the side of the affected eye to receive irrigating solution. If patient is able, ask him/her to support the basin.	Gravity aids flow of solution.
10. Expose lower conjunctival sac and hold upper lid open with your nondominant hand.	Solution is directed only into lower conjunctival sac because the cornea is sensitive and easily injured. This also prevents reflex blinking.
11. Fill the irrigation syringe with the prescribed fluid. **Hold irrigation syringe about 2.5 cm (1 inch) from eye. Direct flow of solution from inner to outer canthus along the conjunctival sac.**	This minimizes the risk for injury to the cornea. Directing solution toward the outer canthus helps to prevent the spread of contamination from the eye to the lacrimal sac, the lacrimal duct, and the nose.
12. Irrigate until the solution is clear or all the solution has been used. **Use only enough force to remove secretions gently from the conjunctiva. Avoid touching any part of the eye with the irrigating tip.**	Directing solutions with force may cause injury to the tissues of the eye as well as to the conjunctiva. Touching the eye is uncomfortable for the patient and may cause damage to the cornea.
13. Pause the irrigation and have the patient close the eye periodically during the procedure.	Movement of the eye when the lids are closed helps to move secretions from the upper to the lower conjunctival sac.

ACTION	RATIONALE
14. Dry the periorbital area after irrigation with gauze sponge. Offer a towel to the patient if face and neck are wet.	Leaving the skin moist after irrigation is uncomfortable for the patient.
15. Remove gloves. Assist the patient to a comfortable position.	This ensures patient comfort.
16. Remove additional PPE, if used. Perform hand hygiene.	Removing PPE properly reduces the risk for infection transmission and contamination of other items. Hand hygiene prevents the spread of microorganisms.
17. Evaluate the patient's response to the medication within an appropriate time frame.	The patient needs to be evaluated for therapeutic and adverse effects from the medication.

EVALUATION
- Patient's eye has been irrigated successfully.
- Patient understands the rationale for the procedure and is able to comply with the procedure.
- Patient's eye is not injured.
- Patient experiences minimal discomfort.

DOCUMENTATION
- Document the procedure, site, the type of solution and volume used, length of time irrigation performed, pre- and post-procedure assessments, characteristics of any drainage, and the patient's response to the treatment.

SKILL 72 FALL PREVENTION

Falls are associated with physical and psychological trauma, especially in older adults. Fall-related injuries are often serious and can be fatal. Falls are caused by and associated with multiple factors.

Primary causes of falls include:
- Change in balance or gait disturbance
- Muscle weakness
- Dizziness, syncope, and vertigo

- Cardiovascular changes, such as postural hypotension
- Change in vision or vision impairment
- Physical environment/environmental hazards
- Acute illness
- Neurologic disease, such as dementia or depression
- Language disorders that impair communication
- Polypharmacy

Many of these causes are within the realm of nursing responsibility. Identifying at-risk patients is crucial to planning appropriate interventions to prevent a fall. The combination of an assessment tool with a care/intervention plan sets the stage for best practice (AGS, 2012b; AGS & BGS, 2010; Gray-Micelli, 2012; and Hendrich, 2007). Accurate assessment and use of appropriate multifactorial fall interventions leads to maximum prevention (Degelau et al., 2012). Fall-risk assessment is discussed in the following assessment section. Providing patient education and a safer patient environment can reduce the incidence and severity of falls. The ultimate goal is to reduce the physical and psychological trauma experienced by patients and their significant others.

DELEGATION CONSIDERATIONS

After assessment of fall risk by the RN, activities related to the prevention of falls may be delegated to nursing assistive personnel (NAP) or unlicensed assistive personnel (UAP), as well as to licensed practical/vocational nurses (LPN/LVNs). The decision to delegate must be based on careful analysis of the patient's needs and circumstances, as well as the qualifications of the person to whom the task is being delegated. Refer to the Delegation Guidelines in Appendix A.

EQUIPMENT

- Fall-risk assessment tool, if available
- PPE, as indicated

- Additional intervention tools, as appropriate (refer to sample intervention equipment in this skill)

ASSESSMENT

- At a minimum, fall-risk assessment needs to occur on admission to the facility, following a change in the patient's condition, after a fall, and when the patient is transferred. If it is determined that the patient is at risk for falling, regular assessment must continue.
- Assess the patient and the medical record for factors that increase the patient's risk for falling. The use of an objective, systematic fall assessment is made easier by the use of a fall assessment tool.
- Assess for a history of falls. If the patient has experienced a previous fall, assess the circumstances surrounding the fall and any associated symptoms.
- Review the patient's medication history and medication record for medications that may increase the risk for falls. Assess for the

following additional risk factors for falls (AGS & BGS, 2010; Gray-Micelli, 2012; Hendrich, 2007; Titler, et al., 2011):

- Lower extremity muscle weakness
- Gait or balance deficit
- Restraint use
- Use of an assistive device
- Presence of intravenous therapy
- Impaired activities of daily living
- Age older than 75 years
- Altered elimination
- History of falls
- Administration of high-risk drugs, such as narcotic analgesics, antiepileptics, benzodiazepines, and drugs with anticholinergic effects
- Use of four or more medications
- Depression
- Visual deficit
- Arthritis
- History of cerebrovascular accident
- Cognitive impairment
- Secondary diagnosis/chronic disease

NURSING DIAGNOSIS

- Risk for Falls
- Risk for Injury
- Impaired Physical Mobility

OUTCOME IDENTIFICATION AND PLANNING

- Patient does not experience a fall and remains free of injury.
- Patient's environment is free from hazards.
- Patient and/or caregiver demonstrates an understanding of appropriate interventions to prevent falls.
- Patient uses assistive devices correctly.
- Patient uses safe transfer procedures.
- Appropriate precautions are implemented related to the use of medications that increase the risk for falls.

IMPLEMENTATION

ACTION	RATIONALE
1. Perform hand hygiene and put on PPE, if indicated.	Hand hygiene and PPE prevent the spread of microorganisms. PPE is required based on transmission precautions.

ACTION	RATIONALE
2. Identify the patient. Assess fall risk as outlined above.	Identifying the patient ensures the right patient receives the intervention and helps prevent errors. Fall-risk assessment aids in providing appropriate fall-prevention interventions for the individual patient.
3. Explain the rationale for fall prevention interventions to the patient and family/significant others.	Explanation helps reduce anxiety and promotes compliance and understanding.
4. Include the patient's family and/or significant others in the plan of care.	This promotes continuity of care and cooperation.
5. Provide adequate lighting. Use a night light during sleeping hours.	Good lighting reduces accidental tripping over and bumping into objects that may not be seen. Night light provides illumination in an unfamiliar environment.
6. Remove excess equipment, supplies, furniture, and other objects from rooms and walkways. Pay particular attention to high traffic areas and the route to the bathroom.	All are possible hazards.
7. Orient patient and significant others to new surroundings, including use of the telephone, call bell, patient bed, and room illumination. Indicate the location of the patient's bathroom.	Knowledge of proper use of equipment relieves anxiety and promotes compliance.
8. Provide a 'low bed' to replace regular hospital bed.	To be considered a 'low hospital bed' the frame of the bed must be lower so that the height of the mattress deck off the floor is between 6.5" and 10.5". This low height, as determined by the FDA, reduces the risk of fall-related injuries from bed.
9. Use floor mats if patient is at risk for serious injury.	Floor mats cushion fall and may prevent serious injury in patients at risk, such as those with osteoporosis (Gray-Micelli, 2012).

ACTION	RATIONALE
10. Provide nonskid footwear and/or walking shoes.	Nonskid footwear prevents slipping and walking shoes improve balance when ambulating or transferring.
11. Institute a toileting regimen and/or continence program, if appropriate.	Toileting on a regular basis decreases risk for falls.
12. Provide a bedside commode and/or urinal/bedpan, if appropriate. Ensure that it is near the bed at all times.	This prevents falls related to incontinence or trying to get to the bathroom.
13. Ensure that the call bell, bedside table, telephone, and other personal items are within the patient's reach at all times.	This prevents the patient from having to overreach for device or items, and/or possibly attempt ambulation or transfer unassisted.
14. Confer with primary care provider regarding appropriate exercise and physical therapy.	Exercise programs, such as muscle strengthening, balance training, and walking plans, decrease falls and fall-related injuries (AGS & BGS, 2010).
15. Confer with primary care provider regarding appropriate mobility aids, such as a cane or walker.	Mobility aids can help improve balance and steady the patient's gait.
16. Confer with primary care provider regarding the use of bone-strengthening medications, such as calcium, vitamin D, and drugs to prevent/treat osteoporosis.	Bone strengthening has been suggested to reduce fracture rates with falls (AGS & BGS, 2010).
17. Encourage the patient to rise or change position slowly and sit for several minutes before standing.	Gradual position changes reduce the risk of falls related to orthostatic hypotension.
18. Evaluate the appropriateness of elastic stockings for lower extremities.	Elastic stockings minimize venous pooling and promote venous return.
19. Review medications for potential hazards.	Certain medications and combinations of medications have been associated with increased risk for falls.
20. Keep the bed in the lowest position. If elevated to provide care (to reduce caregiver strain), ensure that it is lowered when care is completed.	Keeping bed in lowest position reduces the risk of a fall-related injury.

ACTION	RATIONALE
21. Make sure locks on the bed or wheelchair are secured at all times.	Locking prevents the bed or wheelchair from moving out from under the patient.
22. Use bed rails according to facility policy, when appropriate.	Inappropriate bed-rail use has been associated with patient injury and increased fall risk. Side rails may be considered a restraint when used to prevent an ambulatory patient from getting out of bed.
23. Anticipate patient needs and provide assistance with activities instead of waiting for the patient to ask.	Patients whose needs are met sustain fewer falls.
24. Consider the use of an electronic personal alarm or pressure sensor alarm for the bed or chair.	The alarm helps alert staff to unassisted changes in position by the patient.
25. Discuss the possibility of appropriate family member(s) staying with patient.	The presence of a family member provides familiarity and companionship.
26. Consider the use of patient attendant or sitter.	Attendant or sitter can provide companionship and supervision.
27. Increase the frequency of patient observation and surveillance. Utilize 1- or 2-hour nursing rounds, including pain assessment, toileting assistance, patient comfort, making sure personal items are in reach, and meeting patient needs.	Patient care rounds/nursing rounds can reduce patient falls (Kessler et al., 2012; Olrich et al., 2012; Meade et al., 2006; Weisgram & Raymond, 2008).
28. Remove PPE, if used. Perform hand hygiene.	Removing PPE properly reduces the risk for infection transmission and contamination of other items. Hand hygiene prevents transmission of microorganisms.

EVALUATION

- Patient remains free of falls and injury.
- Interventions to minimize risk factors that might precipitate a fall are implemented.

- Patient's environment is free from hazards.
- Patient and/or caregiver demonstrates an understanding of appropriate interventions to prevent falls.
- Patient uses assistive devices correctly.
- Patient uses safe transfer procedures.
- Appropriate precautions are implemented related to use of medications that increase the risk for falls.

DOCUMENTATION

- Document patient fall-risk assessment. Include appropriate interventions to reduce fall risk in nursing care plan. Document patient and family teaching relative to fall-risk reduction.
- Document interventions included in care.

SKILL 73 APPLYING A FECAL INCONTINENCE DEVICE

A fecal incontinence device is used to protect the perianal skin from excoriation due to repeated exposure to liquid stool. This device reduces perineal skin damage by diverting liquid stool into a collection bag (Zimmaro Bliss & Norton, 2010). A skin barrier may be applied before the device to protect the patient's skin and improve adhesion. If excoriation is already present, the skin barrier should be applied before applying a device.

DELEGATION CONSIDERATIONS

Application of a fecal incontinence device may be delegated to nursing assistive personnel (NAP) or to unlicensed assistive personnel (UAP) who have received appropriate training. Application of a fecal incontinence device may be delegated to licensed practical/vocational nurses (LPN/LVNs). The decision to delegate must be based on careful analysis of the patient's needs and circumstances, as well as the qualifications of the person to whom the task is being delegated. Refer to the Delegation Guidelines in Appendix A.

EQUIPMENT

- Fecal incontinence device
- Disposable gloves
- Additional PPE, as indicated
- Washcloth, skin cleanser, and towel
- Drainage (Foley) bag
- Scissors (optional)
- Skin protectant or barrier
- Bath blanket

ASSESSMENT

- Assess the amount and consistency of stool being passed. Note the frequency of bowel movements.

• Inspect the perianal area for any excoriation, wounds, or hemorrhoids.

NURSING DIAGNOSIS
• Bowel Incontinence
• Risk for Impaired Skin Integrity
• Impaired Skin Integrity

OUTCOME IDENTIFICATION AND PLANNING
• Patient expels feces into the device and maintains intact perianal
skin.
• Patient demonstrates a decrease in the amount and severity of exco-
riation.
• Patient verbalizes decreased discomfort.
• Patient remains free of any signs and symptoms of infection.

IMPLEMENTATION

ACTION	RATIONALE
1. Gather equipment.	Assembling equipment provides for an organized approach to the task.
2. Perform hand hygiene and put on PPE, if indicated.	Hand hygiene and PPE prevent the spread of microorganisms. PPE is required based on transmission precautions.
3. Identify the patient.	Identifying the patient ensures the right patient receives the intervention and helps prevent errors.
4. Close the curtains around the bed and close the door to the room, if possible. Explain what you are going to do and why you are going to do it to the patient.	This ensures the patient's privacy. Explanation relieves anxiety and facilitates cooperation. Discussion promotes cooperation and helps to minimize anxiety.
5. Assemble equipment on overbed table within reach.	Arranging items nearby is convenient, saves time, and avoids unnecessary stretching and twisting of muscles on the part of the nurse.

ACTION	RATIONALE
6. Adjust the bed to a comfortable working height, usually elbow height of the caregiver (VISN 8 Patient Safety Center, 2009). Position the patient on the left side (Sims' position), as dictated by patient comfort and condition. Fold top linen back just enough to allow access to the patient's rectal area. Drape the patient with the bath blanket, as necessary, to maintain privacy and provide warmth. Place a waterproof pad under the patient's hip.	Having the bed at the proper height prevents back and muscle strain. Sims' position facilitates access into the rectum. Folding back the linen in this manner minimizes unnecessary exposure and promotes the patient's comfort and warmth. The waterproof pad will protect the bed.
7. Put on gloves. Cleanse perianal area. Pat dry thoroughly.	Gloves protect the nurse from microorganisms in feces. Skin must be dry for device to adhere securely.
8. Trim perianal hair with scissors, if needed.	It may be uncomfortable if the perianal hair is pulled by adhesive from the fecal device. Trimming with scissors minimizes the risk for infection compared with shaving.
9. Apply the skin protectant or barrier and allow it to dry. Skin protectant may be contraindicated for use with some devices. Check manufacturer's recommendations before use.	Skin protectant aids in device adhesion and protects skin from irritation and injury from the adhesive. Skin must be dry for device to adhere securely.
10. If necessary, enlarge the opening in the adhesive skin barrier to fit the patient's anatomy. Do not cut beyond the printed line on the barrier. Remove paper backing from adhesive of device.	Cutting away too much of the adhesive backing will result in poor adhesion to the patient's skin. Removing the paper backing is necessary so that the device can adhere to the skin.
11. With nondominant hand, separate buttocks. Apply fecal device to anal area with	Opening should be over anus so that stool empties into bag and does not stay on patient's skin,

ACTION	RATIONALE
dominant hand, ensuring that the bag opening is over anus (Figure 1). Hold the device in place for 30 seconds to achieve good adhesion.	which could lead to skin breakdown. The device is effective only if it is properly positioned and adhered securely.

FIGURE 1 Applying device over anal opening.

12. Release buttocks. Attach connector of fecal incontinence device to drainage bag. Hang drainage bag below level of the patient.	Bag must be dependent for stool to drain into bag.
13. Remove gloves. Return the patient to a comfortable position. Make sure the linens under the patient are dry. Ensure that the patient is covered.	Removing contaminated gloves prevents spread of microorganisms. Promotes patient comfort.
14. Raise side rail. Lower bed height and adjust head of bed to a comfortable position.	Promotes patient safety.
15. Remove additional PPE, if used. Perform hand hygiene.	Removing PPE properly reduces the risk for infection transmission and contamination of other items. Hand hygiene prevents the spread of microorganisms.

EVALUATION

- Patient expels feces into the device and maintains intact perianal skin.
- Patient demonstrates a decrease in the amount and severity of excoriation.
- Patient verbalizes decreased discomfort.
- Patient remains free of any signs and symptoms of infection.

DOCUMENTATION

- Document the date and time the fecal device was applied; appearance of perianal area; color of stool; intake and output (amount of stool out); and the patient's reaction to the procedure.

SKILL 74 | CARING FOR A PATIENT WITH A FIBER OPTIC INTRACRANIAL CATHETER

Intracranial pressure (ICP), the pressure inside the cranium, is the result of blood, tissue, and cerebrospinal fluid circulating in the ventricles and subarachnoid space (Moreda et al., 2009). ICP monitoring is used to assess cerebral perfusion. When ICP increases, as a result of conditions such as a mass (e.g., a tumor), bleeding into the brain or fluid around the brain, or swelling within the brain matter itself, neurologic consequences may range from minor to severe, including death (Hill et al., 2012). Normal ICP is less than 15 mm Hg. Elevated ICP, intracranial hypertension, is a sustained ICP of 20 mm Hg or more (Schimpf, 2012; Barker, 2008).

Fiber optic catheters are one method used to monitor intracranial pressure (ICP). Fiber optic catheters directly monitor ICP using an intracranial transducer located in the tip of the catheter. A miniature transducer in the catheter tip is coupled by a long, continuous wire or fiber optic cable to an external electronic module. This device can be inserted into the lateral ventricle, subarachnoid space, subdural space, brain parenchyma, or under a bone flap. The dura is perforated, and the transducer probe is threaded through the cerebral tissue to the desired depth and fixed in position (Hickey, 2009). These devices are not fluid-filled systems, eliminating the problems associated with an external transducer and pressure tubing, such as an external ventriculostomy (Skill 182). The monitor provides continuous information (Cecil et al., 2011). Fiber optic catheters can be used to monitor the ICP and cerebral perfusion pressure (CPP). Some versions of catheters can also be used to drain cerebral spinal fluid (CSF). These devices are calibrated by the manufacturer and zero-balanced only once at the time of insertion.

ICP and blood pressure measurements are used to calculate cerebral perfusion pressure (CPP) the pressure needed to perfuse the blood upward to the brain against gravity (Barker, 2008). ICP monitoring also provides information about intracranial adaptive capacity, the ability of the brain to tolerate stimulation or increase in intracranial volume without an increase in pressure through waveform assessment (AANN, 2011; Barker, 2008; Hinkle & Cheever, 2014). CPP is calculated by finding the difference between the mean arterial pressure (MAP) and the ICP.

DELEGATION CONSIDERATIONS

The care of a patient with a fiber optic intracranial catheter may not be delegated to nursing assistive personnel (NAP) or to unlicensed assistive personnel (UAP). Depending on the state's nurse practice act and the organization's policies and procedures, care for these patients may be delegated to licensed practical/vocational nurses (LPN/LVNs). The decision to delegate must be based on careful analysis of the patient's needs and circumstances, as well as the qualifications of the person to whom the task is being delegated. Refer to the Delegation Guidelines in Appendix A.

EQUIPMENT
- PPE, as indicated

ASSESSMENT
- Perform a neurologic assessment. Assess the patient's level of consciousness. If the patient is awake, assess the patient's orientation to person, place, and time. If the patient's level of consciousness is decreased, note the patient's ability to respond and to be aroused. Inspect pupil size and response to light. Pupils should be equal and round and should react to light bilaterally. Any changes in level of consciousness or pupillary response may suggest a neurologic problem. If the patient can move the extremities, assess strength of hands and feet. A change in strength or a difference in strength on one side compared with the other may indicate a neurologic problem.
- Assess vital signs, because changes in vital signs can reflect a neurologic problem.
- Assess the patient's pain level. The patient may be experiencing pain at the fiber optic catheter insertion site.

NURSING DIAGNOSIS
- Risk for Infection
- Risk for Ineffective Cerebral Tissue Perfusion
- Risk for Injury
- Pain

OUTCOME IDENTIFICATION AND PLANNING
- Patient maintains intracranial pressure at less than 15 mm Hg and cerebral perfusion pressure at 60 to 90 mm Hg (Hickey, 2014).
- Patient is free from infection.
- Patient is free from pain.
- Patient and significant others understand the need for the ventriculostomy.

IMPLEMENTATION

ACTION	RATIONALE
1. Review the medical orders for specific information about monitoring parameters.	The nurse needs to know the most recent order for acceptable ICP and CPP values.

ACTION	RATIONALE
2. Perform hand hygiene and put on PPE, if indicated.	Hand hygiene and PPE prevent the spread of microorganisms. PPE is required based on transmission precautions.
3. Identify the patient.	Identifying the patient ensures the right patient receives the intervention and helps prevent errors.
4. Close the curtains around the bed and close the door to the room, if possible. Explain what you are going to do and why you are going to do it to the patient.	This ensures the patient's privacy. Explanation relieves anxiety and facilitates cooperation.
5. Assess the patient for any changes in neurologic status.	Patients with ventriculostomies are at risk for problems with the neurologic system.
6. Assess ICP, MAP, and CPP at least hourly. Note ICP value and waveforms as shown on the monitor. If there is an increase in the ICP, the value should be obtained more often, as often as every 15 minutes (AANN, 2011). Note drainage amount, color, clarity, as appropriate.	Frequent assessment provides valuable indicators for identifying subtle trends that may suggest developing problems. Some versions of catheters can also be used to drain cerebral spinal fluid (CSF).
7. Care for the insertion site according to the facility's policy. Maintain the system using strict sterile technique. Assess the site for any signs of infection, such as drainage, redness, or warmth. Ensure the catheter is secured at site per facility policy.	Site care varies, possibly ranging from leaving the site open to air to applying antibiotic ointment and gauze. Site care aids in reducing the risk for infection. Sterile technique helps to prevent infection (Barker, 2008). Securing the catheters after insertion prevents dislodgement and breakage of the device.
8. Calculate the CPP, if necessary. Calculate the difference between the systemic MAP and the ICP.	CPP is an estimate of the adequacy of the blood supply to the brain.

ACTION	RATIONALE
9. Remove PPE, if used. Perform hand hygiene.	Removing PPE properly reduces the risk for infection transmission and contamination of other items. Hand hygiene prevents the spread of microorganisms.

EVALUATION

- Patient demonstrates a CPP and an ICP within identified parameters.
- Patient remains free from infection.
- Patient understands the need for the catheter and monitoring.
- Patient reports no pain.

DOCUMENTATION

- Document the following information: neurologic assessment; ICP and CPP; vital signs; pain; appearance of insertion site.

SKILL 75 ADMINISTERING A TUBE FEEDING

Depending on the patient's physical and psychosocial condition and nutritional requirements, a feeding through the nasogastric (NG) tube or other GI tube might be ordered. The steps for administering feedings are similar regardless of the tube used. Feeding can be provided on an intermittent or continuous basis. Intermittent feedings are delivered at regular intervals, using gravity for instillation or a feeding pump to administer the formula over a set period of time. Intermittent feedings might also be given as a bolus, using a syringe to instill the formula quickly in one large amount. Intermittent feedings are the preferred method, introducing the formula over a set period of time via gravity or pump. If the order calls for continuous feeding, an external feeding pump is needed to regulate the flow of formula. Continuous feedings permit gradual introduction of the formula into the GI tract, promoting maximal absorption. However, there is a risk of both reflux and aspiration with this method. Feeding intolerance is less likely to occur with smaller volumes. Hanging smaller amounts of feeding also reduces the risk for bacteria growth and contamination of feeding at room temperature (when using open systems).

The procedure below describes using open systems and a feeding pump; the skill variation at the end of the skill describes using a closed system.

DELEGATION CONSIDERATIONS

The administration of a tube feeding is not usually delegated to nursing assistive personnel (NAP) or to unlicensed assistive personnel (UAP) in the acute care setting. The administration of a tube feeding in some settings may be delegated to NAP or UAP who have received appropriate training, after assessment of tube placement and patency by the registered nurse. Depending on the state's nurse practice act and the organization's policies and procedures, the administration of a tube feeding may be delegated to licensed practical/vocational nurses (LPN/ LVNs). The decision to delegate must be based on careful analysis of the patient's needs and circumstances, as well as the qualifications of the person to whom the task is being delegated. Refer to the Delegation Guidelines in Appendix A.

EQUIPMENT

- Prescribed tube feeding formula at room temperature
- Feeding bag or prefilled tube feeding set
- Stethoscope
- Nonsterile gloves
- Additional PPE, as indicated
- Alcohol preps
- Disposable pad or towel
- Asepto or Toomey syringe
- Enteral feeding pump (if ordered)
- Rubber band
- Clamp (Hoffman or butterfly)
- IV pole
- Water for irrigation and hydration, as needed
- pH paper
- Tape measure, or other measuring device

ASSESSMENT

- Assess the abdomen by inspecting for presence of distention, auscultate for bowel sounds, and palpate the abdomen for firmness or tenderness. If the abdomen is distended, consider measuring the abdominal girth at the umbilicus.
- If the patient reports any tenderness or nausea, exhibits any rigidity or firmness of the abdomen, and if bowel sounds are absent, confer with primary care provider before administering the tube feeding. Assess for patient and/or family understanding, if appropriate, for the rationale for the tube feeding and address any questions or concerns expressed by the patient and family members. Consult primary care provider, if needed, for further explanation.

NURSING DIAGNOSIS

- Risk for Aspiration
- Deficient Knowledge
- Imbalanced Nutrition, Less than Body Requirements

OUTCOME IDENTIFICATION AND PLANNING

- Patient will receive the tube feeding without complaints of nausea, episodes of vomiting, gastric distention, or diarrhea.

- Patient demonstrates an increase in weight.
- Patient exhibits no signs and symptoms of aspiration.
- Patient verbalizes knowledge related to tube feeding.

IMPLEMENTATION

ACTION	RATIONALE
1. Gather equipment. Check amount, concentration, type, and frequency of tube feeding in the patient's medical record. Check formula expiration date.	This provides for an organized approach to the task. Checking ensures that correct feeding will be administered. Outdated formula may be contaminated.
2. Perform hand hygiene and put on PPE, if indicated.	Hand hygiene and PPE prevent the spread of microorganisms. PPE is required based on transmission precautions.
3. Identify the patient.	Identifying the patient ensures the right patient receives the intervention and helps prevent errors.
4. Explain the procedure to the patient and why this intervention is needed. Answer any questions as needed.	Explanation facilitates patient cooperation.
5. Assemble equipment on overbed table within reach.	Organization facilitates performance of the task.
6. Close the patient's bedside curtain or door. Raise the bed to a comfortable working position, usually elbow height of the caregiver (VISN 8, 2009). Perform key abdominal assessments as described above.	Closing curtains or door provides for patient privacy. Having the bed at the proper height prevents back and muscle strain. Due to changes in the patient's condition, assessment is vital before initiating the intervention.
7. **Position the patient with head of bed (HOB) elevated at least 30 to 45 degrees or as near normal position for eating as possible.**	This position minimizes possibility of aspiration into the trachea. Patients who are considered at high risk for aspiration should be assisted to at least a 45-degree position.
8. Put on gloves. Unpin the tube from the patient's	Gloves prevent contact with blood and body fluids. The tube

ACTION	RATIONALE
gown. Verify the position of the marking on the tube at the nostril. Measure length of exposed tube and compare with the documented length.	should be marked with an indelible marker at the nostril. This marking should be assessed each time the tube is used to ensure the tube has not become displaced. Tube length should be checked and compared with this initial measurement, in conjunction with pH measurement and visual assessment of aspirate. An increase in the length of the exposed tube may indicate dislodgement (AACN, 2010b; Bourgault et al., 2007; Hinkle & Cheever, 2014).
9. Attach syringe to end of tube and aspirate a small amount of stomach contents, as described in Skill 111.	The tube is in the stomach if its contents can be aspirated: pH of aspirate can then be tested to determine gastric placement. If unable to obtain a specimen, reposition the patient and flush the tube with 30 mL of air. This action may be necessary several times. Current literature recommends that the nurse ensures proper placement of the NG tube by relying on multiple methods and not on one method alone.
10. Check the pH as described in Skill 111.	Current research demonstrates that the use of pH is predictive of correct placement. The pH of gastric contents is acidic (less than 5.5). If the patient is taking an acid-inhibiting agent, the range may be 4.0 to 6.0. The pH of intestinal fluid is 7.0 or higher. The pH of respiratory fluid is 6.0 or higher. This method will not effectively differentiate between intestinal fluid and pleural fluid.
	Testing for pH before the next feeding in intermittent feedings is conducted since the stomach has been emptied of the feeding formula. However, if the patient

ACTION	RATIONALE
	is receiving continuous feedings, the pH measurement is not as useful, since the formula raises the pH.
11. Visualize aspirated contents, checking for color and consistency.	Gastric fluid can be green, with particles, off-white, or brown if old blood is present. Intestinal aspirate tends to look clear or straw-colored to a deep golden-yellow color. Also, intestinal aspirate may be greenish-brown if stained with bile. Respiratory or tracheobronchial fluid is usually off-white to tan and may be tinged with mucus. A small amount of blood-tinged fluid may be seen immediately after NG insertion.
12. If it is not possible to aspirate contents; assessments to check placement are inconclusive; the exposed tube length has changed; or there are any other indications that the tube is not in place, check placement by x-ray.	The x-ray is considered the most reliable method for identifying the position of the NG tube.
13. After multiple steps have been taken to ensure that the feeding tube is located in the stomach or small intestine, **aspirate all gastric contents with the syringe and measure to check for gastric residual—the amount of feeding remaining in the stomach.** Return the residual based on facility policy. Proceed with feeding if amount of residual does not exceed agency policy or the limit indicated in the medical record.	Checking for residual before each feeding or every 4 to 6 hours during a continuous feeding according to institutional policy is implemented to identify delayed gastric emptying. High gastric residual volumes (200 to 250 mL or greater) can be associated with high risk for aspiration and aspiration-related pneumonia (Bourgault et al., 2007; Metheny, 2008). Some experts now recommend that the patient's pattern of residual is more important than the amount (ASPEN, 2011; Bourgault et al.; Metheny). Feedings should be held if residual volumes exceed 200 mL on two successive

ACTION	RATIONALE
	assessments (ASPEN). Research findings are inconclusive on the benefit of returning gastric volumes to the stomach or intestine to avoid fluid or electrolyte imbalance, which has been accepted practice. Consult facility policy concerning this practice.
14. Flush tube with 30 mL of water for irrigation. Disconnect syringe from tubing and cap end of tubing while preparing the formula feeding equipment. Remove gloves.	Flushing tube prevents occlusion (ASPEN, 2011; Bourgault et al., 2007; Metheny, 2008). Capping the tube deters the entry of microorganisms and prevents leakage onto the bed linens.
15. Put on gloves before preparing, assembling, and handling any part of the feeding system.	Gloves prevent contact with blood and body fluids and deter transmission of contaminants to feeding equipment and/or formula.
16. Administer feeding. **When Using a Feeding Bag (Open System):**	
a. Label bag and/or tubing with date and time. Hang bag on IV pole and adjust to about 12 inches above the stomach. Clamp tubing.	Labeling date and time of first use allows for disposal within 24 hours, to deter growth of microorganisms. Proper feeding bag height reduces risk of formula being introduced too quickly.
b. Check the expiration date of the formula. Cleanse top of feeding container with a disinfectant before opening it. Pour formula into feeding bag and allow solution to run through tubing. Close clamp.	Cleansing container top with alcohol minimizes risk for contaminants entering feeding bag. Formula displaces air in tubing.
c. Attach feeding setup to feeding tube, open clamp, and regulate drip according to the medical order, or allow feeding to run in over 30 minutes.	Introducing formula at a slow, regular rate allows the stomach to accommodate to the feeding and decreases GI distress.

ACTION	RATIONALE
d. Add 30 to 60 mL (1 to 2 oz.) of water for irrigation to feeding bag when feeding is almost completed and allow it to run through the tube.	Water rinses the feeding from the tube and helps to keep it patent.
e. Clamp tubing immediately after water has been instilled. Disconnect feeding setup from feeding tube. Clamp tube and cover end with cap.	Clamping the tube prevents air from entering the stomach. Capping the tube deters entry of microorganisms and covering end of tube protects patient and linens from fluid leakage from tube.

When Using a Large Syringe (Open System):

ACTION	RATIONALE
a. Remove plunger from 30- or 60-mL syringe.	Introducing the formula at a slow, regular rate allows the stomach to accommodate to the feeding and decreases GI distress. The higher the syringe is held, the faster the formula flows.
b. Attach syringe to feeding tube, pour premeasured amount of tube feeding formula into syringe, open clamp, and allow food to enter tube. Regulate rate, fast or slow, by height of the syringe. **Do not push formula with syringe plunger.**	Water rinses the feeding from the tube and helps to keep it patent.
c. Add 30 to 60 mL (1 to 2 oz.) of water for irrigation to syringe when feeding is almost completed, and allow it to run through the tube.	
d. When syringe has emptied, hold syringe high and disconnect from tube. Clamp tube and cover end with cap.	By holding syringe high, the formula will not backflow out of tube and onto patient. Clamping the tube prevents air from entering the stomach. Capping end of tube deters entry of microorganisms. Covering the end protects patient and linens from fluid leakage from tube.

ACTION	RATIONALE

When Using an Enteral Feeding Pump:

a. Close flow-regulator clamp on tubing and fill feeding bag with prescribed formula. Amount used depends on agency policy. Place label on container with patient's name, date, and time the feeding was hung.

Closing clamp prevents formula from moving through tubing until nurse is ready. Labeling date and time of first use allows for disposal within 24 hours, to deter growth of microorganisms.

b. Hang feeding container on IV pole. Allow solution to flow through tubing.

This prevents air from being forced into the stomach or intestines.

c. Connect to feeding pump following manufacturer's directions. Set rate. Maintain the patient in the upright position throughout the feeding. If the patient needs to lie flat temporarily, pause the feeding. Resume the feeding after the patient's position has been changed back to at least 30 to 45 degrees.

Feeding pumps vary. Some of the newer pumps have built-in safeguards that protect the patient from complications. Safety features include cassettes that prevent free-flow of formula, automatic tube flush, safety tips that prevent accidental attachment to an IV setup, and various audible and visible alarms. Feedings are started at full strength rather than diluted, which was recommended previously. A smaller volume, 10 to 40 mL, of feeding infused per hour and gradually increased has been shown to be more easily tolerated by patients.

d. **Check placement of tube and gastric residual every 4 to 6 hours.**

Checking placement (Steps 9–12) verifies that the tube has not moved out of the stomach. Checking gastric residual (Step 13) monitors absorption of the feeding and prevents distention, which could lead to aspiration.

17. Observe the patient's response during and after tube feeding and assess the abdomen at least once a shift.

Pain or nausea may indicate stomach distention, which may lead to vomiting. Physical signs, such as abdominal distention and firmness or regurgitation of tube feeding, may indicate intolerance.

ACTION	RATIONALE
18. **Have patient remain in upright position for at least 1 hour after feeding.**	This position minimizes risk for backflow and discourages aspiration, if any reflux or vomiting should occur.
19. Remove equipment and return patient to a position of comfort. Remove gloves. Raise side rail and lower bed.	Promotes patient comfort and safety. Removing gloves properly reduces the risk for infection transmission and contamination of other items.
20. Put on gloves. Wash and clean equipment or replace according to agency policy. Remove gloves.	This prevents contamination and deters spread of microorganisms. Reusable systems are cleansed with soap and water with each use and replaced every 24 hours. Refer to agency's policy and manufacturer's guidelines for specifics on equipment care.
21. Remove additional PPE, if used. Perform hand hygiene.	Removing PPE properly reduces the risk for infection transmission and contamination of other items. Hand hygiene prevents transmission of microorganisms.

EVALUATION

- Patient receives the ordered tube feeding without complaints of nausea, episodes of vomiting, gastric distension, or diarrhea.
- Patient demonstrates an increase in weight.
- Patient remains free of any signs and symptoms of aspiration.
- Patient voices knowledge related to tube feeding.

DOCUMENTATION

- Document the type of NG tube or gastrostomy/jejunostomy tube that is present. Record the criteria that were used to confirm proper placement before feeding was initiated, such as the tube length in inches or centimeters compared to the length on initial insertion. Document the aspiration of gastric contents and pH of the gastric contents when intermittent feeding is used. Note the components of the abdominal assessment, such as observation of the abdomen, presence of distention or firmness, and presence of bowel sounds. Include subjective data, such as any reports from the patient of abdominal pain or nausea or any other patient response. Record the amount of gastric residual volume that was obtained. Document the position of the patient, the type of feeding, and the method and the amount of feeding. Include any relevant patient teaching.

Prefilled tube-feeding sets, which are considered closed systems, are frequently used to provide patient nourishment. Closed systems contain sterile feeding solutions in ready-to-hang containers. This method reduces the opportunity for bacterial contamination of the feeding formula. In general, these pre-filled feedings are administered via an enteral pump.

1. Check amount, concentration, type, and frequency of tube feeding in the patient's medical record.

2. Gather all equipment, checking the feeding solution and container for correct solution and expiration date. Label with patient's name, type of solution, and prescribed rate.

3. Perform hand hygiene. Put on PPE, as indicated.

4. Identify the patient and explain the procedure.

5. Put on gloves.

6. Ensure the correct placement of the feeding tube by checking marking on tube at nose (if NG tube), length of exposed tube, aspiration of stomach contents, and for gastric or intestinal pH.

7. Check for residual amount of feeding in the stomach and return residual, as ordered.

8. Flush tube with 30 mL of water.

9. Put on nonsterile gloves: remove screw on cap and attach administration setup with drip chamber and tubing.

10. Hang feeding container on IV pole and connect to feeding pump, allowing solution to flow through tubing, following manufacturer's directions.

11. Attach the feeding setup to the patient's feeding tube.

12. Open the clamp of the patient's feeding tube.

13. Turn on the pump.

14. Set the pump at the prescribed rate of flow and remove the nonsterile gloves.

15. Observe the patient's response during the tube feeding.

16. Continue to assess the patient for signs and symptoms of gastrointestinal distress, such as nausea, abdominal distention, or absence of bowel sounds.

17. Have the patient remain in the upright position throughout the feeding and for at least 1 hour after feeding. If patient's position needs to be changed to a supine position or turned in bed, pause the feeding pump during this time.

18. After the prescribed amount of feeding has been administrated or according to agency policy, turn off the pump, put on nonsterile

Using a Prefilled Tube-Feeding Set (Closed System)   *continued*

gloves, clamp the feeding tube, and disconnect it from the feeding set tube, capping the end of the feeding set.

19. Draw up 30 to 60 mL of water using a syringe.

20. Attach the syringe to the feeding tube; unclamp the feeding tube and instill the 30 to 60 mL of water into it.

21. Clamp the feeding tube.

22. Remove equipment, according to facility policy.

23. Provide for any patient needs.

24. Remove gloves and additional PPE, if used. Perform hand hygiene.

SKILL 76   CARING FOR A GASTROSTOMY TUBE

When long-term enteral feeding is required, an enterostomal tube may be placed through an opening created into the stomach (gastrostomy) or into the jejunum (jejunostomy). Placement of a tube into the stomach can be accomplished by a surgeon or gastroenterologist via a percutaneous endoscopic gastrostomy (PEG) or a surgically (open or laparoscopically) placed gastrostomy tube. PEG tube insertion is often used because, unlike a traditional, surgically placed gastrostomy tube, it usually does not require general anesthesia. Use of a PEG tube or other type of gastrostomy tube requires an intact, functional GI tract. Providing care at the insertion site is a nursing responsibility. Site care is the same for a jejunostomy (enterostomal tube placed through an opening created into the jejunum).

DELEGATION CONSIDERATIONS

The care of a gastrostomy tube, in the postoperative period, is not delegated to nursing assistive personnel (NAP) or to unlicensed assistive personnel (UAP) in the acute care setting. The care of a healed gastrostomy tube site in some settings may be delegated to NAP or UAP who have received appropriate training, after assessment of tube by the registered nurse. Depending on the state's nurse practice act and the organization's policies and procedures, the care of a gastrostomy tube may be delegated to licensed practical/vocational nurses (LPN/LVNs). The decision to delegate must be based on careful analysis of the patient's needs and circumstances, as well as the qualifications of the person to whom the task is being delegated. Refer to the Delegation Guidelines in Appendix A.

EQUIPMENT

- Nonsterile gloves
- Additional PPE, as indicated
- Washcloth, towel, and soap
- Cotton-tipped applicators
- Sterile saline solution
- Gauze (if needed)

ASSESSMENT

- Assess gastrostomy or jejunostomy tube site, noting any drainage, skin breakdown, or erythema.
- Measure the length of exposed tube, comparing it with the initial measurement after insertion. Alternately, mark the tube at the skin with indelible marker; mark should be at skin level at the insertion site.
- Check to ensure that the tube is securely stabilized and has not become dislodged. Also, assess the tension of the tube. If there is not enough tension, the tube may leak gastric or intestinal drainage around exit site. If the tension is too great, the internal anchoring device may erode through the skin.

NURSING DIAGNOSIS

- Imbalanced Nutrition, Less than Body Requirements
- Impaired Skin Integrity
- Risk for Infection

OUTCOME IDENTIFICATION AND PLANNING

- Patient ingests an adequate diet and exhibits no signs and symptoms of irritation, excoriation, or infection at the tube insertion site.
- Patient verbalizes little discomfort related to tube placement.
- Patient will be able to verbalize the care needed for the gastrostomy tube.

IMPLEMENTATION

ACTION	RATIONALE
1. Gather equipment. Verify the medical order or facility policy and procedure regarding site care.	Assembling the equipment provides for an organized approach to the task. Verification ensures the patient receives the correct intervention.
2. Perform hand hygiene and put on PPE, if indicated.	Hand hygiene and PPE prevent the spread of microorganisms. PPE is required based on transmission precautions.
3. Identify the patient.	Identifying the patient ensures the right patient receives the intervention and helps prevent errors.

ACTION	RATIONALE
4. Explain the procedure to the patient and why this intervention is needed. Answer any questions, as needed.	Explanation facilitates patient cooperation.
5. Assess the patient for presence of pain at the tube insertion site. If pain is present, offer the patient analgesic medication per the medical order and wait for medication absorption before beginning insertion site care.	Feeding tubes can be uncomfortable, especially the first few days after insertion. Analgesic medication may permit the patient to tolerate the insertion site care more easily. After the first few days, it has been reported that the need for pain medication decreases.
6. Pull the patient's bedside curtain. Assemble equipment on the bedside table, within reach. Raise bed to a comfortable working position, usually elbow height of the caregiver (VISN 8, 2009).	Provides for privacy. Assembling equipment provides for an organized approach to the task. Appropriate working height facilitates comfort and proper body mechanics for the nurse.
7. Put on gloves. If gastrostomy tube is new and still has sutures holding it in place, dip a cotton-tipped applicator into sterile saline solution and gently clean around the insertion site, removing any crust or drainage. **Avoid adjusting or lifting the external disk for the first few days after placement, except to clean the area.** If the gastric tube insertion site has healed and the sutures are removed, wet a washcloth and apply a small amount of soap onto washcloth. Gently cleanse around the insertion, removing any crust or drainage. Rinse site, removing all soap.	Cleaning new site with sterile saline solution prevents the introduction of microorganisms into the wound. Crust and drainage can harbor bacteria and lead to skin breakdown. Removing soap helps to prevent skin irritation. If able, the patient may shower and cleanse the site with soap and water.
8. **Pat skin around insertion site dry.**	Drying the skin thoroughly prevents skin breakdown.

ACTION	RATIONALE
9. If the sutures have been removed, gently rotate the guard or external bumper 90 degrees at least once a day. Assess that the guard or external bumper is not digging into the surrounding skin. Avoid placing any tension on the tube.	Rotation of the guard or external bumper prevents skin breakdown and pressure ulcers. The risk of dislodgement is decreased when the tube has an external anchoring or bumper device.
10. Leave the site open to air unless there is drainage. If drainage is present, place one thickness of a precut gauze pad or drain sponge under the external bumper and change, as needed, to keep the area dry. Use a skin protectant or barrier cream to prevent skin breakdown.	The digestive enzymes from the gastric secretions may cause skin breakdown. Under normal conditions, expect only a minimal amount of drainage on a feeding tube dressing. Increased amounts of drainage should be explored for cause such as a possible gastric fluid leak.
11. Remove gloves. Lower the bed and assist the patient to a position of comfort, as needed.	Removing gloves reduces the risk for infection transmission and contamination of other items. Lowering bed and assisting patient ensure patient safety and comfort.
12. Remove additional PPE, if used. Perform hand hygiene.	Removing PPE properly reduces the risk for infection transmission and contamination of other items. Hand hygiene prevents transmission of microorganisms.

EVALUATION

- Patient exhibits a clean, dry, intact gastrostomy tube site without evidence of irritation, excoriation, breakdown, or infection.
- Patient verbalizes no pain when guard is rotated.
- Patient participates in care measures.

DOCUMENTATION

- Document the care that was given, including the substance used to cleanse the tube site. Record the condition of the site, including the surrounding skin. Note if any drainage was present, recording the amount and color. Note the rotation of the guard. Comment on the patient's response to the care, if the patient experienced any pain, and if an analgesic was given. Record any patient instruction that was given.

PUTTING ON STERILE GLOVES AND REMOVING SOILED GLOVES

When applying and wearing sterile gloves, keep hands above waist level and away from nonsterile surfaces. Replace gloves if they develop an opening or tear; the integrity of the material becomes compromised; or the gloves come in contact with any nonsterile surface or nonsterile item.

DELEGATION CONSIDERATIONS

Procedures requiring the use of sterile gloves and other sterile items are not delegated to nursing assistive personnel (NAP) or unlicensed assistive personnel (UAP). Depending on the state's nurse practice act and the organization's policies and procedures, these procedures may be delegated to licensed practical/vocational nurses (LPN/LVNs). The decision to delegate must be based on careful analysis of the patient's needs and circumstances, as well as the qualifications of the person to whom the task is being delegated. Refer to the Delegation Guidelines in Appendix A.

EQUIPMENT

- Sterile gloves of the appropriate size
- PPE, as indicated

ASSESSMENT

- Assess the situation to determine the necessity for sterile gloves.
- Check the patient's medical record for information about a possible latex allergy.
- Question the patient about any history of allergy, including latex allergy or sensitivity, and signs and symptoms that have occurred. If the patient has a latex allergy, anticipate the need for latex-free gloves.

NURSING DIAGNOSIS

- Risk for Infection
- Ineffective Protection
- Risk for Latex Allergy Response

OUTCOME IDENTIFICATION AND PLANNING

- The gloves are applied and removed without contamination.
- The patient remains free of exposure to infectious microorganisms.
- The patient does not exhibit signs and symptoms of a latex allergy response.

IMPLEMENTATION

ACTION	RATIONALE
1. Perform hand hygiene and put on PPE, if indicated.	Hand hygiene and PPE prevent the spread of microorganisms. PPE is required based on transmission precautions.
2. Identify the patient. Explain the procedure to the patient.	Patient identification validates the correct patient and correct procedure. Discussion and explanation help allay anxiety and prepare the patient for what to expect.
3. Check that the sterile glove package is dry and unopened. Also note expiration date, making sure that the date is still valid.	Moisture contaminates a sterile package. Expiration date indicates the period that the package remains sterile.
4. Place sterile glove package on clean, dry surface at or above your waist.	Moisture could contaminate the sterile gloves. Any sterile object held below the waist is considered contaminated.
5. Open the outside wrapper by carefully peeling the top layer back. Remove inner package, handling only the outside of it.	This maintains sterility of gloves in inner packet.
6. Place the inner package on the work surface with the side labeled 'cuff end' closest to the body.	Allows for ease of glove application.
7. Carefully open the inner package. Fold open the top flap, then the bottom and sides. **Take care not to touch the inner surface of the package or the gloves.**	The inner surface of the package is considered sterile. The outer 1-inch border of the inner package is considered contaminated. The sterile gloves are exposed with the cuff end closest to the nurse.
8. With the thumb and forefinger of the nondominant hand, grasp the folded cuff of the glove for the dominant hand, touching only	Unsterile hand touches only inside of glove. Outside remains sterile.

ACTION	RATIONALE

the exposed inside of the glove (Figure 1).

FIGURE 1 Grasping cuff of glove for dominant hand.

9. Keeping the hands above the waistline, lift and hold the glove up and off the inner package with fingers down. **Be careful it does not touch any unsterile object.**

Glove is contaminated if it touches any unsterile objects.

10. Carefully insert dominant hand palm up into glove and pull on glove. Leave the cuff folded until the opposite hand is gloved.

Attempting to turn upward with unsterile hand may result in contamination of sterile glove.

11. Hold the thumb of the gloved hand outward. Place the fingers of the gloved hand inside the cuff of the remaining glove (Figure 2). Lift it from the wrapper, taking care not to touch anything with the gloves or hands.

Thumb is less likely to become contaminated if held outward. Sterile surface touching sterile surface prevents contamination.

FIGURE 2 Sliding fingers under cuff of glove for nondominant hand.

ACTION	RATIONALE

12. Carefully insert nondominant hand into glove. Pull the glove on, taking care that the skin does not touch any of the outer surfaces of the gloves.

Sterile surface touching sterile surface prevents contamination.

13. **Slide the fingers of one hand under the cuff of the other and fully extend the cuff down the arm, touching only the sterile outside of the glove (Figure 3). Repeat for the remaining hand.**

Sterile surface touching sterile surface prevents contamination.

FIGURE 3 Sliding fingers of one hand under cuff of other hand and extending cuff down the arm.

14. Adjust gloves on both hands if necessary, **touching only sterile areas with other sterile areas.**

Sterile surface touching sterile surface prevents contamination.

15. Continue with procedure as indicated.

Removing Soiled Gloves

16. Use dominant hand to grasp the opposite glove **near cuff end on the outside exposed area.** Remove it by pulling it off, inverting it as it is pulled, keeping the contaminated area on the inside. Hold the removed glove in the remaining gloved hand.

Contaminated area does not come in contact with hands or wrists.

17. Slide fingers of ungloved hand between the remaining glove and the wrist. **Take care to avoid touching**

Contaminated area does not come in contact with hands or wrists.

ACTION	RATIONALE
the outside surface of the **glove.** Remove it by pulling it off, inverting it as it is pulled, keeping the contaminated area on the inside, and securing the first glove inside the second.	
18. Discard gloves in appropriate container. Remove additional PPE, if used. Perform hand hygiene.	Proper disposal and removal of PPE reduces the risk for infection transmission and contamination of other items. Hand hygiene prevents the spread of microorganisms.

EVALUATION

• Gloves are applied and removed without contamination.
• Patient remains free of exposure to potential infection-causing microorganisms.
• Patient does not exhibit signs and symptoms of a latex-allergy response.

DOCUMENTATION

• It is not usually necessary to document the addition of sterile items to a sterile field. However, document the use of sterile technique performed for any procedure using sterile technique.

SKILL 78 APPLYING AND REMOVING GRADUATED COMPRESSION STOCKINGS

Graduated compression stockings are often used for patients at risk for deep-vein thrombosis (DVT) and pulmonary embolism, and to help prevent phlebitis. Manufactured by several companies, graduated compression stockings are made of elastic material and are available in either knee-high or thigh-high length. By applying pressure, graduated compression stockings increase the velocity of blood flow in the superficial and deep veins and improve venous valve function in the legs, promoting venous return to the heart. A physician's order is required for their use.

Be prepared to apply the stockings in the morning before the patient is out of bed and while the patient is supine. If the patient is sitting or has been up and about, have the patient lie down with legs and feet elevated for at least 15 minutes before applying the stockings. Otherwise, the leg vessels are congested with blood, reducing the effectiveness of the stockings.

DELEGATION CONSIDERATIONS

The application and removal of graduated compression stockings may be delegated to nursing assistive personnel (NAP) or to unlicensed assistive personnel (UAP), as well as to licensed practical/vocational nurses (LPN/LVNs). The decision to delegate must be based on careful analysis of the patient's needs and circumstances, as well as the qualifications of the person to whom the task is being delegated. Refer to the Delegation Guidelines in Appendix A.

EQUIPMENT

- Elastic graduated compression stockings in ordered length in correct size. See Assessment for appropriate measurement procedure.
- Measuring tape
- Talcum powder (optional)
- Skin cleanser, basin, towel
- PPE, as indicated

ASSESSMENT

- Assess the skin condition and neurovascular status of the legs. Report any abnormalities before continuing with the application of the stockings.
- Assess patient's legs for any redness, swelling, warmth, tenderness, or pain that may indicate a DVT. If any of these symptoms are noted, notify the physician before applying stockings.
- Measure the patient's legs to obtain the correct size stocking. For knee-high length: Measure around the widest part of the calf and the leg length from the bottom of the heel to the back of the knee, at the bend. For thigh-high length: Measure around the widest part of the calf and the thigh. Measure the length from the bottom of the heel to the gluteal fold. Follow the manufacturer's specifications to select the correct sized stockings. Each leg should have a correctly fitted stocking; if measurements differ, then two different sizes of stocking need to be ordered to ensure correct fitting on each leg (Walker & Lamont, 2008).

NURSING DIAGNOSIS

- Ineffective Peripheral Tissue Perfusion
- Risk for Impaired Skin Integrity
- Deficient Knowledge

OUTCOME IDENTIFICATION AND PLANNING

- Stockings are applied and removed with minimal discomfort to the patient.
- Edema will decrease in the lower extremities.
- Patient will understand the rationale for stocking application.
- Patient will remain free of DVT.

IMPLEMENTATION

ACTION	RATIONALE
1. Review the medical record and medical orders to determine the need for graduated compression stockings.	Reviewing the medical record and order validates the correct patient and correct procedure.
2. Perform hand hygiene. Put on PPE, as indicated.	Hand hygiene and PPE prevent the spread of microorganisms. PPE is required based on transmission precautions.
3. Identify the patient. Explain what you are going to do and the rationale for use of elastic stockings.	Patient identification validates the correct patient and correct procedure. Discussion and explanation allay anxiety and prepare the patient for what to expect.
4. Close the curtains around the bed and close the door to the room, if possible.	This ensures the patient's privacy.
5. Adjust the bed to a comfortable working height, usually elbow height of the caregiver (VISN 8 Patient Safety Center, 2009).	Having the bed at the proper height prevents back and muscle strain.
6. Assist patient to supine position. If patient has been sitting or walking, have him or her lie down with legs and feet well elevated for at least 15 minutes before applying stockings.	Dependent position of legs encourages blood to pool in the veins, reducing the effectiveness of the stockings if they are applied to congested blood vessels.
7. Expose legs one at a time. Wash and dry legs, if necessary. Powder the leg lightly unless patient has a respiratory problem, dry skin, or sensitivity to the powder. If the skin is dry, a lotion may be used. Powders and lotions are not recommended by some manufacturers; check the package material for manufacturer specifications.	Helps maintain patient's privacy. Powder and lotion reduce friction and make application of stockings easier.

ACTION	RATIONALE

8. Stand at the foot of the bed. Place hand inside stocking and grasp heel area securely. Turn stocking inside-out to the heel area, leaving the foot inside the stocking leg.

Inside-out technique provides for easier application; bunched elastic material can compromise extremity circulation.

9. With the heel pocket down, ease the stocking foot over the foot and heel (Figure 1). Check that patient's heel is centered in heel pocket of stocking.

Wrinkles and improper fit interfere with circulation.

FIGURE 1 Putting foot of stocking onto patient.

10. Using your fingers and thumbs, carefully grasp edge of stocking and pull it up smoothly over ankle and calf, toward the knee. Make sure it is distributed evenly.

Easing the stocking carefully into position ensures proper fit of the stocking to the contour of the leg. Even distribution prevents interference with circulation.

11. Pull forward slightly on toe section. If the stocking has a toe window, make sure it is properly positioned. Adjust if necessary to ensure material is smooth.

Ensures toe comfort and prevents interference with circulation.

12. If the stockings are knee-length, make sure each stocking top is 1 to 2 inches below the patella. Make sure the stocking does not roll down.

Prevents pressure and interference with circulation. Rolling stockings may have a constricting effect on veins.

13. If applying thigh-length stocking, continue the application. Flex the patient's leg. Stretch the stocking over the knee.

This ensures even distribution.

ACTION	RATIONALE
14. Pull the stocking over the thigh until the top is 1 to 3 inches below the gluteal fold (Figure 2). Adjust the stocking, as necessary, to distribute the fabric evenly. Make sure the stocking does not roll down.	Prevents excessive pressure and interference with circulation. Rolling stockings may have a constricting effect on veins.

FIGURE 2 Pulling the stocking up over the thigh.

ACTION	RATIONALE
15. Remove equipment and return patient to a position of comfort. Remove gloves. Raise side rail and lower bed. Place call bell and other essential items within reach.	Promotes patient comfort and safety. Removing gloves properly reduces the risk for infection transmission and contamination of other items. Having the call bell and other essential items within reach promotes safety.
16. Remove any other PPE, if used. Perform hand hygiene.	Removing PPE properly reduces the risk for infection transmission and contamination of other items. Hand hygiene prevents the spread of microorganisms.

Removing Stockings

ACTION	RATIONALE
17. To remove stocking, grasp top of stocking with your thumb and fingers and smoothly pull stocking off inside-out to heel. Support foot and ease stocking over it.	This preserves the elasticity and contour of the stocking. It allows assessment of circulatory status and condition of skin on lower extremity and for skin care.

EVALUATION

- Stockings are applied and removed, as indicated.
- Patient exhibits a decrease in peripheral edema.
- Patient can state the reason for using the stockings, and give an accurate return demonstration, as indicated.

DOCUMENTATION
- Document the patient's leg measurements as a baseline. Document the application of the stockings, size stocking applied, skin and leg assessment, and neurovascular assessment.

SKILL 79 PERFORMING HAND HYGIENE USING AN ALCOHOL-BASED HANDRUB

Alcohol-based handrubs can be used in the health care setting; they take less time to use than traditional handwashing. When using these products, check the product labeling for correct amount of product needed. Alcohol-based handrubs (CDC, 2002; IHI, 2011):
- May be used if hands are not visibly soiled, or have not come in contact with blood or body fluids
- May be used before inserting urinary catheters, peripheral vascular catheters, or invasive devices that do not require surgical placement; before donning sterile gloves prior to an invasive procedure (e.g., inserting a central intravascular catheter); and if moving from a contaminated body site to a clean body site during patient care
- Should be used before and after each patient contact, or contact with surfaces in the patient's environment, and after removing gloves
- Significantly reduce the number of microorganisms on skin; alcohol-based handrubs are fast acting and cause less skin irritation.

DELEGATION CONSIDERATIONS

The application and use of hand hygiene is appropriate for all health care providers.

EQUIPMENT
- Alcohol-based handrub
- Oil-free lotion (optional)

ASSESSMENT
- Assess hands for any visible soiling or contact with blood or body fluids.
- Alcohol-based handrubs can be used if hands are not visibly soiled, or have not come in contact with blood or body fluids.
- Wash hands with soap and water before eating and after using the restroom.
- If hands are visibly soiled, or have been in contact with blood or body fluids, even if there is no visible soiling, proceed with washing the hands with soap and water.

NURSING DIAGNOSIS
- Risk for Infection

OUTCOME IDENTIFICATION AND PLANNING

- Transient microorganisms will be eliminated from the hands.
- Other outcomes may be appropriate, depending on the specific nursing diagnosis identified for the patient.

IMPLEMENTATION

ACTION	RATIONALE
1. Remove jewelry, if possible, and secure in a safe place. A plain wedding band may remain in place.	Removal of jewelry facilitates proper cleansing. Microorganisms may accumulate in settings of jewelry. If jewelry was worn during patient care, it should be left on during handwashing.
2. Check the product labeling for correct amount of product needed.	Amount of product required to be effective varies from manufacturer to manufacturer, but is usually 1 to 3 mL.
3. Apply the correct amount of product to the palm of one hand. Rub hands together, covering all surfaces of hands and fingers, and between fingers. Also clean the fingertips and the area beneath the fingernails.	Adequate amount of product is required to cover hand surfaces thoroughly. All surfaces must be treated to prevent disease transmission.
4. Rub hands together until they are dry (at least 15 seconds).	Drying ensures antiseptic effect.
5. Use oil-free lotion on hands, if desired.	Oil-free lotion helps to keep the skin soft and prevents chapping. It is best applied after patient care is complete and from a small, personal container. Oil-based lotions should be avoided because they can cause deterioration of gloves.

EVALUATION

- Transient microorganisms are eliminated from the hands.

DOCUMENTATION

The performance of hand hygiene using an alcohol-based handrub is not generally documented.

Handwashing, as opposed to hand hygiene with an alcohol-based rub, is required (CDC, 2002):
- When hands are visibly dirty
- When hands are visibly soiled with (or in contact with) blood or other body fluids
- Before eating and after using the restroom
- If exposure to certain organisms, such as those causing anthrax or *Clostridium difficile,* is known or suspected. (Other agents, such as alcohol-based hand rubs, have poor activity against these organisms.)

DELEGATION CONSIDERATIONS

The application and use of hand hygiene is appropriate for all health care providers.

EQUIPMENT

- Antimicrobial or non-antimicrobial soap (if in bar form, soap must be placed on a soap rack)
- Paper towels
- Oil-free lotion (optional)

ASSESSMENT

- Assess for any of the above requirements for handwashing. If no requirements are fulfilled, the caregiver has the option of decontaminating hands with soap and water or using an alcohol-based hand rub.

NURSING DIAGNOSIS

- Risk for Infection

OUTCOME IDENTIFICATION AND PLANNING

- Hands will be free of visible soiling and transient microorganisms will be eliminated. Other outcomes may be appropriate, depending on the specific nursing diagnosis identified for the patient.

IMPLEMENTATION

ACTION	RATIONALE
1. Gather the necessary supplies. Stand in front of the sink. Do not allow your clothing to touch the sink during the washing procedure.	The sink is considered contaminated. Clothing may carry organisms from place to place.

ACTION	RATIONALE
2. Remove jewelry, if possible, and secure in a safe place. A plain wedding band may remain in place.	Removal of jewelry facilitates proper cleansing. Microorganisms may accumulate in settings of jewelry. If jewelry was worn during care, it should be left on during handwashing.
3. Turn on water and adjust force. Regulate the temperature until the water is warm.	Water splashed from the contaminated sink will contaminate clothing. Warm water is more comfortable and is less likely to open pores and remove oils from the skin. Organisms can lodge in roughened and broken areas of chapped skin.
4. Wet the hands and wrist area. Keep hands lower than elbows to allow water to flow toward fingertips.	Water should flow from the cleaner area toward the more contaminated area. Hands are more contaminated than forearms.
5. Use about 1 teaspoon liquid soap from dispenser or rinse bar of soap and lather thoroughly. Cover all areas of hands with the soap product. Rinse soap bar again and return to soap rack without touching the rack.	Rinsing the soap before and after use removes the lather, which may contain microorganisms.
6. With firm rubbing and circular motions, wash the palms and backs of the hands, each finger, the areas between the fingers, and the knuckles, wrists, and forearms. **Wash at least 1 inch above area of contamination.** If hands are not visibly soiled, wash to 1 inch above the wrists.	Friction caused by firm rubbing and circular motions helps to loosen dirt and organisms that can lodge between the fingers, in skin crevices of knuckles, on the palms and backs of the hands, and on the wrists and forearms. Cleaning less contaminated areas (forearms and wrists) after hands are clean prevents spreading microorganisms from the hands to the forearms and wrists.
7. Continue this friction motion for at least 20 seconds.	Length of handwashing is determined by degree of contamination. Hands that are visibly soiled need a longer scrub.

ACTION	RATIONALE
8. Use fingernails of the opposite hand or a clean orangewood stick to clean under fingernails.	Area under nails has a high microorganism count, and organisms may remain under the nails, where they can grow and be spread to other persons.
9. Rinse thoroughly with water flowing toward fingertips.	Running water rinses microorganisms and dirt into the sink.
10. Pat hands dry with a paper towel, beginning with the fingers and moving upward toward forearms, and discard it immediately. Use another clean towel to turn off the faucet. Discard towel immediately without touching other clean hand.	Patting the skin dry prevents chapping. Dry hands first because they are considered the cleanest and least contaminated area. Turning the faucet off with a clean paper towel protects the clean hands from contact with a soiled surface.
11. Use oil-free lotion on hands, if desired.	Oil-free lotion helps to keep the skin soft and prevents chapping. It is best to apply after patient care is complete and from a small, personal container. Oil-based lotions should be avoided because they can cause deterioration of gloves.

EVALUATION

- Hands are free of visible soiling and transient microorganisms are eliminated.

DOCUMENTATION

- The performance of handwashing is not generally documented.

SKILL 81 APPLYING AN EXTERNAL HEATING PAD

Heat applications accelerate the inflammatory response, promoting healing. Heat is also used to reduce muscle tension, and to relieve muscle spasm and joint stiffness. Heat also helps relieve pain. It is used to treat infections, surgical wounds, inflammation, arthritis, joint pain, muscle pain, and chronic pain.

Heat is applied by moist and dry methods. The medical order should include the type of application, the body area to be treated, the frequency of application, and the length of time for the applications. Water used for heat applications needs to be at the appropriate temperature to avoid skin damage: 115°F to 125°F for older children and adults and 105°F to 110°F for infants, young children, older adults, and patients with diabetes or those who are unconscious.

Common types of external heating devices include Aquathermia pads (one brand) and crushable, microwaveable hot packs. Aquathermia pads are used in health care agencies and are safer to use than heating pads. The temperature setting for an Aquathermia pad should not exceed 105°F to 109.4°F, depending on facility policy. Microwaveable packs are easy and inexpensive to use, but have several disadvantages. They may leak and pose a danger from burns related to improper use. They are used most often in the home setting.

DELEGATION CONSIDERATIONS

The application of an external heating pad may be delegated to nursing assistive personnel (NAP) or unlicensed assistive personnel (UAP), as well as to licensed practical/vocational nurses (LPN/LVNs). The decision to delegate must be based on careful analysis of the patient's needs and circumstances, as well as the qualifications of the person to whom the task is being delegated. Refer to the Delegation Guidelines in Appendix A.

EQUIPMENT

- Aquathermia heating pad (or other brand) with electronic unit
- Distilled water
- Cover for the pad, if not part of pad
- Gauze bandage or tape to secure the pad
- Bath blanket
- PPE, as indicated

ASSESSMENT

- Assess the situation to determine the appropriateness for the application of heat.
- Assess the patient's physical and mental status and the condition of the body area to be treated with heat.
- Confirm the medical order for heat therapy, including frequency, type of therapy, body area to be treated, and length of time for the application.
- Check the equipment to be used, including the condition of cords, plugs, and heating elements. Look for fluid leaks. Once the equipment is turned on, make sure there is a consistent distribution of heat and the temperature is within safe limits.

NURSING DIAGNOSIS

- Chronic Pain
- Acute Pain
- Risk for Impaired Skin Integrity

OUTCOME IDENTIFICATION AND PLANNING

- Patient experiences increased comfort.
- Patient experiences decreased muscle spasms.
- Patient exhibits improved wound healing.
- Patient demonstrates a reduction in inflammation.
- Patient remains free from injury.

IMPLEMENTATION

ACTION	RATIONALE
1. Review the medical order for the application of heat therapy, including frequency, type of therapy, body area to be treated, and length of time for the application. Gather necessary supplies.	Reviewing the order and plan of care validates the correct patient and correct procedure. Preparation promotes efficient time management and organized approach to the task.
2. Perform hand hygiene and put on PPE, if indicated.	Hand hygiene and PPE prevent the spread of microorganisms. PPE is required based on transmission precautions.
3. Identify the patient.	Identifying the patient ensures the right patient receives the intervention and helps prevent errors.
4. Assemble equipment on overbed table within reach.	Organization facilitates performance of task.
5. Close the curtains around the bed and close the door to room, if possible. Explain what you are going to do and why you are going to do it to the patient.	This ensures the patient's privacy. Explanation relieves anxiety and facilitates cooperation.
6. Adjust bed to comfortable working height, usually elbow height of the caregiver (VISN 8, 2009).	Having the bed at the proper height prevents back and muscle strain.
7. Assist the patient to a comfortable position that provides easy access to the area where the heat will be applied; use a bath blanket to cover any other exposed area.	Patient positioning and use of a bath blanket provide for comfort and warmth.

ACTION	RATIONALE
8. Assess the condition of the skin where the heat is to be applied.	Assessment supplies baseline data for post-treatment comparison and identifies conditions that may contraindicate the application.
9. Check that the water in the electronic unit is at the appropriate level. Fill the unit two-thirds full or to the fill mark, with distilled water, if necessary. Check the temperature setting on the unit to ensure it is within the safe range.	Sufficient water in the unit is necessary to ensure proper function of the unit. Tap water leaves mineral deposits in the unit. Checking the temperature setting helps to prevent skin or tissue damage.
10. Attach pad tubing to the electronic unit tubing.	Allows flow of warmed water through the heating pad.
11. Plug in the unit and warm the pad before use. Apply the heating pad to the prescribed area. Secure with gauze bandage or tape.	Plugging in the pad readies it for use. Heat travels by conduction from one object to another. Gauze bandage or tape holds the pad in position; **do not use pins, as they may puncture and damage the pad.**
12. **Assess the condition of the skin and the patient's response to the heat at frequent intervals, according to facility policy. Do not exceed the prescribed length of time for the application of heat.**	Maximum vasodilation and therapeutic effects from the application of heat occur within 20 to 30 minutes. Using heat for more than 45 minutes results in tissue congestion and vasoconstriction, known as the rebound phenomenon. Also, prolonged heat application may result in an increased risk of burns.
13. Remove gloves and discard. Remove all remaining equipment; place the patient in a comfortable position, with side rails up and bed in the lowest position.	Proper removal of gloves prevents spread of microorganisms. Proper patient and bed positioning promotes safety and comfort.
14. Remove additional PPE, if used. Perform hand hygiene.	Removing PPE properly reduces the risk for infection transmission and contamination of other items. Hand hygiene prevents the spread of microorganisms.

ACTION	RATIONALE
15. Monitor the time the heating pad is in place to prevent burns and skin/tissue damage. Monitor the condition of the patient's skin and the patient's response at frequent intervals.	Extended use of heat results in an increased risk for burns from the heat. Impaired circulation may affect the patient's sensitivity to heat.
16. Remove the pad after the prescribed amount of time (up to 30 minutes). Reassess the patient and area of application, noting the effect and presence of adverse effects.	Removal reduces risk of injury due to prolonged heat application. Heat applications are used to promote healing; reduce muscle tension; relieve muscle spasm, joint stiffness, and pain; and treat infections, surgical wounds, inflammation, arthritis, joint pain, muscle pain, and chronic pain. Assessment provides input as to the effectiveness of the treatment.

EVALUATION

• Patient exhibits increased comfort, decreased muscle spasm, decreased pain, improved wound healing, and/or decreased inflammation.
• Patient remains free of injury.

DOCUMENTATION

• Document the rationale for application of heat therapy. If the patient is receiving heat therapy for pain, document the assessment of pain pre- and post-intervention. Specify the type of heat therapy and location where it is applied, as well as length of time applied. Record the condition of the skin, noting any redness or irritation before the heat application and after the application. Document the patient's reaction to the heat therapy. Record any appropriate patient or family education.

SKILL 82

Hemodialysis, a method of removing fluid and wastes from the body, requires access to the patient's vascular system. This is done via the insertion of a catheter into a large vein, typically a central venous catheter inserted into the chest (short-term or long-term access) or the creation of a fistula or graft (long-term access). If a catheter is used, it is cared for in the same manner as a central venous access device (see Skill 32). An arteriovenous fistula is a surgically created passage that connects an artery and vein. An arteriovenous graft is a surgically created connection between an artery and vein using a synthetic material. Accessing a hemodialysis arteriovenous graft or fistula should be done only by specially trained health care team members.

DELEGATION CONSIDERATIONS

The assessment of and care for a hemodialysis access is not delegated to nursing assistive personnel (NAP) or to unlicensed assistive personnel (UAP). Depending on the state's nurse practice act and the organization's policies and procedures, these procedures may be delegated to licensed practical/vocational nurses (LPN/LVNs). The decision to delegate must be based on careful analysis of the patient's needs and circumstances, as well as the qualifications of the person to whom the task is being delegated. Refer to the Delegation Guidelines in Appendix A.

EQUIPMENT
- Stethoscope
- PPE, as indicated

ASSESSMENT
- Ask the patient how much he or she knows about caring for the site. Ask the patient to describe important observations to be made.
- Note the location of the access site. Assess the site for signs of infection, including inflammation, edema, and drainage; and for healing of the incision.
- Assess for patency by assessing for presence of bruit and thrill (refer to explanation in Step 4, below).

NURSING DIAGNOSIS
- Deficient Knowledge
- Risk for Injury

OUTCOME IDENTIFICATION AND PLANNING
- Graft or fistula remains patent.
- Patient verbalizes appropriate care measures and observations to be made.
- Patient demonstrates appropriate care measures.

IMPLEMENTATION

ACTION	RATIONALE

1. Perform hand hygiene and put on PPE, if indicated.

   Hand hygiene and PPE prevent the spread of microorganisms. PPE is required based on transmission precautions.

2. Identify the patient.

   Identifying the patient ensures the right patient receives the intervention and helps prevent errors.

3. Close the curtains around the bed and close the door to the room, if possible. Explain what you are going to do, and why you are going to do it, to the patient.

   This ensures the patient's privacy. Explanation relieves anxiety and facilitates cooperation. Discussion promotes cooperation and helps to minimize anxiety.

4. Question the patient about the presence of muscle weakness and cramping; changes in temperature; sensations, such as numbness, tingling, pain, burning, itchiness; and pain.

   Aids in determining the patency of the hemodialysis access, as well as the presence of complications.

5. Inspect the area over the access site for continuity of skin color. Inspect for any redness, warmth, tenderness, edema, rash, blemishes, bleeding, tremors, and twitches. Inspect the muscle strength, and the patient's ability to perform range of motion in the extremity/body part with the hemodialysis access.

   Inspection aids in determining the patency of the hemodialysis access, as well as the status of the patient's circulatory, neurologic and muscular function; and presence of infection. Compare with the opposite body area/part.

6. Palpate over the access site, feeling for a thrill or vibration. Palpate pulses above and below the site. Palpate the continuity of the skin temperature along and around the extremity. Check capillary refill in fingers or toes of extremity with the fistula or graft.

   Palpation aids in determining the patency of the hemodialysis access, as well as the status of the patient's circulatory, neurologic and muscular function; and presence of infection. Compare with the opposite body area/part.

ACTION	RATIONALE
7. Auscultate over the access site with bell of stethoscope, listening for a bruit or vibration.	Palpation aids in determining the patency of the hemodialysis access.
8. Ensure that a sign is placed over the head of the bed informing the health care team which arm is affected. **Do not measure blood pressure, perform a venipuncture, or start an IV on the access arm.**	The affected arm should not be used for any other procedures, such as obtaining blood pressure, which could lead to clotting of the graft or fistula. Venipuncture or IV access could lead to an infection of the affected arm and could cause the loss of the graft or fistula.
9. Instruct the patient not to sleep with the arm with the access site under the head or body.	This could lead to clotting of the fistula or graft.
10. Instruct the patient not to lift heavy objects with, or put pressure on, the arm with the access site. Advise the patient not to carry heavy bags (including purses) on the shoulder of that arm.	This could lead to clotting of the fistula or graft.
11. Remove PPE, if used. Perform hand hygiene.	Removing PPE properly reduces the risk for infection transmission and contamination of other items. Hand hygiene prevents the spread of microorganisms.

EVALUATION

- Access site has an audible bruit and a palpable thrill.
- Site is intact without signs of adverse complications or pain.
- Patient verbalizes appropriate information about caring for the access site and observations to report.

DOCUMENTATION

- Document assessment findings, including the presence or absence of a bruit and thrill.
- Document any patient education and patient response.

A hypothermia blanket, or cooling pad, is a blanket-sized aquathermia pad that conducts a cooled solution, usually distilled water, through coils in a plastic blanket or pad. Placing a patient on a hypothermia blanket or pad helps to lower body temperature. The nurse monitors the patient's body temperature and can reset the blanket setting accordingly. The blanket also can be preset to maintain a specific body temperature; the device continually monitors the patient's body temperature using a temperature probe (which is inserted rectally or in the esophagus, or placed on the skin) and adjusts the temperature of the circulating liquid accordingly.

DELEGATION CONSIDERATIONS

The application of a hypothermia pad is not delegated to nursing assistive personnel (NAP) or to unlicensed assistive personnel (UAP). The measurement of a patient's body temperature while a hypothermia pad is in use may be delegated to nursing assistive personnel (NAP) or to unlicensed assistive personnel (UAP). Depending on the state's nurse practice act and the organization's policies and procedures, the application of a hypothermia pad may be delegated to a licensed practical/vocational nurse (LPN/LVN). The decision to delegate must be based on careful analysis of the patient's needs and circumstances, as well as the qualifications of the person to whom the task is being delegated. Refer to the Delegation Guidelines in Appendix A.

EQUIPMENT

- Disposable cooling blanket or pad
- Electronic control panel
- Distilled water to fill the device, if necessary
- Thermometer, if needed to monitor the patient's temperature
- Sphygmomanometer
- Stethoscope
- Temperature probe, if needed
- Thin blanket or sheet
- Towels
- Clean gloves
- Additional PPE, as indicated

ASSESSMENT

- Assess the patient's condition, including current body temperature, to determine the need for the cooling blanket.
- Consider alternative measures to help lower the patient's body temperature before implementing the blanket.
- Verify the medical order for the application of a hypothermia blanket.
- Assess the patient's vital signs, neurologic status, peripheral circulation, and skin integrity.
- Assess the equipment to be used, including the condition of cords, plugs, and cooling elements. Look for fluid leaks. Once the

equipment is turned on, make sure there is a consistent distribution of cooling.

NURSING DIAGNOSIS

- Risk for Injury
- Risk for Impaired Skin Integrity
- Hyperthermia
- Hypothermia
- Risk for Imbalanced Body Temperature
- Ineffective Thermoregulation

OUTCOME IDENTIFICATION AND PLANNING

- Patient maintains the desired body temperature.
- Patient does not experience shivering.
- Patient's vital signs are within normal limits.
- Patient does not experience alterations in skin integrity, neurologic status, peripheral circulation, or fluid and electrolyte status and edema.

IMPLEMENTATION

ACTION	RATIONALE
1. Review the medical order for the application of the hypothermia blanket. Obtain consent for the therapy per facility policy.	Reviewing the order validates the correct patient and correct procedure.
2. Perform hand hygiene and put on PPE, if indicated.	Hand hygiene and PPE prevent the spread of microorganisms. PPE is required based on transmission precautions.
3. Identify the patient. Determine if the patient has had any previous adverse reaction to hypothermia therapy.	Identifying the patient ensures the right patient receives the intervention and helps prevent errors. Individual differences exist in tolerating specific therapies.
4. Assemble equipment on the overbed table within reach.	Organization facilitates performance of task.
5. Close curtains around the bed and close the door to the room, if possible. Explain what you are going to do and why you are going to do it to the patient.	This ensures the patient's privacy. Explanation relieves anxiety and facilitates cooperation.

ACTION	RATIONALE
6. Check that the water in the electronic unit is at the appropriate level. Fill the unit two thirds full with distilled water, or to the fill mark, if necessary. Check the temperature setting on the unit to ensure it is within the safe range.	Sufficient water in the unit is necessary to ensure proper function of the unit. Tap water leaves mineral deposits in the unit. Checking the temperature setting helps to prevent skin or tissue damage.
7. Assess the patient's vital signs, neurologic status, peripheral circulation, and skin integrity.	Assessment supplies baseline data for comparison during therapy and identifies conditions that may contraindicate the application.
8. Adjust bed to comfortable working height, usually elbow height of the care giver (VISN 8 Patient Safety Center, 2009).	Having the bed at the proper height prevents back and muscle strain.
9. Make sure the patient's gown has cloth ties, not snaps or pins.	Cloth ties minimize the risk of cold injury.
10. Apply lanolin or a mixture of lanolin and cold cream to the patient's skin where it will be in contact with the blanket.	These agents help protect the skin from cold.
11. Turn on the blanket and make sure the cooling light is on. Verify that the temperature limits are set within the desired safety range.	Turning on the blanket prepares it for use. Keeping temperature within the safety range prevents excessive cooling.
12. Cover the hypothermia blanket with a thin sheet or bath blanket.	A sheet or blanket protects the patient's skin from direct contact with the cooling surface, reducing the risk for injury.
13. Position the blanket under the patient so that the top edge of the pad is aligned with the patient's neck.	The blanket's rigid surface may be uncomfortable. The cold may lead to tissue breakdown.
14. Put on gloves. Lubricate the rectal probe and insert it into the patient's rectum unless contraindicated. Or tuck the skin probe deep into the patient's axilla and tape it in place. For patients who are	The probe allows continuous monitoring of the patient's core body temperature. Rectal insertion may be contraindicated in patients with a low white blood cell or platelet count.

ACTION	RATIONALE
comatose or anesthetized, use an esophageal probe. Remove gloves. Attach the probe to the control panel for the blanket.	
15. Wrap the patient's hands and feet in gauze if ordered, or if the patient desires. For male patients, elevate the scrotum off the cooling blanket with towels.	These actions minimize chilling, promote comfort, and protect sensitive tissues from direct contact with cold.
16. Place the patient in a comfortable position. Lower the bed. Dispose of any other supplies appropriately.	Repositioning promotes patient comfort and safety.
17. Recheck the thermometer and settings on the control panel.	Rechecking verifies that the blanket temperature is maintained at a safe level.
18. Remove any additional PPE, if used. Perform hand hygiene.	Removing PPE properly reduces the risk for infection transmission and contamination of other items. Hand hygiene prevents the spread of microorganisms.
19. **Turn and position the patient regularly (every 30 minutes to 1 hour).** Keep linens free from condensation. Reapply cream, as needed. Observe the patient's skin for change in color, changes in lips and nail beds, edema, pain, and sensory impairment.	Turning and repositioning prevent alterations in skin integrity and provide for assessment of potential skin injuries.
20. **Monitor vital signs and perform a neurologic assessment, per facility policy, usually every 15 minutes, until the body temperature is stable.** In addition, monitor the patient's fluid and electrolyte status.	Continuous monitoring provides evaluation of the patient's response to the therapy and permits early identification and intervention if adverse effects occur.
21. Observe for signs of shivering, including verbalized sensations, facial	Shivering increases heat production, and is often controlled with medications.

ACTION	RATIONALE

muscle twitching, hyper-
ventilation, or twitching of
extremities.

22. Assess the patient's level of comfort.

Hypothermia therapy can cause discomfort. Prompt assessment and action can prevent injuries.

23. Turn off the blanket according to facility policy, usually
when the patient's body
temperature reaches 1 degree
above the desired temperature. **Continue to monitor
the patient's temperature
until it stabilizes.**

Body temperature can continue
to fall after this therapy.

EVALUATION

• Patient maintains the desired body temperature and other vital signs within acceptable parameters.
• Patient remains free from shivering.
• Patient does not experience alterations in skin integrity, neurologic status, peripheral circulation, or fluid and electrolyte status, and edema.

DOCUMENTATION

• Document assessments, such as vital signs, neurologic, peripheral circulation, and skin integrity status, before use of hypothermia blanket. Record verification of medical order and that the procedure was explained to the patient. Document the control settings, time of application and removal, and the route of the temperature monitoring. Include the application of lanolin cream to the skin as well as the frequency of position changes. Document the patient's response to the therapy using agency flow sheet, especially noting a decrease in temperature, and discomfort assessment. Record the possible use of medication to reduce shivering or other discomforts. Include any pertinent patient and family teaching.

SKILL 84 | TEACHING A PATIENT TO USE AN INCENTIVE SPIROMETER

Incentive spirometry provides visual reinforcement for deep breathing by the patient. It assists the patient to breathe slowly and deeply, and to sustain maximal inspiration, while providing immediate positive reinforcement. Incentive spirometry encourages the patient to maximize lung inflation and prevent or reduce atelectasis. Optimal gas exchange is supported and secretions can be cleared and expectorated.

DELEGATION CONSIDERATIONS

Patient teaching related to the use of an incentive spirometer is not delegated to nursing assistive personnel (NAP), to unlicensed assistive personnel (UAP), or to licensed practical/vocational nurses (LPN/LVNs). Depending on the state's nurse practice act and the organization's policies and procedures, the LPN/LVN may reinforce and encourage the use of the incentive spirometer by the patient. The decision to delegate must be based on careful analysis of the patient's needs and circumstances, as well as the qualifications of the person to whom the task is being delegated. Refer to the Delegation Guidelines in Appendix A.

EQUIPMENT

- Incentive spirometer
- Stethoscope
- Folded blanket or pillow for splinting of chest or abdominal incision, if appropriate
- PPE, as indicated

ASSESSMENT

- Assess the patient for pain and administer pain medication, as prescribed, if deep breathing may cause pain. Presence of pain may interfere with learning and performing required activities.
- Assess lung sounds before and after use to establish a baseline and to determine the effectiveness of incentive spirometry. Incentive spirometry encourages patients to take deep breaths, and lung sounds may be diminished before using the incentive spirometer.
- Assess vital signs and oxygen saturation to provide baseline data to evaluate patient response. Oxygen saturation may increase due to reinflation of alveoli.

NURSING DIAGNOSIS

- Ineffective Breathing Pattern
- Risk for Infection
- Acute Pain
- Deficient Knowledge

OUTCOME IDENTIFICATION AND PLANNING

- Patient accurately demonstrates the procedure for using the spirometer.
- Patient demonstrates increased oxygen saturation level.
- Patient reports adequate control of pain during use.
- Patient demonstrates increased lung expansion with clear breath sounds.

IMPLEMENTATION

ACTION	RATIONALE
1. Review the patient's health record for any health problems that would affect the patient's oxygenation status.	Identifying influencing factors aids in interpretation of results.
2. Bring necessary equipment to the bedside stand or over-bed table.	Bringing everything to the bedside conserves time and energy. Arranging items nearby is convenient, saves time, and avoids unnecessary stretching and twisting of muscles on the part of the nurse.
3. Perform hand hygiene and put on PPE, if indicated.	Hand hygiene and PPE prevent the spread of microorganisms. PPE is required based on transmission precautions.
4. Identify the patient.	Identifying the patient ensures the right patient receives the intervention and helps prevent errors.
5. Close the curtains around the bed and close the door to the room, if possible. Explain what you are going to do and why you are going to do it to the patient. Using the chart provided with the device by the manufacturer, note the patient's inspiration target, based on the patient's height and age.	This ensures the patient's privacy. Explanation relieves anxiety and facilitates cooperation. Target for inspiration is based on the patient's height and age and provides an individualized target for each patient.
6. Assist the patient to an upright or semi-Fowler's	Upright position facilitates lung expansion. Dentures may inhibit

ACTION	RATIONALE

position, if possible. Remove dentures if they fit poorly. Assess the patient's level of pain. Administer pain medication, as prescribed, if needed. Wait the appropriate amount of time for the medication to take effect. **If the patient has recently undergone abdominal or chest surgery, place a pillow or folded blanket over a chest or abdominal incision for splinting.**

the patient from taking deep breaths if the patient is concerned that dentures may fall out. Pain may decrease the patient's ability to take deep breaths. Deep breaths may cause the patient to cough. Splinting the incision supports the area and helps reduce pain from the incision.

7. Demonstrate how to steady the device with one hand and hold the mouthpiece with the other hand (Figure 1). If the patient cannot use hands, assist the patient with the incentive spirometer.

This allows the patient to remain upright, visualize the volume of each breath, and stabilize the device.

FIGURE 1 Patient using incentive spirometer.

8. Instruct the patient to exhale normally and then place lips securely around the mouthpiece.

Patient should fully empty lungs so that maximum volume may be inhaled. A tight seal allows for maximum use of the device.

9. **Instruct the patient to inhale slowly and as deeply as possible through the mouthpiece without using nose (if desired, a nose clip may be used).**

Inhaling through the nose would provide an inaccurate measurement of inhalation volume.

10. When the patient cannot inhale anymore, **the patient should hold his or her breath and count to three.**

Holding breath for 3 seconds helps the alveoli to re-expand. Volume on incentive spirometry should increase with practice.

ACTION	RATIONALE
Check position of gauge to determine progress and level attained. If patient begins to cough, splint an abdominal or chest incision.	
11. Instruct the patient to remove lips from mouthpiece and exhale normally. **If patient becomes light-headed during the process, tell him or her to stop and take a few normal breaths before resuming incentive spirometry.**	Deep breaths may change the CO_2 level, leading to light-headedness.
12. Encourage the patient to perform incentive spirometry 5 to 10 times every 1 to 2 hours, if possible.	This helps to reinflate the alveoli and prevent atelectasis due to hypoventilation.
13. Clean the mouthpiece with water and shake to dry. Remove PPE, if used. Perform hand hygiene.	Cleaning equipment deters the spread of microorganisms and contaminants. Removing PPE properly reduces the risk for infection transmission and contamination of other items. Hand hygiene prevents the spread of microorganisms.

EVALUATION

- Patient demonstrates the steps for use of the incentive spirometer correctly and exhibits lung sounds that are clear and equal in all lobes.
- Patient demonstrates an increase in oxygen saturation levels.
- Patient verbalizes adequate pain control and the importance of, and need for, incentive spirometry.

DOCUMENTATION

- Document that the incentive spirometer was used by the patient, the number of repetitions, and the average volume reached. Document patient teaching and patient response, if appropriate. If the patient coughs, document whether the cough is productive or nonproductive. If productive cough is present, include the characteristics of the sputum, including consistency, amount, and color.

SKILL 85 ADMINISTERING MEDICATION VIA A DRY POWDER INHALER

Dry powder inhalers (DPIs) are another type of delivery method for inhaled medications. The medication is supplied in a powder form, either in a small capsule or disk inserted into the DPI, or in a compartment inside the DPI. DPIs are breath activated. A quick breath by the patient activates the flow of medication, eliminating the need to coordinate activating the inhaler (spraying the medicine) while inhaling the medicine. However, the drug output and size distribution of the aerosol from a DPI is more or less dependent on the flow rate through the device, so the patient must be able to take a powerful, deep inspiration (Rubin, 2010). Many types of DPIs are available, with distinctive operating instructions. Some have to be loaded with a dose of medication each time they are used and some hold a number of preloaded doses. It is important to understand the particular instructions both for the medication and for particular delivery device being used.

DELEGATION CONSIDERATIONS

The administration of medication via a dry powder inhaler is not delegated to nursing assistive personnel (NAP) or to unlicensed assistive personnel (UAP). Depending on the state's nurse practice act and the organization's policies and procedures, administration of medication using a dry powder inhaler may be delegated to licensed practical/vocational nurses (LPN/LVNs). The decision to delegate must be based on careful analysis of the patient's needs and circumstances, as well as the qualifications of the person to whom the task is being delegated. Refer to the Delegation Guidelines in Appendix A.

EQUIPMENT

- Stethoscope
- DPI and appropriate medication
- Computer-generated Medication Administration Record
- (CMAR) or Medication Administration Record (MAR)
- PPE, as indicated

ASSESSMENT

- Assess respiratory rate, rhythm, and depth to establish a baseline.
- Assess lung sounds before and after use to establish a baseline and determine the effectiveness of the medication.
- If appropriate, assess oxygen saturation level before medication administration.
- Assess the patient's ability to manage the DPI.
- Verify patient name, dose, route, and time of administration.
- Assess the patient's knowledge and understanding of the medication's purpose and action.

NURSING DIAGNOSIS

- Deficient Knowledge
- Risk for Activity Intolerance
- Ineffective Breathing Pattern

OUTCOME IDENTIFICATION AND PLANNING

- Patient receives the medication.
- Patient demonstrates improved lung expansion and breath sounds.
- Patient's respiratory status is within acceptable parameters.
- Patient verbalizes an understanding of medication purpose and action.
- Patient demonstrates correct use of the DPI.

IMPLEMENTATION

ACTION	RATIONALE
1. Gather equipment. Check each medication order against the original order in the medical record, according to facility policy. Clarify any inconsistencies. Check the patient's chart for allergies.	This comparison helps to identify errors that may have occurred when orders were transcribed. The primary care provider's order is the legal record of medication orders for each facility.
2. Know the actions, special nursing considerations, safe dose ranges, purpose of administration, and adverse effects of the medications to be administered. Consider the appropriateness of the medication for this patient.	This knowledge aids the nurse in evaluating the therapeutic effect of the medication in relation to the patient's disorder and can also be used to educate the patient about the medication.
3. Perform hand hygiene.	Hand hygiene prevents the spread of microorganisms.
4. Move the medication cart to the outside of the patient's room or prepare for administration in the medication area.	Organization facilitates error-free administration and saves time.
5. Unlock the medication cart or drawer. Enter pass code and scan employee identification, if required.	Locking the cart or drawer safeguards each patient's medication supply. Hospital accrediting organizations require medication

ACTION	RATIONALE
	carts to be locked when not in use. Entering pass code and scanning ID allows only authorized users into the system and identifies the user for documentation by the computer.
6. **Prepare medications for one patient at a time.**	This prevents errors in medication administration.
7. Read the CMAR/MAR and select the proper medication from the patient's medication drawer or unit stock.	This is the *first* check of the label.
8. Compare the label with the CMAR/MAR. Check expiration dates and perform calculations, if necessary. Scan the bar code on the package, if required.	This is the *second* check of the label. Verify calculations with another nurse to ensure safety, if necessary.
9. **Depending on facility policy, the third check of the label may occur at this point. If so, when all medications for one patient have been prepared, recheck the labels with the CMAR/MAR before taking the medications to the patient.**	This *third* check ensures accuracy and helps to prevent errors. *Note:* Many facilities require the *third* check to occur at the bedside, after identifying the patient and before administration.
10. Lock the medication cart before leaving it.	Locking the cart or drawer safeguards the patient's medication supply. Hospital accrediting organizations require medication carts to be locked when not in use.
11. Transport medications to the patient's bedside carefully, and keep the medications in sight at all times.	Careful handling and close observation prevent accidental or deliberate disarrangement of medications.
12. **Ensure that the patient receives the medications at the correct time.**	Check agency policy, which may allow for administration within a period of 30 minutes before or 30 minutes after the designated time.

ACTION	RATIONALE

13. Perform hand hygiene and put on PPE, if indicated.

Hand hygiene and PPE prevent the spread of microorganisms. PPE is required based on transmission precautions.

14. **Identify the patient.** **Compare the information with the CMAR/MAR. The patient should be identified using at least two methods (The Joint Commission, 2013):**

Identifying the patient ensures the right patient receives the medications and helps prevent errors. The patient's room number or physical location is not used as an identifier (The Joint Commission, 2013). Replace the identification band if it is missing or inaccurate in any way.

   a. Check the name on the patient's identification band.

   b. Check the identification number on the patient's identification band.

   c. Check the birth date on the patient's identification band.

   d. Ask the patient to state his or her name and birth date, based on facility policy.

This requires a response from the patient, but illness and strange surroundings often cause patients to be confused.

15. **Complete necessary assessments before administering medications. Check the patient's allergy bracelet or ask the patient about allergies. Explain what you are going to do, and the reason for doing it, to the patient.**

Assessment is a prerequisite to administration of medications.

16. Scan the patient's bar code on the identification band, if required.

Provides an additional check to ensure that the medication is given to the right patient.

17. **Based on facility policy, the third check of the label may occur at this point. If so, recheck the labels with the CMAR/MAR before administering the medications to the patient.**

Many facilities require the *third* check to occur at the bedside, after identifying the patient and before administration. If facility policy directs the *third* check at this time, this *third* check ensures accuracy and helps to prevent errors.

ACTION	RATIONALE
18. Remove the mouthpiece cover or remove the device from storage container. Load a dose into the device as directed by the manufacturer, if necessary. Alternately, activate the inhaler, if necessary, according to manufacturer's directions.	This is necessary to deliver the medication.
19. Have the patient breathe out slowly and completely, without breathing into the DPI.	This allows for deeper inhalation with the medication dose. Moisture from the patient's breath can clog the inhaler.
20. **Instruct the patient to place teeth over, and seal lips around, the mouthpiece. Do not block the opening with the tongue or teeth.**	Prevents medication from escaping and allows for a tight seal, ensuring maximal dosing of medication. Blocking of opening interferes with medication delivery.
21. **Instruct patient to breathe in quickly and deeply through the mouth, for longer than 2 to 3 seconds.**	Activates the flow of medication. Deep inhalation allows for maximal distribution of medication to lung tissue.
22. Remove inhaler from mouth. Instruct patient to hold the breath for 5 to 10 seconds, or as long as possible, and then to exhale slowly through pursed lips.	This allows better distribution and longer absorption time for the medication.
23. Wait 1 to 5 minutes, as prescribed, before administering the next puff.	This ensures that both puffs are absorbed as much as possible. Bronchodilation after the first puff allows for deeper penetration by subsequent puffs.
24. After the prescribed number of puffs has been administered, have the patient replace the cap or storage container.	By replacing the cap, the patient is preventing any dust or dirt from entering the inhaler and being propelled into the bronchioles with later doses or from clogging the inhaler.
25. Have the patient gargle and rinse with tap water after using DPI, as necessary. Clean the DPI according to the manufacturer's directions.	Rinsing is necessary when using inhaled steroids, because oral fungal infections can occur. Rinsing removes medication residue from the mouth. Medication buildup in the device

ACTION	RATIONALE
	can affect how the medication is delivered, as well as attract bacteria.
26. Remove gloves and additional PPE, if used. Perform hand hygiene.	Removing PPE properly reduces the risk for infection transmission and contamination of other items. Hand hygiene prevents the spread of microorganisms.
27. Document the administration of the medication immediately after administration. See Documentation section below.	Timely documentation helps to ensure patient safety.
28. Evaluate the patient's response to medication within an appropriate time frame. **Reassess lung sounds, oxygen saturation level, and respirations.**	The patient needs to be evaluated for therapeutic and adverse effects from the medication. Lung sounds and oxygen saturation level may improve after DPI use. Respirations may decrease after DPI use.

EVALUATION

- Patient demonstrates improved lung sounds and ease of breathing.
- Patient demonstrates correct use of the DPI and verbalizes correct information about medication therapy associated with DPI use.

DOCUMENTATION

- Document the administration of the medication immediately after administration, including date, time, dose, and route of administration on the CMAR/MAR or record using the required format. If using a bar-code system, medication administration is automatically recorded when the bar code is scanned. PRN medications require documentation of the reason for administration. Prompt recording avoids the possibility of accidentally repeating the administration of the drug. Document respiratory rate, oxygen saturation, if applicable, lung assessment, and the patient's response to the treatment, if appropriate. If the drug was refused or omitted, record this in the appropriate area on the medication record and notify the primary care provider. This verifies the reason medication was omitted and ensures that the primary care provider is aware of the patient's condition.

SKILL 86 — ADMINISTERING MEDICATION VIA A METERED-DOSE INHALER (MDI)

Many medications for respiratory problems are delivered via the respiratory system. A metered-dose inhaler (MDI) is a handheld inhaler that uses an aerosol spray or mist to deliver a controlled dose of medication with each compression of the canister. The medication is then absorbed rapidly through the lung tissue, resulting in local and systemic effects.

DELEGATION CONSIDERATIONS

The administration of medication via a metered-dose inhaler is not delegated to nursing assistive personnel (NAP) or to unlicensed assistive personnel (UAP). Depending on the state's nurse practice act and the organization's policies and procedures, administration of a metered-dose inhaler may be delegated to licensed practical/vocational nurses (LPN/LVNs). The decision to delegate must be based on careful analysis of the patient's needs and circumstances, as well as the qualifications of the person to whom the task is being delegated. Refer to the Delegation Guidelines in Appendix A.

EQUIPMENT

- Stethoscope
- Medication in an MDI
- Spacer or holding chamber (optional, but recommended for many medications)
- Computerized-generated Medication Administration Record (CMAR) or Medication Administration Record (MAR)
- PPE, as indicated

ASSESSMENT

- Assess respiratory rate, rhythm, and depth to establish a baseline.
- Assess lung sounds before and after use to establish a baseline and determine the effectiveness of the medication. Frequently, patients will have wheezes or coarse lung sounds before medication administration.
- If ordered, assess oxygen saturation level before medication administration. The oxygenation level usually increases after the medication is administered.
- Verify patient name, dose, route, and time of administration.
- Assess the patient's ability to manage an MDI; young and older patients may have dexterity problems.
- Assess the patient's knowledge and understanding of the medication's purpose and action.

NURSING DIAGNOSIS

- Ineffective Airway Clearance
- Impaired Gas Exchange
- Deficient Knowledge

OUTCOME IDENTIFICATION AND PLANNING

- Patient receives the medication.
- Patient demonstrates improved lung expansion and breath sounds.
- Patient's respiratory status is within acceptable parameters.
- Patient verbalizes an understanding of medication purpose and action; and patient demonstrates correct use of an MDI.

IMPLEMENTATION

ACTION	RATIONALE
1. Gather equipment. Check each medication order against the original order in the medical record, according to facility policy. Clarify any inconsistencies. Check the patient's chart for allergies.	This comparison helps to identify errors that may have occurred when orders were transcribed. The primary care provider's order is the legal record of medication orders for each facility.
2. Know the actions, special nursing considerations, safe dose ranges, purpose of administration, and adverse effects of the medications to be administered. Consider the appropriateness of the medication for this patient.	This knowledge aids the nurse in evaluating the therapeutic effect of the medication in relation to the patient's disorder and can also be used to educate the patient about the medication.
3. Perform hand hygiene.	Hand hygiene prevents the spread of microorganisms.
4. Move the medication cart to the outside of the patient's room or prepare for administration in the medication area.	Organization facilitates error-free administration and saves time.
5. Unlock the medication cart or drawer. Enter pass code and scan employee identification, if required.	Locking the cart or drawer safeguards each patient's medication supply. Hospital accrediting organizations require medication carts to be locked when not in use. Entering pass code and scanning ID allows only authorized users into the computer system and identifies the user for documentation by the computer.

ACTION	RATIONALE
6. **Prepare medications for one patient at a time.**	This prevents errors in medication administration.
7. Read the CMAR/MAR and select the proper medication from the patient's medication drawer or unit stock.	This is the *first* check of the label.
8. Compare the label with the CMAR/MAR. Check expiration dates and perform calculations, if necessary. Scan the bar code on the package, if required.	This is the *second* check of the label. Verify calculations with another nurse to ensure safety, if necessary.
9. **Depending on facility policy, the third check of the label may occur at this point. If so, when all medications for one patient have been prepared, recheck the labels with the CMAR/MAR before taking the medications to the patient.**	This *third* check ensures accuracy and helps to prevent errors. *Note:* Many facilities require the *third* check to occur at the bedside, after identifying the patient and before administration.
10. Lock the medication cart before leaving it.	Locking the cart or drawer safeguards the patient's medication supply. Hospital accrediting organizations require medication carts to be locked when not in use.
11. Transport medications to the patient's bedside carefully, and keep the medications in sight at all times.	Careful handling and close observation prevent accidental or deliberate disarrangement of medications.
12. **Ensure that the patient receives the medications at the correct time.**	Check agency policy, which may allow for administration within a period of 30 minutes before or 30 minutes after the designated time.
13. Perform hand hygiene and put on PPE, if indicated.	Hand hygiene and PPE prevent the spread of microorganisms. PPE is required based on transmission precautions.

ACTION	RATIONALE

14. **Identify the patient.** **Compare the information with the CMAR/MAR. The patient should be identified using at least two methods** (The Joint Commission, 2013):

Identifying the patient ensures the right patient receives the medications and helps prevent errors. The patient's room number or physical location is not used as an identifier (The Joint Commission, 2013). Replace the identification band if it is missing or inaccurate in any way.

a. Check the name on the patient's identification band.

b. Check the identification number on the patient's identification band.

c. Check the birth date on the patient's identification band.

d. Ask the patient to state his or her name and birth date, based on facility policy.

This requires a response from the patient, but illness and strange surroundings often cause patients to be confused.

15. **Complete necessary assessments before administering medications. Check the patient's allergy bracelet or ask the patient about allergies. Explain what you are going to do and the reason for doing it to the patient.**

Assessment is a prerequisite to administration of medications. Explanation relieves anxiety and facilitates cooperation.

16. Scan the patient's bar code on the identification band, if required.

Provides an additional check to ensure that the medication is given to the right patient.

17. **Based on facility policy, the third check of the label may occur at this point. If so, recheck the labels with the CMAR/MAR before administering the medications to the patient.**

Many facilities require the *third* check to occur at the bedside, after identifying the patient and before administration. If facility policy directs the *third* check at this time, this *third* check ensures accuracy and helps to prevent errors.

18. Remove the mouthpiece cover from the MDI and the spacer. Attach the MDI to the spacer. (See accompanying Skill Variation for using an MDI without a spacer.)

The use of a spacer is preferred because it traps the medication and aids in delivery of the correct dose.

ACTION	RATIONALE
19. Shake the inhaler and spacer well.	The medication and propellant may separate when the canister is not in use. Shaking well ensures that the patient is receiving the correct dosage of medication.
20. Have patient place the spacer's mouthpiece into mouth, grasping securely with teeth and lips. Have patient breathe normally through the spacer.	Medication should not leak out around the mouthpiece.
21. Patient should depress the canister, releasing one puff into the spacer, then inhale slowly and deeply through the mouth.	The spacer will hold the medication in suspension for a short period so that the patient can receive more of the prescribed medication than if it had been projected into the air. Breathing slowly and deeply distributes the medication deep into the airways.
22. **Instruct patient to hold his or her breath for 5 to 10 seconds, or as long as possible, and then to exhale slowly through pursed lips.**	This allows better distribution and longer absorption time for the medication.
23. **Wait 1 to 5 minutes, as prescribed, before administering the next puff, as prescribed.**	This ensures that both puffs are absorbed as much as possible. Bronchodilation after the first puff allows for deeper penetration by subsequent puffs.
24. After the prescribed number of puffs has been administered, have patient remove the MDI from the spacer and replace the caps on both MDI and spacer.	By replacing the caps, the patient is preventing any dust or dirt from entering and being propelled into the bronchioles with later doses.
25. Have the patient gargle and rinse with tap water after using an MDI, as necessary. Clean the MDI according to the manufacturer's directions.	Rinsing removes medication residue from the mouth. Rinsing is necessary when using inhaled steroids because oral fungal infections can occur. The buildup of medication in the device can attract bacteria and affect how the medication is delivered.

ACTION	RATIONALE
26. Remove gloves and additional PPE, if used. Perform hand hygiene.	Removing PPE properly reduces the risk for infection transmission and contamination of other items. Hand hygiene prevents the spread of microorganisms.
27. Document the administration of the medication immediately after administration. See Documentation section below.	Timely documentation helps to ensure patient safety.
28. Evaluate the patient's response to the medication within an appropriate time frame. **Reassess lung sounds, oxygen saturation level, and respirations.**	The patient needs to be evaluated for therapeutic and adverse effects from the medication. Lung sounds and oxygen saturation level may improve after MDI use. Respiratory rate may decrease after MDI use.

EVALUATION

- Medication is administered successfully using the MDI.
- Patient demonstrates improved lung sounds and ease of breathing.
- Patient demonstrates correct use of the MDI.
- Patient verbalizes correct information about medication therapy associated with MDI use.

DOCUMENTATION

- Document the administration of the medication immediately after administration, including date, time, dose, and route of administration on the CMAR/MAR or record using the required format. If using a bar-code system, medication administration is recorded automatically when the bar code is scanned. PRN medications require documentation of the reason for administration. Prompt recording avoids the possibility of accidentally repeating the administration of the drug. Document respiratory rate, oxygen saturation, if applicable, lung assessment, and the patient's response to the treatment, if appropriate. If the drug was refused or omitted, record this in the appropriate area on the medication record and notify the primary care provider. This verifies the reason medication was omitted and ensures that the primary care provider is aware of the patient's condition.

SKILL VARIATION | Using an MDI Without a Spacer

Prepare medication as outlined in steps 1–12 above (Skill 86).

1. Perform hand hygiene and put on PPE, if indicated.

2. Identify the patient. The patient should be identified using two methods.

3. Close the door to the room or pull the bedside curtain.

4. **Complete necessary assessments before administering medications. Check allergy bracelet or ask patient about allergies. Explain the purpose and action of the medication to the patient.**

5. Scan the patient's bar code on the identification band, if required.

6. Based on facility policy, the third check of the label may occur at this point. If so, recheck the labels with the CMAR/MAR before administering the medications to the patient.

7. Remove the cap from the MDI. Shake the inhaler well.

8. Have the patient take a deep breath and exhale.

9. Have the patient hold the inhaler 1 to 2 inches away from the mouth. Have the patient begin to inhale slowly and deeply, depress the medication canister, and continue to inhale for a full breath.

10. Instruct the patient to hold the breath for 5 to 10 seconds, or as long as possible, and then to exhale slowly through pursed lips.

11. Wait 1 to 5 minutes, as prescribed, before administering the next puff.

12. After the prescribed number of puffs has been administered, have patient replace the cap on the MDI.

13. Remove additional PPE, if used. Perform hand hygiene.

14. Document administration of the medication on the CMAR/MAR immediately after administering the medication.

15. Evaluate the patient's response to the medication within an appropriate time frame. Reassess lung sounds, oxygen saturation level, if ordered, and respirations.

Intradermal injections are administered into the dermis, just below the epidermis. The intradermal route has the longest absorption time of all parenteral routes. For this reason, intradermal injections are used for sensitivity tests, such as tuberculin and allergy tests, and local anesthesia. The advantage of the intradermal route for these tests is that the body's reaction to substances is easily visible, and degrees of reaction are discernible by comparative study.

Sites commonly used are the inner surface of the forearm and the upper back, under the scapula. Equipment used for an intradermal injection includes a tuberculin syringe calibrated in tenths and hundredths of a milliliter and a 0.25- to 0.5-inch, 25- or 27-gauge needle. The dosage given intradermally is small, usually less than 0.5 mL. The angle of administration for an intradermal injection is 5 to 15 degrees.

DELEGATION CONSIDERATIONS

The administration of an intradermal injection is not delegated to nursing assistive personnel (NAP) or to unlicensed assistive personnel (UAP). Depending on the state's nurse practice act and the organization's policies and procedures, the administration of an intradermal injection may be delegated to licensed practical/vocational nurses (LPN/LVNs). The decision to delegate must be based on careful analysis of the patient's needs and circumstances, as well as the qualifications of the person to whom the task is being delegated. Refer to the Delegation Guidelines in Appendix A.

EQUIPMENT

- Prescribed medication
- Sterile syringe, usually a tuberculin syringe calibrated in tenths and hundredths, and needle, 1/4- to 1/2-inch, 25- or 27-gauge
- Antimicrobial swab
- Disposable gloves
- Small gauze square
- Computer-generated Medication Administration Record (CMAR) or Medication Administration Record (MAR)
- PPE, as indicated

ASSESSMENT

- Assess the patient for any allergies.
- Check expiration date before administering medication.
- Assess the appropriateness of the drug for the patient.
- Review assessment and laboratory data that may influence drug administration.
- Assess the site on the patient where the injection is to be given. Avoid areas of broken or open skin. Avoid areas that are highly pigmented, and those that have lesions, bruises, or scars and are hairy.

- Assess the patient's knowledge of the medication. This may provide an opportune time for patient education.
- Verify the patient's name, dose, route, and time of administration.

NURSING DIAGNOSIS

- Deficient Knowledge
- Risk for Infection
- Risk for Injury

OUTCOME IDENTIFICATION AND PLANNING

- Appearance of a wheal at the injection site.
- Patient refrains from rubbing the site.
- Patient's anxiety is decreased.
- Patient does not experience adverse effects.
- Patient understands and complies with the medication regimen.

IMPLEMENTATION

ACTION	RATIONALE
1. Gather equipment. Check each medication order against the original order in the medical record according to facility policy. Clarify any inconsistencies. Check the patient's chart for allergies.	This comparison helps to identify errors that may have occurred when orders were transcribed. The primary care provider's order is the legal record of medication orders for each facility.
2. Know the actions, special nursing considerations, safe dose ranges, purpose of administration, and adverse effects of the medications to be administered. Consider the appropriateness of the medication for this patient.	This knowledge aids the nurse in evaluating the therapeutic effect of the medication in relation to the patient's disorder and can also be used to educate the patient about the medication.
3. Perform hand hygiene.	Hand hygiene deters the spread of microorganisms.
4. Move the medication cart to the outside of the patient's room or prepare for administration in the medication area.	Organization facilitates error-free administration and saves time.

ACTION	RATIONALE
5. Unlock the medication cart or drawer. Enter pass code and scan employee identification, if required.	Locking the cart or drawer safeguards each patient's medication supply. Hospital accrediting organizations require medication carts to be locked when not in use. Entering pass code and scanning ID allows only authorized users into the system and identifies the user for documentation by the computer.
6. **Prepare medications for one patient at a time.**	This prevents errors in medication administration.
7. Read the CMAR/MAR and select the proper medication from unit stock or the patient's medication drawer.	This is the *first* check of the label.
8. Compare the label with the CMAR/MAR. Check expiration dates and perform calculations, if necessary. Scan the bar code on the package, if required.	This is the *second* check of the label. Verify calculations with another nurse to ensure safety.
9. If necessary, withdraw the medication from an ampule or vial as described in Skills 103 and 104.	
10. **Depending on facility policy, the third check of the label may occur at this point. If so, when all medications for one patient have been prepared, recheck the labels with the CMAR/MAR before taking the medications to the patient.**	This *third* check ensures accuracy and helps to prevent errors. *Note:* Many facilities require the *third* check to occur at the bedside, after identifying the patient and before administration.
11. Lock the medication cart before leaving it.	Locking the cart or drawer safeguards the patient's medication supply. Hospital accrediting organizations require medication carts to be locked when not in use.
12. Transport medications to the patient's bedside carefully, and keep the medications in sight at all times.	Careful handling and close observation prevent accidental or deliberate disarrangement of medications.

ACTION	RATIONALE
13. **Ensure that the patient receives the medications at the correct time.**	Check agency policy, which may allow for administration within a period of 30 minutes before or 30 minutes after the designated time.
14. Perform hand hygiene and put on PPE, if indicated.	Hand hygiene and PPE prevent the spread of microorganisms. PPE is required based on transmission precautions.
15. **Identify the patient.** Compare the information with the CMAR/MAR. **The patient should be identified using at least two methods** (The Joint Commission, 2013): 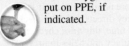	Identifying the patient ensures the right patient receives the medications and helps prevent errors. The patient's room number or physical location is not used as an identifier (The Joint Commission, 2013). Replace the identification band if it is missing or inaccurate in any way.
a. Check the name on the patient's identification band.	
b. Check the identification number on the patient's identification band.	
c. Check the birth date on the patient's identification band.	
d. Ask the patient to state his or her name and birth date, based on facility policy.	This requires a response from the patient, but illness and strange surroundings often cause patients to be confused.
16. Close the door to the room or pull the bedside curtain.	This provides patient privacy.
17. **Complete necessary assessments before administering medications. Check allergy bracelet or ask the patient about allergies. Explain the purpose and action of the medication to the patient.**	Assessment is a prerequisite to administration of medications. Explanation provides rationale, increases knowledge, and reduces anxiety.

ACTION	RATIONALE
18. Scan the patient's bar code on the identification band, if required.	Provides an additional check to ensure that the medication is given to the right patient.
19. **Based on facility policy, the third check of the label may occur at this point. If so, recheck the labels with the CMAR/MAR before administering the medications to the patient.**	Many facilities require the *third* check to occur at the bedside, after identifying the patient and before administration. If facility policy directs the *third* check at this time, this *third* check ensures accuracy and helps to prevent errors.
20. Put on clean gloves.	Gloves help prevent exposure to contaminants.
21. Select an appropriate administration site. Assist the patient to the appropriate position for the site chosen. Drape, as needed, to expose only site area to be used.	Appropriate site prevents injury and allows for accurate reading of the test site at the appropriate time. Draping provides privacy and warmth.
22. Cleanse the site with an antimicrobial swab while wiping with a firm, circular motion and moving outward from the injection site. Allow the skin to dry.	Pathogens on the skin can be forced into the tissues by the needle. Moving from the center outward prevents contamination of the site. Allowing skin to dry prevents introducing alcohol into the tissue, which can be irritating and uncomfortable.
23. Remove the needle cap with the nondominant hand by pulling it straight off.	This technique lessens the risk of an accidental needlestick.
24. Use the nondominant hand to spread the skin taut over the injection site.	Taut skin provides an easy entrance into intradermal tissue.
25. Hold the syringe in the dominant hand, between the thumb and forefinger with the bevel of the needle up.	Using the dominant hand allows for easy, appropriate handling of the syringe. Having the bevel up allows for smooth piercing of the skin and introduction of medication into the dermis.
26. Hold the syringe at a 5- to 15-degree angle from the site. Place the needle almost flat against the patient's skin	The dermis is entered when the needle is held as nearly parallel to the skin as possible and is inserted about ⅛ inch.

ACTION	RATIONALE

(Figure 1), bevel side up, and insert the needle into the skin. Insert the needle only about ⅛ inch with entire bevel under the skin.

FIGURE 1 Inserting the needle almost level with the skin.

27. Once the needle is in place, steady the lower end of the syringe. Slide your dominant hand to the end of the plunger.

Prevents injury and inadvertent advancement or withdrawal of needle.

28. Slowly inject the agent while watching for a small wheal or blister to appear (Figure 2).

The appearance of a wheal indicates the medication is in the dermis.

FIGURE 2 Observing for wheal while injecting medication.

29. Withdraw the needle quickly at the same angle that it was inserted. Do not recap the used needle. Engage the safety shield or needle guard.

Withdrawing the needle quickly and at the angle at which it entered the skin minimizes tissue damage and discomfort for the patient. Safety shield or needle guard prevents accidental needlestick injury.

30. **Do not massage the area after removing needle. Tell the patient not to rub or scratch the site. If necessary,**

Massaging the area where an intradermal injection is given may spread the medication to underlying subcutaneous tissue.

ACTION	RATIONALE
gently blot the site with a dry gauze square. **Do not apply pressure or rub the site.**	
31. Assist the patient to a position of comfort.	This provides for the well-being of the patient.
32. Discard the needle and syringe in the appropriate receptacle.	Proper disposal of the needle prevents injury.
33. Remove gloves and additional PPE, if used. Perform hand hygiene.	Removing PPE properly reduces the risk for infection transmission and contamination of other items. Hand hygiene prevents the spread of microorganisms.
34. Document the administration of the medication immediately after administration. See Documentation section below.	Timely documentation helps to ensure patient safety.
35. Evaluate the patient's response to the medication within an appropriate time frame.	The patient needs to be evaluated for therapeutic and adverse effects from the medication.
36. Observe the area for signs of a reaction at determined intervals after administration. Inform the patient of the need for inspection.	With many intradermal injections, you need to look for a localized reaction in the area of the injection at the appropriate interval(s) determined by the type of medication and purpose. Explaining this to the patient increases compliance.

EVALUATION
- Wheal is present at the site of injection.
- Patient refrains from rubbing the site.
- Patient's anxiety is decreased.
- Patient did not experience adverse effects.
- Patient verbalizes an understanding of, and complies with, the medication regimen.

DOCUMENTATION
- Record each medication administered on the CMAR/MAR or record using the required format, including date, time, and the site

of administration, immediately after administration. Some facilities recommend circling the injection site with ink. Circling the injection site easily identifies the intradermal injection site and allows for future careful observation of the exact area. If using a bar-code system, medication administration is automatically recorded when the bar code is scanned. PRN medications require documentation of the reason for administration. Prompt recording avoids the possibility of accidentally repeating the administration of the drug. If the drug was refused or omitted, record this in the appropriate area on the medication record and notify the primary care provider. This verifies the reason medication was omitted and ensures that the primary care provider is aware of the patient's condition.

SKILL 88 | ADMINISTERING AN INTRAMUSCULAR INJECTION

Intramuscular injections deliver medication through the skin and subcutaneous tissues into certain muscles. Muscles have a larger and a greater number of blood vessels than subcutaneous tissue, allowing faster onset of action than with subcutaneous injections. An intramuscular injection is chosen when a reasonably rapid systemic uptake of the drug is needed by the body and when a relatively prolonged action is required. Some medications administered intramuscularly are formulated to have a longer duration of effect. The deposit of medication creates a depot at the injection site, designed to deliver slow, sustained release over hours, days, or weeks.

To administer an intramuscular injection correctly and effectively, choose the right equipment, select the appropriate location, use the correct technique, and deliver the correct dose. Inject the medication into the denser part of the muscle fascia below the subcutaneous tissues. This is ideal because skeletal muscles have fewer pain-sensing nerves than subcutaneous tissue and can absorb larger volumes of solution because of the rapid uptake of the drug into the bloodstream via the muscle fibers (Hunter, 2008).

It is important to choose the right needle length for a particular intramuscular injection. Needle length should be based on the site for injection and the patient's age. Patients who are obese may require a longer needle, and emaciated patients may require a shorter needle. Appropriate gauge is determined by the medication being administered. Generally, biologic agents and medications in aqueous solutions should be administered with a 20- to 25-gauge needle. Medications in oil-based solutions should be administered with an 18- to 25-gauge needle. Many medications come in prefilled syringe units. If a needle is provided on the prefilled unit, ensure that the needle on the unit is the appropriate length for the patient and situation.

Site/Age	Needle Length
Vastus lateralis	$5/8''$ to $1\frac{1}{4}''$
Deltoid (children)	$5/8''$ to $1\frac{1}{4}''$
Deltoid (adults)	$1''$ to $1\frac{1}{2}''$
Ventrogluteal (adults)	$1\frac{1}{2}''$

(Adapted from Centers for Disease Control and Prevention (CDC). (2012). The pink book: Appendices. Epidemiology and prevention of vaccine preventable diseases (11th ed.). Appendix D; CDC. (2008). Needle length and injection site of intramuscular injections; and Nicoll, L., & Hesby, A. (2002). Intramuscular injection: An integrative research review and guideline for evidence-based practice. Applied Nursing Research, 16(2), 149–162.)

To avoid complications, be able to identify anatomic landmarks and site boundaries. Consider the age of the patient, medication type, and medication volume when selecting an intramuscular injection site. Rotate the sites used to administer intramuscular medications when therapy requires repeated injections. Whatever pattern of rotating sites is used, a description of it should appear in the patient's plan of nursing care. Depending on the site selected, it may be necessary to reposition the patient. Administer the intramuscular injection so that the needle is perpendicular to the patient's body. This ensures it is given using an injection angle between 72 and 90 degrees (Katsma & Katsma, 2000).

The medication volume that can be administered intramuscularly varies based on the intended site. Generally, 1 to 4 mL is the accepted volume range, with no more than 1 to 2 mL given at the deltoid site. The less-developed muscles of children and older people limit the intramuscular injection to 1 to 2 mL.

According to the CDC (2012) and current review of evidence (Crawford & Johnson, 2012), aspiration is not required for intramuscular injections. Some literature suggests aspiration *may* be indicated when administering large molecule medications such as penicillin (Crawford & Johnson, 2012). Consult facility policy and manufacturer recommendations to ensure safe administration.

DELEGATION CONSIDERATIONS

The administration of an intramuscular injection is not delegated to nursing assistive personnel (NAP) or to unlicensed assistive personnel (UAP). Depending on the state's nurse practice act and the organization's policies and procedures, the administration of an intramuscular injection may be delegated to licensed practical/vocational nurses (LPN/LVNs). The decision to delegate must be based on careful analysis of the patient's needs and circumstances, as well as the qualifications of the person to whom the task is being delegated. Refer to the Delegation Guidelines in Appendix A.

EQUIPMENT

- Gloves
- Additional PPE, as indicated
- Medication
- Sterile syringe and needle of appropriate size and gauge
- Antimicrobial swab
- Small gauze square
- Computer-generated Medication Administration Record (CMAR) or Medication Administration Record (MAR)

ASSESSMENT

- Assess the patient for any allergies.
- Check the expiration date before administering the medication.
- Assess the appropriateness of the drug for the patient.
- Verify patient name, dose, route, and time of administration.
- Review assessment and laboratory data that may influence drug administration.
- Assess the site on the patient where the injection is to be given. Avoid any site that is bruised, tender, hard, swollen, inflamed, or scarred.
- Assess the patient's knowledge of the medication. If the patient has deficient knowledge about the medication, this may be the appropriate time to begin education about it.
- If the medication may affect the patient's vital signs, assess them before administration.
- If the medication is intended for pain relief, assess the patient's pain before and after administration.

NURSING DIAGNOSIS

- Acute Pain
- Risk for Injury
- Anxiety

OUTCOME IDENTIFICATION AND PLANNING

- Patient receives the medication via the intramuscular route.
- Patient's anxiety is decreased.
- Patient does not experience adverse effects.
- Patient understands and complies with the medication regimen.

IMPLEMENTATION

ACTION	RATIONALE
1. Gather equipment. Check each medication order against the original order in the medical record according to facility policy. Clarify any inconsistencies. Check the patient's chart for allergies.	This comparison helps to identify errors that may have occurred when orders were transcribed. The primary care provider's order is the legal record of medication orders for each facility.
2. Know the actions, special nursing considerations, safe dose ranges, purpose of administration, and adverse effects of the medications to be administered. Consider the appropriateness of the medication for this patient.	This knowledge aids the nurse in evaluating the therapeutic effect of the medication in relation to the patient's disorder and can also be used to educate the patient about the medication.

ACTION	RATIONALE
3. Perform hand hygiene.	Hand hygiene prevents the spread of microorganisms.
4. Move the medication cart to the outside of the patient's room or prepare for administration in the medication area.	Organization facilitates error-free administration and saves time.
5. Unlock the medication cart or drawer. Enter pass code and scan employee identification, if required.	Locking the cart or drawer safeguards each patient's medication supply. Hospital accrediting organizations require medication carts to be locked when not in use. Entering pass code and scanning ID allows only authorized users into the system and identifies the user for documentation by the computer.
6. **Prepare medications for one patient at a time.**	This prevents errors in medication administration.
7. Read the CMAR/MAR and select the proper medication from unit stock or the patient's medication drawer.	This is the *first* check of the label.
8. Compare the label with the CMAR/MAR. Check expiration dates and perform calculations, if necessary. Scan the bar code on the package, if required.	This is the *second* check of the label. Verify calculations with another nurse to ensure safety, if necessary.
9. If necessary, withdraw medication from an ampule or vial as described in Skills 103 and 104.	
10. **Depending on facility policy, the third check of the label may occur at this point. If so, when all medications for one patient have been prepared, recheck the labels with the CMAR/MAR before taking the medications to the patient.**	This *third* check ensures accuracy and helps to prevent errors. *Note:* Many facilities require the *third* check to occur at the bedside, after identifying the patient and before administration.

ACTION	RATIONALE
11. Lock the medication cart before leaving it.	Locking the cart or drawer safeguards the patient's medication supply. Hospital accrediting organizations require medication carts to be locked when not in use.
12. Transport medications to the patient's bedside carefully, and keep the medications in sight at all times.	Careful handling and close observation prevent accidental or deliberate disarrangement of medications.
13. **Ensure that the patient receives the medications at the correct time.**	Check agency policy, which may allow for administration within a period of 30 minutes before or 30 minutes after the designated time.
14. Perform hand hygiene and put on PPE, if indicated.	Hand hygiene and PPE prevent the spread of microorganisms. PPE is required based on transmission precautions.
15. **Identify the patient.** **Compare the information with the CMAR/MAR. The patient should be identified using at least two methods** (The Joint Commission, 2013):	Identifying the patient ensures the right patient receives the medications and helps prevent errors. The patient's room number or physical location is not used as an identifier (The Joint Commission, 2013). Replace the identification band if it is missing or inaccurate in any way.
a. Check the name on the patient's identification band.	
b. Check the identification number on the patient's identification band.	
c. Check the birth date on the patient's identification band.	
d. Ask the patient to state his or her name and birth date, based on facility policy.	This requires a response from the patient, but illness and strange surroundings often cause patients to be confused.

ACTION	RATIONALE
16. Close the door to the room or pull the bedside curtain.	This provides patient privacy.
17. **Complete necessary assessments before administering medications. Check the patient's allergy bracelet or ask the patient about allergies. Explain the purpose and action of the medication to the patient.**	Assessment is a prerequisite to administration of medications. Explanation provides rationale, increases knowledge, and reduces anxiety.
18. Scan the patient's bar code on the identification band, if required.	Provides an additional check to ensure that the medication is given to the right patient.
19. **Based on facility policy, the third check of the label may occur at this point. If so, recheck the labels with the CMAR/MAR before administering the medications to the patient.**	Many facilities require the *third* check to occur at the bedside, after identifying the patient and before administration. If facility policy directs the *third* check at this time, this *third* check ensures accuracy and helps to prevent errors.
20. Put on clean gloves.	Gloves help prevent exposure to contaminants.
21. Select an appropriate administration site.	Selecting the appropriate site prevents injury.
22. Assist the patient to the appropriate position for the site chosen. Drape, as needed, to expose only the site area being used.	Appropriate positioning for the site chosen prevents injury. Draping helps maintain the patient's privacy.
23. Identify the appropriate landmarks for the site chosen.	Good visualization is necessary to establish the correct site location and to avoid tissue damage.
24. Cleanse the area around the injection site with an antimicrobial swab. Use a firm, circular motion while moving outward from the injection site. Allow the area to dry.	Pathogens on the skin can be forced into the tissues by the needle. Moving from the center outward prevents contamination of the site. Allowing skin to dry prevents introducing alcohol into the tissue, which can be irritating and uncomfortable.
25. Remove the needle cap by pulling it straight off. Hold	This technique lessens the risk of an accidental needlestick

ACTION	RATIONALE

the syringe in your dominant hand between the thumb and forefinger.

and also prevents inadvertently unscrewing the needle from the barrel of the syringe.

26. Displace the skin in a Z-track manner. Pull the skin down or to one side about 1 inch (2.5 cm) with your nondominant hand and hold the skin and tissue in this position.

Z-track technique is recommended for all intramuscular injections to ensure medication does not leak back along the needle track and into the subcutaneous tissue (Nicoll & Hesby, 2002; Zimmerman, 2010). This technique reduces pain and discomfort, particularly for patients receiving injections over an extended period. The Z-track method is also suggested for older patients who have decreased muscle mass. Some agents, such as iron, are best given via the Z-track method due to the irritation and discoloration associated with this agent.

27. Quickly dart the needle into the tissue so that the needle is perpendicular to the patient's body. This should ensure that the medication is administered using an injection angle between 72 and 90 degrees.

A quick injection is less painful. Inserting the needle at a 72- to 90-degree angle facilitates entry into muscle tissue.

28. As soon as the needle is in place, use the thumb and forefinger of your nondominant hand to hold the lower end of the syringe. Slide your dominant hand to the end of the plunger. Inject the solution slowly (10 sec/mL of medication).

Moving the syringe could cause damage to the tissues and inadvertent administration into an incorrect area. Rapid injection of the solution creates pressure in the tissues, resulting in discomfort. According to the CDC (2012) and current review of evidence (Crawford & Johnson, 2012), aspiration is not required for intramuscular injections. Some literature suggests aspiration *may* be indicated when administering large molecule medications such as penicillin (Crawford & Johnson, 2012). Consult facility policy and manufacturer recommendations to ensure safe administration.

ACTION	RATIONALE
29. Once the medication has been instilled, wait 10 seconds before withdrawing the needle.	Allows medication to begin to diffuse into the surrounding muscle tissue (Nicoll & Hesby, 2002).
30. Withdraw the needle smoothly and steadily at the same angle at which it was inserted, supporting tissue around the injection site with your nondominant hand.	Slow withdrawal of the needle pulls the tissues and causes discomfort. Applying counter traction around the injection site helps to prevent pulling on the tissue as the needle is withdrawn. Removing the needle at the same angle at which it was inserted minimizes tissue damage and discomfort for the patient.
31. Apply gentle pressure at the site with a dry gauze. **Do not massage the site.**	Light pressure causes less trauma and irritation to the tissues. Massaging can force medication into subcutaneous tissues.
32. Do not recap the used needle. Engage the safety shield or needle guard, if present. Discard the needle and syringe in the appropriate receptacle.	Proper disposal of the needle prevents injury.
33. Assist the patient to a position of comfort.	This provides for the well-being of the patient.
34. Remove gloves and additional PPE, if used. Perform hand hygiene.	Removing PPE properly reduces the risk for infection transmission and contamination of other items. Hand hygiene prevents the spread of microorganisms.
35. Document the administration of the medication immediately after administration. See Documentation section below.	Timely documentation helps to ensure patient safety.
36. Evaluate the patient's response to the medication within the appropriate time frame. Assess site, if possible, within 2 to 4 hours after administration.	The patient needs to be evaluated for therapeutic and adverse effects from the medication. Visualization of the site allows for assessment of any untoward effects.

EVALUATION

• Patient receives the medication via the intramuscular route.
• Patient's anxiety is decreased.
• Patient does not experience adverse effects or injury.
• Patient understands and complies with the medication regimen.

DOCUMENTATION

• Record each medication given on the CMAR/MAR or record using
  the required format, including date, time, and the site of administration, immediately after administration. If using a bar-code system,
  medication administration is automatically recorded when the bar
  code is scanned. PRN medications require documentation of the
  reason for administration. Prompt recording avoids the possibility
  of accidentally repeating the administration of the drug. If the drug
  was refused or omitted, record this in the appropriate area on the
  medication record and notify the primary care provider. This verifies
  the reason medication was omitted and ensures that the primary care
  provider is aware of the patient's condition.

SKILL 89 | ADMINISTERING A SUBCUTANEOUS INJECTION

Subcutaneous injections are administered into the adipose tissue layer
just below the epidermis and dermis. This tissue has few blood vessels,
so drugs administered here have a slow, sustained rate of absorption into
the capillaries.

It is important to choose the right equipment to ensure depositing the
medication into the intended tissue layer and not the underlying muscle. Equipment used for a subcutaneous injection includes a syringe of
appropriate volume for the amount of drug being administered. An insulin injection pen may be used for subcutaneous injection of insulin. A
25- to 30-gauge, ⅜- to 1-inch needle can be used; ⅜- and ⅝-inch needles
are most commonly used for subcutaneous injections. Choose the needle length based on the amount of subcutaneous tissue present, which
is based on the patient's body weight and build (Annersten & Willman,
2005). Some medications are packaged in prefilled cartridges with a
needle attached. Confirm that the provided needle is appropriate for the
patient before use. If not, the medication will have to be transferred to
another syringe and the appropriate needle attached.

Review the specifics of the particular medication before administrating
it to the patient. Various sites may be used for subcutaneous injections,
including the outer aspect of the upper arm, the abdomen (from below
the costal margin to the iliac crests), the anterior aspects of the thigh, the
upper back, and the upper ventral gluteal area. Absorption rates differ at
different sites. Injections in the abdomen are absorbed most rapidly; ones

in the arms are absorbed somewhat more slowly; those in the thighs, even more slowly; and those in the upper ventral or dorsogluteal areas have the slowest absorption (American Diabetes Association [ADA], 2004).

Subcutaneous injections are administered at a 45- to 90-degree angle. Choose the angle of needle insertion based on the amount of subcutaneous tissue present and the length of the needle. Generally, insert the shorter, ⅜-inch, needle at a 90-degree angle and the longer, ⅝-inch needle at a 45-degree angle. Recommendations differ regarding pinching or bunching of a skin fold for administration. Pinching is advised for thinner patients and when a longer needle is used, to lift the adipose tissue away from underlying muscle and tissue. If pinching is used, once the needle is inserted, release the skin to avoid injecting into compressed tissue.

Aspiration, or pulling back on the plunger to check that a blood vessel has been entered, is not necessary and has not proved to be a reliable indicator of needle placement. The likelihood of injecting into a blood vessel is small (Crawford & Johnson, 2012). The American Diabetes Association (2004) has stated that routine aspiration is not necessary when injecting insulin. Aspiration is definitely contraindicated with administration of heparin because this action can result in hematoma formation.

Usually, no more than 1 mL of solution is given subcutaneously. Giving larger amounts adds to the patient's discomfort and may predispose to poor absorption. It is necessary to rotate sites or areas for injection if the patient is to receive frequent injections. This helps to prevent buildup of fibrous tissue and permits complete absorption of the medication.

DELEGATION CONSIDERATIONS

The administration of a subcutaneous injection is not delegated to nursing assistive personnel (NAP) or to unlicensed assistive personnel (UAP). Depending on the state's nurse practice act and the organization's policies and procedures, the administration of a subcutaneous injection may be delegated to licensed practical/vocational nurses (LPN/LVNs). The decision to delegate must be based on careful analysis of the patient's needs and circumstances, as well as the qualifications of the person to whom the task is being delegated. Refer to the Delegation Guidelines in Appendix A.

EQUIPMENT

- Prescribed medication
- Sterile syringe and needle. Needle size depends on the medication to be administered and patient body type (see previous discussion).
- Antimicrobial swab
- Non-latex, disposable gloves
- Small gauze square
- Computer-generated Medication Administration Record (CMAR) or Medication Administration Record (MAR)
- PPE, as indicated

ASSESSMENT

- Assess the patient for any allergies.
- Check expiration date before administering medication.

- Assess the appropriateness of the drug for the patient.
- Verify patient name, dose, route, and time of administration.
- Review assessment and laboratory data that may influence drug administration.
- Assess the site on the patient where the injection is to be given. Avoid sites that are bruised, tender, hard, swollen, inflamed, or scarred. These conditions could affect absorption or cause discomfort and injury (Hunter, 2008).
- Assess the patient's knowledge of the medication. If the patient has deficient knowledge about the medication, this may be the appropriate time to begin education about it.
- If the medication may affect the patient's vital signs, assess them before administration.
- If the medication is for pain relief, assess the patient's pain before and after administration.

NURSING DIAGNOSIS
- Deficient Knowledge
- Risk for Injury
- Acute Pain

OUTCOME IDENTIFICATION AND PLANNING
- Patient receives the medication via the subcutaneous route.
- Patient's anxiety is decreased.
- Patient does not experience adverse effects.
- Patient understands and complies with the medication regimen.

IMPLEMENTATION

ACTION	RATIONALE
1. Gather equipment. Check each medication order against the original order in the medical record, according to facility policy. Clarify any inconsistencies. Check the patient's chart for allergies.	This comparison helps to identify errors that may have occurred when orders were transcribed. The primary care provider's order is the legal record of medication orders for each facility.
2. Know the actions, special nursing considerations, safe dose ranges, purpose of administration, and adverse effects of the medications to be administered. Consider the appropriateness of the medication for this patient.	This knowledge aids the nurse in evaluating the therapeutic effect of the medication in relation to the patient's disorder and can also be used to educate the patient about the medication.

ACTION	RATIONALE
3. Perform hand hygiene.	Hand hygiene prevents the spread of microorganisms.
4. Move the medication cart to the outside of the patient's room or prepare for administration in the medication area.	Organization facilitates error-free administration and saves time.
5. Unlock the medication cart or drawer. Enter pass code and scan employee identification, if required.	Locking the cart or drawer safeguards each patient's medication supply. Hospital accrediting organizations require medication carts to be locked when not in use. Entering pass code and scanning ID allows only authorized users into the computer system and identifies the user for documentation by the computer.
6. **Prepare medications for one patient at a time.**	This prevents errors in medication administration.
7. Read the CMAR/MAR and select the proper medication from unit stock or the patient's medication drawer.	This is the *first* check of the label.
8. Compare the label with the CMAR/MAR. Check expiration dates and perform calculations, if necessary. Scan the bar code on the package, if required.	This is the *second* check of the label. Verify calculations with another nurse to ensure safety, if necessary.
9. If necessary, withdraw medication from an ampule or vial as described in Skills 103 and 104.	
10. **Depending on facility policy, the third check of the label may occur at this point. If so, when all medications for one patient have been prepared, recheck the labels with the CMAR/ MAR before taking the medications to the patient.**	This *third* check ensures accuracy and helps to prevent errors. *Note:* Many facilities require the *third* check to occur at the bedside, after identifying the patient and before administration.

ACTION	RATIONALE
11. Lock the medication cart before leaving it.	Locking the cart or drawer safeguards the patient's medication supply. Hospital accrediting organizations require medication carts to be locked when not in use.
12. Transport medications to the patient's bedside carefully, and keep the medications in sight at all times.	Careful handling and close observation prevent accidental or deliberate disarrangement of medications.
13. **Ensure that the patient receives the medications at the correct time.**	Check agency policy, which may allow for administration within a period of 30 minutes before or 30 minutes after the designated time.
14. Perform hand hygiene and put on PPE, if indicated.	Hand hygiene and PPE prevent the spread of microorganisms. PPE is required based on transmission precautions.
15. **Identify the patient. Compare the information with the CMAR/MAR. The patient should be identified using at least two methods** (The Joint Commission, 2013):	Identifying the patient ensures the right patient receives the medications and helps prevent errors. The patient's room number or physical location is not used as an identifier (The Joint Commission, 2013). Replace the identification band if it is missing or inaccurate in any way.
a. Check the name on the patient's identification band.	
b. Check the identification number on the patient's identification band.	
c. Check the birth date on the patient's identification band.	
d. Ask the patient to state his or her name and birth date, based on facility policy.	This requires a response from the patient, but illness and strange surroundings often cause patients to be confused.

ACTION	RATIONALE
16. Close the door to the room or pull the bedside curtain.	This provides patient privacy.
17. **Complete necessary assessments before administering medications. Check the patient's allergy bracelet or ask the patient about allergies. Explain the purpose and action of the medication to the patient.**	Assessment is a prerequisite to administration of medications. Explanation provides rationale, increases knowledge, and reduces anxiety.
18. Scan the patient's bar code on the identification band, if required.	Scanning provides an additional check to ensure that the medication is given to the right patient.
19. **Based on facility policy, the third check of the label may occur at this point. If so, recheck the labels with the CMAR/MAR before administering the medications to the patient.**	Many facilities require the *third* check to occur at the bedside, after identifying the patient and before administration. If facility policy directs the *third* check at this time, this *third* check ensures accuracy and helps to prevent errors.
20. Put on clean gloves.	Gloves help prevent exposure to contaminants.
21. Select an appropriate administration site.	Appropriate site prevents injury and allows for accurate reading of the test site at the appropriate time.
22. Assist the patient to the appropriate position for the site chosen. Drape, as needed, to expose only site area to be used.	Appropriate site prevents injury. Draping helps maintain the patient's privacy.
23. Identify the appropriate landmarks for the site chosen.	Good visualization is necessary to establish the correct site location and to avoid tissue damage.
24. Cleanse the area around the injection site with an antimicrobial swab. Use a firm, circular motion while moving outward from the injection site. Allow the area to dry.	Pathogens on the skin can be forced into the tissues by the needle. Moving from the center outward prevents contamination of the site. Allowing skin to dry prevents introducing alcohol into the tissue, which is irritating and uncomfortable.

ACTION	RATIONALE
25. Remove the needle cap with the nondominant hand, pulling it straight off.	The cap protects the needle from contact with microorganisms. This technique lessens the risk of an accidental needlestick.
26. Grasp and bunch the area surrounding the injection site or spread the skin taut at the site.	Decision to create a skin fold is based on the nurse's assessment of the patient and needle length used. Pinching is advised for thinner patients and when a longer needle is used, to lift the adipose tissue away from underlying muscle and tissue. If pinching is used, once the needle is inserted, release the skin to avoid injecting into compressed tissue. If skin is pulled taut, it provides easy, less painful entry into the subcutaneous tissue.
27. Hold the syringe in the dominant hand between the thumb and forefinger. Inject the needle quickly at a 45- to 90-degree angle.	Inserting the needle quickly causes less pain to the patient. Subcutaneous tissue is abundant in well-nourished, well-hydrated people and spare in emaciated, dehydrated, or very thin persons. For a person with little subcutaneous tissue, it is best to insert the needle at a 45-degree angle.
28. After the needle is in place, release the tissue. If you have a large skin fold pinched up, ensure that the needle stays in place as the skin is released. Immediately move your nondominant hand to steady the lower end of the syringe. Slide your dominant hand to the end of the plunger. Avoid moving the syringe.	Injecting the solution into compressed tissues results in pressure against nerve fibers and creates discomfort. If there is a large skin fold, the skin may retract away from the needle. The nondominant hand secures the syringe. Moving the syringe could cause damage to the tissues and inadvertent administration into an incorrect area.
29. Inject the medication slowly (at a rate of 10 sec/mL).	Rapid injection of the solution creates pressure in the tissues, resulting in discomfort.
30. Withdraw the needle quickly at the same angle at which it	Slow withdrawal of the needle pulls the tissues and causes

ACTION	RATIONALE
was inserted, while supporting the surrounding tissue with your nondominant hand.	discomfort. Applying counter traction around the injection site helps to prevent pulling on the tissue as the needle is withdrawn. Removing the needle at the same angle at which it was inserted minimizes tissue damage and discomfort for the patient.
31. Using a gauze square, apply gentle pressure to the site after the needle is withdrawn. **Do not massage the site.**	Massaging the site can damage underlying tissue and increase the absorption of the medication. Massaging after heparin administration can contribute to hematoma formation. Massaging after an insulin injection may contribute to unpredictable absorption of the medication.
32. Do not recap the used needle. Engage the safety shield or needle guard. Discard the needle and syringe in the appropriate receptacle.	Safety shield or needle guard prevents accidental needlestick. Proper disposal of the needle prevents injury.
33. Assist the patient to a position of comfort.	This provides for the well-being of the patient.
34. Remove gloves and additional PPE, if used. Perform hand hygiene.	Removing PPE properly reduces the risk for infection transmission and contamination of other items. Hand hygiene prevents the spread of microorganisms.
35. Document the administration of the medication immediately after administration. See Documentation section below.	Timely documentation helps to ensure patient safety.
36. Evaluate the patient's response to the medication within the appropriate time frame for the particular medication.	The patient needs to be evaluated for therapeutic and adverse effects from the medication.

EVALUATION

• Patient receives the medication via the subcutaneous route.
• Patient's anxiety is decreased.

- Patient does not experience adverse effects.
- Patient understands and complies with the medication regimen.

DOCUMENTATION

- Record each medication given on the CMAR/MAR or record using the required format, including date, dose, time, and the site of administration, immediately after administration. If using a bar-code system, medication administration is automatically recorded when the bar code is scanned. PRN medications require documentation of the reason for administration. Prompt recording avoids the possibility of accidentally repeating the administration of the drug. If the drug was refused or omitted, record this in the appropriate area on the medication record and notify the primary care provider. This verifies the reason medication was omitted and ensures that the primary care provider is aware of the patient's condition.

SKILL 90 — ADMINISTERING A CONTINUOUS SUBCUTANEOUS INFUSION: APPLYING AN INSULIN PUMP

Some medications, such as insulin and morphine, may be administered continuously via the subcutaneous route. Continuous subcutaneous insulin infusion (CSII or insulin pump) allows for multiple preset rates of insulin delivery. This system uses a small, computerized reservoir that delivers insulin via tubing through a small plastic cannula or needle inserted into the subcutaneous tissue. The pump is programmed to deliver multiple preset rates of insulin. The settings can be adjusted for exercise and illness, and bolus dose delivery can be timed in relation to meals. It is recommended that the site is changed every 2 to 3 days to prevent tissue damage or absorption problems (American Association of Diabetes Educators, 2008). Advantages of continuous subcutaneous medication infusion include the longer rate of absorption via the subcutaneous route and convenience for the patient. There are many different manufacturers of insulin pumps. Nurses need to be familiar with the particular pump in use by their patient and to refer to the specific manufacturer's recommendations for use.

DELEGATION CONSIDERATIONS

The administration of a continuous subcutaneous infusion using an insulin pump is not delegated to nursing assistive personnel (NAP) or to unlicensed assistive personnel (UAP). Depending on the state's nurse practice act and the organization's policies and procedures, the management of an insulin pump in some settings may be delegated to licensed practical/vocational nurses (LPN/LVNs) who have received appropriate training. The decision to delegate must be based on careful analysis of the patient's needs and circumstances, as well as the qualifications of the person to whom the task is being delegated. Refer to the Delegation Guidelines in Appendix A.

EQUIPMENT

- Insulin pump
- Pump syringe and vial of insulin or prefilled cartridge, as ordered
- Sterile infusion set
- Insertion (triggering) device
- Needle (24- or 22-gauge, or blunt-ended needle)
- Antimicrobial swabs
- Sterile non-occlusive dressing
- Computer-generated Medication Administration Record (CMAR) or Medication Administration Record (MAR)
- Disposable gloves
- Additional PPE, as indicated

ASSESSMENT

- Assess the patient for any allergies.
- Check the expiration date before administering the medication.
- Assess the appropriateness of the drug for the patient.
- Review assessment and laboratory data that may influence drug administration.
- Verify patient name, dose, route, and time of administration.
- Assess the infusion site. Typical infusion sites include those areas used for subcutaneous insulin injection.
- Assess the area where the pump is to be applied. Do not place the pump on skin that is irritated or broken down.
- Assess the patient's knowledge of the medication. If the patient has a knowledge deficit about the medication, this may be the appropriate time to begin education about it.
- Assess the patient's blood glucose level as appropriate or as ordered.

NURSING DIAGNOSIS

- Deficient Knowledge
- Risk for Unstable Blood Glucose Level
- Risk for Infection

OUTCOME IDENTIFICATION AND PLANNING

- Device is applied successfully and medication is administered correctly.
- Patient understands the rationale for the pump use and mechanism of action.
- Patient experiences no allergy response.
- Patient's skin remains intact.
- Pump is applied using aseptic technique.
- Patient does not experience unstable blood glucose levels or adverse effect.

IMPLEMENTATION

ACTION	RATIONALE
1. Gather equipment. Check each medication order against the original order in the medical record, according to facility policy. Clarify any inconsistencies. Check the patient's chart for allergies.	This comparison helps to identify errors that may have occurred when orders were transcribed. The primary care provider's order is the legal record of medication orders for each facility.
2. Know the actions, special nursing considerations, safe dose ranges, purpose of administration, and adverse effects of the medications to be administered. Consider the appropriateness of the medication for this patient.	This knowledge aids the nurse in evaluating the therapeutic effect of the medication in relation to the patient's disorder and can also be used to educate the patient about the medication.
3. Perform hand hygiene.	Hand hygiene prevents the spread of microorganisms.
4. Move the medication cart to the outside of the patient's room or prepare for administration in the medication area.	Organization facilitates error-free administration and saves time.
5. Unlock the medication cart or drawer. Enter pass code and scan employee identification, if required.	Locking the cart or drawer safeguards each patient's medication supply. Hospital accrediting organizations require medication carts to be locked when not in use. Entering pass code and scanning ID allows only authorized users into the system and identifies the user for documentation by the computer.
6. **Prepare medications for one patient at a time.**	This prevents errors in medication administration.
7. Read the CMAR/MAR and select the proper medication from unit stock or the patient's medication drawer.	This is the *first* check of the label.
8. Compare the label with the CMAR/MAR. Check	This is the *second* check of the label. Verify calculations with

ACTION	RATIONALE
expiration dates and perform calculations, if necessary. Scan the bar code on the package, if required.	another nurse to ensure safety, if necessary.
9. Attach a blunt-ended needle or a small-gauge needle to a syringe. Follow Skill 104 to prepare insulin from a vial, if necessary. Prepare enough insulin to last the patient 2 to 3 days, plus 30 units for priming tubing. If using prepackaged insulin syringe or cartridge, remove from packaging.	Patient will wear pump for up to 3 days without changing syringe or tubing.
10. Depending on facility policy, the third check of the label may occur at this point. If so, when all medications for one patient have been prepared, recheck the labels with the CMAR/MAR before taking the medications to the patient.	This *third* check ensures accuracy and helps to prevent errors. *Note:* Many facilities require the *third* check to occur at the bedside, after identifying the patient and before administration.
11. Lock the medication cart before leaving it.	Locking the cart or drawer safeguards the patient's medication supply. Hospital accrediting organizations require medication carts to be locked when not in use.
12. Transport medications to the patient's bedside carefully, and keep the medications in sight at all times.	Careful handling and close observation prevent accidental or deliberate disarrangement of medications.
13. Ensure that the patient receives the medications at the correct time.	Check agency policy, which may allow for administration within a period of 30 minutes before or 30 minutes after the designated time.
14. Perform hand hygiene and put on PPE, if indicated.	Hand hygiene and PPE prevent the spread of microorganisms. PPE is required based on transmission precautions.

ACTION	RATIONALE

15. Identify the patient. Compare the information with the CMAR/MAR. The patient should be identified using at least two methods (The Joint Commission, 2013):

Identifying the patient ensures the right patient receives the medications and helps prevent errors. The patient's room number or physical location is not used as an identifier (The Joint Commission, 2013). Replace the identification band if it is missing or inaccurate in any way.

   a. Check the name on the patient's identification band.

   b. Check the identification number on the patient's identification band.

   c. Check the birth date on the patient's identification band.

   d. Ask the patient to state his or her name and birth date, based on facility policy.

This requires a response from the patient, but illness and strange surroundings often cause patients to be confused.

16. Close the door to the room or pull the bedside curtain.

This provides patient privacy.

17. Complete necessary assessments before administering medications. Check the patient's allergy bracelet or ask the patient about allergies. Explain the purpose and action of the medication to the patient.

Assessment is a prerequisite to administration of medications. Explanation provides rationale, increases knowledge, and reduces anxiety.

18. Scan the patient's bar code on the identification band, if required.

Provides an additional check to ensure that the medication is given to the right patient.

19. Based on facility policy, the third check of the label may occur at this point. If so, recheck the labels with the CMAR/MAR before administering the medications to the patient.

Many facilities require the *third* check to occur at the bedside, after identifying the patient and before administration. If facility policy directs the *third* check at this time, this *third* check ensures accuracy and helps to prevent errors.

ACTION	RATIONALE

20. Perform hand hygiene. Put on gloves.

Hand hygiene prevents the spread of microorganisms. Gloves prevent contact with blood and body fluids.

21. Remove the cap from the syringe or insulin cartridge. Attach sterile tubing to the syringe or insulin cartridge. Open the pump and place the syringe or cartridge in compartment according to manufacturer's directions. Close the pump.

Tubing must be attached correctly and syringe must be placed in pump correctly for insulin delivery.

22. Initiate priming of the tubing, according to manufacturer's directions. Program the pump according to manufacturer's recommendations following primary care provider's orders. **Check for any bubbles in the tubing.**

Removing all the air from the tubing and correct programming of pump ensures the patient receives the correct dose of insulin.

23. Activate the delivery device. Place the needle between prongs of the insertion device with the sharp edge facing out. Push insertion set down until a click is heard.

To ensure correct placement of insulin pump needle, an insertion device must be used.

24. Select an appropriate administration site.

Appropriate site prevents injury.

25. Assist the patient to the appropriate position for the site chosen. Drape, as needed, to expose only site area to be used.

Appropriate site prevents injury. Draping maintains privacy and warmth.

26. Identify the appropriate landmarks for the site chosen.

Good visualization is necessary to establish the correct site location and to avoid tissue damage.

27. Cleanse area around injection site with antimicrobial swab. Use a firm, circular motion while moving outward from insertion site. Allow antiseptic to dry.

Pathogens on the skin can be forced into the tissues by the needle. Moving from the center outward prevents contamination of the site. Allowing skin to dry prevents introducing alcohol into

ACTION	RATIONALE
	the tissue, which can be irritating and uncomfortable.
28. Remove paper from adhesive backing. Remove the needle guard. Pinch skin at insertion site, press insertion device on site, and press release button to insert needle. Remove triggering device.	To ensure delivery of insulin into subcutaneous tissue, a skin fold is made with a pinch *before* insertion of the medication.
29. Apply the sterile occlusive dressing over the insertion site, if not part of insertion device. Attach the pump to patient's clothing, as desired.	Dressing prevents contamination of site. Pump can be dislodged easily if not attached securely to patient.
30. Assist the patient to a position of comfort.	This provides for the well-being of the patient.
31. Discard the needle and syringe in the appropriate receptacle.	Proper disposal of the needle prevents injury.
32. Remove gloves and additional PPE, if used. Perform hand hygiene.	Removing PPE properly reduces the risk for infection transmission and contamination of other items. Hand hygiene prevents the spread of microorganisms.
33. Document the administration of the medication immediately after administration. See Documentation section below.	Timely documentation helps to ensure patient safety.
34. Evaluate the patient's response to the medication within the appropriate time frame. Monitor the patient's blood glucose levels, as appropriate, or as ordered.	Patient needs to be evaluated to ensure that the pump is delivering the drug appropriately. The patient needs to be evaluated for therapeutic and adverse effects from the medication.

EVALUATION

- Patient receives insulin from the attached pump successfully without hypo- or hyperglycemic effects noted.
- Patient understands the rationale for the pump attachment.
- Patient experiences no allergy response.
- Patient's skin remains intact.

- Patient remains infection free.
- Patient experiences no or minimal pain.

DOCUMENTATION

- Document the application of the pump, the type of insulin used, pump settings, insertion site, and any teaching done with the patient on the CMAR/MAR or record using the required format, including date, time, and the site of administration, immediately after administration. If using a bar-code system, medication administration is automatically recorded when the bar code is scanned. PRN medications require documentation of the reason for administration. Prompt recording avoids the possibility of accidentally repeating the administration of the drug. If the drug was refused or omitted, record this in the appropriate area on the medication record and notify the primary care provider. This verifies the reason medication was omitted and ensures that the primary care provider is aware of the patient's condition.

SKILL 91 CHANGING AN IV SOLUTION CONTAINER AND ADMINISTRATION SET

Intravenous fluid administration frequently involves multiple bags or bottles of fluid infusion. Verify the amount and type of solution to be administered, as well as the prescribed infusion rate. The nurse is responsible for critically evaluating all patient orders prior to administration. Any concerns regarding the type or amount of therapy prescribed should be immediately and clearly communicated to the prescribing practitioner. The nurse must understand the patient's need for IV therapy, the type of solution to be used, its desired effect, and potential adverse reactions and effects. Follow the facility's policies and guidelines to determine if the infusion should be administered by electronic infusion device or by gravity.

DELEGATION CONSIDERATIONS

The changing of an IV solution container and administration set is not delegated to nursing assistive personnel (NAP) or to unlicensed assistive personnel (UAP). Depending on the state's nurse practice act and the organization's policies and procedures, these procedures may be delegated to licensed practical/vocational nurses (LPN/LVNs). The decision to delegate must be based on careful analysis of the patient's needs and circumstances, as well as the qualifications of the person to whom the task is being delegated. Refer to the Delegation Guidelines in Appendix A.

EQUIPMENT

For solution container change:
- IV solution, as prescribed
- MAR/CMAR
- Time tape and/or label (for IV container)
- PPE, as indicated

For tubing change:
- Administration set
- Label for administration set (for next change date)
- Sterile gauze
- Nonallergenic tape
- IV securement/stabilization device, as appropriate
- Clean gloves
- Additional PPE, as indicated
- Alcohol or other disinfectant wipes

ASSESSMENT

- Review the patient's record for baseline data, such as vital signs, intake and output balance, and pertinent laboratory values, such as serum electrolytes.
- Assess the appropriateness of the solution for the patient.
- Review assessment and laboratory data that may influence solution administration.
- Inspect the IV site. The dressing should be intact, adhering to the skin on all edges. Check for any leaks or fluid under or around the dressing. Inspect the tissue around the IV entry site for swelling, coolness, or pallor. These are signs of fluid infiltration into the tissue around the IV catheter. Also inspect the site for redness, swelling, and warmth. These signs might indicate the development of phlebitis or an inflammation of the blood vessel at the site. Ask the patient if he or she is experiencing any pain or discomfort related to the IV line. Pain or discomfort can be a sign of infiltration, extravasation, phlebitis, thrombophlebitis, and infection related to IV therapy.

NURSING DIAGNOSIS

- Deficient Fluid Volume
- Risk for Infection
- Impaired Skin Integrity

OUTCOME IDENTIFICATION AND PLANNING

- Prescribed IV infusion continues without interruption and no infusion complications are identified.

IMPLEMENTATION

ACTION	RATIONALE
1. Verify the IV solution order on the MAR/CMAR with	This ensures that the correct IV solution and rate of infusion,

ACTION	RATIONALE
the medical order. Consider the appropriateness of the prescribed therapy in relation to the patient. Clarify any inconsistencies. Check the patient's chart for allergies. Check for color, leaking, and expiration date. Know the purpose of the IV administration, and medications if ordered. Gather necessary supplies.	and/or medication will be administered. The nurse is responsible for critically evaluating all patient orders prior to administration. Any concerns regarding the type or amount of therapy prescribed should be immediately and clearly communicated to the prescribing practitioner. This knowledge and skill is essential for safe and accurate IV and medication administration. Preparation promotes efficient time management and an organized approach to the task.
2. Perform hand hygiene and put on PPE, if indicated.	Hand hygiene and PPE prevent the spread of microorganisms. PPE is required based on transmission precautions.
3. Identify the patient.	Identifying the patient ensures the right patient receives the intervention and helps prevent errors.
4. Close the curtains around the bed and close the door to the room, if possible. Explain what you are going to do and why you are going to do it to the patient. Ask the patient about allergies to medications or tape, as appropriate.	This ensures the patient's privacy. Explanation relieves anxiety and facilitates cooperation. Possible allergies may exist related to IV solution additive or tape.
5. Compare IV container label with the MAR/CMAR. Remove IV bag from outer wrapper, if indicated. Check expiration dates. Scan bar code on container, if necessary. Compare patient identification band with the MAR/CMAR. Alternately, label solution container with the patient's name, solution type, additives, date, and time.	Checking label with MAR/CMAR ensures the correct IV solution will be administered. Identifying the patient ensures the right patient receives the medications and helps prevent errors. Time strip allows for quick visual reference by the nurse to monitor infusion accuracy.

ACTION	RATIONALE

Complete a time strip for the infusion and apply to IV container.

6. Maintain aseptic technique when opening sterile packages and IV solution. Remove administration set from package. Apply label to tubing reflecting the day/date for next set change, per facility guidelines.

Asepsis is essential for preventing the spread of microorganisms. Labeling tubing ensures adherence to facility policy regarding administration set changes and reduces risk of spread of microorganisms.

To Change IV Solution Container

7. If using an electronic infusion device, pause the device or put on "hold." Close the slide clamp on the administration set closest to the drip chamber. If using gravity infusion, close the roller clamp on the administration set.

The action of the infusion device needs to be paused while the solution container is changed. Closing the clamps prevents the fluid in the drip chamber from emptying and air from entering the tubing during the procedure.

8. Carefully remove the cap on the entry site of the new IV solution container and expose the entry site, **taking care not to touch the exposed entry site.**

Touching the opened entry site on the IV container results in contamination and the container would have to be discarded.

9. Lift empty container off IV pole and invert it. Quickly remove the spike from the old IV container, **being careful not to contaminate it.** Discard old IV container.

Touching the spike on the administration set results in contamination and the tubing would have to be discarded.

10. Using a twisting and pushing motion, insert the administration set spike into the entry site of the IV container. Alternately, follow the manufacturer's directions for insertion. Hang the container on the IV pole.

Inserting the spike punctures the seal in the IV container and allows access to contents.

11. Alternately, hang the new IV fluid container on an open hook on the IV pole.

Touching the opened entry site on the IV container or the administration set spike results in

ACTION	RATIONALE
Carefully remove the cap on the entry site of the new IV solution container and expose the entry site, **taking care not to touch the exposed entry site.** Lift empty container off the IV pole and invert it. Quickly remove the spike from the old IV container, **being careful not to contaminate it.** Discard old IV container. Using a twisting and pushing motion, insert the administration set spike into the entry port of the new IV container as it hangs on the IV pole.	contamination and both would have to be discarded. Inserting the spike punctures the seal in the IV container and allows access to contents.
12. If using an electronic infusion device, open the slide clamp, check the drip chamber of the administration set, verify the flow rate programmed in the infusion device, and turn the device to "run" or "infuse."	Verifying the rate and device settings ensures the patient receives the correct volume of the solution.
13. If using gravity infusion, slowly open the roller clamp on the administration set and count the drops. Adjust until the correct drop rate is achieved.	Opening the clamp regulates the flow rate into the drip chamber. Verifying the rate ensures patient receives the correct volume of solution.

To Change IV Solution Container and Administration Set

14. Prepare the IV solution and administration set. Refer to Skill 129, Steps 6–10.	
15. Hang the IV container on an open hook on the IV pole. Close the clamp on the existing IV administration set. Also, close the clamp on the short extension tubing connected to the IV catheter in the patient's arm.	Clamping the existing IV tubing prevents leakage of fluid from the administration set after it is disconnected. Clamping the tubing on the extension set prevents introduction of air into the extension tubing.

ACTION	RATIONALE
16. If using an electronic infusion device, remove the current administration set from the device. Following manufacturer's directions, insert a new administration set into the infusion device.	Administration set has to be removed in order to insert new tubing into device.
17. Put on gloves. Remove the current infusion tubing from the access cap on the short extension IV tubing. Using an antimicrobial swab, cleanse access cap on extension tubing. Remove the end cap from the new administration set. Insert the end of the administration set into the access cap. Loop the administration set tubing near the entry site, and anchor with tape (nonallergenic) close to the site.	Cleansing the cap or port reduces the risk of contamination. Inserting the administration set allows initiation of the fluid infusion. The weight of the tubing is sufficient to pull it out of the vein if it is not well anchored. Nonallergenic tape is less likely to tear fragile skin.
18. Open the clamp on the extension tubing. Open the clamp on the administration set.	Opening clamps allows solution to flow to patient.
19. If using an electronic infusion device, open the slide clamp, check the drip chamber of the administration set, verify the flow rate programmed in the infusion device, and turn the device to "run" or "infuse."	Verifying the rate and device settings ensures the patient receives the correct volume of solution.
20. If using gravity infusion, slowly open the roller clamp on the administration set and count the drops. Adjust until the correct drop rate is achieved.	Opening the clamp regulates flow rate into the drip chamber. Verifying the rate ensures the patient receives the correct volume of solution.
21. Remove equipment. Ensure patient's comfort. Remove gloves. Lower bed, if not in lowest position.	Promotes patient comfort and safety. Removing gloves properly reduces the risk for infection transmission and contamination of other items.

ACTION	RATIONALE
22. Remove additional PPE, if used. Perform hand hygiene.	Removing PPE properly reduces the risk for infection transmission and contamination of other items. Hand hygiene prevents transmission of microorganisms.
23. Return to check flow rate and observe IV site for infiltration and/or other complications 30 minutes after starting infusion, and at least hourly thereafter. Ask the patient if he or she is experiencing any pain or discomfort related to the IV infusion.	Continued monitoring is important to maintain the correct flow rate. Early detection of problems ensures prompt intervention.

EVALUATION

- IV solution container and administration set are changed.
- IV infusion continues without interruption.
- No infusion complications are identified.

DOCUMENTATION

- Document the type of IV solution and the rate of infusion (often done in the CMAR/MAR); and the assessment of the access site. Record the patient's reaction to the procedure and pertinent patient teaching, such as alerting the nurse if the patient experiences any pain from the IV or notices any swelling at the site. Document the IV fluid solution on the intake and output record.

SKILL 92   MONITORING AN IV SITE AND INFUSION

The nurse is responsible for monitoring the infusion rate and the IV site. This is routinely done as part of the initial patient assessment and at the beginning of a work shift. In addition, IV sites are checked at specific intervals and each time an IV medication is given, as dictated by the facility's policies. It is common to check IV sites every hour, but it is important to be familiar with the requirements of your facility. Monitoring the infusion rate is a very important part of the patient's overall management. If the patient does not receive the prescribed rate, he or she may experience a fluid volume deficit. In contrast, if the patient is administered too much fluid over a period of time, he or she may experience fluid volume overload. Other responsibilities involve checking the IV site for possible complications and assessing for both the desired effects of an IV infusion as well as potential adverse reactions to IV therapy.

DELEGATION CONSIDERATIONS

The monitoring of an IV site and infusion is not delegated to nursing assistive personnel (NAP) or to unlicensed assistive personnel (UAP). Depending on the state's nurse practice act and the organization's policies and procedures, these procedures may be delegated to licensed practical/vocational nurses (LPN/LVNs). The decision to delegate must be based on careful analysis of the patient's needs and circumstances, as well as the qualifications of the person to whom the task is being delegated. Refer to the Delegation Guidelines in Appendix A.

EQUIPMENT
- PPE, as indicated

ASSESSMENT
- Inspect the IV infusion solution for any particulates and check the IV label. Confirm it is the solution ordered.
- Assess the current rate of flow by verifying the settings on the electronic infusion device or timing the drops if it is a gravity infusion.
- Check the tubing for kinks or anything that might clamp or interfere with the flow of the solution.
- Inspect the IV site. The dressing should be intact, adhering to the skin on all edges. Check for any leaks or fluid under or around the dressing.
- Inspect the tissue around the IV entry site for swelling, coolness, or pallor. These are signs of fluid infiltration into the tissue around the IV catheter. Also inspect the site for redness, swelling, and warmth. These signs might indicate the development of phlebitis or an inflammation of the blood vessel at the site. Ask the patient if he or she is experiencing any pain or discomfort related to the IV line. Pain or discomfort can be a sign of infiltration, extravasation, phlebitis, thrombophlebitis, and infection related to IV therapy.
- Assess fluid intake and output.
- Assess the patient's knowledge of IV therapy.

NURSING DIAGNOSIS
- Excess Fluid Volume
- Deficient Fluid Volume
- Risk for Infection

OUTCOME IDENTIFICATION AND PLANNING
- Patient remains free from complications and demonstrates signs and symptoms of fluid balance.

IMPLEMENTATION

ACTION	RATIONALE
1. Verify IV solution order on the MAR/CMAR with the medical order. Consider the appropriateness of the prescribed therapy in relation to the patient. Clarify any inconsistencies. Check the patient's chart for allergies. Check for color, leaking, and expiration date. Know purpose of the IV administration and medications, if ordered.	This ensures that the correct IV solution and rate of infusion, and/or medication will be administered. The nurse is responsible for critically evaluating all patient orders. Any concerns regarding the type or amount of therapy prescribed should be immediately and clearly communicated to the prescribing practitioner. This knowledge and skill is essential for safe and accurate IV and medication administration.
2. **Monitor IV infusion every hour or per facility policy. More frequent checks may be necessary if medication is being infused.**	Promotes safe administration of IV fluids and medication.
3. Perform hand hygiene and put on PPE, if indicated.	Hand hygiene and PPE prevent the spread of microorganisms. PPE is required based on transmission precautions.
4. Identify the patient.	Identifying the patient ensures the right patient receives the intervention and helps prevent errors.
5. Close the curtains around the bed and close the door to the room, if possible. Explain what you are going to do and why you are doing it to the patient.	This ensures the patient's privacy. Explanation relieves anxiety and facilitates cooperation.
6. If an electronic infusion device is being used, check settings, alarm, and indicator lights. Check set infusion rate. Note position of fluid in IV container in relation to time tape. Teach patient about the alarm features on the electronic infusion device.	Observation ensures that infusion control device and the alarm are functioning. Lack of knowledge about "alarms" may create anxiety for patient.

ACTION	RATIONALE
7. If IV is infusing via gravity, check the drip chamber and time the drops.	This ensures that the flow rate is correct. Use a watch with a second hand for counting the drops in regulating a gravity drip IV infusion.
8. Check tubing for anything that might interfere with the flow. Be sure clamps are in the open position.	Any kink or pressure on tubing may interfere with the flow.
9. Observe dressing for leakage of IV solution.	Leakage may occur at the connection of the tubing with the hub of the needle or the catheter and allow for loss of IV solution.
10. Inspect the site for swelling, leakage at the site, coolness, or pallor, which may indicate infiltration. Ask if patient is experiencing any pain or discomfort. If any of these symptoms are present, the IV will need to be removed and restarted at another site. Check facility policy for treating infiltration.	Catheter may become dislodged from the vein, and IV solution may flow into subcutaneous tissue.
11. Inspect the site for redness, swelling, and heat. Palpate for induration. Ask if patient is experiencing pain. These findings may indicate phlebitis. Notify the primary care provider if phlebitis is suspected. IV will need to be discontinued and restarted at another site. Check facility policy for treatment of phlebitis.	Chemical irritation or mechanical trauma causes injury to the vein and can lead to phlebitis. Phlebitis is the most common complication related to IV therapy (Ingram & Lavery, 2005).
12. Check for local manifestations (redness, pus, warmth, induration, and pain) that may indicate an infection is present at the site. Also check for systemic manifestations (chills, fever, tachycardia, hypotension) that may accompany local	Poor aseptic technique may allow bacteria to enter the needle, catheter insertion site, or tubing connection and may occur with manipulation of equipment.

ACTION	RATIONALE

infection at the site. If signs of infection are present, discontinue the IV and notify the primary care provider. Be careful not to disconnect IV tubing when putting on patient's hospital gown or assisting the patient with movement.

13. Be alert for additional complications of IV therapy, such as fluid overload bleeding.

Infusing too much IV solution results in an increased volume of circulating fluid volume.

a. Fluid overload can result in signs of cardiac and/or respiratory failure. Monitor intake and output and vital signs. Assess for edema and auscultate lung sounds. Ask if patient is experiencing any shortness of breath.

Older patients are most at risk for this complication due to possible decrease in cardiac and/or renal functions.

b. Check for bleeding at the site.

Bleeding may be caused by anticoagulant medication. Bleeding at the site is most likely to occur when the IV is discontinued.

14. If appropriate, instruct patient to call for assistance if any discomfort is noted at site, solution container is nearly empty, flow has changed in any way, or if the electronic pump alarm sounds.

This facilitates patient cooperation and safe administration of IV solution.

15. Remove PPE, if used. Perform hand hygiene.

Removing PPE properly reduces the risk for infection transmission and contamination of other items. Hand hygiene prevents transmission of microorganisms.

EVALUATION

• Patient remains free of complications related to IV therapy, exhibits patent IV site, and the IV solution infuses at the prescribed flow rate.

DOCUMENTATION

- Document the type of IV solution as well as the infusion rate.
  Note the insertion site location and site assessment. Document the
  patient's reaction to the IV therapy as well as the absence of sub-
  jective reports that he or she is not experiencing any pain or other
  discomfort, such as coolness or heat associated with the infusion.
  Additionally, record that the patient is not demonstrating any other
  IV complications, such as signs or symptoms of fluid overload.
  Document the IV fluid solution on the intake and output record.

SKILL 93   TEACHING LEG EXERCISES

During surgery, venous blood return from the legs slows. In addition,
some patient positions used during surgery decrease venous return.
Thrombophlebitis, deep vein thrombosis (DVT), and the risk for emboli
are potential complications from circulatory stasis in the legs. Leg
exercises increase venous return through flexion and contraction of the
quadriceps and gastrocnemius muscles. It is important to individualize
leg exercises to patient needs, physical condition, primary care provider
preference, and facility protocol.

DELEGATION CONSIDERATIONS

Preoperative assessment and teaching is not delegated to nursing assistive personnel (NAP) or to unlicensed assistive personnel (UAP).
Depending on the state's nurse practice act and the organization's policies and procedures, preoperative teaching may be delegated to licensed
practical/vocational nurses (LPN/LVNs) after an assessment of education needs by the registered nurse. The decision to delegate must be
based on careful analysis of the patient's needs and circumstances, as
well as the qualifications of the person to whom the task is being delegated. Refer to the Delegation Guidelines in Appendix A.

EQUIPMENT

- PPE, as indicated

ASSESSMENT

- Identify patients who are considered at greater risk, such as those
  with chronic disease; patients who are obese or have underlying
  cardiovascular disease; patients who have decreased mobility; and
  patients who are at risk for decreased compliance with postoperative activities, such as those with alterations in cognitive function.
  Depending on the particular at-risk patient, specific assessments and
  interventions may be warranted.

- Assess the patient's current level of knowledge regarding leg exercises.

NURSING DIAGNOSIS

- Deficient Knowledge
- Risk for Ineffective Cerebral Tissue Perfusion
- Impaired Physical Mobility

OUTCOME IDENTIFICATION AND PLANNING

- Patient and/or significant other verbalizes an understanding of the instructions and is able to demonstrate the activity.

ACTION	RATIONALE

level of knowledge regarding leg exercises. If the patient has had surgery before, ask about this experience.

teaching. Previous surgical experience may impact preoperative/postoperative care positively or negatively, depending on this experience.

6. Explain the rationale for performing leg exercises.

Explanation facilitates patient cooperation. An understanding of rationale may contribute to increased compliance.

7. Teach regarding leg exercises and explain their purpose.

Leg exercises assist in preventing muscle weakness, promote venous return, and decrease complications related to venous stasis.

a. Assist or ask the patient to sit up (semi-Fowler's position) and explain to the patient that you will first demonstrate, and then coach him or her to exercise one leg at a time.

b. Straighten the patient's knee, raise the foot, extend the lower leg, and hold this position for a few seconds. Lower the entire leg. Practice this exercise with the other leg.

c. Assist or ask the patient to point the toes of both legs toward the foot of the bed, then relax them. Next, flex or pull the toes toward the chin.

d. Assist or ask the patient to keep legs extended and to make circles with both ankles, first circling to the left and then to the right. Instruct the patient to repeat these exercises three times. Instruct the patient to perform leg exercises every 2 to 4 hours when awake after surgery.

ACTION	RATIONALE
8. Validate the patient's understanding of the information. Ask the patient for a return demonstration. Ask the patient if he or she has any questions. Encourage the patient to practice the activities and ask questions, if necessary.	Validation facilitates the patient's understanding of information and performance of activities.
9. Remove PPE, if used. Perform hand hygiene.	Removing PPE properly reduces the risk for infection transmission and contamination of other items. Hand hygiene prevents the spread of microorganisms.

EVALUATION

- Patient and/or significant other verbalizes an understanding of the instructions related to leg exercises and is able to demonstrate the activities.

DOCUMENTATION

- Document the components of teaching related to leg exercises that were reviewed with the patient and family, if present. Record the patient's ability to demonstrate the leg exercises and response to the teaching; note if any follow-up instruction needs to be performed.

SKILL 94 LOGROLLING A PATIENT

The "logrolling" technique is a maneuver that involves moving the patient's body as one unit so that the spine is kept in alignment, without twisting or bending. This technique is commonly used to reposition patients who have had spinal or back surgery or who have suffered back or neck injuries. The use of logrolling when repositioning the patient helps to maintain neck and spine alignment. If the patient is being logrolled due to a neck injury, do not use a fluffy pillow under the patient's head. However, the patient may need a cervical collar in place for the move (see Skill 35). A bath blanket or small pillow under the head may be used to keep the spinal column straight. The patient's neck should remain straight during the procedure and after positioning. Do not twist the patient's head, spine, shoulders, knees, or hips while logrolling. Three caregivers, or more as appropriate, are needed to accomplish the maneuver safely. Do not try to logroll the patient without sufficient help.

DELEGATION CONSIDERATIONS

The use of the logrolling technique may be delegated to nursing assistive personnel (NAP) or to unlicensed assistive personnel (UAP), as well as to licensed practical/vocational nurses (LPN/LVNs). The decision to delegate must be based on careful analysis of the patient's needs and circumstances, as well as the qualifications of the person to whom the task is being delegated. Refer to the Delegation Guidelines in Appendix A.

EQUIPMENT

- At least two additional people to help
- Friction-reducing sheet to facilitate smooth movement, if not already in place; a draw sheet may be substituted if a friction-reducing sheet is not available
- Bath blanket or small pillow for under the head, if indicated
- Small pillow for placement between the legs
- Wedge pillow or two pillows for behind the patient's back
- PPE, as indicated

ASSESSMENT

- Assess for conditions that would contraindicate logrolling, such as unstable neurologic status or severe pain.
- Assess the patient's baseline neurologic status. Assess for paresthesias and pain.
- Assess for the need to use a cervical collar (see Skill 35).
- Assess the patient's pain. If the patient is experiencing pain, consider medicating the patient before repositioning.

NURSING DIAGNOSIS

- Risk for Injury
- Impaired Physical Mobility
- Risk for Impaired Skin Integrity
- Impaired Skin Integrity

OUTCOME IDENTIFICATION AND PLANNING

- Patient's spine remains in proper alignment, thereby reducing the risk for injury.
- Patient verbalizes relief of pain.
- Patient maintains joint mobility.
- Patient remains free of alterations in skin and tissue integrity.

IMPLEMENTATION

ACTION	RATIONALE
1. Review the medical record and nursing plan of care for activity orders and conditions that may influence the patient's ability to move or to be positioned. Assess for tubes, IV lines, incisions, or equipment that may alter the positioning procedure. Identify any movement limitations.	Reviewing the medical record and care plan validates the correct patient and correct procedure. Checking for equipment and limitations reduces the risk for injury during the transfer.
2. Perform hand hygiene and put on PPE, if indicated.	Hand hygiene and PPE prevent the spread of microorganisms. PPE is required based on transmission precautions.
3. Identify the patient.	Identifying the patient ensures the right patient receives the intervention and helps prevent errors.
4. Close the curtains around the bed and close the door to the room, if possible. Explain the purpose of the logrolling technique and what you are going to do to the patient, even if the patient is not conscious. Answer any questions.	This ensures the patient's privacy. Explanation relieves anxiety and facilitates cooperation.
5. Place the bed at an appropriate and comfortable working height, usually elbow height of the caregiver (VISN 8 Patient Safety Center, 2009).	Having the bed at the proper height prevents back and muscle strain.
6. Position at least one caregiver on one side of the bed and the two other caregivers on the opposite side of the bed. Position one caregiver at the top of the bed, at the patient's head. Place the bed in flat position. Lower the side rails. Place a small pillow between the patient's knees.	Using three or more people to turn the patient helps ensure that the spinal column will remain in straight alignment. A pillow placed between the knees helps keep the spinal column aligned.

ACTION	RATIONALE
7. If a friction-reducing sheet is not in place under the patient, take the time to place one now, to facilitate future movement of the patient.	Use of a friction-reducing sheet facilitates smooth movement in unison and minimizes pulling on the patient's body. A drawsheet may be used if friction-reducing sheets are not available.
8. If the patient can move the arms, ask the patient to cross the arms on the chest. Roll or fanfold the friction-reducing sheet close to the patient's sides and grasp it. In unison, gently slide the patient to the side of the bed opposite to that which the patient will be turned.	Crossing arms across the chest keeps the arms out of the way while rolling the patient. This also encourages the patient not to help by pulling on the side rails. Moving the patient to the side opposite to that which the patient will be turned prevents the patient from being uncomfortably close to the side rail. If the patient is large, more assistants may be needed to prevent injury to the patient.
9. Make sure the friction-reducing sheet under the patient is straight and wrinkle free.	Friction-reducing sheet should be wrinkle free to prevent skin breakdown. Rolling it strengthens the sheet and helps the nurse hold on to the sheet.
10. If necessary, reposition personnel to ensure two stand on the side of the bed to which the patient is turning. The third helper stands on the other side. **Grasp the friction-reducing sheet at hip and shoulder level.**	Proper positioning of personnel provides even division of support and pulling forces on the patient to maintain alignment.
11. Have everyone face the patient. On a predetermined signal, turn the patient by holding the friction-reducing sheet taut to support the body. The caregiver at the patient's head should firmly hold the patient's head on either side, directly above the ears, as appropriate. **Turn the patient as a unit in one smooth motion toward the side of the bed**	Holding the patient's head stabilizes the cervical spine. The patient's spine should not twist during the turn. The spine should move as one unit.

ACTION	RATIONALE
with the two nurses. The patient's head, shoulders, spine, hips, and knees should turn simultaneously.	
12. Once the patient has been turned, use pillows to support the patient's neck, back, buttocks, and legs in straight alignment in a side-lying position. Raise the side rails, as appropriate.	The pillows or wedge provides support and ensure continued spinal alignment after turning.
13. Stand at the foot of the bed and assess the spinal column. It should be straight, without any twisting or bending. Place the bed in the lowest position. Ensure that the call bell and telephone are within reach. Replace covers. Lower bed height.	Inspection of the spinal column ensures that the patient's back is not twisted or bent. Lowering the bed ensures patient safety.
14. Reassess the patient's neurologic status and comfort level.	Reassessment helps to evaluate the effects of movement on the patient.
15. Remove PPE, if used. Perform hand hygiene.	Removing PPE properly reduces the risk for infection transmission and contamination of other items. Hand hygiene prevents transmission of microorganisms.

EVALUATION
- Patient remains free of injury during and after turning and exhibits proper spinal alignment in the side-lying position.
- Patient states that pain was minimal on turning.
- Patient demonstrates adequate joint mobility.
- Patient exhibits no signs or symptoms of skin breakdown.

DOCUMENTATION
- Document the time of the patient's change of position, use of supports, and any pertinent observations, including neurologic and skin assessments. Document the patient's tolerance of the position change. Many facilities provide areas on bedside flow sheets to document repositioning.

SKILL 95 ADMINISTERING ORAL MEDICATIONS

Drugs given orally are intended for absorption in the stomach and small intestine. The oral route is the most commonly used route of administration. It is usually the most convenient and comfortable route for the patient. After oral administration, drug action has a slower onset and a more prolonged, but less potent, effect than other routes.

DELEGATION CONSIDERATIONS

The administration of oral medications is not delegated to nursing assistive personnel (NAP) or to unlicensed assistive personnel (UAP) in the acute care setting. The administration of specified oral medications to stable patients in some long-term care settings may be delegated to nursing assistive personnel (NAP) or unlicensed assistive personnel (UAP) who have received appropriate training. Depending on the state's nurse practice act and the organization's policies and procedures, the administration of oral medications may be delegated to licensed practical/vocational nurses (LPN/LVNs). The decision to delegate must be based on careful analysis of the patient's needs and circumstances, as well as the qualifications of the person to whom the task is being delegated. Refer to the Delegation Guidelines in Appendix A.

EQUIPMENT

- Medication in disposable cup or oral syringe
- Liquid (e.g., water, juice) with straw, if not contraindicated
- Medication cart or tray
- Computer-generated Medication Administration Record (CMAR) or Medication Administration Record (MAR)
- PPE, as indicated

ASSESSMENT

- Assess the appropriateness of the drug for the patient.
- Review medical history, allergy, assessment, and laboratory data that may influence drug administration.
- Assess the patient's ability to swallow medications; check the gag reflex, if indicated. If the patient cannot swallow, is NPO, does not have gag reflex, or is experiencing nausea or vomiting, withhold the medication, notify the primary care provider, and complete proper documentation.
- Assess the patient's knowledge of the medication. If the patient has a knowledge deficit about the medication, this may be the appropriate time to begin education about the medication.
- If the medication may affect the patient's vital signs, assess them before administration.
- If the medication is for pain relief, assess the patient's pain level before and after administration.
- Verify the patient name, dose, route, and time of administration.

NURSING DIAGNOSIS

- Impaired Swallowing
- Deficient Knowledge
- Risk for Aspiration

OUTCOME IDENTIFICATION AND PLANNING

- Patient will swallow the medication.
- Patient will experience the desired effect from the medication.
- Patient will not aspirate.
- Patient does not experience adverse effects.
- Patient understands and complies with the medication regimen.

IMPLEMENTATION

ACTION	RATIONALE
1. Gather equipment. Check each medication order against the original in the medical record, according to facility policy. Clarify any inconsistencies. Check the patient's medical record for allergies.	This comparison helps to identify errors that may have occurred when orders were transcribed. The primary care provider's order is the legal record of medication orders for each facility.
2. Know the actions, special nursing considerations, safe dose ranges, purpose of administration, and adverse effects of the medications to be administered. Consider the appropriateness of the medication for this patient.	This knowledge aids the nurse in evaluating the therapeutic effect of the medication in relation to the patient's disorder and can also be used to educate the patient about the medication.
3. Perform hand hygiene.	Hand hygiene prevents the spread of microorganisms.
4. Move the medication cart to the outside of the patient's room or prepare for administration in the medication area.	Organization facilitates error-free administration and saves time.
5. Unlock the medication cart or drawer. Enter pass code into the computer and scan employee identification, if required.	Locking the cart or drawer safeguards each patient's medication supply. Hospital accrediting organizations require medication carts to be locked when not in use. Entering pass code and

ACTION	RATIONALE
	scanning ID allows only authorized users into the computer system and identifies the user for documentation by the computer.
6. **Prepare medications for one patient at a time.**	This prevents errors in medication administration.
7. Read the CMAR/MAR and select the proper medication from the unit stock or patient's medication drawer.	This is the *first* check of the medication label.
8. Compare the medication label with the CMAR/MAR. Check expiration dates and perform calculations, if necessary. Scan the bar code on the package, if required.	This is the *second* check of the label. Verify calculations with another nurse to ensure safety, if necessary.
9. Prepare the required medications:	
a. *Unit dose packages:* Place unit dose-packaged medications in a disposable cup. **Do not open the wrapper until at the bedside.** Keep opioids and medications that require special nursing assessments in a separate container.	Wrapper is kept intact because the label is needed for an additional safety check. Special assessments may be required before giving certain medications. These may include assessing vital signs and checking laboratory test results.
b. *Multidose containers:* When removing tablets or capsules from a multidose bottle, pour the necessary number into the bottle cap and then place the tablets or capsules in a medication cup. Break only scored tablets, if necessary, to obtain the proper dosage. Do not touch tablets or capsules with hands.	Pouring medication into the cap allows for easy return of excess medication to the bottle. Pouring tablets or capsules into your hand is unsanitary.
c. *Liquid medication in multidose bottle:* When pouring liquid medications out of a multidose bottle, hold the bottle so the label is against the palm. Use	Liquid that may drip onto the label makes the label difficult to read. Accuracy is possible when the appropriate measuring device is used and then read accurately.

ACTION	RATIONALE
the appropriate measuring device when pouring liquids, and read the amount of medication at the bottom of the meniscus at eye level. Wipe the lip of the bottle with a paper towel.	
10. **Depending on facility policy, the third check of the label may occur at this point. If so, when all medications for one patient have been prepared, recheck the labels with the CMAR/MAR before taking the medications to the patient.**	This *third* check ensures accuracy and helps to prevent errors. *Note:* Many facilities require the *third* check to occur at the bedside, after identifying the patient and before administration.
11. Replace any multidose containers in the patient's drawer or unit stock. **Lock the medication cart before leaving it.**	Locking the cart or drawer safeguards the patient's medication supply. Hospital accrediting organizations require medication carts to be locked when not in use.
12. Transport medications to the patient's bedside carefully, and keep the medications in sight at all times.	Careful handling and close observation prevent accidental or deliberate disarrangement of medications.
13. **Ensure that the patient receives the medications at the correct time.**	Check agency policy, which may allow for administration within a period of 30 minutes before or 30 minutes after the designated time.
14. Perform hand hygiene and put on PPE, if indicated.	Hand hygiene and PPE prevent the spread of microorganisms. PPE is required based on transmission precautions.
15. **Identify the patient. Compare the information with the CMAR/MAR. The patient should be identified using at least two methods** (The Joint Commission, 2013):	Identifying the patient ensures the right patient receives the medications and helps prevent errors. The patient's room number or physical location is not used as an identifier (The Joint Commission, 2013). Replace the identification band if it is missing or inaccurate in any way.

ACTION	RATIONALE
a. Check the name on the patient's identification band.	
b. Check the identification number on the patient's identification band.	
c. Check the birth date on the patient's identification band.	
d. Ask the patient to state his or her name and birth date, based on facility policy.	This requires a response from the patient, but illness and strange surroundings often cause patients to be confused.
16. **Complete necessary assessments before administering medications. Check the patient's allergy bracelet or ask the patient about allergies. Explain the purpose and action of each medication to the patient.**	Assessment is a prerequisite to administration of medications.
17. Scan the patient's bar code on the identification band, if required.	The bar code provides an additional check to ensure that the medication is given to the right patient.
18. **Based on facility policy, the third check of the medication label may occur at this point. If so, recheck the labels with the CMAR/MAR before administering the medications to the patient.**	Many facilities require the *third* check to occur at the bedside, after identifying the patient and before administration. If facility policy directs the *third* check at this time, this *third* check ensures accuracy and helps prevent errors.
19. Assist the patient to an upright or lateral (side-lying) position.	Swallowing is facilitated by proper positioning. An upright or side-lying position protects the patient from aspiration.
20. Administer medications:	
a. Offer water or other permitted fluids with pills, capsules, tablets, and some liquid medications.	Liquids facilitate swallowing of solid drugs. Some liquid drugs are intended to adhere to the pharyngeal area, in which case liquid is not offered with the medication.

EVALUATION

- Patient swallows the medication and does not aspirate.
- Patient verbalizes an understanding of the medication.
- Patient experiences the desired effect from the medication and does not experience adverse effects.

DOCUMENTATION

- Record each medication immediately after it is administered on the CMAR/MAR or record using the required format. Include the date and time of administration. If using a bar-code system, medication administration is automatically recorded when the bar code is scanned. PRN medications require documentation of the reason for administration. Prompt recording avoids the possibility of accidentally repeating the administration of the drug. If the drug was refused or omitted, record this in the appropriate area on the medication record and notify the primary care provider. This verifies the reason medication was omitted and ensures that the primary care provider is aware of the patient's condition. Recording administration of an opioid may require additional documentation on a controlled-substance record, stating drug count and other specific information. A record of fluid intake and output measurement is required.

SKILL 96 | ADMINISTERING MEDICATIONS VIA A GASTRIC TUBE

Patients with a gastrointestinal tube (nasogastric, nasointestinal, percutaneous endoscopic gastrostomy [PEG], or jejunostomy [J] tube) often receive medication through the tube. Use liquid medications, when possible, because they are readily absorbed and less likely to cause tube occlusions. Certain solid dosage medications can be crushed and combined with liquid. Crush each pill one at a time to a fine powder and mix with 15 to 30 mL of water before delivery through the tube, keeping each medication separate from the others. Also, certain capsules may be opened, emptied into liquid, and administered through the tube. **Not all medications can be crushed or altered; long-acting and slow-release drugs are examples of medications that cannot be crushed.** Check manufacturer's recommendations and/or with a pharmacist to verify. Keep the package label with the medication cup for future comparison of information.

DELEGATION CONSIDERATIONS

The administration of medications via a gastric tube is not delegated to nursing assistive personnel (NAP) or to unlicensed assistive personnel (UAP). Depending on the state's nurse practice act and the organization's policies and procedures, the administration of medications via a gastric tube may be delegated to licensed practical/vocational nurses (LPN/LVNs). The decision to delegate must be based on careful analysis of the patient's needs and circumstances, as well as the qualifications of the person to whom the task is being delegated. Refer to the Delegation Guidelines in Appendix A.

EQUIPMENT

- Irrigation set (60-mL syringe and irrigation container)
- Medications
- Water (gastrostomy tubes) or sterile water (nasogastric [NG] tubes), according to facility policy
- Gloves
- Additional PPE, as indicated

ASSESSMENT

- Research each medication to be given, especially for mode of action, side effects, nursing implications, ability to be crushed, and whether the medication should be given with or without food.
- Verify patient name, dose, route, and time of administration.
- Assess patient's knowledge of the medication and the reason for its administration.

- Auscultate the abdomen for evidence of bowel sounds. Palpate the abdomen for tenderness and distention.
- Ascertain the time of the patient's last bowel movement and measure abdominal girth, if appropriate.

NURSING DIAGNOSIS

- Deficient Knowledge
- Risk for Injury
- Impaired Swallowing

OUTCOME IDENTIFICATION AND PLANNING

- Patient receives the medication via the tube and experiences the intended effect of the medication.
- Patient verbalizes knowledge of the medications given.
- Patient remains free from adverse effects and injury.
- Gastrointestinal tube remains patent.

ACTION	RATIONALE
5. Unlock the medication cart or drawer. Enter pass code into the computer and scan employee identification, if required.	Locking the cart or drawer safeguards each patient's medication supply. Hospital accrediting organizations require medication carts to be locked when not in use. Entering pass code and scanning ID allows only authorized users into the computer system and identifies the user for documentation by the computer.
6. **Prepare medications for one patient at a time.**	This prevents errors in medication administration.
7. Read the CMAR/MAR and select the proper medication from the unit stock or patient's medication drawer.	This is the *first* check of the label.
8. Compare the label with the CMAR/MAR. Check expiration dates and perform calculations, if necessary. Scan the bar code on the package, if required.	This is the *second* check of the label. Verify calculations with another nurse to ensure safety, if necessary.
9. Check to see if medications to be administered come in a liquid form. **If pills or capsules are to be given, check with pharmacy or drug reference to verify the ability to crush tablets or open capsules.**	To prevent the tube from becoming clogged, all medications should be given in liquid form whenever possible. Medications in extended-release formulations should not be crushed before administration.
10. Prepare medication.

Pills: Using a pill crusher, crush each pill one at a time. Dissolve the powder with water or other recommended liquid in a liquid medication cup, keeping each medication separate from the others. Keep the package label with the medication cup, for future comparison of information.

Liquid: When pouring liquid medications from a multidose bottle, hold the bottle | Some medications require dissolution in liquid other than water. The label is needed for an additional safety check. Some medications require pre-administration assessments.

Liquid that may drip onto the label makes the label difficult to read. Accuracy is possible when the appropriate measuring device is used and then read accurately. |

ACTION	RATIONALE
with the label against the palm. Use the appropriate measuring device when pouring liquids, and read the amount of medication at the bottom of the meniscus at eye level. Wipe the lip of the bottle with a paper towel.	
11. **Depending on facility policy, the third check of the label may occur at this point. If so, when all medications for one patient have been prepared, recheck the labels with the CMAR/MAR before taking the medications to the patient.**	This *third* check ensures accuracy and helps to prevent errors. *Note:* Many facilities require the *third* check to occur at the bedside, after identifying the patient and before administration.
12. Replace any multidose containers in the patient's drawer or unit stock. **Lock the medication cart before leaving it.**	Locking the cart or drawer safeguards the patient's medication supply. Hospital accrediting organizations require medication carts to be locked when not in use.
13. Transport medications to the patient's bedside carefully, and keep the medications in sight at all times.	Careful handling and close observation prevent accidental or deliberate disarrangement of medications.
14. **Ensure that the patient receives the medications at the correct time.**	Check agency policy, which may allow for administration within a period of 30 minutes before or 30 minutes after designated time.
15. Perform hand hygiene and put on PPE, if indicated.	Hand hygiene and PPE prevent the spread of microorganisms. PPE is required based on transmission precautions.
16. **Identify the patient. Compare the information with the CMAR/MAR.** The patient should be identified using at least	Identifying the patient ensures the right patient receives the medications and helps prevent errors. The patient's room number or physical location is not used as an identifier (The Joint

ACTION	RATIONALE
two methods (The Joint Commission, 2013):	Commission, 2013). Replace the identification band if it is missing or inaccurate in any way.
a. Check the name on the patient's identification band.	
b. Check the identification number on the patient's identification band.	
c. Check the birth date on the patient's identification band.	
d. Ask the patient to state his or her name and birth date, based on facility policy.	This requires a response from the patient, but illness and strange surroundings often cause patients to be confused.
17. **Complete necessary assessments before administering medications. Check the patient's allergy bracelet or ask the patient about allergies. Explain what you are going to do, and the reason for doing it, to the patient.**	Assessment is a prerequisite to administration of medications. Explanation relieves anxiety and facilitates cooperation.
18. Scan the patient's bar code on the identification band, if required.	This provides an additional check to ensure that the medication is given to the right patient.
19. **Based on facility policy, the third check of the label may occur at this point. If so, recheck the labels with the CMAR/MAR before administering the medications to the patient.**	Many facilities require the *third* check to occur at the bedside, after identifying the patient and before administration. If facility policy directs the *third* check at this time, this *third* check ensures accuracy and helps to prevent errors.
20. Assist the patient to the high Fowler's position, unless contraindicated.	This reduces the risk of aspiration.
21. Put on gloves.	Gloves prevent contact with mucous membranes and body fluids.
22. If patient is receiving continuous tube feedings, pause the tube-feeding pump.	If the pump is not stopped, tube feeding will flow out of the tube and onto the patient.

ACTION	RATIONALE
23. Pour the water into the irrigation container. Measure 30 mL of water. Apply clamp on feeding tube, if present. Alternately, pinch gastric tube below port with fingers, or position stopcock to correct direction. Open port on gastric tube delegated to medication administration or disconnect tubing for feeding from gastric tube and place cap on end of feeding tubing.	Fluid is ready for flushing of the tube. Applying clamp, folding the tube over and clamping, or the correct positioning of the stopcock prevents any backflow of gastric drainage. Covering end of feeding tubing prevents contamination.
24. **Check tube placement, depending on type of tube and facility policy.**	Tube placement must be confirmed before administering anything through the tube to avoid inadvertent instillation in the respiratory tract.
25. Note the amount of any residual. Replace residual back into stomach, based on facility policy.	Research findings are inconclusive on the benefit of returning gastric volumes to the stomach or intestine to avoid fluid or electrolyte imbalance, which has been accepted practice. Consult agency policy concerning this practice (Bourgault et al., 2007; Keithley & Swanson, 2004; Metheny, 2008).
26. Apply clamp on feeding tube, if present. Alternately, pinch the gastric tube below port with fingers, or position stop-cock to correct direction. Remove 60-mL syringe from gastric tube. Remove the plunger of the syringe. Reinsert the syringe in the gastric tube without the plunger. Pour 30 mL of water into the syringe. **Unclamp the tube and allow the water to enter the stomach via gravity infusion.**	Clamping prevents backflow of gastric drainage. Flushing the tube ensures that all the residual is cleared from the tube.
27. Administer the first dose of medication by pouring it into the syringe. Follow with a	Flushing between medications prevents any possible interactions between the medications.

ACTION	RATIONALE
5- to 10-mL water flush between medication doses. Follow the last dose of medication with 30 to 60 mL of water flush.	Flushing at the end maintains tube patency, prevents blockage by medication particles, and ensures all doses enter the stomach.
28. Clamp the tube, remove the syringe, and replace the feeding tubing. If a stopcock is used, position it to correct direction. If a tube medication port was used, cap the port. Unclamp the gastric tube and restart tube feeding, if appropriate for medications administered.	Some medications require the holding of the tube feeding for a certain period of time after administration. Consult a drug reference or a pharmacist.
29. Remove gloves. Assist the patient to a comfortable position. If receiving a tube feeding, the head of the bed must remain elevated at least 30 degrees.	Ensures patient comfort. Keeping the head of the bed elevated helps prevent aspiration.
30. Remove additional PPE, if used. Perform hand hygiene.	Removing PPE properly reduces the risk for infection transmission and contamination of other items. Hand hygiene prevents the spread of microorganisms.
31. Document the administration of the medication immediately after administration. See Documentation section below.	Timely documentation helps to ensure patient safety.
32. Evaluate the patient's response to the medication within the appropriate time frame.	The patient needs to be evaluated for therapeutic and adverse effects from the medication.

EVALUATION

- Patient receives the prescribed medications and experiences the intended effects of the medications administered.
- Patient demonstrates a patent and functioning gastric tube.
- Patient verbalizes knowledge of the medications given, and remains free from adverse effects and injury.

DOCUMENTATION

- Document the administration of the medication immediately after administration, including date, time, dose, and route of administration on the CMAR/MAR or record using the required format. If using a bar-code system, medication administration is automatically recorded when the bar code is scanned. PRN medications require documentation of the reason for administration. Prompt recording avoids the possibility of accidentally repeating the administration of the drug. Record the amount of gastric residual, if appropriate. Record the amount of liquid given on the intake and output record. If the drug was refused or omitted, record this in the appropriate area on the medication record and notify the primary care provider. This verifies the reason medication was omitted and ensures that the primary care provider is aware of the patient's condition.

SKILL 97 ADMINISTERING MEDICATION VIA A SMALL-VOLUME NEBULIZER

Many medications prescribed for respiratory problems may be delivered via the respiratory system using a small-volume nebulizer. Nebulizers disperse fine particles of liquid medication into the deeper passages of the respiratory tract, where absorption occurs. The treatment continues until all the medication in the nebulizer cup has been inhaled.

DELEGATION CONSIDERATIONS

The administration of medication via a nebulizer is not delegated to nursing assistive personnel (NAP) or to unlicensed assistive personnel (UAP). Depending on the state's nurse practice act and the organization's policies and procedures, administration of medication using a nebulizer may be delegated to licensed practical/vocational nurses (LPN/LVNs). The decision to delegate must be based on careful analysis of the patient's needs and circumstances, as well as the qualifications of the person to whom the task is being delegated. Refer to the Delegation Guidelines in Appendix A.

EQUIPMENT

- Stethoscope
- Medication
- Nebulizer tubing and chamber
- Air compressor or oxygen hookup
- Sterile saline (if not premeasured)
- Computer-generated Medication Administration Record (CMAR) or Medication Administration Record (MAR)
- PPE, as indicated

ASSESSMENT

- Assess respiratory rate, rhythm, and depth to establish a baseline.
- Assess lung sounds before and after use to establish a baseline and determine the effectiveness of the medication. Often, patients have wheezes or coarse lung sounds before medication administration.
- If ordered, assess patient's oxygen saturation level before medication administration. The oxygen saturation level may increase after the medication has been administered.
- Verify patient name, dose, route, and time of administration.
- Assess the patient's knowledge and understanding of the medication's purpose and action.

NURSING DIAGNOSIS

- Ineffective Airway Clearance
- Impaired Gas Exchange
- Ineffective Breathing Pattern

OUTCOME IDENTIFICATION AND PLANNING

- Patient receives the medication.
- Patient exhibits improved lung sounds and respiratory effort.
- Patient demonstrates the steps for nebulizer use.
- Patient verbalizes an understanding of medication purpose and action.

IMPLEMENTATION

ACTION	RATIONALE
1. Gather equipment. Check each medication order against the original order in the medical record, according to facility policy. Clarify any inconsistencies. Check the patient's chart for allergies.	This comparison helps to identify errors that may have occurred when orders were transcribed. The primary care provider's order is the legal record of medication orders for each facility.
2. Know the actions, special nursing considerations, safe dose ranges, purpose of administration, and adverse effects of the medications to be administered. Consider the appropriateness of the medication for this patient.	This knowledge aids the nurse in evaluating the therapeutic effect of the medication in relation to the patient's disorder and can also be used to educate the patient about the medication.

ACTION	RATIONALE
3. Perform hand hygiene.	Hand hygiene prevents the spread of microorganisms.
4. Move the medication cart to the outside of the patient's room or prepare for administration in the medication area.	Organization facilitates error-free administration and saves time.
5. Unlock the medication cart or drawer. Enter pass code and scan employee identification, if required.	Locking the cart or drawer safeguards each patient's medication supply. Hospital accrediting organizations require medication carts to be locked when not in use. Entering pass code and scanning ID allows only authorized users into the system and identifies the user for documentation by the computer.
6. **Prepare medications for one patient at a time.**	This prevents errors in medication administration.
7. Read the CMAR/MAR and select the proper medication from unit stock or the patient's medication drawer.	This is the *first* check of the label.
8. Compare the label with the CMAR/MAR. Check expiration dates and perform calculations, if necessary. Scan the bar code on the package, if required.	This is the *second* check of the label. Verify calculations with another nurse to ensure safety, if necessary.
9. **Depending on facility policy, the third check of the label may occur at this point. If so, when all medications for one patient have been prepared, recheck the labels with the CMAR/MAR before taking the medications to the patient.**	This *third* check ensures accuracy and helps to prevent errors. *Note:* Many facilities require the *third* check to occur at the bedside, after identifying the patient and before administration.
10. Lock the medication cart before leaving it.	Locking the cart or drawer safeguards the patient's medication supply. Hospital accrediting

ACTION	RATIONALE

organizations require medication carts to be locked when not in use.

11. Transport medications to the patient's bedside carefully, and keep the medications in sight at all times.

Careful handling and close observation prevent accidental or deliberate disarrangement of medications.

12. **Ensure that the patient receives the medications at the correct time.**

Check agency policy, which may allow for administration within a period of 30 minutes before or 30 minutes after the designated time.

13. Perform hand hygiene and put on PPE, if indicated.

Hand hygiene and PPE prevent the spread of microorganisms. PPE is required based on transmission precautions.

14. **Identify the patient. Compare the information with the CMAR/MAR. The patient should be identified using at least two methods** (The Joint Commission, 2013):

Identifying the patient ensures the right patient receives the medications and helps prevent errors. The patient's room number or physical location is not used as an identifier (The Joint Commission, 2013). Replace the identification band if it is missing or inaccurate in any way.

   a. Check the name on the patient's identification band.

   b. Check the identification number on the patient's identification band.

   c. Check the birth date on the patient's identification band.

   d. Ask the patient to state his or her name and birth date, based on facility policy.

This requires a response from the patient, but illness and strange surroundings often cause patients to be confused.

15. **Complete necessary assessments before administering medications. Check the patient's allergy bracelet or**

Assessment is a prerequisite to administration of medications. Explanation relieves anxiety and facilitates cooperation.

ACTION	RATIONALE

ask the patient about allergies. Explain what you are going to do, and the reason for doing it, to the patient.

16. Scan the patient's bar code on the identification band, if required.

Scanning provides an additional check to ensure that the medication is given to the right patient.

17. Based on facility policy, the third check of the label may occur at this point. If so, recheck the labels with the CMAR/MAR before administering the medications to the patient.

Many facilities require the *third* check to occur at the bedside, after identifying the patient and before administration. If facility policy directs the *third* check at this time, this *third* check ensures accuracy and helps to prevent errors.

18. Remove the nebulizer cup from the device and open it. Place premeasured unit-dose medication in the bottom section of the cup or use a dropper to place a concentrated dose of medication in the cup. Add prescribed diluent, if required.

To get enough volume to make a fine mist, normal saline may need to be added to the concentrated medication.

19. Screw the top portion of the nebulizer cup back in place and attach the cup to the nebulizer. Attach one end of tubing to the stem on the bottom of the nebulizer cuff and the other end to the air compressor or oxygen source.

Air or oxygen must be forced through the nebulizer to form a fine mist.

20. Turn on the air compressor or oxygen. Check that a fine medication mist is produced by opening the valve. Have the patient place the mouthpiece into the mouth and grasp securely with teeth and lips.

If there is no fine mist, make sure that medication has been added to the cup and that the tubing is connected to the air compressor or oxygen outlet. Adjust flow meter if necessary.

21. Instruct the patient to inhale slowly and deeply through the mouth. A nose clip may be necessary if

While the patient inhales and holds the breath, the medication comes in contact with the respiratory tissue and is absorbed.

ACTION	RATIONALE
the patient is also breathing through the nose. Hold each breath for a slight pause, before exhaling.	The longer the breath is held, the more medication can be absorbed.
22. Continue this inhalation technique until all medication in the nebulizer cup has been aerosolized (usually about 15 minutes). Once the fine mist decreases in amount, gently flick the sides of the nebulizer cup.	Once the fine mist stops, the medication is no longer being aerosolized. By gently flicking the cup sides, any medication that is stuck to the sides is knocked into the bottom of the cup, where it can become aerosolized.
23. Have the patient gargle and rinse with tap water after using the nebulizer, as necessary. Clean the nebulizer according to the manufacturer's directions.	Rinsing is necessary when using inhaled steroids, because oral fungal infections can occur. Rinsing removes medication residue from the mouth. The buildup of medication in the device can affect how the medication is delivered, as well as attract bacteria.
24. Remove gloves and additional PPE, if used. Perform hand hygiene.	Removing PPE properly reduces the risk for infection transmission and contamination of other items. Hand hygiene prevents the spread of microorganisms.
25. Document the administration of the medication immediately after administration. See Documentation section below.	Timely documentation helps to ensure patient safety.
26. Evaluate patient's response to the medication within an appropriate time frame. **Reassess lung sounds, oxygen saturation level, and respirations.**	The patient needs to be evaluated for therapeutic and adverse effects from the medication. Lung sounds and oxygen saturation level may improve after nebulizer use. Respirations may decrease after nebulizer use.

EVALUATION

- Patient receives the medication and exhibits improved lung sounds and respiratory effort.
- Patient demonstrates correct steps for use, and verbalizes an understanding, of the need for the medication.

DOCUMENTATION

- Document the administration of the medication immediately after administration, including date, time, dose, and route of administration on the CMAR/MAR or record using the required format. If using a bar-code system, medication administration is automatically recorded when the bar code is scanned. PRN medications require documentation of the reason for administration. Prompt recording avoids the possibility of accidentally repeating the administration of the drug. Document respiratory rate, oxygen saturation, if applicable, lung assessment, and the patient's response to the treatment, if appropriate. If the drug was refused or omitted, record this in the appropriate area on the medication record and notify the primary care provider. This verifies the reason medication was omitted and ensures that the primary care provider is aware of the patient's condition.

SKILL 98 | ADMINISTERING A PIGGYBACK INTERMITTENT INTRAVENOUS INFUSION OF MEDICATION

With intermittent IV infusion, the drug is mixed with a small amount of the IV solution, such as 50 to 100 mL, and administered over a short period at the prescribed interval (e.g., every 4 hours). The administration is most often performed using an IV infusion pump, which requires the nurse to program the infusion rate into the pump. "Smart (computerized) pumps" are being used by many facilities for IV infusions, including intermittent infusions. Smart pumps also require programming of infusion rates by the nurse, but also are able to identify dosing limits and practice guidelines to aid in safe administration. Administration may also be achieved by gravity infusion, which requires the nurse to calculate the infusion rate in drops per minute. The best practice, however, is to use an IV infusion pump.

The IV piggyback delivery system requires the intermittent or additive solution to be placed higher than the primary solution container. An extension hook provided by the manufacturer provides for easy lowering of the main IV container. The port on the primary IV line has a back-check valve that automatically stops the flow of the primary solution, allowing the secondary or piggyback solution to flow when connected. Because manufacturers' designs vary, it is important to check the directions carefully for the systems used in the facility. The nurse is responsible for calculating and regulating the infusion with an infusion pump or manually adjusting the flow rate of the IV intermittent infusion. Needleless devices (recommended by the CDC and the Occupational Safety and Health Administration [OSHA]) prevent needlesticks and provide access to the primary venous line. Either a blunt-ended cannula or a recessed connection port may be used to connect intermittent IV infusions.

DELEGATION CONSIDERATIONS

The administration of medications by intermittent IV infusion is not delegated to nursing assistive personnel (NAP) or to unlicensed assistive personnel (UAP). Depending on the state's nurse practice act and the organization's policies and procedures, the administration of specified IV medications in some settings may be delegated to licensed practical/vocational nurses (LPN/LVNs) who have received appropriate training. The decision to delegate must be based on careful analysis of the patient's needs and circumstances, as well as the qualifications of the person to whom the task is being delegated. Refer to the Delegation Guidelines in Appendix A.

EQUIPMENT

- Medication prepared in labeled small-volume bag
- Short secondary infusion tubing (microdrip or macrodrip)
- IV pump
- Needleless connector, if required, based on facility system
- Antimicrobial swab
- Metal or plastic hook
- IV pole
- Date label for tubing
- Computer-generated Medication Administration Record (CMAR) or Medication Administration Record (MAR)
- PPE, as indicated

ASSESSMENT

- Assess the patient for any allergies.
- Check the expiration date before administering the medication.
- Assess the appropriateness of the drug for the patient.
- Assess the compatibility of the ordered medication, diluent, and the infusing IV fluid.
- Review assessment and laboratory data that may influence drug administration.
- Verify patient name, dose, route, and time of administration.
- Assess the patient's knowledge of the medication. If the patient has a knowledge deficit about the medication, this may be the appropriate time to begin education about the medication.
- If the medication may affect the patient's vital signs, assess them before administration.
- Assess the IV insertion site, noting any swelling, coolness, leakage of fluid at site, redness, or pain.

NURSING DIAGNOSIS

- Risk for Allergy Response
- Risk for Infection
- Risk for Injury

OUTCOME IDENTIFICATION AND PLANNING

- Medication is delivered via the intravenous route using sterile technique.
- Medication is delivered to the patient in a safe manner and at the appropriate infusion rate.
- Patient experiences no allergy response.
- Patient remains infection free.
- Patient understands and complies with the medication regimen.

IMPLEMENTATION

ACTION	RATIONALE
1. Gather equipment. Check each medication order against the original order in the medical record, according to facility policy. Clarify any inconsistencies. Check the patient's chart for allergies.	This comparison helps to identify errors that may have occurred when orders were transcribed. The primary care provider order is the legal record of medication orders for each facility.
2. Know the actions, special nursing considerations, safe dose ranges, purpose of administration, and adverse effects of the medications to be administered. Consider the appropriateness of the medication for this patient.	This knowledge aids the nurse in evaluating the therapeutic effect of the medication in relation to the patient's disorder and can also be used to educate the patient about the medication.
3. Perform hand hygiene.	Hand hygiene prevents the spread of microorganisms.
4. Move the medication cart to the outside of the patient's room or prepare for administration in the medication area.	Organization facilitates error-free administration and saves time.
5. Unlock the medication cart or drawer. Enter pass code and scan employee identification, if required.	Locking the cart or drawer safeguards each patient's medication supply. Hospital accrediting organizations require medication carts to be locked when not in use. Entering pass code and scanning ID allows only authorized users into the system and identifies the user for documentation by the computer.

ACTION	RATIONALE
6. Prepare medications for one patient at a time.	This prevents errors in medication administration.
7. Read the CMAR/MAR and select the proper medication from unit stock or the patient's medication drawer.	This is the *first* check of the label.
8. Compare the label with the CMAR/MAR. Check expiration dates. Confirm the prescribed or appropriate infusion rate. Calculate the drip rate if using gravity system. Scan the bar code on the package, if required.	This is the *second* check of the label. Verify calculations with another nurse to ensure safety, if necessary. Infusing medication at an appropriate rate prevents injury.
9. Depending on facility policy, the third check of the label may occur at this point. If so, when all medications for one patient have been prepared, recheck the labels with the CMAR/MAR before taking the medications to the patient.	This *third* check ensures accuracy and helps to prevent errors. *Note:* Many facilities require the *third* check to occur at the bedside, after identifying the patient and before administration.
10. Lock the medication cart before leaving it.	Locking the cart or drawer safeguards the patient's medication supply. Hospital accrediting organizations require medication carts to be locked when not in use.
11. Transport medications to the patient's bedside carefully, and keep the medications in sight at all times.	Careful handling and close observation prevent accidental or deliberate disarrangement of medications.
12. Ensure that the patient receives the medications at the correct time.	Check facility policy, which may allow for administration within a period of 30 minutes before or 30 minutes after the designated time.
13. Perform hand hygiene and put on PPE, if indicated.	Hand hygiene and PPE prevent the spread of microorganisms. PPE is required based on transmission precautions.

ACTION	RATIONALE

14. Identify the patient. 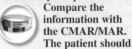 **Compare the information with the CMAR/MAR.** The patient should be identified using at least two methods (The Joint Commission, 2013):

Identifying the patient ensures the right patient receives the medications and helps prevent errors. The patient's room number or physical location is not used as an identifier (The Joint Commission, 2013). Replace the identification band if it is missing or inaccurate in any way.

  a. Check the name on the patient's identification band.

  b. Check the identification number on the patient's identification band.

  c. Check the birth date on the patient's identification band.

  d. Ask the patient to state his or her name and birth date, based on facility policy.

This requires a response from the patient, but illness and strange surroundings often cause patients to be confused.

15. Close the door to the room or pull the bedside curtain.

This provides patient privacy.

16. Complete necessary assessments before administering medications. Check the patient's allergy bracelet or ask the patient about allergies. Explain the purpose and action of the medication to the patient.

Assessment is a prerequisite to administration of medications. Explanation provides rationale, increases knowledge, and reduces anxiety.

17. Scan the patient's bar code on the identification band, if required.

Scanning provides an additional check to ensure that the medication is given to the right patient.

18. Based on facility policy, the third check of the label may occur at this point. If so, recheck the labels with the CMAR/MAR before administering the medications to the patient.

Many facilities require the *third* check to occur at the bedside, after identifying the patient and before administration. If facility policy directs the *third* check at this time, this *third* check ensures accuracy and helps to prevent errors.

ACTION	RATIONALE
19. Assess the IV site for the presence of inflammation or infiltration.	IV medication must be given directly into a vein for safe administration.
20. Close the clamp on the short secondary infusion tubing. Using aseptic technique, remove the cap on the tubing spike and the cap on the port of the medication container, taking care to avoid contaminating either end.	Closing the clamp prevents fluid from entering the system until the nurse is ready. Maintaining sterility of the tubing and the medication port prevents contamination.
21. Attach infusion tubing to the medication container by inserting the tubing spike into the port with a firm push and twisting motion, taking care to avoid contaminating either end.	Maintaining sterility of tubing and medication port prevents contamination.
22. Hang piggyback container on IV pole, positioning it higher than primary IV according to manufacturer's recommendations. Use metal or plastic hook to lower primary IV fluid container.	Position of containers influences the flow of IV fluid into the primary setup.
23. Place label on tubing with appropriate date.	Tubing for piggyback setup may be used for 48 to 96 hours, depending on agency policy. Label allows for tracking of the next date to change.
24. Squeeze drip chamber on tubing and release. Fill to the line or about half full. Open clamp and prime tubing. Close clamp. Place needleless connector on the end of the tubing, using sterile technique, if required.	This removes air from the tubing and preserves the sterility of the setup.
25. Use an antimicrobial swab to clean the access port or stopcock above the roller clamp on the primary IV infusion tubing.	This deters entry of microorganisms when the piggyback setup is connected to the port. Backflow valve in the primary line secondary port stops flow of primary infusion while piggyback solution

ACTION	RATIONALE
	is infusing. Once completed, backflow valves open and flow of primary solution resumes.
26. Connect piggyback setup to the access port or stopcock. If using, turn the stopcock to the open position.	Needleless systems and stopcock setup eliminate the need for a needle and are recommended by the CDC.
27. Open clamp on the secondary tubing. Set rate for secondary infusion on infusion pump and begin infusion. If using gravity infusion, use the roller clamp on the primary infusion tubing to regulate the flow at the prescribed delivery rate. Monitor medication infusion at periodic intervals.	Backflow valve in the primary line secondary port stops flow of primary infusion while piggyback solution is infusing. Once completed, backflow valves open and flow of primary solution resumes. It is important to verify the safe administration rate for each drug to prevent adverse effects.
28. Clamp tubing on piggyback set when solution is infused. Follow facility policy regarding disposal of equipment.	Most facilities allow the reuse of tubing for 48 to 96 hours. This reduces risk for contaminating primary IV setup.
29. Raise primary IV fluid container to original height. **Check primary infusion rate on infusion pump. If using gravity infusion, readjust flow rate of primary IV.**	Most infusion pumps automatically restart primary infusion at previous rate after secondary infusion is completed. If using gravity infusion, piggyback medication administration may interrupt normal flow rate of primary IV. Rate readjustment may be necessary.
30. Remove PPE, if used. Perform hand hygiene.	Removing PPE properly reduces the risk for infection transmission and contamination of other items. Hand hygiene prevents the spread of microorganisms.
31. Document the administration of the medication immediately after administration. See Documentation section below. Document the volume of fluid administered on the intake and output record, if necessary.	Timely documentation helps to ensure patient safety.

ACTION	RATIONALE
32. Evaluate the patient's response to the medication within an appropriate time frame. Monitor IV site at periodic intervals.	The patient needs to be evaluated for therapeutic and adverse effects from the medication.

EVALUATION

- Medication is delivered via the IV route using sterile technique.
- Medication is delivered to the patient in a safe manner and at the appropriate infusion rate.
- Patient experiences no allergy response.
- Patient remains infection free.
- Patient understands and complies with the medication regimen.

DOCUMENTATION

- Document the administration of the medication immediately after administration, including date, time, dose, route of administration, site of administration, and rate of administration on the CMAR/MAR or record using the required format. If using a bar-code system, medication administration is automatically recorded when the bar code is scanned. PRN medications require documentation of the reason for administration. Prompt recording avoids the possibility of accidentally repeating the administration of the drug. If the drug was refused or omitted, record this in the appropriate area on the medication record and notify the primary care provider. This verifies the reason medication was omitted and ensures that the primary care provider is aware of the patient's condition. Document the volume of fluid administered on the intake and output record, if necessary.

SKILL 99   ADMINISTERING AN INTERMITTENT INTRAVENOUS INFUSION OF MEDICATION VIA A MINI-INFUSION PUMP

With intermittent IV infusion, the drug is mixed with a small amount of the IV solution, and administered over a short period at the prescribed interval (e.g., every 4 hours). The mini-infusion pump (syringe pump) for intermittent infusion is battery or electrical operated and allows medication mixed in a syringe to be connected to the primary line and delivered by mechanical pressure applied to the syringe plunger.

"Smart (computerized) pumps" are being used by many facilities for IV infusions, including intermittent infusions. Smart pumps also require programming of infusion rates by the nurse, but also are able to identify dosing limits and practice guidelines to aid in safe administration. Needleless devices (recommended by the CDC and the Occupational Safety and Health Administration [OSHA]) prevent needlesticks and provide access to the primary venous line. Either a blunt-ended cannula or a recessed connection port may be used to connect intermittent IV infusions.

DELEGATION CONSIDERATIONS

The administration of medications by intermittent IV infusion is not delegated to nursing assistive personnel (NAP) or to unlicensed assistive personnel (UAP). Depending on the state's nurse practice act and the organization's policies and procedures, the administration of specified IV medications in some settings may be delegated to licensed practical/vocational nurses (LPN/LVNs) who have received appropriate training. The decision to delegate must be based on careful analysis of the patient's needs and circumstances, as well as the qualifications of the person to whom the task is being delegated. Refer to the Delegation Guidelines in Appendix A.

EQUIPMENT

- Medication prepared in labeled syringe
- Mini-infusion pump and tubing
- Needleless connector, if required, based on facility system
- Antimicrobial swab
- Date label for tubing
- Computer-generated Medication Administration Record (CMAR) or Medication Administration Record (MAR)
- PPE, as indicated

ASSESSMENT

- Assess the patient for any allergies.
- Check the expiration date before administering medication.
- Assess the appropriateness of the drug for the patient.
- Assess the compatibility of the ordered medication, diluent, and the infusing IV fluid.
- Review assessment and laboratory data that may influence drug administration.
- Verify patient name, dose, route, and time of administration.
- Assess the patient's knowledge of the medication. If the patient has a knowledge deficit about the medication, this may be the appropriate time to begin education about the medication.
- If the medication may affect the patient's vital signs, assess them before administration.
- Assess the IV insertion site, noting any swelling, coolness, leakage of fluid at site, redness, or pain.

NURSING DIAGNOSIS
- Risk for Allergy Response
- Risk for Injury
- Risk for Infection

OUTCOME IDENTIFICATION AND PLANNING
- Medication is delivered via the IV route using sterile technique.
- Medication is delivered to the patient in a safe manner and at the appropriate infusion rate.
- Patient experiences no allergy response.
- Patient remains infection free.
- Patient understands and complies with the medication regimen.

IMPLEMENTATION

ACTION	RATIONALE
1. Gather equipment. Check each medication order against the original order in the medical record according to facility policy. Clarify any inconsistencies. Check the patient's chart for allergies.	This comparison helps to identify errors that may have occurred when orders were transcribed. The primary care provider's order is the legal record of medication orders for each facility. Compatibility of medication and solution prevents complications.
2. Know the actions, special nursing considerations, safe dose ranges, purpose of administration, and adverse effects of the medications to be administered. Consider the appropriateness of the medication for this patient.	This knowledge aids the nurse in evaluating the therapeutic effect of the medication in relation to the patient's disorder and can also be used to educate the patient about the medication.
3. Perform hand hygiene.	Hand hygiene prevents the spread of microorganisms.
4. Move the medication cart to the outside of the patient's room or prepare for administration in the medication area.	Organization facilitates error-free administration and saves time.
5. Unlock the medication cart or drawer. Enter pass code and scan employee identification, if required.	Locking the cart or drawer safeguards each patient's medication supply. Hospital accrediting organizations require medication

ACTION	RATIONALE
	carts to be locked when not in use. Entering pass code and scanning ID allows only authorized users into the system and identifies the user for documentation by the computer.
6. **Prepare medications for one patient at a time.**	This prevents errors in medication administration.
7. Read the CMAR/MAR and select the proper medication from unit stock or the patient's medication drawer.	This is the *first* check of the label.
8. Compare the label with the CMAR/MAR. Check expiration dates. Confirm the prescribed or appropriate infusion rate. Scan the bar code on the package, if required.	This is the *second* check of the label. Verify calculations with another nurse to ensure safety, if necessary. Infusing medication at appropriate rate prevents injury.
9. **Depending on facility policy, the third check of the label may occur at this point. If so, when all medications for one patient have been prepared, recheck the labels with the CMAR/MAR before taking the medications to the patient.**	This *third* check ensures accuracy and helps to prevent errors. *Note:* Many facilities require the *third* check to occur at the bedside, after identifying the patient and before administration.
10. Lock the medication cart before leaving it.	Locking the cart or drawer safeguards the patient's medication supply. Hospital accrediting organizations require medication carts to be locked when not in use.
11. Transport medications to the patient's bedside carefully, and keep the medications in sight at all times.	Careful handling and close observation prevent accidental or deliberate disarrangement of medications.
12. **Ensure that the patient receives the medications at the correct time.**	Check agency policy, which may allow for administration within a period of 30 minutes before or 30 minutes after the designated time.

ACTION	RATIONALE

13. Perform hand hygiene and put on PPE, if indicated.

Hand hygiene and PPE prevent the spread of microorganisms. PPE is required based on transmission precautions.

14. **Identify the patient. Compare the information with the CMAR/MAR. The patient should be identified using at least two methods (The Joint Commission, 2013):**

Identifying the patient ensures the right patient receives the medications and helps prevent errors. The patient's room number or physical location is not used as an identifier (The Joint Commission, 2013). Replace the identification band if it is missing or inaccurate in any way.

a. Check the name on the patient's identification band.

b. Check the identification number on the patient's identification band.

c. Check the birth date on the patient's identification band.

d. Ask the patient to state his or her name and birth date, based on facility policy.

This requires a response from the patient, but illness and strange surroundings often cause patients to be confused.

15. Close the door to the room or pull the bedside curtain.

Provides patient privacy.

16. **Complete necessary assessments before administering medications. Check the patient's allergy bracelet or ask the patient about allergies. Explain the purpose and action of the medication to the patient.**

Assessment is a prerequisite to administration of medications. Explanation provides rationale, increases knowledge, and reduces anxiety.

17. Scan the patient's bar code on the identification band, if required.

Provides an additional check to ensure that the medication is given to the right patient.

18. **Based on facility policy, the third check of the label may occur at this point. If**

Many facilities require the *third* check to occur at the bedside, after identifying the patient and before

ACTION	RATIONALE
so, recheck the labels with the CMAR/MAR before administering the medications to the patient.	administration. If facility policy directs the *third* check at this time, this *third* check ensures accuracy and helps to prevent errors.
19. Assess the IV site for the presence of inflammation or infiltration.	IV medication must be given directly into a vein for safe administration.
20. Using aseptic technique, remove the cap on the tubing and the cap on the syringe, taking care not to contaminate either end.	Maintaining sterility of tubing and medication port prevents contamination.
21. Attach infusion tubing to the syringe, taking care not to contaminate either end.	Maintaining sterility of tubing and medication port prevents contamination.
22. Place label on tubing with appropriate date.	Tubing for piggyback setup may be used for 48 to 96 hours, depending on facility policy. Label allows for tracking of the next date to change.
23. Fill tubing with medication by applying gentle pressure to syringe plunger. Place needleless connector on the end of the tubing, using sterile technique, if required.	This removes air from tubing and maintains sterility.
24. Insert syringe into mini-infusion pump according to manufacturer's directions.	Syringe must fit securely in pump apparatus for proper operation.
25. Use antimicrobial swab to clean the access port or stopcock below the roller clamp on the primary IV infusion tubing, usually the port closest to the IV insertion site.	This deters entry of microorganisms when the piggyback setup is connected to the port. Proper connection allows IV medication to flow into the primary line.
26. Connect the secondary infusion to the primary infusion at the cleansed port.	Allows for delivery of medication.
27. Program the pump to the appropriate rate and begin infusion. Set the alarm if recommended by the manufacturer.	Pump delivers medication at a controlled rate. Alarm is recommended for use with IV lock apparatus.

ACTION	RATIONALE
28. Clamp tubing on secondary set when solution is infused. Remove secondary tubing from access port and cap, or replace connector with a new, capped one, if reusing. Follow facility policy regarding disposal of equipment.	Many facilities allow reuse of tubing for 48 to 96 hours. Replacing connector or needle with a new, capped one maintains system sterility.
29. Check rate of primary infusion.	Administration of secondary infusion may interfere with primary infusion rate.
30. Remove PPE, if used. Perform hand hygiene.	Removing PPE properly reduces the risk for infection transmission and contamination of other items. Hand hygiene prevents the spread of microorganisms.
31. Document the administration of the medication immediately after administration. See Documentation section below. Document the volume of fluid administered on the intake and output record, if necessary.	Timely documentation helps to ensure patient safety.
32. Evaluate the patient's response to the medication within appropriate time frame. Monitor IV site at periodic intervals.	The patient needs to be evaluated for therapeutic and adverse effects from the medication.

EVALUATION

- Medication is delivered via the IV route using sterile technique.
- Medication is delivered to the patient in a safe manner and at the appropriate infusion rate.
- Patient experiences no allergy response.
- Patient remains infection free.
- Patient understands and complies with the medication regimen.

DOCUMENTATION

- Document the administration of the medication immediately after administration, including date, time, dose, route of administration, site of administration, and rate of administration on the CMAR/MAR or record using the required format. If using a bar-code system, medication administration is automatically recorded when the bar code is scanned. PRN medications require documentation of the reason for administration. Prompt recording avoids the possibility of accidentally repeating the administration of the drug. If the drug was refused or omitted, record this in the appropriate area on the medication record and notify the primary care provider. This verifies the reason medication was omitted and ensures that the primary care provider is aware of the patient's condition. Document the volume of fluid administered on the intake and output record, if necessary.

SKILL 100 ADMINISTERING AN INTERMITTENT INTRAVENOUS INFUSION OF MEDICATION VIA A VOLUME-CONTROL ADMINISTRATION SET

With intermittent IV infusion, the drug is mixed with a small amount of the IV solution (e.g., 50 to 100 mL) and administered over a short period at the prescribed interval (e.g., every 4 hours). The administration is most often performed using an IV infusion pump, which requires the nurse to program the infusion rate into the pump. "Smart (computerized) pumps" are being used by many facilities for IV infusions, including intermittent infusions. Smart pumps also require programming of infusion rates by the nurse, but also are able to identify dosing limits and practice guidelines to aid in safe administration. Administration may also be achieved by gravity infusion, which requires the nurse to calculate the infusion rate in drops per minute. The best practice, however, is to use an intravenous infusion pump.

This skill discusses using a volume-control administration set for intermittent IV infusion. The medication is diluted with a small amount of solution and administered through the patient's IV line. This type of equipment may be used for infusing solutions into children, critically ill patients, and older patients when the fluid volume to be infused is a concern. Needleless devices (recommended by the CDC and the Occupational Safety and Health Administration [OSHA]) prevent needlesticks and provide access to the primary venous line. Either a blunt-ended cannula or a recessed connection port may be used to connect intermittent IV infusions.

DELEGATION CONSIDERATIONS

The administration of medications by intermittent IV infusion is not delegated to nursing assistive personnel (NAP) or to unlicensed assistive personnel (UAP). Depending on the state's nurse practice act and the organization's policies and procedures, the administration of specified

IV medications in some settings may be delegated to licensed practical/vocational nurses (LPN/LVNs) who have received appropriate training. The decision to delegate must be based on careful analysis of the patient's needs and circumstances, as well as the qualifications of the person to whom the task is being delegated. Refer to the Delegation Guidelines in Appendix A.

EQUIPMENT
- Prescribed medication
- Syringe with a needless device or blunt needle, if required, based on facility system
- Volume-control set (Volutrol, Buretrol, Burette)
- Needleless connector or stopcock, if required
- Infusion pump, if needed
- Antimicrobial swab
- Date label for tubing
- Medication label
- Computer-generated Medication Administration Record (CMAR) or Medication Administration Record (MAR)
- PPE, as indicated

ASSESSMENT
- Assess the patient for any allergies.
- Check the expiration date before administering the medication.
- Assess the appropriateness of the drug for the patient.
- Assess the compatibility of the ordered medication, diluent, and the infusing IV fluid.
- Review assessment and laboratory data that may influence drug administration.
- Assess the patient's knowledge of the medication. If the patient has a knowledge deficit about the medication, this may be the appropriate time to begin education about the medication.
- If the medication may affect the patient's vital signs, assess them before administration.
- Assess the IV insertion site, noting any swelling, coolness, leakage of fluid at site, redness, or pain.

NURSING DIAGNOSIS
- Risk for Allergy Response
- Risk for Injury
- Risk for Infection

OUTCOME IDENTIFICATION AND PLANNING
- Medication is delivered via the IV route using sterile technique.
- Medication is delivered to the patient in a safe manner and at the appropriate infusion rate.
- Patient experiences no allergy response.
- Patient remains infection free.
- Patient understands and complies with the medication regimen.

IMPLEMENTATION

ACTION	RATIONALE
1. Gather equipment. Check the medication order against the original order in the medical record according to facility policy. Clarify any inconsistencies. Check the patient's chart for allergies. Verify the compatibility of the medication and IV fluid.	This comparison helps to identify errors that may have occurred when orders were transcribed. The primary care provider's order is the legal record of medication orders for each facility.
2. Know the actions, special nursing considerations, safe dose ranges, purpose of administration, and adverse effects of the medications to be administered. Consider the appropriateness of the medication for this patient.	This knowledge aids the nurse in evaluating the therapeutic effect of the medication in relation to the patient's disorder and can also be used to educate the patient about the medication.
3. Perform hand hygiene.	Hand hygiene prevents the spread of microorganisms.
4. Move the medication cart to the outside of the patient's room or prepare for administration in the medication area.	Organization facilitates error-free administration and saves time.
5. Unlock the medication cart or drawer. Enter pass code and scan employee identification, if required.	Locking the cart or drawer safeguards each patient's medication supply. Hospital accrediting organizations require medication carts to be locked when not in use. Entering pass code and scanning ID allows only authorized users into the computer system and identifies the user for documentation by the computer.
6. **Prepare medication for one patient at a time.**	This prevents errors in medication administration.
7. Read the CMAR/MAR and select the proper medication from unit stock or the patient's medication drawer.	This is the *first* check of the label.

ACTION	RATIONALE
8. Compare the label with the CMAR/MAR. Check expiration dates and perform calculations, if necessary. Confirm the prescribed or appropriate infusion rate. Calculate the drip rate if using a gravity system. Scan the bar code on the package, if required. Check the infusion rate.	This is the *second* check of the label. Verify calculations with another nurse to ensure safety, if necessary. Delivers the correct dose of medication as prescribed.
9. If necessary, withdraw medication from an ampule or vial as described in Skills 103 and 104. Attach needleless connector or blunt needle to end of syringe, if necessary.	Allows for entry into the volume-control administration set chamber.
10. **Depending on facility policy, the third check of the label may occur at this point. If so, when all medications for one patient have been prepared, recheck the label with the CMAR/MAR before taking the medications to the patient.**	This *third* check ensures accuracy and helps to prevent errors. *Note:* Many facilities require the *third* check to occur at the bedside, after identifying the patient and before administration.
11. Prepare medication label, including name of medication, dose, total volume, including diluent, and time of administration.	Allows for accurate identification of medication.
12. Lock the medication cart before leaving it.	Locking the cart or drawer safeguards the patient's medication supply. Hospital accrediting organizations require medication carts to be locked when not in use.
13. Transport medications and equipment to the patient's bedside carefully, and keep the medications in sight at all times.	Careful handling and close observation prevent accidental or deliberate disarrangement of medications. Having equipment available saves time and facilitates performance of the task.

ACTION	RATIONALE
14. **Ensure that the patient receives the medications at the correct time.**	Check facility policy, which may allow for administration within a period of 30 minutes before or 30 minutes after the designated time.
15. Perform hand hygiene and put on PPE, if indicated.	Hand hygiene and PPE prevent the spread of microorganisms. PPE is required based on transmission precautions.
16. **Identify the patient. Compare the information with the CMAR/MAR. The patient should be identified using at least two methods** (The Joint Commission, 2013):	Identifying the patient ensures the right patient receives the medications and helps prevent errors. The patient's room number or physical location is not used as an identifier (The Joint Commission, 2013). Replace the identification band if it is missing or inaccurate in any way.
a. Check the name on the patient's identification band.	
b. Check the identification number on the patient's identification band.	
c. Check the birth date on the patient's identification band.	
d. Ask the patient to state his or her name and birth date, based on facility policy.	This requires a response from the patient, but illness and strange surroundings often cause patients to be confused.
17. Close the door to the room or pull the bedside curtain.	This provides patient privacy.
18. **Complete necessary assessments before administering medications. Check the patient's allergy bracelet or ask the patient about allergies. Explain the purpose and action of the medication to the patient.**	Assessment is a prerequisite to administration of medications. Explanation provides rationale, increases knowledge, and reduces anxiety.

ACTION	RATIONALE
19. Scan the patient's bar code on the identification band, if required.	Provides an additional check to ensure that the medication is given to the right patient.
20. **Based on facility policy, the third check of the label may occur at this point. If so, recheck the labels with the CMAR/MAR before administering the medications to the patient.**	Many facilities require the *third* check to occur at the bedside, after identifying the patient and before administration. If facility policy directs the *third* check at this time, this *third* check ensures accuracy and helps to prevent errors.
21. Assess IV site for presence of inflammation or infiltration.	IV medication must be given directly into a vein for safe administration.
22. Fill the volume-control administration set with the prescribed amount of IV fluid by opening the clamp between IV solution and the volume-control administration set. Follow manufacturer's instructions and fill with prescribed amount of IV solution. Close clamp.	This dilutes the medication in a minimal amount of solution. Reclamping prevents the continued addition of fluid to the volume to be mixed with the medication.
23. Check to ensure the air vent on the volume-control administration set chamber is open.	Air vent allows fluid in the chamber to flow at a regular rate.
24. Use an antimicrobial swab to clean the access port on the volume-control administration set chamber.	This deters entry of microorganisms when the syringe enters the chamber.
25. Attach the syringe with a twisting motion into the access port while holding the syringe steady. Alternately, insert the needleless device or blunt needle into the port. Inject the medication into the chamber. Gently rotate the chamber.	This ensures that medication is evenly mixed with the solution.
26. Attach the medication label to the volume-control device.	This identifies contents of the set and prevents medication error.

ACTION	RATIONALE
27. Use an antimicrobial swab to clean the access port or stopcock below the roller clamp on the primary IV infusion tubing, usually the port closest to the IV insertion site.	This deters entry of microorganisms when the piggyback setup is connected to the port. Proper connection allows IV medication to flow into primary line.
28. Connect the secondary infusion to the primary infusion at the cleansed port.	This allows for delivery of medication.
29. The volume-control administration set may be placed on an infusion pump with the appropriate dose programmed into the pump. Alternately, use the roller clamp on the volume-control administration set tubing to adjust the infusion to the prescribed rate.	Delivery over a 30- to 60-minute interval is a safe method of administering IV medication.
30. Discard the syringe in the appropriate receptacle.	Proper disposal prevents injury.
31. Clamp tubing on secondary set when solution is infused. Remove secondary tubing from access port and cap or replace connector with a new, capped one, if reusing. Follow facility policy regarding disposal of equipment.	Many facilities allow reuse of tubing for 48 to 96 hours. Replacing connector or needle with a new, capped one maintains sterility of system.
32. Check rate of primary infusion.	Administration of a secondary infusion may interfere with the primary infusion rate.
33. Remove PPE, if used. Perform hand hygiene.	Removing PPE properly reduces the risk for infection transmission and contamination of other items. Hand hygiene prevents the spread of microorganisms.
34. Document the administration of the medication immediately after administration. See Documentation section below. Document the volume of fluid administered on the intake and output record, if necessary.	Timely documentation helps to ensure patient safety.

ACTION	RATIONALE
35. Evaluate the patient's response to the medication within appropriate time frame. Monitor IV site at periodic intervals.	The patient needs to be evaluated for therapeutic and adverse effects from the medication. Visualization of the site also allows for assessment of any untoward effects.

EVALUATION

- Medication is delivered via the IV route using sterile technique.
- Medication is delivered to the patient in a safe manner and at the appropriate infusion rate.
- Patient experiences no allergy response.
- Patient remains infection free.
- Patient understands and complies with the medication regimen.

DOCUMENTATION

- Document the administration of the medication immediately after administration, including date, time, dose, route of administration, site of administration, and rate of administration on the CMAR/ MAR or record using the required format. If using a bar-code system, medication administration is automatically recorded when bar code is scanned. PRN medications require documentation of the reason for administration. Prompt recording avoids the possibility of accidentally repeating the administration of the drug. If the drug was refused or omitted, record this in the appropriate area on the medication record and notify the primary care provider. This verifies the reason medication was omitted and ensures that the primary care provider is aware of the patient's condition. Document the volume of fluid administered on the intake and output record, if necessary.

SKILL 101 ADMINISTERING MEDICATIONS BY INTRAVENOUS BOLUS OR PUSH THROUGH AN INTRAVENOUS INFUSION

A medication can be administered via the intravenous (IV) route as an IV bolus or push. This involves a single injection of a concentrated solution directly into an IV line. Drugs given by IV push are used for intermittent dosing or to treat emergencies. The drug is administered very slowly over at least 1 minute. This can be done manually or by using a syringe pump. Confirm exact administration times by consulting a pharmacist or drug reference. Needleless devices prevent needlesticks and provide access to the intravenous line. Either a blunt-ended cannula or a recessed connection port may be used to administer the medication.

DELEGATION CONSIDERATIONS

The administration of medications by intravenous bolus is not delegated to nursing assistive personnel (NAP) or to unlicensed assistive personnel (UAP). Depending on the state's nurse practice act and the organization's policies and procedures, the administration of specified intravenous medications in some settings may be delegated to licensed practical/vocational nurses (LPN/LVNs) who have received appropriate training. The decision to delegate must be based on careful analysis of the patient's needs and circumstances, as well as the qualifications of the person to whom the task is being delegated. Refer to the Delegation Guidelines in Appendix A.

EQUIPMENT

- Antimicrobial swab
- Watch with second hand, or stopwatch
- Disposable gloves
- Additional PPE, as indicated
- Prescribed medication
- Syringe with a needleless device or 23- to 25-gauge,
- 1-inch needle (follow facility policy)
- Syringe pump, if necessary
- Computer-generated Medication Administration Record (CMAR) or Medication Administration Record (MAR)

ASSESSMENT

- Assess the patient for any allergies.
- Check the expiration date before administering the medication.
- Assess the appropriateness of the drug for the patient.
- Assess the compatibility of the ordered medication and the IV fluid.
- Review assessment and laboratory data that may influence drug administration.
- Verify the patient's name, dose, route, and time of administration.
- Assess the patient's IV site, noting any swelling, coolness, leakage of fluid from the IV site, or pain.
- Assess the patient's knowledge of the medication. If the patient has a knowledge deficit about the medication, this may be the appropriate time to begin education about the medication.
- If the medication may affect the patient's vital signs, assess them before administration.
- If the medication is for pain relief, assess the patient's pain before and after administration.

NURSING DIAGNOSIS

- Risk for Injury
- Risk for Allergy Response
- Risk for Infection

OUTCOME IDENTIFICATION AND PLANNING

- Medication is given safely via the IV route.
- Patient experiences no adverse effects.
- Patient experiences no allergy response.
- Patient is knowledgeable about the medication in the bolus.
- Patient remains infection free.
- Patient has no, or decreased, anxiety.

IMPLEMENTATION

ACTION	RATIONALE
1. Gather equipment. Check medication order against the original order in the medical record, according to facility policy. Clarify any inconsistencies. Check the patient's chart for allergies. Verify the compatibility of the medication and IV fluid. Check a drug resource to clarify whether the medication needs to be diluted before administration. Check the administration rate.	This comparison helps to identify errors that may have occurred when orders were transcribed. The primary care provider's order is the legal record of medication orders for each facility. Compatibility of medication and solution prevents complications. Delivers the correct dose of medication as prescribed.
2. Know the actions, special nursing considerations, safe dose ranges, purpose of administration, and adverse effects of the medications to be administered. Consider the appropriateness of the medication for this patient.	This knowledge aids the nurse in evaluating the therapeutic effect of the medication in relation to the patient's disorder and can also be used to educate the patient about the medication.
3. Perform hand hygiene. 	Hand hygiene prevents the spread of microorganisms.
4. Move the medication cart to the outside of the patient's room or prepare for administration in the medication area.	Organization facilitates error-free administration and saves time.
5. Unlock the medication cart or drawer. Enter pass code	Locking the cart or drawer safeguards each patient's medication

ACTION	RATIONALE
and scan employee identification, if required.	supply. Hospital accrediting organizations require medication carts to be locked when not in use. Entering pass code and scanning ID allows only authorized users into the system and identifies the user for documentation by the computer.
6. **Prepare medication for one patient at a time.**	This prevents errors in medication administration.
7. Read the CMAR/MAR and select the proper medication from unit stock or the patient's medication drawer.	This is the *first* check of the label.
8. Compare the label with the CMAR/MAR. Check expiration dates and perform calculations, if necessary. Scan the bar code on the package, if required.	This is the *second* check of the label. Verify calculations with another nurse to ensure safety, if necessary.
9. If necessary, withdraw medication from an ampule or vial as described in Skills 103 and 104.	
10. **Depending on facility policy, the third check of the label may occur at this point. If so, when all medications for one patient have been prepared, recheck the labels with the CMAR/MAR before taking the medications to the patient.**	This *third* check ensures accuracy and helps to prevent errors. *Note:* Many facilities require the *third* check to occur at the bedside, after identifying the patient and before administration.
11. Lock the medication cart before leaving it.	Locking the cart or drawer safeguards the patient's medication supply. Hospital accrediting organizations require medication carts to be locked when not in use.
12. Transport medications and equipment to the patient's bedside carefully, and keep the medications in sight at all times.	Careful handling and close observation prevent accidental or deliberate disarrangement of medications. Having equipment available saves time and facilitates performance of the task.

ACTION	RATIONALE
13. Ensure that the patient receives the medications at the correct time.	Check agency policy, which may allow for administration within a period of 30 minutes before or 30 minutes after the designated time.
14. Perform hand hygiene and put on PPE, if indicated.	Hand hygiene and PPE prevent the spread of microorganisms. PPE is required based on transmission precautions.
15. Identify the patient. Compare the information with the CMAR/MAR. The patient should be identified using at least two methods (The Joint Commission, 2013):	Identifying the patient ensures the right patient receives the medications and helps prevent errors. The patient's room number or physical location is not used as an identifier (The Joint Commission, 2013). Replace the identification band if it is missing or inaccurate in any way.
a. Check the name on the patient's identification band.	
b. Check the identification number on the patient's identification band.	
c. Check the birth date on the patient's identification band.	
d. Ask the patient to state his or her name and birth date, based on facility policy.	This requires a response from the patient, but illness and strange surroundings often cause patients to be confused.
16. Close the door to the room or pull the bedside curtain.	This provides patient privacy.
17. Complete necessary assessments before administering medications. Check the patient's allergy bracelet or ask the patient about allergies. Explain the purpose and action of the medication to the patient.	Assessment is a prerequisite to administration of medications. Explanation provides rationale, increases knowledge, and reduces anxiety.
18. Scan the patient's bar code on the identification band, if required.	Provides an additional check to ensure that the medication is given to the right patient.

ACTION	RATIONALE
19. Based on facility policy, the third check of the label may occur at this point. If so, recheck the label with the CMAR/MAR before administering the medications to the patient.	Many facilities require the *third* check to occur at the bedside, after identifying the patient and before administration. If facility policy directs the *third* check at this time, this *third* check ensures accuracy and helps to prevent errors.
20. Assess IV site for presence of inflammation or infiltration.	IV medication must be given directly into a vein for safe administration.
21. If IV infusion is being administered via an infusion pump, pause the pump.	Pausing prevents infusion of fluid during bolus administration and activation of pump occlusion alarms.
22. Put on clean gloves.	Gloves prevent contact with blood and body fluids.
23. Select injection port on tubing that is closest to venipuncture site. Clean port with antimicrobial swab.	Using port closest to the needle insertion site minimizes dilution of medication. Cleaning deters entry of microorganisms when port is punctured.
24. Uncap syringe. Steady port with your nondominant hand while inserting syringe into center of port.	This supports the injection port and lessens the risk for accidentally dislodging the IV or entering the port incorrectly.
25. Move your nondominant hand to the section of IV tubing just above the injection port. Fold the tubing between your fingers.	This temporarily stops flow of gravity IV infusion and prevents medication from backing up tubing.
26. Pull back slightly on plunger just until blood appears in tubing.	This ensures injection of medication into the bloodstream.
27. **Inject the medication at the recommended rate.**	This delivers the correct amount of medication at the proper interval according to manufacturer's directions.
28. Release the tubing. Remove the syringe. Do not recap the used needle, if used. Engage the safety shield or needle guard, if present.	Proper disposal of the needle prevents injury.

ACTION	RATIONALE
Release the tubing and allow the IV fluid to flow. Discard the needle and syringe in the appropriate receptacle.	
29. Check IV fluid infusion rate. Restart infusion pump, if appropriate.	Injection of bolus may alter fluid infusion rate, if infusing by gravity.
30. Remove gloves and additional PPE, if used. Perform hand hygiene.	Removing PPE properly reduces the risk for infection transmission and contamination of other items. Hand hygiene prevents the spread of microorganisms.
31. Document the administration of the medication immediately after administration. See Documentation section below.	Timely documentation helps to ensure patient safety.
32. Evaluate the patient's response to the medication within the appropriate time frame.	The patient needs to be evaluated for therapeutic and adverse effects from the medication.

EVALUATION

• Medication is safely administered via IV bolus.
• Patient's anxiety is decreased.
• Patient does not experience adverse effects.
• Patient understands and complies with the medication regimen.

DOCUMENTATION

• Document the administration of the medication immediately after administration, including date, time, dose, route of administration, site of administration, and rate of administration on the CMAR/MAR or record using the required format. If using a bar-code system, medication administration is automatically recorded when the bar code is scanned. PRN medications require documentation of the reason for administration. Prompt recording avoids the possibility of accidentally repeating the administration of the drug. If the drug was refused or omitted, record this in the appropriate area on the medication record and notify the primary care provider. This verifies the reason medication was omitted and ensures that the primary care provider is aware of the patient's condition.

SKILL 102 | MIXING MEDICATIONS FROM TWO VIALS IN ONE SYRINGE

Preparation of medications in one syringe depends on how the medication is supplied. When using a single-dose vial and a multidose vial, air is injected into both vials and the medication in the multidose vial is drawn into the syringe first. This prevents the contents of the multidose vial from being contaminated with the medication in the single-dose vial. The CDC recommends that medications packaged as multiuse vials be assigned to a single patient whenever possible (CDC, 2011b). In addition, it is recommended that the top of the vial be cleaned before each entry, and that a new sterile needle and syringe are used before each entry.

When considering mixing two medications in one syringe, you must ensure that the two drugs are compatible. Be aware of drug incompatibilities when preparing medications in one syringe. Certain medications, such as diazepam (Valium), are incompatible with other drugs in the same syringe. Incompatible drugs may become cloudy or form a precipitate in the syringe. Such medications are discarded and prepared again in separate syringes. Other drugs have limited compatibility and should be administered within 15 minutes of preparation. Mixing more than two drugs in one syringe is not recommended. If it must be done, contact the pharmacist to determine the compatibility of the three drugs, as well as the compatibility of their pH values and the preservatives that may be present in each drug. A drug-compatibility table should be available to nurses who are preparing medications.

Insulin, with many types available for use, is an example of a medication that may be combined together in one syringe for injection. Insulins vary in their onset and duration of action and are classified as rapid acting, short acting, intermediate acting, and long acting. Before administering any insulin, be aware of the onset time, peak, and duration of effects, and ensure that proper food is available. Be aware that some insulins, such as Lantus and Levemir, cannot be mixed with other insulins. Refer to a drug reference for a listing of the different types of insulin and action specific to each type. Insulin dosages are calculated in units. The scale commonly used is U100, which is based on 100 units of insulin contained in 1 mL of solution.

DELEGATION CONSIDERATIONS

The preparation of medication from two vials is not delegated to nursing assistive personnel (NAP) or to unlicensed assistive personnel (UAP). Depending on the state's nurse practice act and the organization's policies and procedures, the preparation of medication from two vials may be delegated to licensed practical/vocational nurses (LPN/LVNs). The decision to delegate must be based on careful analysis of the patient's needs and circumstances, as well as the qualifications of the person to whom the task is being delegated. Refer to the Delegation Guidelines in Appendix A.

EQUIPMENT

The preparation of two types of insulin in one syringe is used as the example in the following procedure.
- Two vials of medication (insulin in this example)
- Sterile syringe (insulin syringe in this example)
- Antimicrobial swabs
- Computer-generated Medication Administration Record (CMAR) or Medication Administration Record (MAR)

ASSESSMENT

- Determine the compatibility of the two medications. Not all insulin can be mixed together. For example, Lantus and Levemir cannot be mixed with another insulin.
- Assess the contents of each vial of insulin. It is very important to be familiar with the particular drug's properties to be able to assess the quality of the medication in the vial before withdrawal. Unmodified preparations of insulin typically appear as clear substances, so they should be without particles or foreign matter. Modified preparations of insulin are typically suspensions, so they do not appear as clear substances.
- Check the expiration date before administering the medication.
- Assess the appropriateness of the drug for the patient.
- Review the assessment and laboratory data that may influence drug administration. Check the patient's blood glucose level, if appropriate, before administering the insulin.
- Verify patient name, dose, route, and time of administration.

NURSING DIAGNOSIS

- Risk for Infection
- Deficient Knowledge
- Risk for Injury

OUTCOME IDENTIFICATION AND PLANNING

- Accurate withdrawal of the medication into a syringe in a sterile manner.
- Proper dose is prepared.

IMPLEMENTATION

ACTION	RATIONALE
1. Gather equipment. Check medication order against the original order in the medical record, according to facility policy.	This comparison helps to identify errors that may have occurred when orders were transcribed. The primary care provider's order is the legal record

ACTION	RATIONALE
	of medication orders for each facility.
2. Know the actions, special nursing considerations, safe dose ranges, purpose of administration, and adverse effects of the medications to be administered. Consider the appropriateness of the medication for this patient.	This knowledge aids the nurse in evaluating the therapeutic effect of the medication in relation to the patient's disorder and can also be used to educate the patient about the medication.
3. Perform hand hygiene.	Hand hygiene prevents the spread of microorganisms.
4. Move the medication cart to the outside of the patient's room or prepare for administration in the medication area.	Organization facilitates error-free administration and saves time.
5. Unlock the medication cart or drawer. Enter pass code and scan employee identification, if required.	Locking the cart or drawer safeguards each patient's medication supply. Hospital accrediting organizations require medication carts to be locked when not in use. Entering pass code and scanning ID allows only authorized users into the system and identifies the user for documentation by the computer.
6. **Prepare medications for one patient at a time.**	This prevents errors in medication administration.
7. Read the CMAR/MAR and select the proper medications from unit stock or the patient's medication drawer.	This is the *first* check of the label.
8. Compare the labels with the CMAR/MAR. Check expiration dates and perform dosage calculations, if necessary. Scan the bar code on the package, if required.	This is the *second* check of the labels. Verify calculations with another nurse to ensure safety, if necessary.
9. If necessary, remove the cap that protects the rubber stopper on each vial.	The cap protects the rubber top.

ACTION	RATIONALE
10. **If medication is a suspension (e.g., a modified insulin, such as NPH insulin), roll and agitate the vial to mix it well.**	There is controversy regarding how to mix insulin in suspension. Some sources advise rolling the vial; others advise shaking the vial. Consult facility policy. Regardless of the method used, it is essential that the suspension be mixed well to avoid administering an inconsistent dose.
11. **Cleanse the rubber tops with antimicrobial swabs.** Allow the top to dry.	Antimicrobial swab removes surface bacteria contamination. Allowing the alcohol to dry prevents it from entering the vial on the needle.
12. Remove cap from needle by pulling it straight off. Touch the plunger only at the knob. Draw back an amount of air into the syringe that is equal to the dose of modified insulin to be withdrawn.	Pulling the cap off in a straight manner prevents accidental needlestick. Handling the plunger only by the knob ensures sterility of the shaft of the plunger. Before fluid is removed, injection of an equal amount of air is required to prevent the formation of a partial vacuum, because a vial is a sealed container. If not enough air is injected, the negative pressure makes it difficult to withdraw the medication.
13. Hold the modified vial on a flat surface. Pierce the rubber stopper in the center with the needle tip and inject the measured air into the space above the solution. Do not inject air into the solution. Withdraw the needle.	Unmodified insulin should never be contaminated with modified insulin. Placing air in the modified insulin first without allowing the needle to contact the insulin ensures that the second vial-entered (unmodified) insulin is not contaminated by the medication in the other vial. Air bubbled through the solution could result in withdrawal of an inaccurate amount of medication.
14. Draw back an amount of air into the syringe that is equal to the dose of unmodified insulin to be withdrawn.	A vial is a sealed container. Therefore, injection of an equal amount of air (before fluid is removed) is required to prevent the formation of a partial vacuum. If not enough air is

ACTION	RATIONALE
	injected, the negative pressure makes it difficult to withdraw the medication.
15. Hold the unmodified vial on a flat surface. Pierce the rubber stopper in the center with the needle tip and inject the measured air into the space above the solution. Do not inject air into the solution. Keep the needle in the vial.	Air bubbled through the solution could result in withdrawal of an inaccurate amount of medication.
16. Invert the vial of unmodified insulin. Hold the vial in one hand and use the other to withdraw the medication. **Touch the plunger only at the knob. Draw up the prescribed amount of medication while holding the syringe at eye level and vertically.** Turn the vial over and then remove the needle from the vial.	Holding the syringe at eye level facilitates accurate reading, and the vertical position allows easy removal of air bubbles from the syringe. First dose is prepared and is not contaminated by insulin that contains modifiers.
17. Check that there are no air bubbles in the syringe.	The presence of air in the syringe would result in an inaccurate dose of medication.
18. **Check the amount of medication in the syringe with the medication dose and discard any surplus.**	Careful measurement ensures that correct dose is withdrawn.
19. **Recheck the vial label with the CMAR/MAR.**	This is the *third* check to ensure accuracy and to prevent errors. It must be checked now for the first medication in the syringe, as it is not possible to ensure accuracy once a second drug is in the syringe.
20. Calculate the endpoint on the syringe for the combined insulin amount by adding the number of units for each dose together.	Allows for accurate withdrawal of the second dose.
21. Insert the needle into the modified vial and invert it,	Previous addition of air eliminates need to create positive

ACTION	RATIONALE
taking care not to push the plunger and inject medication from the syringe into the vial. Invert vial of modified insulin. Hold the vial in one hand and use the other to withdraw the medication. **Touch the plunger only at the knob. Draw up the prescribed amount of medication while holding the syringe at eye level and vertically. Take care to withdraw only the prescribed amount.** Turn the vial over and then remove the needle from the vial. Carefully recap the needle. Carefully replace the cap over the needle.	pressure. Holding the syringe at eye level facilitates accurate reading. Capping the needle prevents contamination and protects the nurse against accidental needlesticks. A one-handed recap method may be used as long as care is taken to ensure that the needle remains sterile.
22. **Check the amount of medication in the syringe with the medication dose.**	Careful measurement ensures that correct dose is withdrawn.
23. **Depending on facility policy, the third check of the label may occur at this point. If so, recheck the label with the MAR before taking the medications to the patient.**	This *third* check ensures accuracy and helps to prevent errors. *Note:* Many facilities require the *third* check to occur at the bedside, after identifying the patient and before administration.
24. **Label the vials with the date and time opened, and store the vials containing the remaining medication according to facility policy.**	Because the vial is sealed, the medication inside remains sterile and can be used for future injections. Labeling the opened vials with a date and time limits its use after a specific time period. The CDC recommends that medications packaged as multiuse vials be assigned to a single patient whenever possible (CDC, 2011).
25. Lock medication cart before leaving it.	Locking the cart or drawer safeguards the patient's medication supply. Hospital accrediting organizations require medication carts to be locked when not in use.

EVALUATION

- Medication is withdrawn into a syringe in a sterile manner, and the proper dose is prepared.

DOCUMENTATION

- It is not necessary to record the removal of the medication from the ampule. Prompt recording of administration of the medication is required immediately after it is administered.

SKILL 103 | REMOVING MEDICATION FROM AN AMPULE

An ampule is a glass flask that contains a single dose of medication for parenteral administration. Because there is no way to prevent contamination of any unused portion of medication after the ampule is opened, discard any remaining medication if not all the medication is used for the prescribed dose. You must break the thin neck of the ampule to remove the medication.

DELEGATION CONSIDERATIONS

The preparation of medication from an ampule is not delegated to nursing assistive personnel (NAP) or to unlicensed assistive personnel (UAP). Depending on the state's nurse practice act and the organization's policies and procedures, the preparation of medication from an ampule may be delegated to a licensed practical/vocational nurse (LPN/LVN). The decision to delegate must be based on careful analysis of the patient's needs and circumstances, as well as the qualifications of the person to whom the task is being delegated. Refer to the Delegation Guidelines in Appendix A.

EQUIPMENT

- Sterile syringe and filter needle
- Ampule of medication
- Small gauze pad

- Computer-generated Medication Administration Record (CMAR) or Medication Administration Record (MAR)

ASSESSMENT

- Assess the medication in the ampule for any particles or discoloration. Assess the ampule for any cracks or chips.
- Check expiration date before administering the medication.
- Verify patient name, dose, route, and time of administration.
- Assess the appropriateness of the drug for the patient.
- Review assessment and laboratory data that may influence drug administration.

NURSING DIAGNOSIS

- Risk for Infection
- Deficient Knowledge
- Risk for Injury

OUTCOME IDENTIFICATION AND PLANNING

- Medication will be removed in a sterile manner.
- Medication will be free from glass shards.
- Proper dose will be prepared.

IMPLEMENTATION

ACTION	RATIONALE
1. Gather equipment. Check the medication order against the original order in the medical record, according to facility policy. Clarify any inconsistencies. Check the patient's chart for allergies.	This comparison helps to identify errors that may have occurred when orders were transcribed. The primary care provider's order is the legal record of medication orders for each facility.
2. Know the actions, special nursing considerations, safe dose ranges, purpose of administration, and adverse effects of the medications to be administered. Consider the appropriateness of the medication for this patient.	This knowledge aids the nurse in evaluating the therapeutic effect of the medication in relation to the patient's disorder and can also be used to educate the patient about the medication.
3. Perform hand hygiene.	Hand hygiene prevents the spread of microorganisms.
4. Move the medication cart to the outside of the patient's	Organization facilitates error-free administration and saves time.

ACTION	RATIONALE
room or prepare for administration in the medication area.	
5. Unlock the medication cart or drawer. Enter pass code and scan employee identification, if required.	Locking the cart or drawer safeguards each patient's medication supply. Hospital accrediting organizations require medication carts to be locked when not in use. Entering pass code and scanning ID allows only authorized users into the computer system and identifies the user for documentation by the computer.
6. **Prepare medications for one patient at a time.**	This prevents errors in medication administration.
7. Read the CMAR/MAR and select the proper medication from unit stock or the patient's medication drawer.	This is the *first* check of the label.
8. Compare the label with the CMAR/MAR. Check expiration dates and perform calculations, if necessary. Scan the bar code on the package, if required.	This is the *second* check of the label. Verify calculations with another nurse to ensure safety, if necessary.
9. Tap the stem of the ampule or twist your wrist quickly while holding the ampule vertically.	This facilitates movement of medication in the stem to the body of the ampule.
10. Wrap a small gauze pad around the neck of the ampule.	This will protect your fingers from the glass as the ampule is broken.
11. Use a snapping motion to break off the top of the ampule along the scored line at its neck. **Always break away from your body.**	This protects your face and fingers from any shattered glass fragments.
12. Attach filter needle to syringe. Remove the cap from the filter needle by pulling it straight off.	Use of a filter needle prevents the accidental withdrawing of small glass particles with the medication. Pulling the cap off in a straight manner prevents accidental needlestick.

ACTION	RATIONALE
13. Withdraw medication in the amount ordered plus a small amount more (approximately 30% more). **Do not inject air into the solution. While inserting the filter needle into the ampule, be careful not to touch the rim.** Use either of the following methods to withdraw the medication:	By withdrawing an additional small amount of medication, any air bubbles in the syringe can be displaced once the syringe is removed while allowing ample medication to remain in the syringe. The contents of the ampule are not under pressure; therefore, air is unnecessary and will cause the contents to overflow. The rim of the ampule is considered contaminated.
a. Insert the tip of the needle into the ampule, which is upright on a flat surface, and withdraw fluid into the syringe. **Touch the plunger only at the knob.**	Handling the plunger only at the knob will keep the shaft of the plunger sterile.
b. Insert the tip of the needle into the ampule and invert the ampule. Keep the needle centered and not touching the sides of the ampule. Withdraw fluid into syringe. **Touch the plunger only at the knob.**	Surface tension holds the fluids in the ampule when inverted. If the needle touches the sides or is removed and then reinserted into the ampule, surface tension is broken, and fluid runs out. Handling the plunger only at the knob will keep the shaft of the plunger sterile.
14. Wait until the needle has been withdrawn to tap the syringe and expel the air carefully by pushing on the plunger. **Check the amount of medication in the syringe with the medication dose and discard any surplus, according to facility policy.**	Ejecting air into the solution increases pressure in the ampule and can force the medication to spill out over the ampule. Ampules may have overfill. Careful measurement ensures that the correct dose is withdrawn.
15. **Depending on facility policy, the third check of the label may occur at this point. If so, when all medications for one patient have been prepared, recheck the labels with the CMAR/MAR before taking the medications to the patient.**	This *third* check ensures accuracy and helps to prevent errors. *Note:* Many facilities require the *third* check to occur at the bedside, after identifying the patient and before administration.

ACTION	RATIONALE
16. **Engage safety guard on filter needle and remove the needle. Discard the filter needle in a suitable container. Attach appropriate administration device to syringe.**	The filter needle used to draw up medication should not be used to administer the medication. This will prevent any glass shards from entering the patient during administration.
17. Discard the ampule in a suitable container.	Any medication that has not been removed from the ampule must be discarded because sterility of contents cannot be maintained in an opened ampule.
18. Lock the medication cart before leaving it.	Locking the cart or drawer safeguards the patient's medication supply. Hospital accrediting organizations require medication carts to be locked when not in use.
19. Perform hand hygiene.	Hand hygiene deters the spread of microorganisms.
20. Proceed with administration, based on prescribed route.	See appropriate skill for prescribed route.

EVALUATION

• Medication is removed from the ampule in a sterile manner, is free from glass shards, and the proper dose is prepared.

• It is not necessary to record the removal of the medication from the ampule. Prompt recording of administration of the medication is required immediately after it is administered.

A vial is a glass bottle with a self-sealing stopper through which medication is removed. For safety in transporting and storing, the vial top is usually covered with a soft metal cap that can be removed easily. The self-sealing stopper that is then exposed is the means of entrance into the vial. Single-dose vials are used once, and then discarded, regardless of the amount of the drug that is used from the vial. Multidose vials contain several doses of medication and can be used multiple times. The Centers for Disease Control and Prevention (CDC) recommends that medications packaged as multiuse vials be assigned to a single patient whenever possible (CDC, 2011). In addition, it is recommended that the top of the vial be cleaned before each entry, and that a new sterile needle and syringe are used for each entry. The medication contained in a vial can be in liquid or powder form. Powdered forms must be dissolved in an appropriate diluent before administration. The following skill reviews removing liquid medication from a vial. Refer to the accompanying Skill Variation for steps to reconstitute powdered medication.

DELEGATION CONSIDERATIONS

The preparation of medication from a vial is not delegated to nursing assistive personnel (NAP) or to unlicensed assistive personnel (UAP). Depending on the state's nurse practice act and the organization's policies and procedures, the preparation of medication from a vial may be delegated to licensed practical/vocational nurses (LPN/LVNs). The decision to delegate must be based on careful analysis of the patient's needs and circumstances, as well as the qualifications of the person to whom the task is being delegated. Refer to the Delegation Guidelines in Appendix A.

EQUIPMENT

- Sterile syringe and needle or blunt cannula (size depends on medication being administered)
- Vial of medication
- Antimicrobial swab
- Second needle (optional)
- Filter needle (optional)
- Computer-generated Medication Administration Record (CMAR) or Medication Administration Record (MAR)

ASSESSMENT

- Assess the medication in the vial for any discoloration or particles.
- Check expiration date before administering medication.
- Verify patient name, dose, route, and time of administration.
- Assess the appropriateness of the drug for the patient.
- Review assessment and laboratory data that may influence drug administration.

NURSING DIAGNOSIS

- Risk for Infection
- Deficient Knowledge
- Risk for Injury

OUTCOME IDENTIFICATION AND PLANNING

- Withdrawal of the medication into a syringe in a sterile manner.
- Proper dose is prepared.

ACTION	RATIONALE
	users into the system and identifies the user for documentation by the computer.
6. **Prepare medications for one patient at a time.**	This prevents errors in medication administration.
7. Read the CMAR/MAR and select the proper medication from unit stock or the patient's medication drawer.	This is the *first* check of the label.
8. Compare the label with the CMAR/MAR. Check expiration dates and perform calculations, if necessary. Scan the bar code on the package, if required.	This is the *second* check of the label. Verify calculations with another nurse to ensure safety, if necessary.
9. Remove the metal or plastic cap on the vial that protects the rubber stopper.	Cap needs to be removed to access medication in the vial.
10. **Swab the rubber top with the antimicrobial swab and allow to dry.**	Antimicrobial swab removes surface bacteria contamination. Allowing the alcohol to dry prevents it from entering the vial on the needle.
11. Remove the cap from the needle or blunt cannula by pulling it straight off. Touch the plunger only at the knob. Draw back an amount of air into the syringe that is equal to the specific dose of medication to be withdrawn. Some facilities require use of a filter needle when withdrawing premixed medication from multidose vials.	Pulling the cap off in a straight manner prevents accidental needlestick injury. Handling the plunger only at the knob will keep the shaft of the plunger sterile. Because a vial is a sealed container, injection of an equal amount of air (before fluid is removed) is required to prevent the formation of a partial vacuum. If not enough air is injected, the negative pressure makes it difficult to withdraw the medication. Using a filter needle prevents any solid material from being withdrawn through the needle.
12. Hold the vial on a flat surface. Pierce the rubber stopper in the center with the needle tip and inject the	Air bubbled through the solution could result in withdrawal of an inaccurate amount of medication.

ACTION	RATIONALE
measured air into the space above the solution. Do not inject air into the solution.	
13. Invert the vial. **Keep the tip of the needle or blunt cannula below the fluid level.**	This prevents air from being aspirated into the syringe.
14. Hold the vial in one hand and use the other to withdraw the medication. **Touch the plunger only at the knob. Draw up the prescribed amount of medication while holding the syringe vertically and at eye level.**	Handling the plunger only at the knob will keep the shaft of the plunger sterile. Holding the syringe at eye level facilitates accurate reading, and the vertical position makes removal of air bubbles from the syringe easy.
15. If any air bubbles accumulate in the syringe, tap the barrel of the syringe sharply and move the needle past the fluid into the air space to re-inject the air bubble into the vial. Return the needle tip to the solution and continue withdrawal of the medication.	Removal of air bubbles is necessary to ensure an accurate dose of medication.
16. After the correct dose is withdrawn, remove the needle from the vial and carefully replace the cap over the needle. **If a filter needle has been used to draw up the medication, remove it and attach the appropriate administration device.** Some facilities require changing the needle, if one was used to withdraw the medication, before administering the medication.	This prevents contamination of the needle and protects against accidental needlesticks. A one-handed recap method may be used as long as care is taken not to contaminate the needle during the process. A filter needle used to draw up medication should not be used to administer the medication to prevent any solid material from entering the patient. Changing the needle may be necessary because passing the needle through the stopper on the vial may dull the needle. In addition, it ensures the tip of the needle is free from medication residue, significantly reducing pain intensity associated with the injection (Ağaç & Güneş, 2010).

ACTION	RATIONALE
17. **Check the amount of medication in the syringe with the medication dose and discard any surplus.**	Careful measurement ensures that the correct dose is withdrawn.
18. **Depending on facility policy, the third check of the label may occur at this point. If so, when all medications for one patient have been prepared, recheck the labels with the CMAR/MAR before taking the medications to the patient.**	This *third* check ensures accuracy and helps to prevent errors. *Note:* Many facilities require the *third* check to occur at the bedside, after identifying the patient and before administration.
19. **If a multidose vial is being used, label the vial with the date and time opened, and store the vial containing the remaining medication according to facility policy.**	Because the vial is sealed, the medication inside remains sterile and can be used for future injections. Labeling the opened vials with a date and time limits its use after a specific time period.
20. **Lock the medication cart before leaving it.**	Locking the cart or drawer safeguards the patient's medication supply. Hospital accrediting organizations require medication carts to be locked when not in use.
21. Perform hand hygiene.	Hand hygiene deters the spread of microorganisms.
22. Proceed with administration, based on prescribed route.	See appropriate skill for prescribed route.

EVALUATION

- Medication is withdrawn into the syringe in a sterile manner and the proper dose is prepared.

DOCUMENTATION

- It is not necessary to record the removal of the medication from the ampule. Prompt recording of administration of the medication is required immediately after it is administered.

Drugs that are unstable in liquid form are often provided in a dry powder form. The powder must be mixed with the correct amount of appropriate solution to prepare the medication for administration. Verify the correct amount and correct solution type for the specific medication prescribed. This information is found on the vial label, package insert, in a drug reference, an on-line pharmacy source, or from the pharmacist. To reconstitute powdered medication:

1. Gather equipment. Check the medication order against the original order in the medical record, according to agency policy.

2. Know the actions, special nursing considerations, safe dose ranges, purpose of administration, and adverse effects of the medications to be administered. Consider the appropriateness of the medication for this patient.

3. Perform hand hygiene.

4. Move the medication cart to the outside of the patient's room or prepare for administration in the medication area.

5. Unlock the medication cart or drawer. Enter pass code and scan employee identification, if required.

6. **Prepare medications for one patient at a time.**

7. Read the CMAR/MAR and select the proper medication and diluent from unit stock or from the patient's medication drawer. This is the *first* check of the medication label.

8. Compare the labels with the CMAR/MAR. This is the *second* check of the medication label. Check expiration dates and perform calculations, check medication calculation with another nurse. Scan the bar code on the package, if required.

9. Remove the metal or plastic cap on the medication vial and diluent vial that protects the self-sealing stoppers.

10. Swab the self-sealing tops with the antimicrobial swab and allow to dry.

11. **Draw up the appropriate amount of diluent into the syringe.**

12. Insert the needle or blunt cannula through the center of the self-sealing stopper on the powdered medication vial.

13. Inject the diluent into the powdered medication vial.

14. Remove the needle or blunt cannula from the vial and replace cap.

15. **Gently agitate the vial to mix the powdered medication and the diluent completely. Do not shake the vial.**

16. **Draw up the prescribed amount of medication**

Reconstituting Powdered Medication in a Vial *continued*

while holding the syringe vertically and at eye level.

17. After the correct dose is withdrawn, remove the needle from the vial and carefully replace the cap over the needle. If a filter needle has been used to draw up the medication, remove it and attach the appropriate administration device. Some facilities require changing the needle, if one was used to withdraw the medication, before administering the medication.

18. **Check the amount of medication in the syringe**

with the medication dose and discard any surplus.

19. Depending on facility policy, the *third* check of the label may occur at this point. If so, recheck the label with the CMAR/MAR before taking the medications to the patient.

20. Lock the medication cart before leaving it.

21. Perform hand hygiene.

22. Proceed with administration, based on prescribed route.

SKILL 105 | APPLYING A TRANSDERMAL PATCH

The transdermal route is being used more frequently to deliver medication. A disk or patch that contains medication intended for daily use or longer is applied to the patient's skin. Transdermal patches are commonly used to deliver hormones, opioid analgesics, cardiac medications, and nicotine. Medication errors have occurred when patients apply multiple patches at once or fail to remove the overlay on the patch that exposes the skin to the medication. Opioid analgesic patches are associated with the most adverse drug effects. Clear patches have a cosmetic advantage, but they can be difficult to find on the patient's skin when they need to be removed or replaced.

DELEGATION CONSIDERATIONS

The administration of medication via a transdermal patch is not delegated to nursing assistive personnel (NAP) or to unlicensed assistive personnel (UAP). Depending on the state's nurse practice act and the organization's policies and procedures, the administration of a transdermal patch may be delegated to licensed practical/vocational nurses (LPN/LVNs). The decision to delegate must be based on careful analysis of the patient's needs and circumstances, as well as the qualifications of the person to whom the task is being delegated. Refer to the Delegation Guidelines in Appendix A.

EQUIPMENT

- Medication patch
- Disposable gloves
- Scissors (optional)
- Washcloth, soap, and water
- Computer-generated Medication Administration Record
- (CMAR) or Medication Administration Record (MAR)
- Additional PPE, as indicated

ASSESSMENT

- Assess the patient for any allergies.
- Check the expiration date before administering the medication.
- Assess the appropriateness of the drug for the patient.
- Review assessment and laboratory data that may influence drug administration.
- Verify patient name, dose, route, and time of administration.
- Assess the skin at the location where the patch will be applied. Many patches have different and specific instructions for where the patch is to be placed. For example, transdermal patches that contain estrogen cannot be placed on breast tissue.
- Check the manufacturer's instructions for the appropriate location for the patch.
- The site should be clean, dry, and free of hair. Do not place transdermal patches on irritated or broken skin.
- Assess the patient for any old patches. Do not place a new transdermal patch until old patches have been removed.
- Verify the application frequency for the specific medication.
- Assess the patient's knowledge of the medication. If the patient has a knowledge deficit about the medication, this may be the appropriate time to begin education about the medication.
- If the medication may affect the patient's vital signs, assess them before administration.
- If the medication is for pain relief, assess the patient's pain before and after administration.

NURSING DIAGNOSIS

- Risk for Allergy Response
- Risk for Impaired Skin Integrity
- Deficient Knowledge

OUTCOME IDENTIFICATION AND PLANNING

- Medication is delivered via the transdermal route.
- Patient experiences no adverse effect.
- Patient's skin remains free from injury.
- Patient understands and complies with the medication regimen.

IMPLEMENTATION

ACTION	RATIONALE
1. Gather equipment. Check medication order against the original order in the medical record, according to facility policy. Clarify any inconsistencies. Check the patient's chart for allergies.	This comparison helps to identify errors that may have occurred when orders were transcribed. The primary care provider's order is the legal record of medication orders for each facility.
2. Know the actions, special nursing considerations, safe dose ranges, purpose of administration, and adverse effects of the medications to be administered. Consider the appropriateness of the medication for this patient.	This knowledge aids the nurse in evaluating the therapeutic effect of the medication in relation to the patient's disorder and can also be used to educate the patient about the medication.
3. Perform hand hygiene.	Hand hygiene prevents the spread of microorganisms.
4. Move the medication cart to the outside of the patient's room or prepare for administration in the medication area.	Organization facilitates error-free administration and saves time.
5. Unlock the medication cart or drawer. Enter pass code and scan employee identification, if required.	Locking the cart or drawer safeguards each patient's medication supply. Hospital accrediting organizations require medication carts to be locked when not in use. Entering pass code and scanning ID allows only authorized users into the system and identifies the user for documentation by the computer.
6. **Prepare medications for one patient at a time.**	This prevents errors in medication administration.
7. Read the CMAR/MAR and select the proper medication from unit stock or the patient's medication drawer.	This is the *first* check of the label.

ACTION	RATIONALE
8. Compare the label with the CMAR/MAR. Check expiration dates and perform calculations, if necessary. Scan the bar code on the package, if required.	This is the *second* check of the label. Verify calculations with another nurse to ensure safety, if necessary.
9. **Depending on facility policy, the third check of the label may occur at this point. If so, when all medications for one patient have been prepared, recheck the labels with the CMAR/MAR before taking the medications to the patient.**	This *third* check ensures accuracy and helps to prevent errors. *Note:* Many facilities require the *third* check to occur at the bedside, after identifying the patient and before administration.
10. Lock the medication cart before leaving it.	Locking the cart or drawer safeguards the patient's medication supply. Hospital accrediting organizations require medication carts to be locked when not in use.
11. Transport medications to the patient's bedside carefully, and keep the medications in sight at all times.	Careful handling and close observation prevent accidental or deliberate disarrangement of medications.
12. **Ensure that the patient receives the medications at the correct time.**	Check agency policy, which may allow for administration within a period of 30 minutes before or 30 minutes after the designated time.
13. Perform hand hygiene and put on PPE, if indicated.	Hand hygiene and PPE prevent the spread of microorganisms. PPE is required based on transmission precautions.
14. **Identify the patient. Compare the information with the CMAR/MAR. The patient should be identified using at least two methods** (The Joint Commission, 2013):	Identifying the patient ensures the right patient receives the medications and helps prevent errors. The patient's room number or physical location is not used as an identifier (The Joint Commission, 2013). Replace the identification band if it is missing or inaccurate in any way.

ACTION	RATIONALE
a. Check the name on the patient's identification band.	
b. Check the identification number on the patient's identification band.	
c. Check the birth date on the patient's identification band.	
d. Ask the patient to state his or her name and birth date, based on facility policy.	This requires a response from the patient, but illness and strange surroundings often cause patients to be confused.
15. **Complete necessary assessments before administering medications. Check the patient's allergy bracelet or ask the patient about allergies. Explain the purpose and action of each medication to the patient.**	Assessment is a prerequisite to administration of medications.
16. Scan the patient's bar code on the identification band, if required.	This provides an additional check to ensure that the medication is given to the right patient.
17. **Based on facility policy, the third check of the label may occur at this point. If so, recheck the labels with the CMAR/MAR before administering the medications to the patient.**	Many facilities require the *third* check to occur at the bedside, after identifying the patient and before administration. If facility policy directs the *third* check at this time, this *third* check ensures accuracy and helps to prevent errors.
18. Put on gloves.	Gloves protect the nurse when handling the medication on the transdermal patch.
19. Assess the patient's skin where patch is to be placed, looking for any signs of irritation or breakdown. Site should be clean, dry, and free of hair. Rotate application sites.	Transdermal patches should not be placed on skin that is irritated or broken down. Hair can prevent the patch from sticking to the skin. Rotating sites reduces risk for skin irritation.
20. **Remove any old transdermal patches from the patient's skin.** Fold the old patch in half with the adhesive sides sticking together	Leaving old patches on a patient while applying new ones may lead to delivery of a toxic level of the drug. Folding sides together prevents accidental contact with

ACTION	RATIONALE
and discard according to facility policy. Gently wash the area where the old patch was with soap and water.	remaining medication. Washing area with soap and water removes all traces of medication in that area.
21. Remove the patch from its protective covering. Remove the covering on the patch without touching the medication surface. Apply the patch to the patient's skin. Use the palm of your hand to press firmly for about 10 seconds. Do not massage.	Touching the adhesive side may alter the amount of medication left on the patch. Pressing firmly for 10 seconds ensures that the patch stays on the patient's skin. Massaging the site may increase absorption of the medication.
22. Depending on facility policy, initial and write the date and time of administration on a piece of medical tape. Apply the tape to the patient's skin in close proximity to the patch. **Do not write directly on the medication patch.**	Most manufacturers recommend against writing on patches due to insufficient data on the practice. Writing on the patch could damage or tear it. Moreover, if ink is used, it may leach through and come into contact with the medication, and it is not known whether ink might interact with a given medication or impede its delivery.
23. Remove gloves and additional PPE, if used. Perform hand hygiene.	Removing PPE properly reduces the risk for infection transmission and contamination of other items. Hand hygiene prevents the spread of microorganisms.
24. Document the administration of the medication immediately after administration. See Documentation section below.	Timely documentation helps to ensure patient safety.
25. Evaluate the patient's response to the medication within the appropriate time frame.	The patient needs to be evaluated for therapeutic and adverse effects from the medication.

EVALUATION

- Medication is delivered via the transdermal route.
- Patient experiences no adverse effect.
- Patient's skin remains free from injury.
- Patient understands and complies with the medication regimen.

DOCUMENTATION

- Document the administration of the medication immediately after administration, including date, time, dose, route of administration, and site of administration on the CMAR/MAR or record using the required format. If using a bar-code system, medication administration is automatically recorded when the bar code is scanned. PRN medications require documentation of the reason for administration. Prompt recording avoids the possibility of accidentally repeating the administration of the drug. If the drug was refused or omitted, record this in the appropriate area on the medication record and notify the primary care provider. This verifies the reason the medication was omitted and ensures that the primary care provider is aware of the patient's condition.

SKILL 106 — APPLYING MONTGOMERY STRAPS

Montgomery straps are prepared strips of nonallergenic tape with ties inserted through holes at one end. One set of straps is placed on either side of a wound, and the straps are tied like shoelaces to secure the dressings. When it is time to change the dressing, the straps are untied, the wound is cared for, and then the straps are retied to hold the new dressing. Often a skin barrier is applied before the straps to protect the skin. The straps or ties need to be changed only if they become loose or soiled.

Montgomery straps are recommended to secure dressings on wounds that require frequent dressing changes, such as wounds with increased drainage. These straps allow the nurse to perform wound care without the need to remove adhesive strips, such as tape, with each dressing change, thus decreasing the risk of skin irritation and injury.

DELEGATION CONSIDERATIONS

Application of Montgomery Straps is not delegated to nursing assistive personnel (NAP) or to unlicensed assistive personnel (UAP). Depending on the state's nurse practice act and the organization's policies and procedures, this procedure may be delegated to licensed practical/vocational nurses (LPN/LVNs). The decision to delegate must be based on careful analysis of the patient's needs and circumstances, as well as the qualifications of the person to whom the task is being delegated. Refer to the Delegation Guidelines in Appendix A.

EQUIPMENT

- Clean disposable gloves
- Additional PPE, as indicated
- Dressings for wound care, as ordered
- Commercially available Montgomery straps or 2- to 3-inch hypoallergenic tape and strings for ties

- Cleansing solution, usually normal saline
- Gauze pads
- Skin-protectant wipe
- Skin-barrier sheet (hydrocolloidal or nonhydrocolloidal)

ASSESSMENT

- Assess the situation to determine the need for wound cleaning and a dressing change. Assess the integrity of any straps currently in use. Replace loose or soiled straps or ties.
- Confirm any medical orders relevant to wound care and any wound care included in the nursing plan of care.
- Assess the patient's level of comfort and the need for analgesics before wound care. Assess if the patient experienced any pain related to prior dressing changes and the effectiveness of interventions employed to minimize the patient's pain.
- Assess the current dressing to determine if it is intact. Assess for excess drainage or bleeding or saturation of the dressing.
- Inspect the wound and the surrounding tissue. Assess the appearance of the wound for the approximation of wound edges, the color of the wound and surrounding area, and signs of dehiscence. Assess for the presence of sutures, staples, or adhesive closure strips. Note the stage of the healing process and characteristics of any drainage.
- Assess the surrounding skin for color, temperature, and edema, ecchymosis, or maceration.

NURSING DIAGNOSIS

- Impaired Skin Integrity
- Acute Pain
- Delayed Surgical Recovery
- Risk for Infection

OUTCOME IDENTIFICATION AND PLANNING

- Patient's skin is free from irritation and injury.
- Care is accomplished without contaminating the wound area, causing trauma to the wound, and/or causing the patient to experience pain or discomfort.
- Wound continues to show signs of progression of healing.

IMPLEMENTATION

ACTION	RATIONALE
1. Review the medical orders for wound care or the nursing plan of care related to wound care. Gather necessary supplies.	Reviewing the order and plan of care validates the correct patient and correct procedure. Preparation promotes efficient time management and an organized approach to the task.

ACTION	RATIONALE
2. Perform hand hygiene and put on PPE, if indicated.	Hand hygiene and PPE prevent the spread of microorganisms. PPE is required based on transmission precautions.
3. Identify the patient.	Identifying the patient ensures the right patient receives the intervention and helps prevent errors.
4. Assemble equipment on overbed table within reach.	Organization facilitates performance of the task.
5. Close the curtains around the bed and close the door to the room, if possible. Explain what you are going to do and why you are going to do it to the patient.	This ensures the patient's privacy. Explanation relieves anxiety and facilitates cooperation.
6. Assess the patient for possible need for nonpharmacologic pain-reducing interventions or analgesic medication before wound care dressing change. Administer appropriate prescribed analgesic. Allow enough time for the analgesic to achieve its effectiveness before beginning the procedure.	Pain is a subjective experience influenced by past experience. Wound care and dressing changes may cause pain for some patients.
7. Place a waste receptacle at a convenient location for use during the procedure.	Having a waste container handy means that the soiled dressing may be discarded easily, without the spread of microorganisms.
8. Adjust bed to comfortable working height, usually elbow height of the caregiver (VISN 8, 2009).	Having the bed at the proper height prevents back and muscle strain.
9. Assist the patient to a comfortable position that provides easy access to the wound area. Use a bath blanket to cover any exposed area other than the wound. Place a waterproof pad under the wound site.	Patient positioning and use of a bath blanket provide for comfort and warmth. Waterproof pad protects underlying surfaces.

ACTION	RATIONALE
10. Perform wound care and a dressing change as outlined in Skills 55 through 57 and Skill 185, as ordered.	Wound care aids in healing and protects the wound.
11. Put on clean gloves. Clean the skin on either side of the wound with the gauze, moistened with normal saline. Dry the skin.	Gloves prevent the spread of microorganisms. Cleaning and drying the skin prevents irritation and injury.
12. **Apply a skin protectant to the skin where the straps will be placed.**	Skin protectant minimizes the risk for skin breakdown and irritation.
13. Remove gloves.	Tape is easier to handle without gloves. Wound is covered with the dressing.
14. Cut the skin barrier to the size of the tape or strap. Apply the skin barrier to the patient's skin, near the dressing. Apply the sticky side of each tape or strap to the skin barrier sheet, so the openings for the strings are at the edge of the dressing. Repeat for the other side.	Skin barrier prevents skin irritation and breakdown.
15. Thread a separate string through each pair of holes in the straps, if not already in place. Tie one end of the string in the hole. Fasten the other end with the opposing tie, like a shoelace (Figure 1). **Do not secure too tightly.** Repeat according to the	Ties hold the dressing in place. Tying too tightly puts additional stress on the surrounding skin. Recording date and time provides a baseline for changing straps.

FIGURE 1 Tying Montgomery straps.

ACTION	RATIONALE

number of straps needed. If commercially prepared straps are used, tie strings like a shoelace. Note date and time of application on strap.

16. After securing the dressing, label dressing with date and time. Remove all remaining equipment; place the patient in a comfortable position, with side rails up and bed in the lowest position.

Recording date and time provides communication and demonstrates adherence to plan of care. Proper patient and bed positioning promotes safety and comfort.

17. Remove additional PPE, if used. Perform hand hygiene.

Removing PPE properly reduces the risk for infection transmission and contamination of other items. Hand hygiene prevents the spread of microorganisms.

18. Check all wound dressings every shift. More frequent checks may be needed if the wound is more complex or dressings become saturated quickly.

Checking dressings ensures the assessment of changes in patient condition and timely intervention to prevent complications.

19. Replace the ties and straps whenever they are soiled, or every 2 to 3 days. Straps can be reapplied onto skin barrier. Skin barrier can remain in place up to 7 days. Use a silicone-based adhesive remover to help remove the skin barrier.

Replacing soiled ties and straps prevents growth of pathogens. Minimizing removal of skin barrier prevents skin irritation and breakdown. A silicone-based adhesive remover allows for the easy, rapid, and painless removal without the associated problems of skin stripping (Denyer, 2011; Benbow, 2011).

EVALUATION

- Patient's skin is clean, dry, intact, and free from irritation and injury.
- Patient exhibits a clean wound area free of contamination and trauma.
- Patient verbalizes minimal to no pain or discomfort.
- Patient exhibits signs and symptoms indicative of progressive wound healing.

DOCUMENTATION

- Document the procedure, the patient's response, and your assessment of the area before and after application of the Montgomery straps. Record a description of the wound, amount and character of the wound drainage, and an assessment of the surrounding skin. Note the type of dressing that was applied, including the application of skin protectant and a skin barrier. Document that Montgomery straps were applied to secure the dressings. Record the patient's response to the dressing care and associated pain assessment. Include any pertinent patient and family education.

SKILL 107 MOVING A PATIENT UP IN BED WITH THE ASSISTANCE OF ANOTHER CAREGIVER

When a patient needs to be moved up in bed, it is important to avoid injuring yourself and the patient. The patient is at risk for injuries from shearing forces while being moved. Evaluate the patient's condition, any activity restrictions, the patient's ability to assist with positioning and to understand directions, and the patient's body weight to decide how much additional assistance is needed. This is not a one-person task. Safe Patient Handling Algorithm 4 in Skill 173 can assist in making decisions about patient handling and movement. Using assistance, appropriate lifting and repositioning devices, good body mechanics, and correct technique are important to avoid injuries to yourself and the patient. During any patient-handling task, if any caregiver is required to lift more than 35 pounds of a patient's weight, consider the patient to be fully dependent and use assistive devices (Waters, 2007). The procedure below describes moving a patient using a friction-reducing sheet.

DELEGATION CONSIDERATIONS

Moving a patient up in bed may be delegated to nursing assistive personnel (NAP) or to unlicensed assistive personnel (UAP), as well as to licensed practical/vocational nurses (LPN/LVNs). The decision to delegate must be based on careful analysis of the patient's needs and circumstances, as well as the qualifications of the person to whom the task is being delegated. Refer to the Delegation Guidelines in Appendix A.

EQUIPMENT

- Friction-reducing sheet or other friction-reducing device
- Nonsterile gloves, if indicated; other PPE, as indicated
- Additional caregivers to assist, based on assessment
- Full-body sling lift and cover sheet, if necessary, based on assessment

ASSESSMENT

- Assess the situation to determine the need to move the patient up in the bed.
- Review the medical record and nursing plan of care for conditions that may influence the patient's ability to move or to be positioned.
- Assess for tubes, IV lines, incisions, or equipment that may alter the positioning procedure.
- Assess the patient's level of consciousness, ability to understand and follow directions, and ability to assist with moving.
- Assess the patient's weight and your strength to determine the number of caregivers required to assist with the activity. Determine the need for bariatric equipment.
- Assess the patient's skin for signs of irritation, redness, edema, or blanching.

NURSING DIAGNOSIS

- Activity Intolerance
- Risk for Injury
- Impaired Bed Mobility

OUTCOME IDENTIFICATION AND PLANNING

- Patient remains free from injury and maintains proper body alignment.
- Patient reports improved comfort.
- Patient's skin is clean, dry, and intact, and without any redness, irritation, or breakdown.

IMPLEMENTATION

ACTION	RATIONALE
1. Review the medical record and nursing plan of care for conditions that may influence the patient's ability to move or to be positioned. Assess for tubes, IV lines, incisions, or equipment that may alter the positioning procedure. Identify any movement limitations. **Consult patient handling algorithm, if available, to plan appropriate approach to moving the patient.**	Reviewing the order and plan of care validates the correct patient and correct procedure. Identification of limitations and ability and use of an algorithm helps to prevent injury and aids in determining best plan for patient movement.

ACTION	RATIONALE
2. Perform hand hygiene and put on PPE, if indicated.	Hand hygiene and PPE prevent the spread of microorganisms. PPE is required based on transmission precautions.
3. Identify the patient. Explain the procedure to the patient.	Patient identification validates the correct patient and correct procedure. Discussion and explanation help allay anxiety and prepare the patient for what to expect.
4. Close the curtains around the bed and close the door to the room, if possible. Place the bed at an appropriate and comfortable working height, usually elbow height of the caregiver (VISN 8 Patient Safety Center, 2009). Adjust the head of the bed to a flat position or as low as the patient can tolerate. Place the bed in slight Trendelenburg position, if the patient is able to tolerate it.	Closing the door or curtain provides for privacy. Proper bed height helps reduce back strain while you are performing the procedure. Flat positioning helps to decrease the gravitational pull of the upper body. Placing the bed in slight Trendelenburg position aids movement.
5. Remove all pillows from under the patient. Leave one at the head of the bed, leaning upright against the headboard.	Removing pillows from under the patient facilitates movement; placing a pillow at the head of the bed prevents accidental head injury against the top of the bed.
6. Position at least one nurse on either side of the bed, and lower both side rails.	Proper positioning and lowering the side rails facilitate moving the patient and minimize strain on the nurses.
7. If a friction-reducing sheet (or device) is not in place under the patient, place one under the patient's midsection.	A friction-reducing device supports the patient's weight and reduces friction during the repositioning.
8. Ask the patient (if able) to bend his or her legs and put his or her feet flat on the bed to assist with the movement.	Patient can use major muscle groups to push. Even if the patient is too weak to push on the bed, placing the legs in this fashion will assist with movement and prevent skin shearing on the heels.

ACTION	RATIONALE
9. Have the patient fold the arms across the chest. Have the patient (if able) lift the head with chin on chest.	Positioning in this manner provides assistance, reduces friction, and prevents hyperextension of the neck.
10. One nurse should be positioned on each side of the bed, at the patient's midsection with feet spread shoulder width apart and one foot slightly in front of the other.	Doing so positions each nurse opposite the center of the body mass, lowers the center of gravity, and reduces the risk for injury.
11. If available on bed, engage mechanism to make the bed surface firmer for repositioning.	Decreases friction and effort needed to move the patient.
12. Grasp the friction-reducing sheet securely, close to the patient's body.	Having the sheet close to the body brings the patient's center of gravity closer to each nurse and provides for a secure hold.
13. Flex your knees and hips. Tighten your abdominal and gluteal muscles and keep your back straight.	Using the legs' large muscle groups and tightening muscles during transfer prevent back injury.
14. If possible, the patient can assist with the move by pushing with the legs. Shift your weight back and forth from your back leg to your front leg and count to three. On the count of three, move the patient up in bed. Repeat the process, if necessary, to get the patient to the right position.	If the patient assists, the nurses exert less effort. The rocking motion uses the nurses' weight to counteract the patient's weight. Rocking develops momentum, which provides a smooth lift with minimal exertion by the nurses.
15. Assist the patient to a comfortable position and readjust the pillows and supports, as needed. Take bed out of Trendelenburg position and return bed surface to normal setting, if necessary. Raise the side rails. Place the bed in the lowest position. Make sure	Readjusting the bed and adjusting the bed height ensures patient safety and comfort. Having the call bell and essential items readily available helps promote safety.

ACTION	RATIONALE
the call bell and other necessary items are within easy reach.	
16. Clean transfer aids per facility policy, if not indicated for single patient use. Remove gloves or other PPE, if used. Perform hand hygiene.	Proper cleaning of equipment between patient use prevents the spread of microorganisms. Removing PPE properly reduces the risk for infection transmission and contamination of other items. Hand hygiene prevents the spread of microorganisms.

EVALUATION

- Patient is moved up in bed without injury and maintains proper body alignment.
- Patient is comfortable.
- Patient demonstrates intact skin without evidence of any breakdown.

DOCUMENTATION

- Many facilities provide areas on the bedside flow sheet to document repositioning. Document the time the patient's position was changed, use of supports, and any pertinent observations, including skin assessment. Document the patient's tolerance of the position change. Document aids used to facilitate movement.

SKILL 108 PROVIDING NAIL CARE

Care of the nails is important to prevent pain and infection. Long, roughened nails that have not been trimmed or filed may increase the occurrence of traumatic nail injury, such as damage to the nail that may result in the nail plate being torn from the nail bed (Malkin & Berridge, 2009). Poor toenail care may lead to poor mobility. The nurse should document and report to the patient's primary care provider any changes to nail color, such as discoloration of the entire nail or a dark streak under the nail; changes in nail shape, such as curled nails; thinning or thickening of the nails; separation of the nail from the surrounding skin; bleeding around the nails; and redness, swelling or pain around the nails (Mayo Foundation for Medical Education and Research, 2011c).

DELEGATION CONSIDERATIONS

Depending on the organization's policies and procedures, the care of a patient's nails may be delegated to nursing assistive personnel (NAP) or to unlicensed assistive personnel (UAP) after assessment by the registered nurse. The care of a patient's nails may be delegated to licensed practical/vocational nurses (LPN/LVNs). The decision to delegate must be based on careful analysis of the patient's needs and circumstances, as well as the qualifications of the person to whom the task is being delegated. Refer to the Delegation Guidelines in Appendix A.

EQUIPMENT

- Nail file
- Nail clipper
- Cuticle scissors
- Orangewood stick or cuticle stick
- Emollient
- Disposable waterproof pad
- Towel
- Wash basin and skin cleanser, or commercially prepared bathing system
- Disposable gloves
- Additional PPE, if indicated

ASSESSMENT

- Assess the patient's nail care preferences: frequency, time of day, and type of products.
- Assess for any physical activity limitations.
- Assess for conditions that may put the patient at high risk for nail problems, such as diabetes and peripheral vascular disease.
- Assess the color and temperature of fingers and toes. Assess adequacy of pulses to area and capillary refill. Assess the skin of fingers and toes for dryness, cracking, or inflammation.
- Assess the nails and surrounding skin for changes in nail color, changes in nail shape, thinning or thickening of the nails, separation of the nail from the surrounding skin, bleeding around the nails, and redness, swelling, or pain around the nails. Nails should appear intact, smooth, firmly attached to nail bed, pink in color, with white crescent visible at the base. Dark streaks running lengthwise in nails are a normal variation for patients with darker skin tones.
- Assess the patient's ability for self-care of nails or assist with the procedure.

NURSING DIAGNOSIS

- Risk for Injury
- Bathing Self-Care Deficit
- Impaired Physical Mobility

OUTCOME IDENTIFICATION AND PLANNING

- Nails are trimmed and clean with smooth edges and intact cuticles, without evidence of trauma to nails or surrounding skin.
- Patient verbalizes feelings of improved self-esteem.

IMPLEMENTATION

ACTION	RATIONALE
1. Review health record for any limitations in physical activity, or contraindications to the procedure. Confirm presence of medical order for nail care, if required by facility policy.	Identifying limitations prevents patient discomfort and injury. In some settings, a medical order is required for nail care, particularly for a patient with certain health problems.
2. Perform hand hygiene. Put on PPE, as indicated.	Hand hygiene and PPE prevent the spread of microorganisms. PPE is required based on transmission precautions.
3. Identify patient. Explain procedure to the patient.	Identifying the patient ensures the right patient receives the intervention and helps prevent errors. Explanation facilitates cooperation.
4. Assemble equipment on overbed table within reach.	Organization facilitates performance of task.
5. Close the curtains around the bed and close the door to the room, if possible.	Provides for patient privacy.
6. Raise bed to a comfortable working position, usually elbow height of the caregiver (VISN 8 Patient Safety Center, 2009). Lower side rail. Place a towel or waterproof pad under the patient's hand or foot.	Proper bed height helps reduce back strain while performing the procedure. Waterproof pad protects bed linens and surrounding surfaces.
7. Put on gloves. Wash patient's hands or feet, depending on care to be given.	Gloves prevent the spread of microorganisms. Washing removes surface dirt and softens nails and skin, making it easier to trim and care for cuticles (Mayo Foundation for Medical Education and Research, 2011c).
8. Gently clean under the nails using the cuticle or orangewood stick. Wash hand or foot.	Washing removes debris and dirt dislodged from under nails.

ACTION	RATIONALE
9. Clip nail, if necessary. Avoid cutting the whole nail in one attempt. Use the tip of the nail clipper and take small cuts (Malkin & Berridge, 2009). Cut the nail straight across. Do not trim so far down on the sides that the skin and cuticle are injured. **Only file, do not cut, the nails of patients with diabetes or circulatory problems.**	Cutting entire nail in one attempt may lead to splitting the nail. Prevents injury to nail, cuticle, and finger or toe and reduces risk for in-growing nails (Mayo Foundation for Medical Education and Research, 2011a; Mayo Foundation for Medical Education and Research, 2011c; Malkin & Berridge, 2009).
10. File the nail straight across, then round the tips in a gentle curve, to shape the nail. Do not trim so far down on the sides that the skin and cuticle are injured. **Only file, do not cut, the nails of patients with diabetes or circulatory problems.**	Smoothes the nail. Prevents injury to nail, cuticle, and finger or toe and reduces risk for in-growing nails (Mayo Foundation for Medical Education and Research, 2011a; Mayo Foundation for Medical Education and Research, 2011c; Malkin & Berridge, 2009).
11. Remove hangnails, which are broken pieces of cuticle, by carefully trimming them off with cuticle scissors. Avoid injury to tissue with the cuticle scissors.	Removes dead cuticle. Reduces hangnail formation. Tearing of hangnail can cause injury to live tissue.
12. Gently push cuticles back off the nail using the orange-wood stick, or towel.	Keeps cuticles and nails neat and prevents cracking and drying of cuticles.
13. Dry hand or foot thoroughly, taking care to be sure to dry between fingers or toes. Apply an emollient to the hand or foot, rubbing it into the nails and cuticles. Do not moisturize between the toes of patients with peripheral artery disease.	Thorough drying reduces risk of maceration, damage from overly and consistently wet skin. Maceration increases risk for injury from rubbing or friction, and risk for fungal and bacterial infections. Moisturizing between the toes of patients with peripheral artery disease can encourage fungal growth (Mayo Foundation for Medical Education and Research, 2012).
14. Repeat Steps 7–13 for other extremity or extremities.	

ACTION	RATIONALE
15. Remove equipment and return patient to a position of comfort. Remove your gloves. Raise side rail and lower bed.	Promotes patient comfort and safety. Removing gloves properly reduces the risk for infection transmission and contamination of other items.
16. Remove additional PPE, if used. Perform hand hygiene.	Removing PPE properly reduces the risk for infection transmission and contamination of other items. Hand hygiene deters spread of microorganisms.

EVALUATION

- Patient's nails are trimmed and clean with smooth edges and intact cuticles, and are without evidence of trauma to nails or surrounding skin.
- Patient verbalizes feeling refreshed and demonstrates improved self-esteem.

DOCUMENTATION

- Record your assessment, significant observations, and unusual findings, such as broken nails or inflammation. Document any teaching done. Document procedure and patient response. Nail care is often recorded on routine flow sheet.

SKILL 109 ADMINISTERING A NASAL SPRAY

Nasal instillations are used to treat allergies, sinus infections, and nasal congestion. Medications with a systemic effect, such as vasopressin, may also be prepared as a nasal instillation. The nose is normally not a sterile cavity, but because of its connection with the sinuses, it is important to observe medical asepsis carefully when using nasal instillations.

DELEGATION CONSIDERATIONS

The administration of medication using a nasal spray is not delegated to nursing assistive personnel (NAP) or to unlicensed assistive personnel (UAP). Depending on the state's nurse practice act and the organization's policies and procedures, administration of a nasal spray may be delegated to licensed practical/vocational nurses (LPN/LVNs). The decision to delegate must be based on careful analysis of the patient's needs and circumstances, as well as the qualifications of the person to

whom the task is being delegated. Refer to the Delegation Guidelines in Appendix A.

EQUIPMENT
- Medication in nasal spray bottle
- Gloves
- Additional PPE, as indicated
- Tissue
- Computer-generated Medication Administration Record (CMAR) or Medication Administration Record (MAR)

ASSESSMENT
- Assess the nares for redness, erythema, edema, drainage, or tenderness.
- Assess the patient for allergies. Verify patient name, dose, route, and time of administration.
- Assess the patient's knowledge of medication and the procedure. If the patient has a knowledge deficit about the medication, this may be an appropriate time to begin education about the procedure.
- Assess the patient's ability to cooperate with the procedure.

NURSING DIAGNOSIS
- Deficient Knowledge
- Risk for Allergy Response

OUTCOME IDENTIFICATION AND PLANNING
- Medication is administered successfully into the nose.
- Patient understands the rationale for the nose spray.
- Patient experiences no allergy response.
- Patient's skin remains intact.
- Patient experiences minimal discomfort.

IMPLEMENTATION

ACTION	RATIONALE
1. Gather equipment. Check medication order against the original order in the medical record, according to facility policy. Clarify any inconsistencies. Check the patient's chart for allergies.	This comparison helps to identify errors that may have occurred when orders were transcribed. The primary care provider's order is the legal record of medication orders for each facility.
2. Know the actions, special nursing considerations, safe dose ranges, purpose of administration, and adverse effects of the medication to be administered. Consider	This knowledge aids the nurse in evaluating the therapeutic effect of the medication in relation to the patient's disorder and can also be used to educate the patient about the medication.

ACTION	RATIONALE
the appropriateness of the medication for this patient.	
3. Perform hand hygiene.	Hand hygiene prevents the spread of microorganisms.
4. Move the medication cart to the outside of the patient's room or prepare for administration in the medication area.	Organization facilitates error-free administration and saves time.
5. Unlock the medication cart or drawer. Enter pass code and scan employee identification, if required.	Locking the cart or drawer safeguards each patient's medication supply. Hospital accrediting organizations require medication carts to be locked when not in use. Entering pass code and scanning ID allows only authorized users into the system and identifies the user for documentation by the computer.
6. **Prepare medications for one patient at a time.**	This prevents errors in medication administration.
7. Read the CMAR/MAR and select the proper medication from the patient's medication drawer or unit stock.	This is the *first* check of the label.
8. Compare the label with the CMAR/MAR. Check expiration dates and perform calculations, if necessary. Scan the bar code on the package, if required.	This is the *second* check of the label. Verify calculations with another nurse to ensure safety, if necessary.
9. **Depending on facility policy, the third check of the label may occur at this point. If so, when all medications for one patient have been prepared, recheck the labels with the CMAR/MAR before taking the medications to the patient.**	This *third* check ensures accuracy and helps to prevent errors. *Note:* Many facilities require the *third* check to occur at the bedside, after identifying the patient and before administration.

ACTION	RATIONALE
10. Lock the medication cart before leaving it.	Locking the cart or drawer safeguards the patient's medication supply. Hospital accrediting organizations require medication carts to be locked when not in use.
11. Transport medications to the patient's bedside carefully, and keep the medications in sight at all times.	Careful handling and close observation prevent accidental or deliberate disarrangement of medications.
12. **Ensure that the patient receives the medications at the correct time.**	Check agency policy, which may allow for administration within a period of 30 minutes before or 30 minutes after the designated time.
13. Perform hand hygiene and put on PPE, if indicated.	Hand hygiene and PPE prevent the spread of microorganisms. PPE is required based on transmission precautions.
14. **Identify the patient. Compare the information with the CMAR/MAR. The patient should be identified using at least two methods** (The Joint Commission, 2013):	Identifying the patient ensures the right patient receives the medications and helps prevent errors. The patient's room number or physical location is not used as an identifier (The Joint Commission, 2013). Replace the identification band if it is missing or inaccurate in any way.
a. Check the name on the patient's identification band.	
b. Check the identification number on the patient's identification band.	
c. Check the birth date on the patient's identification band.	
d. Ask the patient to state his or her name and birth date, based on facility policy.	This requires a response from the patient, but illness and strange surroundings often cause patients to be confused.

ACTION	RATIONALE
15. **Complete necessary assessments before administering medications. Check the patient's allergy bracelet or ask the patient about allergies. Explain the purpose and action of each medication to the patient.**	Assessment is a prerequisite to administration of medications.
16. Scan the patient's bar code on the identification band, if required.	Provides an additional check to ensure that the medication is given to the right patient.
17. **Based on facility policy, the third check of the label may occur at this point. If so, recheck the labels with the CMAR/MAR before administering the medications to the patient.**	Many facilities require the *third* check to occur at the bedside, after identifying the patient and before administration. If facility policy directs the *third* check at this time, this *third* check ensures accuracy and helps to prevent errors.
18. Put on gloves.	Gloves protect the nurse from potential contact with contaminants and body fluids.
19. Provide the patient with paper tissues and ask the patient to blow his or her nose.	Blowing the nose clears the nasal mucosa prior to medication administration.
20. Have the patient sit up with head tilted back. **Tilting the patient's head should be avoided if the patient has a cervical spine injury.**	Allows the spray to flow into the nares. Tilting the head is contraindicated with cervical spine injury.
21. Instruct the patient to inhale gently through the nose as the spray is being administered or not to inhale gently as the spray is being administered. Your instruction to the patient will depend on the medication being administered. Consult the manufacturer's instructions for each medication.	Inhalation helps to distribute the spray in the nares. Inhalation during administration is not recommended for some medications.
22. Agitate the bottle gently, if required for specific medication. Insert the tip of the nosepiece of the bottle into	Mixes medication thoroughly to ensure a consistent dose of medication.

ACTION	RATIONALE
one nostril. Close the opposite nostril with a finger. Instruct the patient to breathe in gently through the nostril, if required. Compress or activate the bottle to release one spray at the same time the patient breathes in.	
23. Keep the medication container compressed and remove it from the nostril. Release the container from the compressed state. Do not allow the container to return to its original position until it is removed from the patient's nose.	Prevents contamination of the contents of the container.
24. Have the patient hold his or her breath for a few seconds, and then breathe out slowly through the mouth. Repeat in the other nostril, as prescribed or indicated.	Allows medication to remain in contact with mucous membranes of nose.
25. Wipe the outside of the bottle nose piece with a clean dry tissue or cloth and replace the cap. Instruct the patient to avoid blowing his or her nose for 5 to 10 minutes, depending on the medication.	Keeps the end of the bottle clean. Keeps the medication in contact with the mucous membranes of the nose.
26. Remove gloves. Assist the patient to a comfortable position.	This ensures patient comfort.
27. Remove additional PPE, if used. Perform hand hygiene.	Removing PPE properly reduces the risk for infection transmission and contamination of other items. Hand hygiene prevents the spread of microorganisms.
28. Document the administration of the medication immediately after administration. See Documentation section below.	Timely documentation helps to ensure patient safety.

ACTION	RATIONALE
29. Evaluate the patient's response to the procedure and medication within an appropriate time frame.	The patient needs to be evaluated for therapeutic and adverse effects from the medication.

EVALUATION

- Patient receives the nose spray successfully.
- Patient understands the rationale for nose spray.
- Patient experiences no allergy response.
- Patient's skin remains intact.
- Patient experiences minimal discomfort.

DOCUMENTATION

- Document the administration of the medication, including date, time, dose, route of administration, and site of administration, specifically right, left, or both nares, on the CMAR/MAR or record using the required format. If using a bar-code system, medication administration is automatically recorded when the bar code is scanned. PRN medications require documentation of the reason for administration. Prompt recording avoids the possibility of accidentally repeating the administration of the drug. Document pre- and post-administration assessments, characteristics of any drainage, and the patient's response to the treatment, if appropriate. If the drug was refused or omitted, record this in the appropriate area on the medication record and notify the primary care provider. This verifies the reason medication was omitted and ensures that the primary care provider is aware of the patient's condition.

SKILL 110 OBTAINING A NASAL SWAB

A nasal swab provides a sample that can be cultured, which will aid in the diagnosis of infection and detect the carrier state for certain organisms. A nasal swab may be used to diagnose infectious respiratory tract diseases, such as influenza. It is commonly used to detect the presence of organisms, such as *Staphylococcus aureus*, which may colonize on the skin in the nose, skin folds, hairline, perineum, and navel. These organisms often survive in these areas without causing infection, unless the organism invades the skin or deeper tissues (CDC, 2011c). Some strains of *S. aureus* have developed resistance to antibiotics. A nasal swab can be part of the screening process to detect potential infection with drug resistant microorganisms (Higgins, 2008).

DELEGATION CONSIDERATIONS

Obtaining a nasal swab is not delegated to nursing assistive personnel (NAP) or to unlicensed assistive personnel (UAP). Depending on the state's nurse practice act and the organization's policies and procedures, this procedure may be delegated to licensed practical/vocational nurses (LPN/LVNs). The decision to delegate must be based on careful analysis of the patient's needs and circumstances, as well as the qualifications of the person to whom the task is being delegated. Refer to the Delegation Guidelines in Appendix A.

EQUIPMENT

- Nasal swab
- Sterile water (optional)
- Nonsterile gloves
- Goggles and face mask, or face shield
- Additional PPE, as indicated
- Biohazard bag
- Appropriate label for specimen, based on facility policy and procedure

ASSESSMENT

- Assess the patient's understanding of the collection procedure, reason for testing, and ability to cooperate.
- Inspect the patient's nares and for the presence of nasal symptoms, such as discharge, erythema, or congestion.
- Assess for conditions that would contraindicate obtaining a nasal swab, such as injury to the nares or nose, and surgery of nose.

NURSING DIAGNOSIS

- Risk for Infection
- Acute Pain
- Deficient Knowledge

OUTCOME IDENTIFICATION AND PLANNING

- An uncontaminated specimen is obtained without injury to the patient and sent to the laboratory promptly.
- Patient verbalizes an understanding of the rationale for the procedure.
- Patient verbalizes a decrease in anxiety related to specimen collection.

IMPLEMENTATION

ACTION	RATIONALE
1. Verify the order for a nasal swab in the medical record. Gather equipment. Check the expiration date on the swab package.	Verifying the medical order is crucial to ensuring that the proper procedure is administered to the right patient. Assembling equipment provides for an organized

ACTION	RATIONALE
	approach to the task. Swab package is sterile and should not be used past the expiration date.
2. Perform hand hygiene and put on PPE, if indicated.	Hand hygiene and PPE prevent the transmission of microorganisms. PPE is required based on transmission precautions.
3. Identify the patient. 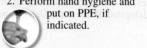	Identifying the patient ensures the right patient receives the intervention and helps prevent errors.
4. Explain the procedure to the patient. Discuss with the patient the need for a nasal swab. Explain to the patient the process by which the specimen will be collected.	Discussion and explanation help to allay some of the patient's anxiety and prepare the patient for what to expect.
5. Check the specimen label with the patient identification bracelet. Label should include the patient's name and identification number, time specimen was collected, route of collection, identification of the person obtaining the sample, and any other information required by facility policy.	Confirmation of patient identification information ensures the specimen is labeled correctly for the right patient.
6. Assemble equipment on overbed table within reach.	Arranging items nearby is convenient, saves time, and avoids unnecessary stretching and twisting of muscles on the part of the nurse.
7. Close curtains around the bed or close the door to the room, if possible.	Closing the door or curtain provides for patient privacy.
8. Put on goggles and face mask, or face shield and nonsterile gloves.	Goggles, face mask, face shield and gloves protect the nurse from exposure to blood or body fluids and prevent the transmission of microorganisms.

ACTION	RATIONALE
9. Ask the patient to tip his or her head back slightly. Assist as necessary.	Tilting the head allows optimal access to the nares, which is where the swab will be inserted.
10. Peel open the swab kit packaging to expose the swab and collection tube. Remove the white plug from the collection tube and discard. Remove the swab from packaging by grasping the exposed end. Take care not to contaminate the swab by touching it to any other surface. Moisten with sterile water, depending on facility policy.	Swab must remain sterile to ensure the specimen is not contaminated. Moistening the end of the swab minimizes discomfort to the patient.
11. Insert swab 2 cm into one naris and rotate against the anterior nasal mucosa for 3 seconds or five rotations, depending on facility policy, and then keep it there for 15 seconds.	Contact with the mucosa is necessary to obtain potential pathogens.
12. Remove the swab and repeat in the second naris, using the same swab.	Repeating in the second naris ensures accurate specimen.
13. Insert the swab fully into the collection tube, taking care not to touch any other surface. The handle end of the swab should fit snugly into the collection tube and the end of swab should be in the culture medium at the distal end of the collection tube. Lightly squeeze the bottom of the collection tube as necessary, depending on type of tube in use in facility, to break the seal on the culture medium.	Swab must remain uncontaminated to ensure accurate results. Full insertion of the swab ensures it will remain in the collection tube. Placement of swab end in culture medium and releasing of the liquid transport medium are necessary to ensure accurate specimen processing.
14. Dispose of used equipment per facility policy. Remove gloves. Perform hand hygiene.	Proper disposal of equipment reduces the transmission of microorganisms. Removing gloves properly reduces the risk

EVALUATION

- Nasal swab is collected without contamination and is sent to the laboratory as soon as possible.
- Patient does not experience injury.
- Patient verbalizes an understanding of the rationale for the specimen collection.
- Patient verbalizes a decrease in anxiety related to the procedure.

DOCUMENTATION

- Record the time the specimen was collected and sent to the laboratory. Document any pertinent assessments of the patient's nares and the presence of nasal symptoms, such as discharge, erythema, or congestion.

INSERTING A NASOGASTRIC (NG) TUBE

The nasogastric (NG) tube is passed through the nose and into the stomach. This type of tube permits the patient to receive nutrition through a tube feeding using the stomach as a natural reservoir for food. Another purpose of an NG tube may be to decompress or to drain unwanted fluid and air from the stomach. This application would be used, for example, to allow the intestinal tract to rest and promote healing after bowel surgery. The NG tube can also be used to monitor bleeding in the gastrointestinal (GI) tract, to remove undesirable substances (lavage) such as poisons, or to help treat an intestinal obstruction.

DELEGATION CONSIDERATIONS

The insertion of an NG tube is not delegated to nursing assistive personnel (NAP) or to unlicensed assistive personnel (UAP). Depending on the state's nurse practice act and the organization's policies and procedures, insertion of an NG tube may be delegated to licensed practical/vocational nurses (LPN/LVNs). The decision to delegate must be based on careful analysis of the patient's needs and circumstances, as well as the qualifications of the person to whom the task is being delegated. Refer to the Delegation Guidelines in Appendix A.

EQUIPMENT

- Nasogastric tube of appropriate size (8–18 French)
- Stethoscope
- Water-soluble lubricant
- Normal saline solution or sterile water, for irrigation, depending on facility policy
- Tongue blade
- Irrigations set, including a Toomey (20–50 mL)
- Flashlight
- Nonallergenic tape (1-inch wide)
- Tissues
- Glass of water with straw
- Topical anesthetic–lidocaine spray or gel (optional)
- Clamp
- Suction apparatus (if ordered)
- Bath towel or disposable pad
- Emesis basin
- Safety pin and rubber band
- Nonsterile, disposable gloves
- Additional PPE, as indicated
- Tape measure, or other measuring device
- Skin barrier
- pH paper

ASSESSMENT

- Assess the patency of the patient's nares by asking the patient to occlude one nostril and breathe normally through the other. Select the nostril through which air passes more easily.
- Assess the patient's history for any recent facial trauma, polyps, blockages, or surgeries. Patients with facial fractures or facial surgeries present a higher risk for misplacement of the tube into the brain. Many facilities require a physician to place NG tubes in these patients.

599

- Inspect the abdomen for distention and firmness; auscultate for bowel sounds or peristalsis and palpate the abdomen for distention and tenderness. If the abdomen is distended, consider measuring the abdominal girth at the umbilicus to establish a baseline.

NURSING DIAGNOSIS

- Imbalanced Nutrition, Less than Body Requirements
- Impaired Swallowing
- Risk for Aspiration

OUTCOME IDENTIFICATION AND PLANNING

- Tube is passed into the patient's stomach without any complications.
- Patient demonstrates weight gain, indicating improved nutrition.
- Patient exhibits no signs and symptoms of aspiration.
- Patient rates pain as decreased from prior to insertion.
- Patient verbalizes an understanding of the reason for NG tube insertion.

IMPLEMENTATION

ACTION	RATIONALE
1. Verify the medical order for insertion of an NG tube. Gather equipment, including selection of the appropriate NG tube.	Ensures the patient receives the correct treatment. Assembling equipment provides for an organized approach to the task. NG tubes should be radiopaque, contain clearly visible markings for measurement, and may have multiple ports for aspiration.
2. Perform hand hygiene and put on PPE, if indicated.	Hand hygiene and PPE prevent the spread of microorganisms. PPE is required based on transmission precautions.
3. Identify the patient.	Identifying the patient ensures the right patient receives the intervention and helps prevent errors.
4. Explain the procedure to the patient, including the rationale why the tube is needed. Discuss the associated discomforts that may be experienced and possible	Explanation facilitates patient cooperation. Some patient surveys report that of all routine procedures, the insertion of an NG tube is considered the most painful. Lidocaine gel or sprays

ACTION	RATIONALE
interventions that may allay this discomfort. Answer any questions, as needed.	are possible options to decrease discomfort during NG tube insertion.
5. Assemble equipment on overbed table within reach.	Arranging items nearby is convenient, saves time, and avoids unnecessary stretching and twisting of muscles on the part of the nurse.
6. Close the patient's bedside curtain or door. Raise the bed to a comfortable working position; usually elbow height of the caregiver (VISN 8, 2009). Assist the patient to high Fowler's position or elevate the head of the bed 45 degrees if the patient is unable to maintain an upright position. Drape chest with bath towel or disposable pad. Have emesis basin and tissues handy.	Closing curtains or door provides for patient privacy. Having the bed at the proper height prevents back and muscle strain. Upright position is more natural for swallowing and protects against bronchial intubation aspiration, if the patient should vomit. Passage of tube may stimulate gagging and tearing of eyes.
7. **Measure the distance to insert the tube by placing the tube tip at the patient's nostril and extending it to tip of earlobe and then to tip of xiphoid process.** Mark tube with an indelible marker.	Measurement ensures that tube will be long enough to enter patient's stomach.
8. Put on gloves. Lubricate tip of tube (at least 2 to 4 inches) with water-soluble lubricant. Apply topical anesthetic to nostril and oropharynx, as appropriate.	Lubrication reduces friction and facilitates passage of the tube into the stomach. Water-soluble lubricant will not cause pneumonia if the tube accidentally enters the lungs. Topical anesthetics act as local anesthetics, reducing discomfort. Consult the physician for an order for a topical anesthetic, such as lidocaine gel or spray, if needed.
9. After selecting the appropriate nostril, ask patient to flex the head back slightly against	Following the normal contour of the nasal passage while inserting the tube reduces irritation and

ACTION	RATIONALE
the pillow. Gently insert the tube into the nostril while directing the tube upward and backward along the floor of the nose. Patient may gag when tube reaches pharynx. Provide tissues for tearing or watering of eyes. Offer comfort and reassurance to the patient.	the likelihood of mucosal injury. The tube stimulates the gag reflex readily. Tears are a natural response as the tube passes into the nasopharynx. Many patients report that gagging and throat discomfort can be more painful than the tube passing through the nostrils.
10. When pharynx is reached, instruct the patient to touch chin to chest. Encourage the patient to sip water through a straw or swallow even if no fluids are permitted. Advance tube in downward and backward direction when patient swallows. Stop when the patient breathes. **If gagging and coughing persist, stop advancing the tube and check placement of tube with tongue blade and flashlight.** If tube is curled, straighten the tube and attempt to advance again. Keep advancing the tube until pen marking is reached. **Do not use force.** Rotate the tube if it meets resistance.	Bringing the head forward helps close the trachea and open the esophagus. Swallowing helps advance the tube, causes the epiglottis to cover the opening of the trachea, and helps to eliminate gagging and coughing. Excessive coughing and gagging may occur if the tube has curled in the back of throat. Forcing the tube may injure mucous membranes.
11. **Discontinue the procedure and remove the tube if there are signs of distress, such as gasping, coughing, cyanosis, and inability to speak or hum.**	The tube is in the airway if the patient shows signs of distress and cannot speak or hum. If after three attempts, NG insertion is unsuccessful, another nurse may try or the patient should be referred to another health care professional.
12. Secure the tube loosely to the nose or cheek until it is determined that the tube is in the patient's stomach:	Securing with tape stabilizes the tube while position is being determined.
a. Attach syringe to end of tube and aspirate a small	The tube is in the stomach if its contents can be aspirated: pH

ACTION	RATIONALE
amount of stomach contents.	of aspirate can then be tested to determine gastric placement. If unable to obtain a specimen, reposition the patient and flush the tube with 30 mL of air. This action may be necessary several times. Current literature recommends that the nurse ensures proper placement of the NG tube by relying on multiple methods and not on one method alone.
b. Measure the pH of aspirated fluid using pH paper or a meter. Place a drop of gastric secretions onto pH paper or place small amount in a plastic cup and dip the pH paper into it. Within 30 seconds, compare the color on the paper with the chart supplied by the manufacturer.	Current research demonstrates that the use of pH is predictive of correct placement. The pH of gastric contents is acidic (less than 5.5). If the patient is taking an acid-inhibiting agent, the range may be 4.0 to 6.0. The pH of intestinal fluid is 7.0 or higher. The pH of respiratory fluid is 6.0 or higher. This method will not effectively differentiate between intestinal fluid and pleural fluid.
c. Visualize aspirated contents, checking for color and consistency.	Gastric fluid can be green with particles, off-white, or brown if old blood is present. Intestinal aspirate tends to look clear or straw-colored to a deep golden-yellow color. Also, intestinal aspirate may be greenish-brown if stained with bile. Respiratory or tracheobronchial fluid is usually off-white to tan and may be tinged with mucus. A small amount of blood-tinged fluid may be seen immediately after NG insertion.
d. Obtain radiograph (x-ray) of placement of tube, based on facility policy (and ordered by physician).	The x-ray is considered the most reliable method for identifying the position of the NG tube.
13. Apply skin barrier to tip and end of nose and allow to dry. Remove gloves and secure tube with a commercially	Skin barrier improves adhesion and protects skin. Constant pressure of the tube against the skin and mucous membranes may

ACTION	RATIONALE
prepared device (follow manufacturer's directions) or tape to patient's nose. To secure with tape:	cause tissue injury. Securing tube prevents migration of the tube inward and outward.
a. Cut a 4-inch piece of tape and split bottom 2 inches or use packaged nose tape for NG tubes.	
b. Place unsplit end over bridge of patient's nose.	
c. Wrap split ends under and around NG tube. **Be careful not to pull tube too tightly against nose.**	
14. Put on gloves. Clamp tube and remove the syringe. Cap the tube or attach tube to suction according to the medical orders.	Suction provides for decompression of stomach and drainage of gastric contents.
15. Measure length of exposed tube. Reinforce marking on tube at nostril with indelible ink. Ask the patient to turn his or her head to the side opposite the nostril in which the tube is inserted. Secure tube to patient's gown by using rubber band or tape and safety pin. For additional support, tape the tube onto patient's cheek using a piece of tape. **If a double-lumen tube (e.g., Salem sump) is used, secure vent above stomach level.** Attach at shoulder level.	Tube length should be checked and compared with this initial measurement, in conjunction with pH measurement and visual assessment of aspirate. An increase in the length of the exposed tube may indicate dislodgement (AACN, 2010b; Bourgault et al., 2007; Hinkle & Cheever, 2014). The tube should be marked with an indelible marker at the nostril. This marking should be assessed each time the tube is used to ensure the tube has not become displaced. Securing prevents tension and tugging on the tube. Turning the head ensures adequate slack in the tubing to prevent tension when the patient turns the head. Securing the double-lumen tube above stomach level prevents seepage of gastric contents and keeps the lumen clear for venting air.

ACTION	RATIONALE
16. Assist with or provide oral hygiene at 2- to 4-hour intervals. Lubricate the lips generously and clean nares and lubricate, as needed. Offer analgesic throat lozenges or anesthetic spray for throat irritation, if needed.	Oral hygiene keeps mouth clean and moist, promotes comfort, and reduces thirst.
17. Remove equipment and return patient to a position of comfort. Remove gloves. Raise side rail and lower bed.	Promotes patient comfort and safety. Removing gloves properly reduces the risk for infection transmission and contamination of other items.
18. Remove additional PPE, if used. Perform hand hygiene.	Removing PPE properly reduces the risk for infection transmission and contamination of other items. Hand hygiene prevents transmission of microorganisms.

EVALUATION

- Patient exhibits a nasogastric tube placed into the stomach without any complications.
- Patient demonstrates weight gain, indicating improved nutrition.
- Patient remains free of any signs and symptoms of aspiration.
- Patient rates pain as decreased from prior to insertion.
- Patient verbalizes an understanding of the reason for NG tube insertion.

DOCUMENTATION

- Document the size and type of NG tube that was inserted and the measurement from tip of the nose to the end of the exposed tube. Also, document the results of the x-ray that was taken to confirm the tube position, if applicable. Record a description of the gastric contents, including the pH of the contents. Document the naris where the tube is placed and the patient's response to the procedure. Include assessment data, both subjective and objective, related to the abdomen. Record the patient teaching that was discussed.

Nasogastric tubes (NGTs) may be inserted to decompress or drain the stomach of fluid or unwanted stomach contents, such as poison, medication, or air, and when conditions are present in which peristalsis is absent. Examples of such conditions include paralytic ileus and intestinal obstruction by tumor or hernia. Nasogastric tubes are also used to allow the gastrointestinal (GI) tract to rest before or after abdominal surgery to promote healing; they are inserted to monitor GI bleeding. Historically, an NG tube has often been used postoperatively as a routine part of care after major abdominal surgery, to rest the intestinal tract and promote healing. However, some research has suggested that the routine use of an NGT after abdominal surgery may serve no beneficial purpose and may actually delay the patient's progress, increasing the time required for flatus to occur and increasing pulmonary complications (Lafon & Lawson, 2012). It is suggested that selective decompression should be reserved for patients with nausea, vomiting, and abdominal distention after surgery (Brennan, 2008; Gannon, 2007; Nelson et al., 2007). The tube is usually attached to suction (intermittent or continuous) when used for these reasons or the tube may be clamped. The tube must be kept free from obstruction or clogging and is usually irrigated every 4 to 6 hours.

To promote patient safety when instilling solutions into a nasogastric tube, tube placement must be verified before administration of any fluids or medications. Radiographic examination, measurement of aspirate pH, visual assessment of aspirate, measurement of tube length and measurement of tube marking, and monitoring of carbon dioxide are used to confirm NGT placement. With the exception of radiographic examination, the use of several of these techniques in conjunction with each other increases the likelihood of correct tube placement. An old technique of auscultation of air injected into an NGT has proved unreliable and may result in tragic consequences if used as an indicator of tube placement (AACN, 2010; Best, 2005; Khair, 2005). Therefore, do not use it to confirm nasogastric tube placement.

DELEGATION CONSIDERATIONS

The irrigation of a nasogastric tube (NGT) is not delegated to nursing assistive personnel (NAP) or to unlicensed assistive personnel (UAP). Depending on the state's nurse practice act and the organization's policies and procedures, irrigation of an NGT may be delegated to licensed practical/vocational nurses (LPN/LVNs). The decision to delegate must be based on careful analysis of the patient's needs and circumstances, as well as the qualifications of the person to whom the task is being delegated. Refer to the Delegation Guidelines in Appendix A.

EQUIPMENT

- NGT connected to continuous or intermittent suction
- Water or normal saline solution for irrigation (based on facility policy)
- Nonsterile gloves
- Additional PPE, as indicated
- Irrigation set (or a 60-mL catheter-tip syringe and cup for irrigating solution)

- Clamp
- Disposable waterproof pad or bath towel
- Emesis basin
- Tape measure, or other measuring device
- pH paper and measurement scale

ASSESSMENT

- Assess abdomen by inspecting for presence of distention, auscultating for bowel sounds, and palpating the abdomen for firmness or tenderness. If the abdomen is distended, consider measuring the abdominal girth at the umbilicus. If the patient reports any tenderness or nausea, or exhibits any rigidity or firmness of the abdomen, confer with the primary care provider.
- If the NGT is attached to suction, assess suction to ensure that it is running at the prescribed pressure.
- Inspect drainage from NGT, including color, consistency, and amount.

NURSING DIAGNOSIS

- Imbalanced Nutrition: Less than Body Requirements
- Risk for Injury
- Risk for Deficient Fluid Volume

OUTCOME IDENTIFICATION AND PLANNING

- Tube will maintain patency with irrigation.
- Patient will not experience any trauma or injury.

IMPLEMENTATION

ACTION	RATIONALE
1. Gather equipment. Verify the medical order or facility policy and procedure regarding frequency of irrigation, solution type, and amount of irrigant. Check expiration dates on irrigating solution and irrigation set.	Assembling equipment provides for an organized approach to the task. Verification ensures the patient receives the correct intervention. Facility policy dictates safe interval for reuse of equipment.

ACTION	RATIONALE

2. Perform hand hygiene and put on PPE, if indicated.

Hand hygiene and PPE prevent the spread of microorganisms. PPE is required based on transmission precautions.

3. Identify the patient.

Identifying the patient ensures the right patient receives the intervention and helps prevent errors.

4. Explain the procedure to the patient and why this intervention is needed. Answer any questions, as needed. Perform key abdominal assessments as described above.

Explanation facilitates patient cooperation. Due to potential changes in a patient's condition, assessment is vital before initiating intervention.

5. Assemble equipment on overbed table within reach.

Organization facilitates performance of the task.

6. Pull the patient's bedside curtain. Raise bed to a comfortable working position, usually elbow height of the caregiver (VISN 8 Patient Safety Center, 2009). Assist patient to 30- to 45-degree position, unless this is contraindicated. Pour the irrigating solution into container.

Provide for privacy. Appropriate working height facilitates comfort and proper body mechanics for the nurse. This position minimizes risk for aspiration. Preparing the irrigation provides for an organized approach to the task.

7. Put on gloves. Place waterproof pad on the patient's chest, under connection of the nasogastric tube and suction tubing. **Check placement of NG tube.** (Refer to Skill 111.)

Gloves prevent contact with body fluids. Waterproof pad protects patient's clothing and bed linens from accidental leakage of gastric fluid. Checking placement before the instillation of fluid is necessary to prevent accidental instillation into the respiratory tract if the tube has become dislodged.

8. Draw up 30 mL of irrigation solution (or amount indicated in the order or policy) into syringe.

This delivers measured amount of irrigant through the tube. Saline solution (isotonic) may be used to compensate for electrolytes lost through nasogastric drainage.

ACTION	RATIONALE
9. Clamp nasogastric tube near connection site. Disconnect tube from suction apparatus and lay on disposable pad or towel, or hold both tubes upright in nondominant hand.	Clamping prevents leakage of gastric fluid.
10. Place tip of syringe in tube. **If Salem sump or double-lumen tube is used, make sure that syringe tip is placed in the drainage port and not in blue air vent.** Hold syringe upright and gently insert the irrigant (or allow solution to flow in by gravity if facility policy or medical order indicates). **Do not force solution into tube.**	Gentle insertion of saline solution (or gravity insertion) is less traumatic to gastric mucosa. The blue air vent acts to decrease pressure built up in the stomach when the Salem sump is attached to suction. It is not to be used for irrigation.
11. **If unable to irrigate tube, reposition patient and attempt irrigation again. Inject 10 to 20 mL of air and aspirate again. If repeated attempts to irrigate tube fail, consult with primary care provider or follow facility policy.**	Tube may be positioned against gastric mucosa, making it difficult to irrigate. Injection of air may reposition end of tube.
12. After irrigant has been instilled, hold end of NGT over irrigation tray or emesis basin. Observe for return flow of NG drainage into available container. Alternately, you may reconnect the NGT to suction and observe the return drainage as it drains into the suction container.	Return flow may be collected in an irrigating tray or other available container and measured. This amount will need to be subtracted from the irrigant to record the true NG drainage. A second method involves subtracting the total irrigant from the shift from the total NG drainage emptied over the entire shift, to find the true NG drainage. Check agency policy for guidelines. Observation determines tube patency and correct operation of suction apparatus.

ACTION	RATIONALE
13. If not already done, reconnect drainage port to suction, if ordered.	Allows for continued removal of gastric contents, as ordered.
14. Inject air into blue air vent after irrigation is complete. Position the blue air vent above the patient's stomach.	Following irrigation, the blue air vent is injected with air to keep it clear. Positioning the blue air vent above the stomach prevents the stomach contents from leaking from the NGT.
15. Remove gloves. Lower the bed and raise side rails, as necessary. Assist the patient to a position of comfort. Perform hand hygiene.	Lowering bed and assisting the patient to a comfortable position promote safety and comfort.
16. Put on gloves. Measure returned solution, if collected outside of suction apparatus. Rinse equipment if it will be reused. Label with the date, patient's name, room number, and purpose (for NGT/ irrigation).	Gloves prevent contact with blood and body fluids. Irrigant placed in tube is considered intake; solution returned is recorded as output. Record on the intake and output record. Rinsing promotes cleanliness, infection control, and prepares equipment for next irrigation.
17. Remove gloves and additional PPE, if used. Perform hand hygiene.	Removing PPE properly reduces the risk for infection transmission and contamination of other items. Hand hygiene prevents transmission of microorganisms.

EVALUATION

- Patient demonstrates a patent and functioning NGT.
- Patient reports no distress with the irrigation.
- Patient remains free of any signs and symptoms of injury or trauma.

DOCUMENTATION

- Document assessment of the patient's abdomen. Record if the patient's NGT is clamped or connected to suction, including the type of suction. Document the color and consistency of the NG drainage. Record the solution type and amount used to irrigate the NGT, as well as ease of irrigation or any difficulty related to the procedure. Record the amount of returned irrigant, if collected outside of the suction apparatus. Alternately, record irrigant amount so it can be subtracted from total NG drainage amount at the end of the shift. Record the patient's response to the procedure and any pertinent teaching points that were reviewed, such as instructions for the patient to contact the nurse for any feelings of nausea, bloating, or abdominal pain.

SKILL 113 REMOVING A NASOGASTRIC TUBE

When the NG tube is no longer necessary for treatment, the primary care provider will order the tube to be removed. The NG tube is removed as carefully as it was inserted, to provide as much comfort as possible for the patient and to prevent complications. When the tube is removed, the patient must hold his or her breath to prevent aspiration of any secretions or fluid left in the tube as it is removed.

DELEGATION CONSIDERATIONS

The removal of a nasogastric (NG) tube is not delegated to nursing assistive personnel (NAP) or to unlicensed assistive personnel (UAP). Depending on the state's nurse practice act and the organization's policies and procedures, removal of an NG tube may be delegated to licensed practical/vocational nurses (LPN/LVNs). The decision to delegate must be based on careful analysis of the patient's needs and circumstances, as well as the qualifications of the person to whom the task is being delegated. Refer to the Delegation Guidelines in Appendix A.

EQUIPMENT

- Tissues
- 50-mL syringe
- Nonsterile gloves
- Additional PPE, as indicated
- Stethoscope
- Disposable plastic bag
- Bath towel or disposable pad
- Normal saline solution for irrigation (optional)
- Emesis basin

ASSESSMENT

- Perform an abdominal assessment by inspecting for presence of distention, auscultating for bowel sounds, and palpating the abdomen for firmness or tenderness. If the abdomen is distended, consider measuring the abdominal girth at the umbilicus. If the patient reports any tenderness or nausea, exhibits any rigidity or firmness with distention, and if bowel sounds are absent, confer with the physician before discontinuing the NG tube.
- Assess any output from the NG tube, noting amount, color, and consistency.

NURSING DIAGNOSIS

• Readiness for Enhanced Nutrition
• Risk for Aspiration

OUTCOME IDENTIFICATION AND PLANNING

• Tube is removed with minimal discomfort to the patient, and the patient maintains an adequate nutritional intake.
• Abdomen remains free from distention and tenderness.

IMPLEMENTATION

ACTION	RATIONALE
1. Check medical record for the order for removal of NG tube.	This ensures correct implementation of primary care provider's order.
2. Perform hand hygiene and put on PPE, if indicated.	Hand hygiene and PPE prevent the spread of microorganisms. PPE is required based on transmission precautions.
3. Identify the patient.	Identifying the patient ensures the right patient receives the intervention and helps prevent errors.
4. Explain the procedure to the patient and why this intervention is warranted. Describe that it will entail a quick few moments of discomfort. Perform key abdominal assessments as described above.	Patient cooperation is facilitated when explanations are provided. Due to changes in a patient's condition, assessment is vital before initiating intervention.
5. Pull the patient's bedside curtain. Raise the bed to a comfortable working position, usually elbow height of the caregiver (VISN 8, 2009). Assist the patient into a 30- to 45-degree position. Place towel or disposable pad across the patient's chest. Give tissues and emesis basin to patient.	Provides for privacy. Appropriate working height facilitates comfort and proper body mechanics for the nurse. Towel or pad protects the patient from contact with gastric secretions. Emesis basin is helpful if patient vomits or gags. Tissues are necessary if patient wants to blow his or her nose when tube is removed.

ACTION	RATIONALE
6. Put on gloves. Discontinue suction and separate tube from suction. Unpin tube from patient's gown and carefully remove adhesive tape from patient's nose.	Gloves prevent contact with blood and body fluids. Disconnecting tube from suction and the patient allows for its unrestricted removal.
7. Check placement (as outlined in Skill 111) and attach syringe and **flush with 10 mL of water or normal saline solution (optional) or clear with 30 to 50 mL of air.**	Air or saline solution clears the tube of secretions, feeding, or debris.
8. Clamp tube with fingers by doubling tube on itself. **Instruct patient to take a deep breath and hold it. Quickly and carefully remove tube while patient holds breath.** Coil the tube in the disposable pad as you remove it from the patient.	Clamping prevents drainage of gastric contents into the pharynx and esophagus. The patient holds breath to prevent accidental aspiration of gastric secretions in tube. Careful removal minimizes trauma and discomfort for patient. Containing the tube in a towel while removing prevents leakage onto the patient.
9. Dispose of tube per facility policy. Remove gloves. Perform hand hygiene.	This prevents contamination with microorganisms.
10. Offer mouth care to the patient and facial tissue to blow nose. Lower the bed and assist the patient to a position of comfort, as needed.	These interventions promote patient comfort.
11. Remove equipment and raise side rail and lower bed.	Promotes patient comfort and safety.
12. Put on gloves and measure the amount of nasogastric drainage in the collection device and record on output flow record, subtracting irrigant fluids if necessary. Add solidifying agent to nasogastric drainage and dispose of drainage according to facility policy.	Irrigation fluids are considered intake. To obtain the true nasogastric drainage, irrigant fluid amounts are subtracted from the total nasogastric drainage. Nasogastric drainage is recorded as part of the output of fluids from the patient. Solidifying agents added to liquid nasogastric drainage facilitate safe biohazard disposal.

ACTION	RATIONALE
13. Remove additional PPE, if used. Perform hand hygiene.	Removing PPE properly reduces the risk for infection transmission and contamination of other items. Hand hygiene prevents transmission of microorganisms.

EVALUATION

- Patient experiences minimal discomfort and pain on NG tube removal.
- Patient's abdomen remains free from distention and tenderness, and the patient verbalizes measures to maintain an adequate nutritional intake.

DOCUMENTATION

- Document assessment of the abdomen. If an abdominal girth reading was obtained, record this measurement. Document the removal of the NG tube from the naris where it had been placed. Note if there is any irritation to the skin of the naris. Record the amount of NG drainage in the suction container on the patient's intake-and-output record as well as the color of the drainage. Record any pertinent teaching, such as instruction to the patient to notify nurse if he or she experiences any nausea, abdominal pain, or bloating.

SKILL 114 INSERTING A NASOPHARYNGEAL AIRWAY

Nasopharyngeal airways (nasal trumpet) are curved, uncuffed, soft plastic tubes inserted into the back of the pharynx through the nose in patients who are breathing spontaneously. The nasal trumpet provides a route from the nares to the pharynx to help maintain a patent airway. These airways may be indicated if the teeth are clenched, the tongue is enlarged, or the patient needs frequent nasopharyngeal suctioning. The appropriate size range for a nasal trumpet for adolescents to adults is 24F to 36F.

DELEGATION CONSIDERATIONS

The insertion of a nasopharyngeal airway is not delegated to nursing assistive personnel (NAP) or to unlicensed assistive personnel (UAP). Depending on the state's nurse practice act and the organization's policies and procedures, the insertion of a nasopharyngeal airway may be delegated to licensed practical/vocational nurses (LPN/LVNs). The decision to delegate must be based on careful analysis of the patient's needs and circumstances, as well as the qualifications of the person to whom the task is being delegated. Refer to the Delegation Guidelines in Appendix A.

EQUIPMENT

- Nasopharyngeal airway of appropriate size
- Disposable gloves
- Suction equipment
- Goggles and mask or face shield (optional)
- Flashlight (optional)
- Additional PPE, as indicated

ASSESSMENT

- Assess patient's lung sounds. If lung sounds are diminished, patient may need nasal airway to keep airway patent. If lung sounds are coarse or wheezing is noted, patient may need the nasal airway to help with suctioning.
- Assess patient's respiratory rate and effort. If the patient is not getting enough air or if the patient needs to be suctioned, the respiratory rate will generally increase and the patient may have retractions, nasal flaring, and grunting.
- Assess the oxygen saturation level. If the patient is not getting enough air or if the patient needs to be suctioned, the oxygen saturation level will generally decrease.
- Assess for the presence of nasal conditions, such as deviated septum or recent nasal or oral surgery, and increased risk for bleeding, such as anticoagulant therapy, which would contraindicate the use of a nasopharyngeal airway.

NURSING DIAGNOSIS

- Risk for Aspiration
- Ineffective Airway Clearance
- Risk for Injury

OUTCOME IDENTIFICATION AND PLANNING

- Patient will maintain a patent airway.
- Patient demonstrates a respiratory rate and depth within normal limits and equal, clear lung sounds bilaterally.

IMPLEMENTATION

ACTION	RATIONALE
1. Gather necessary equipment.	Assembling equipment provides for an organized approach to the task.

ACTION	RATIONALE
2. Perform hand hygiene and put on PPE, if indicated.	Hand hygiene and PPE prevent the spread of microorganisms. PPE is required based on transmission precautions.
3. Identify the patient.	Identifying the patient ensures the right patient receives the intervention and helps prevent errors.
4. Close the curtains around the bed and close the door to the room, if possible.	This ensures the patient's privacy.
5. Explain to the patient what you are going to do and the reason for doing it, even though the patient does not appear to be alert.	Explanation alleviates fears. Even though a patient appears unconscious, the nurse should explain what is happening.
6. Put on disposable gloves; put on goggles and mask or face shield, as indicated.	Gloves and other PPE prevent contact with contaminants and body fluids.
7. Measure the nasopharyngeal airway for correct size. Measure the nasopharyngeal airway by holding the airway on the side of the patient's face. The airway should reach from the tragus of the ear to the nostril plus 1 inch. The diameter should be slightly smaller than the diameter of the nostril.	Correct size ensures correct insertion and fit, allowing for conformation of the airway to the curvature of the palate.
8. Adjust bed to a comfortable working level, usually elbow height of the caregiver (VISN 8 Patient Safety Center, 2009). Lower side rail closest to you. **If the patient is awake and alert, position in semi-Fowler's position. If the patient is not conscious or alert, position in a side-lying position.**	Having the bed at the proper height prevents back and muscle strain. By raising the head of the bed or placing patient in the side-lying position, the nurse is helping to protect the airway if the patient should vomit during the placement of the nasopharyngeal airway.

ACTION	RATIONALE
9. Suction patient, if necessary.	This removes excess secretions and helps maintain patent airway.
10. Lubricate the nasopharyngeal airway generously with the water-soluble lubricant, covering the airway from the tip to the guard rim.	The lubricant helps prevent injury to the mucosa as the airway is inserted.
11. Gently insert the airway into the naris, narrow end first, until the rim is touching the naris. If resistance is met, stop and try other naris.	The airway should not be forced into the naris to prevent injury.
12. Check placement by closing the patient's mouth and place your fingers in front of the tube opening to check for air movement. Assess the pharynx to visualize the tip of the airway behind the uvula. Assess the nose for blanching or skin stretching.	This ensures correct placement and prevents injury. The skin should not be blanched or appear stretched due to the nasopharyngeal airway. If this occurs, a smaller size airway is needed.
13. Remove gloves and raise the bed rail. Place bed in the lowest position. Remove additional PPE, if used. Perform hand hygiene.	Removing PPE properly reduces the risk for infection transmission and contamination of other items. Hand hygiene prevents the spread of microorganisms. Raising side rails and proper bed height provide for patient comfort and safety.
14. Remove the airway, clean in warm soapy water, and place in other naris at least every 8 hours, or according to facility policy. If the patient coughs or gags on insertion, the nasal trumpet may be too long. Assess the pharynx. You should be able to visualize the tip of the airway behind the uvula.	The nasopharyngeal airway may cause tissue trauma and skin breakdown if left in place for too long. Secretions can accumulate on surface and contribute to irritation and tissue trauma.

EVALUATION

- Patient maintains a clear, patent airway with minimal to no secretions.
- Patient exhibits oxygen saturation level within acceptable parameters, or greater than 95%, as well as a respiratory rate within the normal range.

DOCUMENTATION

- Document the placement of the airway, airway size, naris used for insertion, removal/cleaning, assessment before and after intervention, and oxygen saturation level.

SKILL 115 OBTAINING A NASOPHARYNGEAL SWAB

A nasopharyngeal swab provides a sample that can be cultured to aid in the diagnosis of infection and to detect the carrier state for certain organisms. A swab on a flexible wire collects a specimen from the posterior nasopharynx. It is primarily used to detect viral infections. A nasopharyngeal swab is used for detection of *Bordetella pertussis* and *Corynebacterium diphtheriae,* as well as respiratory syncytial virus, *Neisseria meningitis,* methicillin-resistant *Staphylococcus aureus, Haemophilus influenzae,* and viruses causing rhinitis (Azubike et al., 2012).

DELEGATION CONSIDERATIONS

Obtaining a nasopharyngeal swab is not delegated to nursing assistive personnel (NAP) or to unlicensed assistive personnel (UAP). Depending on the state's nurse practice act and the organization's policies and procedures, this procedure may be delegated to licensed practical/vocational nurses (LPN/LVNs). The decision to delegate must be based on careful analysis of the patient's needs and circumstances, as well as the qualifications of the person to whom the task is being delegated. Refer to the Delegation Guidelines in Appendix A.

EQUIPMENT

- Nasopharyngeal swab (flexible wire)
- Penlight
- Tongue depressor
- Facial tissue
- Nonsterile gloves
- Additional PPE, as indicated
- Biohazard bag
- Appropriate label for specimen, based on facility policy and procedure

ASSESSMENT

- Assess the patient's understanding of the collection procedure, reason for testing, and ability to cooperate.
- Assess the patient's nares and for the presence of nasal symptoms, such as discharge, erythema, or congestion. Inspect the patient's nasopharynx.
- Assess for conditions that would contraindicate obtaining a nasopharyngeal swab, such as injury to the nares or nose, and surgery of the nose or throat.

NURSING DIAGNOSIS
- Risk for Infection
- Acute Pain
- Deficient Knowledge

OUTCOME IDENTIFICATION AND PLANNING
- An uncontaminated specimen is obtained without injury to the patient and sent to the laboratory promptly.
- Patient verbalizes an understanding of the rationale for the procedure.
- Patient verbalizes a decrease in anxiety related to specimen collection.

IMPLEMENTATION

ACTION	RATIONALE
1. Verify the order for a nasopharyngeal swab in the medical record. Gather equipment. Check the expiration date on the swab package.	Verifying the medical order is crucial to ensuring that the proper procedure is administered to the right patient. Assembling equipment provides for an organized approach to the task. Swab package is sterile and should not be used past the expiration date.
2. Perform hand hygiene and put on PPE, if indicated.	Hand hygiene and PPE prevent the transmission of microorganisms. PPE is required based on transmission precautions.
3. Identify the patient.	Identifying the patient ensures the right patient receives the intervention and helps prevent errors.
4. Discuss with patient the need for a nasal swab. Explain to patient the process by which the specimen will be collected. Inform the patient that he or she may experience slight discomfort and may gag.	Discussion and explanation help to allay some of the patient's anxiety and prepare the patient for what to expect.
5. Check the specimen label with the patient's identification bracelet. Label should include the patient's name	Confirmation of patient identification information ensures the specimen is labeled correctly for the right patient.

ACTION	RATIONALE
and identification number, time specimen was collected, route of collection, identification of person obtaining the sample, and any other information required by facility policy.	
6. Assemble equipment on overbed table within reach.	Arranging items nearby is convenient, saves time, and avoids unnecessary stretching and twisting of muscles on the part of the nurse.
7. Close curtains around the bed or close the door to the room, if possible.	Closing the door or curtain provides for patient privacy.
8. Put on goggles and face mask, or face shield and nonsterile gloves.	Goggles, face mask, face shield, and gloves protect the nurse from exposure to blood or body fluids and prevent the transmission of microorganisms.
9. Ask the patient to blow his or her nose into facial tissue. Ask the patient to cough into facial tissue, and then to tip his or her head back. Assist, as necessary.	Blowing of nose clears nasal passages and coughing clears the nasopharynx of material that may interfere with accurate sampling. Tilting the head allows optimal access to the nares, where the swab will be inserted.
10. Peel open the swab packaging to expose the swab and collection tube. Remove the cap from the collection tube and discard. Remove the swab from packaging by grasping the exposed end. Take care not to contaminate the swab by touching it to any other surface.	Swab must remain sterile to ensure specimen is not contaminated.
11. Ask the patient to open the mouth. Inspect the back of the patient's throat using the tongue depressor.	The swab must make contact with mucosa to ensure collection of potential pathogens.
12. Continue to observe the nasopharynx and gently insert the swab straight back	Observation of the nasopharynx during collection ensures an accurate specimen is collected.

ACTION	RATIONALE

into the nostril, aiming posteriorly along the floor of the nasal cavity. Insert approximately 6 inches (adult) (approximately the distance from the nose to the ear) to the posterior wall of the nasopharynx (Figure 1). **Do not insert the swab upward. Do not force the swab.** Rotate the swab. Leave the swab in the nasopharynx for 15 to 30 seconds and remove. Take care not to touch the swab to the patient's tongue or sides of the nostrils.

Swab must remain uncontaminated to ensure accurate results.

FIGURE 1 Nasopharyngeal swab inserted to the posterior wall of the nasopharynx.

13. Insert the swab fully into the collection tube, taking care not to touch any other surface. The handle end of the swab should fit snugly into the collection tube and the end of swab should be in the culture medium at the distal end of the collection tube. Lightly squeeze the bottom of the collection tube as necessary, depending on type of tube in use in facility, to break the seal on the culture medium.

Swab must remain uncontaminated to ensure accurate results. Full insertion of the swab ensures it will remain in the collection tube. Placement of the swab end in culture medium and releasing of liquid transport medium is necessary to ensure accurate specimen processing.

ACTION	RATIONALE
14. Dispose of used equipment per facility policy. Remove gloves. Perform hand hygiene.	Proper disposal of equipment reduces the transmission of microorganisms. Removing gloves properly reduces the risk for infection transmission and contamination of other items. Hand hygiene reduces the transmission of microorganisms.
15. Place label on the collection tube per facility policy. Place container in plastic, sealable biohazard bag.	Ensures specimen is labeled correctly for the right patient and ensures proper processing of specimen. Packaging the specimen in a biohazard bag prevents the person transporting the container from coming in contact with the specimen.
16. Remove other PPE, if used. Perform hand hygiene.	Removing PPE properly reduces the risk for infection transmission and contamination of other items. Hand hygiene reduces the transmission of microorganisms.
17. Transport the specimen to the laboratory immediately. If immediate transport is not possible, check with laboratory personnel or policy manual whether refrigeration is contraindicated.	Timely transport ensures accurate results.

EVALUATION

- Nasopharyngeal swab is collected without contamination and sent to the laboratory as soon as possible.
- Patient does not experience injury, verbalizes an understanding of the rationale for the specimen collection, and verbalizes a decrease in anxiety related to the procedure.

DOCUMENTATION

- Record the time the specimen was collected and sent to the laboratory. Document any pertinent assessments of the patient's nares and the presence of nasal symptoms, such as discharge, erythema, or congestion. Record significant assessments of the patient's oral cavity and throat.

Negative-pressure wound therapy (NPWT) (or topical negative pressure [TNP]) promotes wound healing and wound closure through the application of uniform negative pressure on the wound bed. NPWT results in reduction in bacteria in the wound and the removal of excess wound fluid, while providing a moist wound healing environment. The negative pressure results in mechanical tension on the wound tissues, stimulating cell proliferation, blood flow to wounds, and the growth of new blood vessels. An open-cell foam dressing or gauze is applied in the wound. A fenestrated tube is connected to the foam, allowing the application of the negative pressure. The dressing and distal tubing are covered by a transparent, occlusive, air-permeable dressing that provides a seal, allowing the application of the negative pressure. Excess wound fluid is removed through tubing into a collection container. NPWT also acts to pull the wound edges together.

NPWT is used to treat a variety of acute or chronic wounds, wounds with heavy drainage, wounds failing to heal, or wounds healing slowly. Examples of such wounds include pressure ulcers: arterial, venous, and diabetic ulcers; dehisced surgical wounds; infected wounds; skin graft sites; and burns. NPWT is not considered for use in the presence of active bleeding; wounds with exposed blood vessels, organs, or nerves; malignancy in wound tissue; presence of dry/necrotic tissue; or with fistulas of unknown origin (Hess, 2013; Martindell, 2012; Preston, 2008; Thompson, 2008). Cautious use is indicated in the presence of unrelieved pressure, anticoagulant therapy, poor nutritional status, and immunosuppressant therapy (Martindell; Preston). Candidates must be assessed for preexisting bleeding disorders, use of anticoagulants and other medications, or use of supplements that prolong bleeding times, such as aspirin or ginkgo biloba (Malli, 2005; Preston). NPWT dressings are changed every 48 to 72 hours, depending on the manufacturer's specifications and medical orders. Infected wounds may require dressing changes every 12 to 24 hours. The following Skill outlines the procedure for vacuum-assisted closure (V.A.C.) therapy (KCI), as an example of NPWT. There are many manufacturers of negative pressure wound therapy systems. **The nurse should be familiar with the components of, and procedures related to, the particular system in use for an individual patient.**

DELEGATION CONSIDERATIONS

The application of negative-pressure wound therapy is not delegated to nursing assistive personnel (NAP) or to unlicensed assistive personnel (UAP). Depending on the state's nurse practice act and the organization's policies and procedures, the application of negative-pressure wound therapy may be delegated to licensed practical/vocational nurses (LPN/LVNs). The decision to delegate must be based on careful analysis of the patient's needs and circumstances, as well as the qualifications of the person to whom the task is being delegated. Refer to the Delegation Guidelines in Appendix A.

EQUIPMENT

- Negative pressure unit (V.A.C. ATS Unit)
- Evacuation/collection canister
- V.A.C. Foam dressing
- V.A.C. Drape
- T.R.A.C. Pad
- Skin-protectant wipes
- Sterile gauze sponge
- Sterile irrigation set, including a basin, irrigant container, and irrigation syringe
- Sterile irrigation solution as ordered, warmed to body temperature
- Waste receptacle to dispose of contaminated materials
- Sterile gloves (2 pairs)
- Sterile scissors
- Clean disposable gloves
- Gown, mask, eye protection
- Additional PPE, as indicated
- Waterproof pad and bath blanket

ASSESSMENT

- Confirm the medical order for the application of NPWT.
- Check the patient's chart and question the patient about current treatments and medications that may make the application contraindicated.
- Assess the situation to determine the need for a dressing change.
- Confirm any medical orders relevant to wound care and any wound care included in the nursing plan of care.
- Assess the patient's level of comfort and the need for analgesics before wound care. Assess if the patient experienced any pain related to prior dressing changes and the effectiveness of interventions employed to minimize the patient's pain.
- Assess the current dressing to determine if it is intact. Assess for excess drainage or bleeding or saturation of the dressing.
- Inspect the wound and the surrounding tissue. Assess the location, appearance of the wound, stage (if appropriate), drainage, and types of tissue present in the wound. Measure the wound. Note the stage of the healing process and characteristics of any drainage. Assess the surrounding skin for color, temperature, and edema, ecchymosis, or maceration.

NURSING DIAGNOSIS

- Anxiety
- Acute Pain
- Impaired Tissue Integrity
- Disturbed Body Image
- Deficient Knowledge

OUTCOME IDENTIFICATION AND PLANNING

- Therapy is accomplished without contaminating the wound area, causing trauma to the wound, and/or causing the patient to experience pain or discomfort.
- Negative pressure device functions correctly.
- Appropriate and ordered pressure is maintained throughout therapy.
- Wound exhibits progression in healing.

IMPLEMENTATION

ACTION	RATIONALE
1. Review the medical order for the application of NPWT therapy, including the ordered pressure setting for the device. Gather necessary supplies.	Reviewing the order validates the correct patient and correct procedure. Preparation promotes efficient time management and an organized approach to the task.
2. Perform hand hygiene and put on PPE, if indicated.	Hand hygiene and PPE prevent the spread of microorganisms. PPE is required based on transmission precautions.
3. Identify the patient.	Identifying the patient ensures the right patient receives the intervention and helps prevent errors.
4. Assemble equipment on overbed table within reach.	Organization facilitates performance of task.
5. Close the curtains around the bed and close the door to the room if possible. Explain what you are going to do and why you are going to do it to the patient.	This ensures the patient's privacy. Explanation relieves anxiety and facilitates cooperation.
6. Assess the patient for possible need for nonpharmacologic pain-reducing interventions or analgesic medication before wound care dressing change. Administer appropriate prescribed analgesic. Allow enough time for the analgesic to achieve its effectiveness before beginning the procedure.	Pain is a subjective experience influenced by past experience. Wound care and dressing changes may cause pain for some patients.
7. Adjust bed to comfortable working height, usually elbow height of the caregiver (VISN 8, 2009).	Having the bed at the proper height prevents back and muscle strain.
8. Assist the patient to a comfortable position that provides easy access to the	Patient positioning and draping provide for comfort and warmth. Gravity directs the flow of liquid

ACTION	RATIONALE
wound area. Position the patient so the irrigation solution will flow from the clean end of the wound toward the dirty end. Expose the area and drape the patient with a bath blanket, if needed. Put a waterproof pad under the wound area.	from the least contaminated to the most contaminated area. Waterproof pad protects the patient and the bed linens.
9. Have the disposal bag or waste receptacle within easy reach for use during the procedure.	Having a waste container handy allows for easy disposal of the soiled dressings and supplies, without the spread of microorganisms.
10. Using sterile technique, prepare a sterile field and add all the sterile supplies needed for the procedure to the field. Pour warmed, sterile irrigating solution into the sterile container.	Proper preparation ensures that supplies are within easy reach and sterility is maintained. Warmed solution may result in less discomfort.
11. Put on a gown, mask, and eye protection.	Use of PPE is part of *Standard Precautions*. A gown protects your clothes from contamination if splashing should occur. Goggles protect mucous membranes of your eyes from contact with irrigant fluid.
12. Put on clean gloves. Carefully and gently remove the dressing. If there is resistance, use a silicone-based adhesive remover to help remove the drape. **Note the number of pieces of foam removed from the wound. Compare with the documented number from the previous dressing change.**	Gloves protect the nurse from handling contaminated dressings. A silicone-based adhesive remover allows for the easy, rapid, and painless removal without the associated problems of skin stripping (Denyer, 2011; Benbow, 2011). Counting the number of pieces of foam assures the removal of all foam that was placed during the previous dressing change.
13. Discard the dressings in the receptacle. Remove your gloves and put them in the receptacle.	Proper disposal of dressings and used gloves prevents the spread of microorganisms.

ACTION	RATIONALE
14. Put on sterile gloves. Using sterile technique, irrigate the wound (see Skill 185).	Irrigation removes exudate and debris.
15. Clean the area around the wound with normal saline. Dry the surrounding skin with a sterile gauze sponge.	Moisture provides a medium for growth of microorganisms.
16. Assess the wound for appearance, stage, presence of eschar, granulation tissue, epithelialization, undermining, tunneling, necrosis, sinus tract, and drainage. Assess the appearance of the surrounding tissue. Measure the wound.	This information provides evidence about the wound healing process and/or the presence of infection.
17. **Wipe intact skin around the wound with a skin-protectant wipe and allow it to dry well.**	Skin protectant provides a barrier against irritation and breakdown.
18. **Using sterile scissors, cut the foam to the shape and measurement of the wound. Do not cut foam over the wound.** More than one piece of foam may be necessary if the first piece is cut too small. Carefully place the foam in the wound. **Ensure foam-to-foam contact if more than one piece is required. Note the number of pieces of foam placed in the wound.**	Aseptic technique maintains sterility of items to come in contact with wound. Foam should fill the wound but not cover intact surrounding skin. Foam fragments may fall into the wound if cutting is performed over the wound. Foam-to-foam contact allows for even distribution of negative pressure. Recording the number of pieces of foam aids in assuring the removal of all foam with next dressing change.
19. Trim and place the V.A.C. Drape to cover the foam dressing and an additional 3 to 5 cm border of intact periwound tissue. V.A.C. Drape may be cut into multiple pieces for easier handling.	The occlusive air-permeable V.A.C. Drape provides a seal, allowing the application of the negative pressure.
20. Choose an appropriate site to apply the T.R.A.C. Pad.	T.R.A.C. Pad should be placed in the area where the greatest fluid flow and optimal drainage

ACTION	RATIONALE

is anticipated. Avoid placing over bony prominences or within creases in the tissue.

21. Pinch the drape and cut a 2-cm hole through it. Apply the T.R.A.C. Pad. Remove V.A.C. Canister from package and insert into the V.A.C. Therapy Unit until it locks into place. Connect T.R.A.C. Pad tubing to canister tubing and check that the clamps on each tube are open. Turn on the power to the V.A.C. Therapy Unit and select the prescribed therapy setting.

A hole in the drape allows for removal of fluid and/or exudate. The canister provides a collection chamber for drainage.

22. **Assess the dressing to ensure seal integrity. The dressing should be collapsed, shrinking to the foam and skin.**

Shrinkage confirms a good seal, allowing for accurate application of pressure and treatment.

23. Remove and discard gloves.

Proper disposal of gloves prevents the spread of microorganisms.

24. Label dressing with date and time. Remove all remaining equipment; place the patient in a comfortable position, with side rails up and bed in the lowest position.

Recording date and time provides communication and demonstrates adherence to plan of care. Proper patient and bed positioning promotes safety and comfort.

25. Remove PPE, if used. Perform hand hygiene.

Removing PPE properly reduces the risk for infection transmission and contamination of other items. Hand hygiene prevents the spread of microorganisms.

26. Check all wound dressings every shift. More frequent checks may be needed if the wound is more complex or dressings become saturated quickly.

Checking dressings ensures the assessment of changes in patient condition and timely intervention to prevent complications.

EVALUATION

- Application of negative-pressure wound therapy is accomplished without contaminating the wound area, causing trauma to the wound, and/or causing the patient to experience pain or discomfort.
- Negative pressure device functions correctly.
- Appropriate and ordered pressure is maintained throughout therapy.
- Wound exhibits progression in healing.

DOCUMENTATION

- Record your assessment of the wound, including evidence of granulation tissue, presence of necrotic tissue, stage (if appropriate), and characteristics of drainage. Include the appearance of the surrounding skin. Document the cleansing or irrigation of the wound and solution used. Document the application of the NPWT, noting the pressure setting, patency, and seal of the dressing. Describe the color and characteristics of the drainage in the collection chamber. Record pertinent patient and family education and any patient reaction to this procedure, including the presence of pain and effectiveness or ineffectiveness of pain interventions.

SKILL 117   ASSISTING THE PATIENT WITH ORAL CARE

Adequate oral hygiene care is imperative to promote the patient's sense of well-being and prevent deterioration of the oral cavity. Poor oral hygiene is reported to lead to the colonization of the oropharyngeal secretions by respiratory pathogens. Diligent oral hygiene care can improve oral health and limit the growth of pathogens in oropharyngeal secretions, decreasing the incidence of aspiration pneumonia, community-acquired pneumonia, ventilator-associated pneumonia, and other systemic diseases, such as diabetes, heart disease and stroke (Tada & Miura, 2012; CDC, 2011; Durgunde & Cocks, 2011; AACN, 2010). If the patient can assist with mouth care, provide the necessary materials. Teeth should be brushed and flossed twice a day; the mouth should be rinsed after meals. If the patient is unable to perform oral hygiene, make certain that the mouth receives care as often as necessary to keep it clean and moist, as often as every 1 or 2 hours if necessary. This is especially important for patients who cannot drink or are not permitted fluids by mouth.

DELEGATION CONSIDERATIONS

The implementation of oral care may be delegated to nursing assistive personnel (NAP) or to unlicensed assistive personnel (UAP), as well as to licensed practical/vocational nurses (LPN/LVNs).The decision to delegate must be based on careful analysis of the patient's needs and circumstances, as well as the qualifications of the person to whom the task is being delegated. Refer to the Delegation Guidelines in Appendix A.

EQUIPMENT

- Toothbrush
- Toothpaste
- Emesis basin
- Glass with cool water
- Disposable gloves
- Additional PPE, as indicated
- Towel
- Mouthwash (optional)
- Washcloth or paper towel
- Lip lubricant (optional)
- Dental floss

ASSESSMENT

- Assess the patient's oral hygiene preferences: frequency, time of day, and type of hygiene products.
- Assess for any physical activity limitations.
- Assess patient's oral cavity and dentition. Look for any inflammation or bleeding of the gums. Look for ulcers, lesions, and yellow or white patches.
- Assess for signs of dehydration (dry mucosa) and dental decay. Look at the lips for dryness or cracking. Ask the patient if he or she is having pain, dryness, soreness, or difficulty chewing or swallowing.
- Assess patient's ability to perform own care.

NURSING DIAGNOSIS

- Risk for Aspiration
- Impaired Oral Mucous Membrane
- Deficient Knowledge

OUTCOME IDENTIFICATION AND PLANNING

- The patient's mouth and teeth will be clean.
- The patient will exhibit a positive body image.
- The patient will verbalize the importance of oral care.

ACTION	RATIONALE
3. Assemble equipment on overbed table within patient's reach.	Organization facilitates performance of the task.
4. Close the room door or curtains. Place the bed at an appropriate and comfortable working height; usually elbow height of the caregiver (VISN 8 Patient Safety Center, 2009).	Closing the door or curtains provides privacy. Proper bed height helps reduce back strain while performing the procedure.
5. Lower side rail and assist the patient to a sitting position, if permitted, or turn the patient onto side. Place towel across the patient's chest.	The sitting or side-lying position prevents aspiration of fluids into the lungs. The towel protects the patient from dampness.
6. Encourage the patient to brush own teeth according to the following guidelines. Assist, if necessary.	
a. Moisten toothbrush and apply toothpaste to bristles.	Water softens the bristles.
b. Place brush at a 45-degree angle to gum line and brush from gum line to crown of each tooth (Figure 1). Brush outer and inner surfaces. Brush back and forth across biting surface of each tooth.	Facilitates removal of plaque and tartar. The 45-degree angle of brushing permits cleansing of all surface tooth areas.
c. Brush tongue gently with toothbrush.	Removes coating on the tongue. Gentle motion does not stimulate gag reflex.

FIGURE 1 Brushing from the gum line to the crown of each tooth.

ACTION	RATIONALE
d. Have patient rinse vigorously with water and spit into emesis basin. Repeat until clear. Suction may be used as an alternative for removal of fluid and secretions from the mouth.	The vigorous swishing motion helps to remove debris. Suction is appropriate if patient is unable to expectorate well.
7. Assist patient to floss teeth, if appropriate:	Flossing aids in removal of plaque and promotes healthy gum tissue.
a. Remove approximately 6 inches of dental floss from container or use a plastic floss holder. Wrap the floss around the index fingers, keeping about 1 to 1.5 inches of floss taut between the fingers.	The floss must be held taut to get between the teeth.
b. Insert floss gently between teeth, moving it back and forth downward to the gums.	Trauma to the gums can occur if floss is forced between teeth.
c. Move the floss up and down, first on one side of a tooth and then on the side of the other tooth, until the surfaces are clean. Repeat in the spaces between all teeth.	This ensures that the sides of both teeth are cleaned.
d. Instruct patient to rinse mouth well with water after flossing.	Vigorous rinsing helps to remove food particles and plaque that have been loosened by flossing.
8. Offer mouthwash if patient prefers.	Mouthwash leaves a pleasant taste in the mouth.
9. Offer lip balm or petroleum jelly.	Lip balm lubricates lips and prevents drying.
10. Remove equipment. Remove gloves and discard. Raise side rail and lower bed. Assist patient to a position of comfort.	Removing gloves properly reduces the risk for infection transmission and contamination of other items. These actions promote patient comfort and safety.

ACTION	RATIONALE
11. Remove any other PPE, if used. Perform hand hygiene.	Removing PPE properly reduces the risk for infection transmission and contamination of other items. Hand hygiene prevents the spread of microorganisms.

EVALUATION

- Patient receives oral care and experiences little to no discomfort.
- Patient states mouth feels refreshed.
- Patient demonstrates understanding of the reasons for proper oral care.

DOCUMENTATION

- Record oral assessment, significant observations and unusual findings, such as bleeding or inflammation. Document any teaching done. Document procedure and patient response.

SKILL 118 PROVIDING ORAL CARE FOR THE DEPENDENT PATIENT

Physical limitations, such as those associated with aging, often lead to less than adequate oral hygiene. The dexterity required for adequate brushing and flossing may decrease with age, or illness. Patients with cognitive impairment, such as dementia, are also at risk for inadequate oral hygiene (Jablonski et al., 2011). Teeth should be brushed and flossed twice a day; the mouth should be rinsed after meals. If the patient is unable to perform oral hygiene, make certain that the mouth receives care as often as necessary to keep it clean and moist, as often as every 1 or 2 hours, if necessary. Moisten the mouth with water, if allowed, and lubricate the lips often enough to keep the membranes well moistened.

DELEGATION CONSIDERATIONS

The implementation of oral care for a dependent patient may be delegated to nursing assistive personnel (NAP) or to unlicensed assistive personnel (UAP) after assessment by the registered nurse, as well as to licensed practical/vocational nurses (LPN/LVNs). The decision to delegate must be based on careful analysis of the patient's needs and circumstances, as well as the qualifications of the person to whom the task is being delegated. Refer to the Delegation Guidelines in Appendix A.

EQUIPMENT

- Toothbrush
- Toothpaste
- Emesis basin
- Glass with cool water

- Disposable gloves
- Additional PPE, as indicated
- Towel
- Mouthwash (optional)
- Dental floss (optional)
- Denture-cleaning equipment (if necessary)
- Denture cup
- Denture cleaner
- 4 × 4 gauze
- Washcloth or paper towel
- Lip lubricant (optional)
- Sponge toothette
- Irrigating syringe with rubber tip (optional)
- Suction catheter with suction apparatus (optional)

ASSESSMENT

- Assess the patient's oral hygiene preferences: frequency, time of day, and type of hygiene products.
- Assess for any physical activity limitations.
- Assess the patient's level of consciousness and overall ability to assist with oral care and respond to directions.
- Assess the patient's risk for oral hygiene problems.
- Assess the patient's gag reflex.
- Assess patient's oral cavity and dentition. Look for any inflammation or bleeding of the gums. Look for ulcers, lesions, and yellow or white patches.
- Assess for signs of dehydration (dry mucosa) and dental decay. Look at the lips for dryness or cracking. If the patient is conscious and/or cognitively able to respond, ask the patient if he or she is having pain, dryness, soreness, or difficulty chewing or swallowing.

NURSING DIAGNOSIS

- Impaired Oral Mucous Membrane
- Deficient Knowledge
- Risk for Aspiration

OUTCOME IDENTIFICATION AND PLANNING

- The patient's mouth and teeth will be clean.
- The patient will not experience impaired oral mucous membranes.
- The patient will demonstrate improvement in body image.
- The patient will verbalize, if able, an understanding about the importance of oral care.

ACTION	RATIONALE

2. Identify the patient. Explain the procedure to the patient.

Identifying the patient ensures the right patient receives the intervention and helps prevent errors. Explanation facilitates cooperation.

3. Assemble equipment on overbed table within reach.

Organization facilitates performance of task.

4. Close the room door or curtains. Place the bed at an appropriate and comfortable working height, usually elbow height of the caregiver (VISN 8 Patient Safety Center, 2009). Lower one side rail and position the patient on the side, with head tilted forward. Place towel across the patient's chest and emesis basin in position under chin. Put on gloves.

Cleaning another person's mouth is invasive and may be embarrassing (Holman et al., 2005). Closing the door or curtains provides privacy. Proper bed height helps reduce back strain while performing the procedure. The side-lying position with head forward prevents aspiration of fluid into lungs. Towel and emesis basin protects the patient from dampness. Gloves prevent the spread of microorganisms.

5. Gently open the patient's mouth by applying pressure to the lower jaw at the front of the mouth. Remove dentures, if present. (Refer to Skill 49.) Brush the teeth and gums carefully with toothbrush and paste (Figure 1). Lightly brush the tongue.

Toothbrush provides friction necessary to clean areas where plaque and tartar accumulate.

FIGURE 1 Carefully brushing patient's teeth.

6. Use toothette dipped in water to rinse the oral cavity. If desired, insert the rubber tip of the irrigating syringe into patient's mouth and

Rinsing helps clean debris from the mouth. Forceful irrigation may cause aspiration.

ACTION	RATIONALE

rinse gently with a small amount of water (Figure 2). **Position patient's head to allow for return of water or use suction apparatus to remove the water from oral cavity (Figure 3).**

FIGURE 2 Using irrigating syringe and a small amount of water to rinse mouth.

FIGURE 3 Using suction to remove excess fluid.

7. Clean the dentures before replacing. (See Skill 49.)	Cleaning maintains dentures and oral hygiene. Plaque can accumulate on dentures and promote oropharyngeal colonization of pathogens.
8. Apply lubricant to patient's lips.	This prevents drying and cracking of lips.
9. Remove equipment and return patient to a position of comfort. Remove your gloves. Raise side rail and lower bed.	Promotes patient comfort and safety. Removing gloves properly reduces the risk for infection transmission and contamination of other items.
10. Remove additional PPE, if used. Perform hand hygiene.	Removing PPE properly reduces the risk for infection transmission and contamination of other items. Hand hygiene prevents the spread of microorganisms.

EVALUATION
- Patient's oral cavity is clean and free from complications.
- Patient states or demonstrates improved body image.
- If patient is able, he or she verbalizes a basic understanding of the need for oral care.

DOCUMENTATION

- Record oral assessment, significant observations, and unusual findings, such as bleeding or inflammation. Document any teaching done. Document procedure and patient response.

SKILL 119 — INSERTING AN OROPHARYNGEAL AIRWAY

An oropharyngeal airway is a semicircular tube of plastic inserted into the back of the pharynx through the mouth in a patient who is breathing spontaneously. The oropharyngeal airway can help protect the airway of an unconscious patient by preventing the tongue from falling back against the posterior pharynx and blocking it. Once the patient regains consciousness, the oropharyngeal airway is removed. Tape is not used to hold the airway in place because the patient should be able to expel the airway once he or she becomes alert. The nurse can insert this device at the bedside with little to no trauma to the unconscious patient. Oropharyngeal airways may also be used to aid in ventilation during a code situation and to facilitate suctioning an unconscious or semiconscious patient. Alternately, airway support may be provided with a nasopharyngeal airway. (Refer to Skill 114.)

DELEGATION CONSIDERATIONS

The insertion of an oropharyngeal airway is not delegated to nursing assistive personnel (NAP) or to unlicensed assistive personnel (UAP). Depending on the state's nurse practice act and the organization's policies and procedures, the insertion of an oropharyngeal airway may be delegated to licensed practical/vocational nurses (LPN/LVNs). The decision to delegate must be based on careful analysis of the patient's needs and circumstances, as well as the qualifications of the person to whom the task is being delegated. Refer to the Delegation Guidelines in Appendix A.

EQUIPMENT

- Oropharyngeal airway of appropriate size
- Disposable gloves
- Suction equipment
- Goggles and mask or face shield (optional)
- Flashlight (optional)
- Additional PPE, as indicated

ASSESSMENT

- Assess patient's level of consciousness and ability to protect the airway.
- Assess amount and consistency of oral secretions.
- Auscultate lung sounds. If the tongue is occluding the airway, lung sounds may be diminished.

• Assess for loose teeth or recent oral surgery, which may contraindicate the use of an oropharyngeal airway.

NURSING DIAGNOSIS

• Risk for Aspiration
• Ineffective Airway Clearance
• Risk for Injury

OUTCOME IDENTIFICATION AND PLANNING

• Patient will maintain a patent airway and exhibit oxygen saturation within acceptable parameters, or greater than 95%.
• Patient remains free of aspiration and injury.

IMPLEMENTATION

ACTION	RATIONALE
1. Bring necessary equipment to the bedside stand or over-bed table.	Bringing everything to the bedside conserves time and energy. Arranging items nearby is convenient, saves time, and avoids unnecessary stretching and twisting of muscles on the part of the nurse.
2. Perform hand hygiene and put on PPE, if indicated.	Hand hygiene and PPE prevent the spread of microorganisms. PPE is required based on transmission precautions.
3. Identify the patient.	Identifying the patient ensures the right patient receives the intervention and helps prevent errors.
4. Close the curtains around the bed and close the door to the room, if possible.	This ensures the patient's privacy.
5. Explain to the patient what you are going to do and the reason for doing it, even if the patient does not appear to be alert.	Explanation alleviates fears. Even if a patient appears unconscious, the nurse should explain what is happening.
6. Put on disposable gloves; put on goggles and mask or face shield, as indicated.	Gloves and other PPE prevent contact with contaminants and body fluids.

ACTION	RATIONALE
7. Measure the oropharyngeal airway for correct size. Measure the oropharyngeal airway by holding the airway on the side of the patient's face. The airway should reach from the opening of the mouth to the back angle of the jaw.	Correct size ensures correct insertion and fit, allowing for conformation of the airway to the curvature of the palate.
8. **Check mouth for any loose teeth, dentures, or other foreign material. Remove dentures or material if present.**	Prevents aspiration or swallowing of objects. During insertion, the airway may push any foreign objects in the mouth to the back of the throat.
9. Position patient in semi-Fowler's position.	This position facilitates airway insertion and helps prevent the tongue from moving back against the posterior pharynx.
10. Suction the patient, if necessary.	This removes excess secretions and helps maintain a patent airway.
11. Open the patient's mouth by using your thumb and index finger to gently pry teeth apart. **Insert the airway with the curved tip pointing up toward the roof of the mouth (Figure 1).**	This is done to advance the tip of the airway past the tongue, toward the back of the throat.

FIGURE 1 Inserting the airway.

12. Slide the airway across the tongue to the back of the mouth. Rotate the airway 180 degrees as it passes the uvula. The tip should point down and the curvature	This is done to shift the tongue anteriorly, thereby allowing the patient to breathe through and around the airway.

ACTION	RATIONALE
should follow the contour of the roof of the mouth. Use a flashlight to confirm the position of the airway with the curve fitting over the tongue.	
13. Ensure accurate placement and adequate ventilation by auscultating breath sounds.	If the airway is placed correctly, lung sounds should be audible and equal in all lobes.
14. Position the patient on his or her side when the airway is in place.	This position helps keep the tongue out of the posterior pharynx area and helps to prevent aspiration if the unconscious patient should vomit.
15. Remove gloves and additional PPE, if used. Perform hand hygiene.	Removing PPE properly reduces the risk for infection transmission and contamination of other items. Hand hygiene prevents the spread of microorganisms.
16. Remove the airway for a brief period every 4 hours, or according to facility policy. Assess mouth; provide mouth care; and clean the airway according to facility policy before reinserting it.	Tissue irritation and ulceration can result from prolonged use of an airway. Mouth care provides moisture to mucous membranes and helps maintain tissue integrity.

EVALUATION

- Patient exhibits a patent airway with oxygen saturation within acceptable parameters, or greater than 95%.
- Patient remains free of injury and aspiration.

DOCUMENTATION

- Document the placement of the airway, airway size, removal/cleaning, assessment before and after intervention, and oxygen saturation level.

SKILL 120 | CHANGING AND EMPTYING AN OSTOMY APPLIANCE

The word *ostomy* is a term for a surgically formed opening from the inside of an organ to the outside. The intestinal mucosa is brought out to the abdominal wall, and a *stoma,* the part of the ostomy that is attached to the skin, is formed by suturing the mucosa to the skin. An *ileostomy* allows liquid fecal content from the ileum of the small intestine to be eliminated through the stoma. A *colostomy* permits formed feces in the colon to exit through the stoma. Colostomies are further classified by the part of the colon from which they originate. Ostomy appliances or pouches are applied to the opening to collect stool. They should be emptied promptly, usually when they are one-third to one-half full. If they are allowed to fill up, they may leak or become detached from the skin. Ostomy appliances are available in a one-piece (barrier backing already attached to the pouch) or two-piece (separate pouch that fastens to the barrier backing) system. Appliances are usually changed every 3 to 7 days, although they could be changed more often. Proper application minimizes the risk for skin breakdown around the stoma. This skill addresses changing a one-piece appliance. A one-piece appliance consists of a pouch with an integral adhesive section that adheres to the patient's skin. The adhesive flange is generally made from hydrocolloid. The accompanying Skill Variation addresses changing a two-piece appliance.

DELEGATION CONSIDERATIONS

Empting a stoma appliance on an ostomy may be delegated to nursing assistive personnel (NAP) or to unlicensed assistive personnel (UAP), as well as to licensed practical/vocational nurses (LPN/LVNs). Changing a stoma appliance on an ostomy may be delegated to an LPN/LVN. The decision to delegate must be based on careful analysis of the patient's needs and circumstances, as well as the qualifications of the person to whom the task is being delegated. Refer to the Delegation Guidelines in Appendix A.

EQUIPMENT

- Basin with warm water
- Skin cleanser, towel, washcloth
- Toilet tissue or paper towel
- Silicone-based adhesive remover
- Gauze squares
- Washcloth
- Skin protectant, such as SkinPrep
- One-piece ostomy appliance
- Closure clamp, if required, for appliance
- Stoma measuring guide
- Graduated container, toilet or bedpan
- Ostomy belt (optional)
- Disposable gloves
- Additional PPE, as indicated
- Small plastic trash bag
- Waterproof disposable pad

ASSESSMENT

- Assess current ostomy appliance, looking at product style, condition of appliance, and stoma (if bag is clear). Note length of time the appliance has been in place.
- Determine the patient's knowledge of ostomy care.
- After removing the appliance, assess the stoma and the skin surrounding the stoma. Assess any abdominal scars, if surgery was recent.
- Assess the amount, color, consistency, and odor of stool from the ostomy.

NURSING DIAGNOSIS

- Risk for Impaired Skin Integrity
- Deficient Knowledge
- Disturbed Body Image

OUTCOME IDENTIFICATION AND PLANNING

- Stoma appliance is applied correctly to the skin to allow stool to drain freely.
- Patient exhibits a moist red stoma with intact skin surrounding the stoma.
- Patient demonstrates knowledge of how to apply the appliance.
- Patient demonstrates positive coping skills.
- Patient expels stool that is appropriate in consistency and amount for the ostomy location.
- Patient verbalizes positive self-image.

IMPLEMENTATION

ACTION	RATIONALE
1. Gather equipment.	Assembling equipment provides for an organized approach to the task.
2. Perform hand hygiene and put on PPE, if indicated.	Hand hygiene and PPE prevent the spread of microorganisms. PPE is required based on transmission precautions.
3. Identify the patient.	Identifying the patient ensures the right patient receives the intervention and helps prevent errors.
4. Close the curtains around the bed and close the door to the	This ensures the patient's privacy. Explanation relieves

ACTION	RATIONALE
room, if possible. Explain what you are going to do and why you are going to do it to the patient. Encourage the patient to observe or participate, if possible.	anxiety and facilitates cooperation. Discussion promotes cooperation and helps to minimize anxiety. Having the patient observe or assist encourages self-acceptance.
5. Assemble equipment on overbed table within reach.	Arranging items nearby is convenient, saves time, and avoids unnecessary stretching and twisting of muscles on the part of the nurse.
6. Assist the patient to a comfortable sitting or lying position in bed or a standing or sitting position in the bathroom. If the patient is in bed, adjust the bed to a comfortable working height, usually elbow height of the caregiver (VISN 8 Patient Safety Center, 2009). Place waterproof pad under the patient at the stoma site.	Either position should allow the patient to view the procedure in preparation to learn to perform it independently. Lying flat or sitting upright facilitates smooth application of the appliance. Having the bed at the proper height prevents back and muscle strain. A waterproof pad protects linens and patient from moisture.

Emptying an Appliance

ACTION	RATIONALE
7. Put on disposable gloves. Remove clamp and fold end of appliance or pouch upward like a cuff.	Gloves prevent contact with blood, body fluids, and microorganisms. Creating a cuff before emptying prevents additional soiling and odor.
8. Empty contents into bedpan, toilet, or measuring device.	Appliances do not need rinsing because rinsing may reduce appliance's odor barrier.
9. Wipe the lower 2 inches of the appliance or pouch with toilet tissue or paper towel.	Drying the lower section removes any additional fecal material, thus decreasing odor problems.
10. Uncuff edge of appliance or pouch and apply clip or clamp, or secure Velcro closure. Ensure the curve of the clamp follows the curve of the patient's body. Remove gloves. Assist the patient to a comfortable position.	The edge of the appliance or pouch should remain clean. The clamp secures closure. Hand hygiene deters spread of microorganisms. Ensures patient comfort.

ACTION	RATIONALE

11. If appliance is not to be changed, remove additional PPE, if used. Perform hand hygiene.

Removing PPE properly reduces the risk for infection transmission and contamination of other items. Hand hygiene prevents the spread of microorganisms.

Changing an Appliance

12. Place a disposable pad on the work surface. Set up the washbasin with warm water and the rest of the supplies. Place a trash bag within reach.

Protects surface. Organization facilitates performance of procedure.

13. Put on clean gloves. Place waterproof pad under the patient at the stoma site. Empty the appliance as described previously.

Protects linens and patient from moisture. Emptying the contents before removal prevents accidental spillage of fecal material.

14. Start at the top of the appliance and keep the abdominal skin taut. Gently remove pouch faceplate from skin by pushing skin from the appliance rather than pulling the appliance from skin. Apply a silicone-based adhesive remover by spraying or wiping with the remover wipe.

The seal between the surface of the faceplate and the skin must be broken before the faceplate can be removed. Harsh handling of the appliance can damage the skin and impair the development of a secure seal in the future. Silicone-based adhesive remover allows for the rapid and painless removal of adhesives and prevents skin stripping (Rudoni, 2008; Stephen-Haynes, 2008).

15. Place the appliance in the trash bag, if disposable. If reusable, set aside to wash in lukewarm soap and water and allow to air dry after the new appliance is in place.

Thorough cleaning and airing of the appliance reduce odor and deterioration of the appliance. For esthetic and infection-control purposes, discard used appliances appropriately.

16. Use toilet tissue to remove any excess stool from the stoma. Cover stoma with gauze pad. Clean skin around stoma with skin cleanser and water or a cleansing agent and a washcloth. Remove all old adhesive from skin; use an

Toilet tissue, used gently, will not damage the stoma. The gauze absorbs any drainage from the stoma while the skin is being prepared. Cleaning the skin removes excretions and old adhesive and skin protectant. Excretions or a buildup of other substances can irritate and

ACTION	RATIONALE
adhesive remover, as necessary. Do not apply lotion to the peristomal area.	damage the skin. Lotion will prevent a tight adhesive seal.
17. Gently pat area dry. **Make sure skin around stoma is thoroughly dry.** Assess stoma and condition of surrounding skin.	Careful drying prevents trauma to skin and stoma. An intact, properly applied fecal collection device protects skin integrity. Any change in color and size of the stoma may indicate circulatory problems.
18. Apply skin protectant to a 2-inch (5 cm) radius around the stoma, and allow it to dry completely, which takes about 30 seconds.	The skin needs protection from the excoriating effect of the excretion and appliance adhesive. The skin must be perfectly dry before the appliance is placed to get good adherence and to prevent leaks.
19. Lift the gauze squares for a moment and measure the stoma opening, using the measurement guide. Replace the gauze. Trace the same-size opening on the back center of the appliance. Cut the opening 1/8 inch larger than the stoma size. Using a finger, gently smooth the wafer edges after cutting.	The appliance should fit snugly around the stoma, with only 1/8 inch of skin visible around the opening. A faceplate opening that is too small can cause trauma to the stoma. If the opening is too large, exposed skin will be irritated by stool. Wafer edges may be uneven after cutting and could cause irritation to and/or pressure on the stoma.
20. Remove the paper backing from the appliance faceplate. Quickly remove the gauze squares and ease the appliance over the stoma. Gently press onto the skin while smoothing over the surface. Apply gentle, even pressure to the appliance for approximately 30 seconds.	The appliance is effective only if it is properly positioned and adhered securely. Pressure on appliance faceplate allows it to mold to the patient's skin and improve seal (Jones et al., 2011).
21. Close bottom of appliance or pouch by folding the end upward and using the clamp or clip that comes with the product, or secure Velcro closure. Ensure the curve of the clamp follows the curve of the patient's body.	A tightly sealed appliance will not leak and cause embarrassment and discomfort for the patient.

ACTION	RATIONALE
22. Remove gloves. Assist the patient to a comfortable position. Cover the patient with bed linens. Place the bed in the lowest position.	Provides warmth and promotes comfort and safety.
23. Put on clean gloves. Remove or discard equipment and assess the patient's response to the procedure.	Gloves prevent contact with blood, body fluids, and micro-organisms that contaminate the used equipment. The patient's response may indicate acceptance of the ostomy as well as the need for health teaching.
24. Remove gloves and additional PPE, if used. Perform hand hygiene.	Removing PPE properly reduces the risk for infection transmission and contamination of other items. Hand hygiene prevents the spread of microorganisms.

EVALUATION

- The expected outcomes are met when the patient tolerates the procedure without pain and the peristomal skin remains intact without excoriation.
- Odor is contained within the closed system.
- Patient participates in ostomy appliance care, demonstrates positive coping skills, and expels stool that is appropriate in consistency and amount for the location of the ostomy.

DOCUMENTATION

- Document appearance of stoma, condition of peristomal skin, characteristics of drainage (amount, color, consistency, unusual odor), patient's reaction to procedure, and pertinent patient teaching.

SKILL VARIATION **Applying a Two-Piece Appliance**

A two-piece colostomy appliance is composed of a pouch and a separate adhesive faceplate. The faceplate is left in place for a period of time, usually 3 to 7 days. During this period, when the colostomy appliance requires changing, only the bag needs to be replaced. The two main types of two-piece appliance are (1) those that 'click' together and (2) those that 'adhere' together. The clicking Tupperware-type joining action provides extra security because

Applying a Two-Piece Appliance *continued*

there is a sensation when the appliance is secured, which the patient can feel. One problem with this type of system is that those with reduced manual dexterity may find it difficult to secure. Another disadvantage is that it is less discreet because the parts of the appliance that click together are more bulky than the one-piece system. Two-piece appliances with an adhesive system have the advantage that they are more discreet than conventional two-piece systems. They may also be simpler to use for those with poor manual dexterity. A potential disadvantage is that if the adhesive is not joined correctly and forms a crease, then feces or flatus may leak out, causing odor and embarrassment. Regardless of the type of two-piece appliance in use, the procedure to change is basically the same.

1. Gather necessary equipment.
2. Perform hand hygiene and put on PPE, if indicated.

3. Identify the patient.

4. Close the curtains around the bed and close the door to the room, if possible. Explain what you are going to do and why you are going to do it to the patient.

Encourage the patient to observe or participate, if possible.
5. Assemble equipment on overbed table within reach.
6. Assist the patient to a comfortable sitting or lying position in bed or a standing or sitting position in the bathroom.
7. Place a disposable pad on the work surface. Set up the washbasin with warm water and the rest of the supplies. Place a trash bag within reach.
8. Put on gloves. Place waterproof pad under the patient at the stoma site. Empty the appliance as described previously above.
9. Starting at the top of the appliance, gently remove the pouch faceplate while keeping the abdominal skin taut. Apply a silicone-based adhesive remover by spraying or wiping with the remover wipe. Push the skin from the appliance rather than pulling the appliance from the skin.
10. Place the appliance in the trash bag, if disposable. If reusable, set aside to wash in lukewarm soap and water and allow to air dry after the new appliance is in place.
11. Use toilet tissue to remove any excess stool from the stoma. Cover the stoma with gauze pad. Clean skin around the stoma with

continued on page 648

skin cleanser and water
or a cleansing agent and a
washcloth. Remove all old
adhesive from skin; use an
adhesive remover as necessary. Do not apply lotion to
peristomal area.

12. Gently pat area dry. Make
sure skin around the stoma
is thoroughly dry. Assess
the stoma and condition of
surrounding skin.

13. Apply skin protectant to a
2-inch (5 cm) radius around
the stoma, and allow it
to dry completely, which
takes about 30 seconds

14. Lift the gauze squares for
a moment and measure
the stoma opening, using
the measurement guide.
Replace the gauze. Trace
the same-size opening
on the back center of the
appliance faceplate. Cut
the opening 1/8 inch larger
than the stoma size. Use a
finger to gently smooth the
wafer edges after cutting.

15. Remove the backing from
the faceplate. Quickly
remove the gauze squares
and ease the faceplate
over the stoma. Gently
press onto the skin while
smoothing over the surface.
Apply gentle pressure to
the faceplate for approximately 30 seconds.

16. Apply the appliance pouch
to the faceplate following
manufacturer's directions.
If using a 'click' system,

lay the ring on the pouch
over the ring on the faceplate. Ask the patient to
tighten stomach muscles, if
possible. Beginning at one
edge of the ring, push the
pouch ring onto the face-
plate ring. A 'click' should
be heard when the pouch is
secured onto the faceplate.

17. If using an 'adhere' system,
remove the paper back-
ing from the faceplate and
pouch. Starting at one edge,
carefully match the pouch
adhesive with the faceplate
adhesive. Press firmly and
smooth the pouch onto the
faceplate, taking care to
avoid creases.

18. Close bottom of pouch by
folding the end upward and
using the clamp or clip that
comes with the product,
or secure Velcro closure.
Ensure the curve of the
clamp follows the curve of
the patient's body.

19. Remove gloves. Assist the
patient to a comfortable
position. Cover the patient
with bed linens. Place the
bed in the lowest position.

20. Put on clean gloves.
Remove or discard equip-
ment and assess the
patient's response to the
procedure.

21. Remove gloves and
additional PPE, if
used. Perform hand
hygiene.

SKILL 121 ADMINISTERING OXYGEN BY MASK

When a patient requires a higher concentration of oxygen than a nasal cannula can deliver (6 L or 44% oxygen concentration), or is unable or unwilling to maintain nasal cannula, use an oxygen mask. Fit the mask carefully to the patient's face to avoid oxygen leakage. The mask should be comfortably snug, but not tight against the face. Disposable and reusable face masks are available. The most commonly used types of masks are the simple face mask, the partial rebreather mask, the nonrebreather mask, and the Venturi mask.

DELEGATION CONSIDERATIONS

The administration of oxygen by a mask is not delegated to nursing assistive personnel (NAP) or to unlicensed assistive personnel (UAP). Reapplication of the mask during nursing care activities, such as during bathing, may be performed by NAP or UAP. Depending on the state's nurse practice act and the organization's policies and procedures, administration of oxygen by a mask may be delegated to licensed practical/vocational nurses (LPN/LVNs). The decision to delegate must be based on careful analysis of the patient's needs and circumstances, as well as the qualifications of the person to whom the task is being delegated. Refer to the Delegation Guidelines in Appendix A.

EQUIPMENT

- Flow meter connected to oxygen supply
- Humidifier with sterile distilled water, if necessary, for the type of mask prescribed
- Face mask, specified by medical order
- Gauze to pad elastic band (optional)
- PPE, as indicated

ASSESSMENT

- Assess the patient's oxygen saturation level before starting oxygen therapy to provide a baseline for determining the effectiveness of therapy.
- Assess the patient's respiratory status, including respiratory rate, rhythm, effort, and lung sounds. Note any signs of respiratory distress, such as tachypnea, nasal flaring, use of accessory muscles, or dyspnea.

NURSING DIAGNOSIS

- Impaired Gas Exchange
- Ineffective Breathing Pattern
- Ineffective Airway Clearance

OUTCOME IDENTIFICATION AND PLANNING

- Patient exhibits an oxygen saturation level within acceptable parameters.

- Patient will remain free of signs and symptoms of respiratory distress.
- Patient's respiratory status, including respiratory rate and depth, will be in an acceptable range for the patient's age.

IMPLEMENTATION

ACTION	RATIONALE
1. Bring necessary equipment to the bedside stand or overbed table.	Bringing everything to the bedside conserves time and energy. Arranging items nearby is convenient, saves time, and avoids unnecessary stretching and twisting of muscles on the part of the nurse.
2. Perform hand hygiene and put on PPE, if indicated.	Hand hygiene and PPE prevent the spread of microorganisms. PPE is required based on transmission precautions.
3. Identify the patient.	Identifying the patient ensures the right patient receives the intervention and helps prevent errors.
4. Close the curtains around the bed and close the door to the room, if possible.	This ensures the patient's privacy.
5. Explain what you are going to do and the reason for doing it to the patient. Review safety precautions necessary when oxygen is in use.	Explanation relieves anxiety and facilitates cooperation. Oxygen supports combustion; a small spark could cause a fire.
6. Attach face mask to oxygen source (with humidification, if appropriate, for the specific mask). Start the flow of oxygen at the specified rate. For a mask with a reservoir, be sure to allow oxygen to fill the bag before proceeding to the next step.	Oxygen forced through a water reservoir is humidified before it is delivered to the patient, thus preventing dehydration of the mucous membranes. A reservoir bag must be inflated with oxygen because the bag is the oxygen supply source for the patient.
7. Position face mask over the patient's nose and mouth. Adjust the elastic strap so	A loose or poorly fitting mask will result in oxygen loss and decreased therapeutic value.

ACTION	RATIONALE
that the mask fits snugly but comfortably on the face. Adjust to the prescribed flow rate.	Masks may cause a feeling of suffocation, and the patient needs frequent attention and reassurance.
8. If the patient reports irritation or you note redness, use gauze pads under the elastic strap at pressure points to reduce irritation to ears and scalp.	Pads reduce irritation and pressure and protect the skin.
9. Reassess the patient's respiratory status, including respiratory rate, effort, and lung sounds. Note any signs of respiratory distress, such as tachypnea, nasal flaring, use of accessory muscles, or dyspnea.	This helps assess the effectiveness of oxygen therapy.
10. Remove PPE, if used. Perform hand hygiene.	Removing PPE properly reduces the risk for infection transmission and contamination of other items. Hand hygiene prevents the spread of microorganisms.
11. **Remove the mask and dry the skin every 2 to 3 hours if the oxygen is running continuously. Do not use powder around the mask.**	The tight-fitting mask and moisture from condensation can irritate the skin on the face. There is a danger of inhaling powder if it is placed on the mask.

EVALUATION

- Patient exhibits an oxygen saturation level within acceptable parameters.
- Patient demonstrates an absence of respiratory distress and accessory muscle use and exhibits respiratory rate and depth within acceptable parameters.

DOCUMENTATION

- Document type of mask used, amount of oxygen used, oxygen saturation level, lung sounds, and rate/pattern of respirations. Document your assessment before and after intervention.

SKILL 122 | ADMINISTERING OXYGEN BY NASAL CANNULA

A variety of devices are available for delivering oxygen to the patient. Each has a specific function and oxygen concentration. Device selection is based on the patient's condition and oxygen needs. A nasal cannula, also called nasal prongs, is the most commonly used oxygen delivery device. The cannula is a disposable plastic device with two protruding prongs for insertion into the nostrils. The cannula connects to an oxygen source with a flow meter and, many times, a humidifier. It is commonly used because the cannula does not impede eating or speaking and is used easily in the home. Disadvantages of this system are that it can be dislodged easily and can cause dryness of the nasal mucosa. In addition, if a patient breathes through the mouth, it is difficult to determine the amount of oxygen actually being received. A nasal cannula is used to deliver from 1 L/minute to 6 L/minute of oxygen.

DELEGATION CONSIDERATIONS

The administration of oxygen by nasal cannula is not delegated to nursing assistive personnel (NAP) or to unlicensed assistive personnel (UAP). Reapplication of the nasal cannula during nursing care activities, such as during bathing, may be performed by NAP or UAP. Depending on the state's nurse practice act and the organization's policies and procedures, administration of oxygen by nasal cannula may be delegated to licensed practical/vocational nurses (LPN/LVNs). The decision to delegate must be based on careful analysis of the patient's needs and circumstances, as well as the qualifications of the person to whom the task is being delegated. Refer to the Delegation Guidelines in Appendix A.

EQUIPMENT

- Flow meter connected to oxygen supply
- Humidifier with sterile, distilled water (optional for low-flow system)
- Nasal cannula and tubing
- Gauze to pad tubing over ears (optional)
- PPE, as indicated

ASSESSMENT

- Assess the patient's oxygen saturation level before starting oxygen therapy to provide a baseline for evaluating the effectiveness of oxygen therapy.
- Assess the patient's respiratory status, including respiratory rate, rhythm, effort, and lung sounds. Note any signs of respiratory distress, such as tachypnea, nasal flaring, use of accessory muscles, or dyspnea.

NURSING DIAGNOSIS

- Impaired Gas Exchange
- Ineffective Breathing Pattern
- Risk for Activity Intolerance

OUTCOME IDENTIFICATION AND PLANNING

- Patient will exhibit an oxygen saturation level within acceptable parameters.
- Patient will not experience dyspnea.
- Patient will demonstrate effortless respirations in an acceptable range for age group, without evidence of nasal flaring or use of accessory muscles.

IMPLEMENTATION

ACTION	RATIONALE
1. Bring necessary equipment to the bedside stand or overbed table.	Bringing everything to the bedside conserves time and energy. Arranging items nearby is convenient, saves time, and avoids unnecessary stretching and twisting of muscles on the part of the nurse.
2. Perform hand hygiene and put on PPE, if indicated.	Hand hygiene and PPE prevent the spread of microorganisms. PPE is required based on transmission precautions.
3. Identify the patient.	Identifying the patient ensures the right patient receives the intervention and helps prevent errors.
4. Close the curtains around the bed and close the door to the room, if possible.	This ensures the patient's privacy.
5. Explain what you are going to do and the reason for doing it to the patient. Review safety precautions necessary when oxygen is in use.	Explanation relieves anxiety and facilitates cooperation. Oxygen supports combustion; a small spark could cause a fire.
6. Connect nasal cannula to oxygen setup with humidification, if humidification is in use. Adjust flow rate as	Oxygen forced through a water reservoir is humidified before it is delivered to the patient, thus preventing dehydration of the

ACTION	RATIONALE
ordered. Check that oxygen is flowing out of prongs.	mucous membranes. Low-flow oxygen does not require humidification.
7. Place prongs in patient's nostrils. Place tubing over and behind each ear with adjuster comfortably under chin. Alternately, the tubing may be placed around the patient's head, with the adjuster at the back or base of the head. Place gauze pads at ear beneath the tubing, as necessary.	Correct placement of the prongs and fastener facilitates oxygen administration and patient comfort. Pads reduce irritation and pressure and protect the skin.
8. Adjust the fit of the cannula, as necessary. Tubing should be snug but not tight against the skin.	Proper adjustment maintains the prongs in the patient's nose. Excessive pressure from tubing could cause irritation and pressure to the skin.
9. **Encourage patients to breathe through the nose, with the mouth closed.**	Nose breathing provides for optimal delivery of oxygen to the patient. The percentage of oxygen delivered can be reduced in patients who breathe through the mouth.
10. Reassess the patient's respiratory status, including respiratory rate, effort, and lung sounds. Note any signs of respiratory distress, such as tachypnea, nasal flaring, use of accessory muscles, or dyspnea.	Assesses the effectiveness of oxygen therapy.
11. Remove PPE, if used. Perform hand hygiene.	Removing PPE properly reduces the risk for infection transmission and contamination of other items. Hand hygiene prevents the spread of microorganisms.
12. Put on clean gloves. Remove and clean the cannula and assess nares at least every 8 hours, or according to agency recommendations. Check nares for evidence of irritation or bleeding.	The continued presence of the cannula causes irritation and dryness of the mucous membranes.

EVALUATION

- Patient demonstrates an oxygen saturation level within acceptable parameters.
- Patient remains free of dyspnea, nasal flaring, or accessory muscle use and demonstrates respiratory rate and depth within normal range.

DOCUMENTATION

- Document your assessment before and after intervention. Document the amount of oxygen applied, and the patient's respiratory rate, oxygen saturation, and lung sounds.

SKILL 123   USING AN OXYGEN HOOD

Oxygen hoods are generally used to deliver oxygen to infants. They can supply an oxygen concentration up to 80% to 90% (Kyle & Carman, 2013). The oxygen hood, a clear plastic cover, is placed over the infant's head and neck; it allows easy access to the chest and lower body. Continuous pulse oximetry allows for monitoring oxygenation and making adjustments according to the infant's condition (Perry et al., 2010). The infant must be removed from the hood for feeding; obtain an order for oxygen delivery for use during feeding times. Assessment of an infant should include assessment of skin color. A pale or cyanotic patient may not be receiving sufficient oxygen. Assess the patient's respiratory status, including respiratory rate, rhythm, effort, and lung sounds. Assessment should also include assessing the patient for any signs of respiratory distress, such as nasal flaring, grunting, or retractions; oxygen-depleted patients often exhibit these signs. Additional equipment required includes the oxygen hood, oxygen analyzer, and a humidification device.

DELEGATION CONSIDERATIONS

The administration of oxygen using an oxygen hood is not delegated to nursing assistive personnel (NAP) or to unlicensed assistive personnel (UAP). Reapplication of the oxygen hood during nursing care activities, such as during bathing, may be performed by NAP or UAP. Depending on the state's nurse practice act and the organization's policies and procedures, administration of oxygen by an oxygen hood may be delegated to licensed practical/vocational nurses (LPN/LVNs). The decision to delegate must be based on careful analysis of the patient's needs and circumstances, as well as the qualifications of the person to whom the task is being delegated. Refer to the Delegation Guidelines in Appendix A.

EQUIPMENT

- Flow meter connected to oxygen supply
- Humidifier with sterile distilled water, if necessary, for the type of mask prescribed
- Face mask, specified by medical order
- Gauze to pad elastic band (optional)
- PPE, as indicated
- Oxygen hood, oxygen analyzer, and a humidification device

ASSESSMENT

- Assess patient's oxygen saturation level before starting oxygen therapy to provide a baseline for determining the effectiveness of therapy. The primary care provider will usually order a baseline for the pulse oximeter (i.e., deliver oxygen to keep pulse ox greater that 95%).
- Assess patient's respiratory status, including respiratory rate, rhythm, effort, lung sounds. Note any signs of respiratory distress, such as tachypnea, nasal flaring, use of accessory muscles, or dyspnea.

NURSING DIAGNOSIS

- Impaired Gas Exchange
- Ineffective Breathing Pattern
- Ineffective Airway Clearance

OUTCOME IDENTIFICATION AND PLANNING

- Patient exhibits an oxygen saturation level within acceptable parameters.
- Patient will remain free of signs and symptoms of respiratory distress.
- Patient's respiratory status, including respiratory rate and depth, will be in the normal range for the patient's age group.
- Patient's skin will be dry and without evidence of breakdown.

IMPLEMENTATION

ACTION	RATIONALE
1. Bring necessary equipment to the bedside stand or overbed table.	Bringing everything to the bedside conserves time and energy. Arranging items nearby is convenient, saves time, and avoids unnecessary stretching and twisting of muscles on the part of the nurse.
2. Perform hand hygiene and put on PPE, if indicated.	Hand hygiene and PPE prevent the spread of microorganisms. PPE is required based on transmission precautions.

ACTION	RATIONALE
3. Identify the patient.	Identifying the patient ensures the right patient receives the intervention and helps prevent errors.
4. Close the curtains around the bed and close the door to the room, if possible.	This ensures the patient's privacy.
5. Explain what you are going to do and the reason for doing it to the patient and parents/guardians. Review safety precautions necessary when oxygen is in use.	Explanation relieves anxiety and facilitates cooperation. Oxygen supports combustion; a small spark could cause a fire.
6. Calibrate the oxygen analyzer according to manufacturer's directions.	This ensures accurate readings and appropriate adjustments to therapy.
7. Place hood on crib. Connect humidifier to oxygen source in the wall. Connect the oxygen tubing to the hood. Adjust flow rate as ordered by physician. Check that oxygen is flowing into the hood.	Oxygen forced through a water reservoir is humidified before it is delivered to the patient, thus preventing dehydration of the mucous membranes.
8. Turn on analyzer. **Place oxygen analyzer probe in hood.**	The analyzer will give an accurate reading of the oxygen concentration in the hood.
9. Adjust oxygen flow, as necessary, based on sensor readings. Once oxygen levels reach the prescribed amount, place hood over patient's head (Figure 1). The hood should	Patient will receive oxygen once placed under the hood. Pressure and irritation could result in alterations in the infant's skin integrity.

FIGURE 1 Placing oxygen hood over infant's head.

EVALUATION

- Patient exhibits an oxygen saturation level within acceptable parameters.
- Patient demonstrates an absence of respiratory distress and accessory muscle use and exhibits respiratory rate and depth within normal parameters.

DOCUMENTATION

- Document amount of oxygen applied, respiratory rate, oxygen saturation levels, and assessment before and after intervention.

SKILL 124 USING AN OXYGEN TENT

Oxygen tents are often used for children who will not leave a face mask or nasal cannula in place. The oxygen tent gives the patient freedom to move in the bed or crib while cool, highly humidified oxygen is being delivered. However, it is difficult to keep the tent closed because the child may want contact with his or her parents. It is also difficult to maintain a consistent level of oxygen and to deliver oxygen at a rate higher than 30% to 50% (Kyle & Carman, 2013). Frequent assessment of the child's temperature, pajamas, and bedding is necessary because the humidification quickly creates moisture, leading to damp clothing and linens, and, possibly, hypothermia.

DELEGATION CONSIDERATIONS

The application of an oxygen tent is not delegated to nursing assistive personnel (NAP) or to unlicensed assistive personnel (UAP). Depending on the state's nurse practice act and the organization's policies and procedures, the application of an oxygen tent may be delegated to licensed practical/vocational nurses (LPN/LVNs). The decision to delegate must be based on careful analysis of the patient's needs and circumstances, as well as the qualifications of the person to whom the task is being delegated. Refer to the Delegation Guidelines in Appendix A.

EQUIPMENT

- Oxygen source
- Oxygen tent
- Humidifier compatible with tent
- Oxygen analyzer
- Small blankets for blanket rolls
- PPE, as indicated

ASSESSMENT

- Assess the patient's lung sounds. Secretions may cause the patient's oxygen demand to increase.
- Assess the oxygen saturation level. There will usually be an order for a baseline or goal for the oxygen saturation level (i.e., deliver oxygen to keep $SpO_2 \geq 95\%$).
- Assess skin color. A pale or cyanotic patient may not be receiving sufficient oxygen.
- Assess the patient's respiratory status, including respiratory rate, rhythm, and effort.
- Assess the patient for any signs of respiratory distress, such as nasal flaring, grunting, or retractions; oxygen-depleted patients often exhibit these signs.

NURSING DIAGNOSIS

- Impaired Gas Exchange
- Ineffective Breathing Pattern

- Ineffective Airway Clearance
- Risk for Impaired Skin Integrity

OUTCOME IDENTIFICATION AND PLANNING

- Patient exhibits an oxygen saturation level within acceptable parameters.
- Patient will remain free of signs and symptoms of respiratory distress.
- Patient's respiratory status, including respiratory rate and depth, will be in the acceptable range for the patient's age.
- Patient's skin will be warm, dry, and without evidence of breakdown.

IMPLEMENTATION

ACTION	RATIONALE
1. Bring necessary equipment to the bedside stand or overbed table.	Bringing everything to the bedside conserves time and energy. Arranging items nearby is convenient, saves time, and avoids unnecessary stretching and twisting of muscles on the part of the nurse.
2. Perform hand hygiene and put on PPE, if indicated.	Hand hygiene and PPE prevent the spread of microorganisms. PPE is required based on transmission precautions.
3. Identify the patient.	Identifying the patient ensures the right patient receives the intervention and helps prevent errors.
4. Close the curtains around the bed and close the door to the room, if possible.	This ensures the patient's privacy.
5. Explain what you are going to do and the reason for doing it to the patient and parents/guardians. Review safety precautions necessary when oxygen is in use.	Explanation relieves anxiety and facilitates cooperation. Oxygen supports combustion; a small spark could cause a fire.
6. Calibrate the oxygen analyzer according to manufacturer's directions.	Ensures accurate readings and appropriate adjustments to therapy.

ACTION	RATIONALE
7. Place tent over crib or bed. Connect the humidifier to the oxygen source in the wall and connect the tent tubing to the humidifier. Adjust flow rate as ordered by primary care provider. Check that oxygen is flowing into the tent.	Oxygen forced through a water reservoir is humidified before it is delivered to the patient, thus preventing dehydration of the mucous membranes.
8. Turn on analyzer. Place oxygen analyzer probe in tent, out of patient's reach.	The analyzer will give an accurate reading of the concentration of oxygen in the crib or bed.
9. Adjust oxygen as necessary, based on sensor readings. Once oxygen levels reach the prescribed amount, place the patient in the tent.	Patient will receive oxygen once placed in the tent.
10. Roll small blankets like a jelly roll and tuck tent edges under blanket rolls, as necessary.	The blanket helps keep the edges of the tent flap from coming up and letting oxygen out.
11. **Encourage patient and family members to keep tent flap closed.**	Every time the tent flap is opened, oxygen is released.
12. Reassess the patient's respiratory status, including respiratory rate, effort, and lung sounds. Note any signs of respiratory distress, such as tachypnea, nasal flaring, use of accessory muscles, grunting, retractions, or dyspnea.	This assesses the effectiveness of oxygen therapy.
13. Remove PPE, if used. Perform hand hygiene.	Removing PPE properly reduces the risk for infection transmission and contamination of other items. Hand hygiene prevents the spread of microorganisms.
14. **Frequently check bedding and patient's pajamas for moisture. Change as needed to keep the patient dry. Monitor the patient's body temperature at regular intervals.**	The large amount of humidification delivered in an oxygen tent quickly makes cloth moist, which would be uncomfortable for the patient and may affect temperature regulation. The cool environment can cause hypothermia and cold stress (Perry et al., 2010).

EVALUATION

- Patient exhibits an oxygen saturation level within acceptable parameters.
- Patient remains free of dyspnea, nasal flaring, grunting, or use of accessory muscles when breathing.
- Patient's respirations remain in normal range for age and body temperature remains within normal limits.

DOCUMENTATION

- Document amount of oxygen applied; respiratory rate, rhythm, and effort; oxygen saturation level; and your assessment before and after intervention.

SKILL 125 APPLYING AND MONITORING AN EXTERNAL (TRANSCUTANEOUS) PACEMAKER

Temporary cardiac pacing is used to correct life-threatening cardiac dysrhythmias and as an elective procedure, such as to evaluate the need for permanent pacing or after cardiac surgery. A temporary pacemaker consists of an external, battery-powered pulse generator and a lead or electrode system to electrically stimulate heartbeat. Transcutaneous pacing can temporarily supply an electrical current in the heart when electrical conduction is abnormal. This device works by sending an electrical impulse from the pulse generator to the patient's heart by way of two electrodes, which are placed on the front and back of the patient's chest. This stimulates the contraction of cardiac muscle fibers through electrical stimulation (depolarization) of the myocardium. Transcutaneous pacing is quick and effective, but is usually used as short-term therapy until the situation resolves or transvenous or permanent pacing can be initiated.

Transcutaneous pacing can cause significant discomfort. Patient should be made aware of this and adequate sedation is necessary (Morton & Fontaine, 2013).

DELEGATION CONSIDERATIONS

The use of a transcutaneous pacemaker is not delegated to nursing assistive personnel (NAP) or to unlicensed assistive personnel (UAP). Depending on the state's nurse practice act and the organization's policies and procedures, this procedure may be delegated to licensed practical/vocational nurses (LPN/LVNs). The decision to delegate must be based on careful analysis of the patient's needs and circumstances, as well as the qualifications of the person to whom the task is being delegated. Refer to the Delegation Guidelines in Appendix A.

EQUIPMENT

- Transcutaneous noninvasive pacemaker
- Transcutaneous pacing electrodes and cables
- ECG electrodes and cables
- Cardiac monitor
- Medication for analgesia and/or sedation, as prescribed

ASSESSMENT

- Review the patient's medical record and plan of care for information about the patient's need for pacing. Transcutaneous pacing is generally an emergency measure.
- Assess the patient's initial cardiac rhythm, including a rhythm strip and 12-lead ECG.
- Monitor heart rate, respiratory rate, level of consciousness, and skin color. If the patient is pulseless, initiate CPR.

NURSING DIAGNOSIS

- Decreased Cardiac Output
- Deficient Knowledge
- Anxiety
- Risk for Injury

OUTCOME IDENTIFICATION AND PLANNING

- External transcutaneous pacemaker is applied correctly without adverse effect to the patient.
- Patient regains signs of circulation, including the capture of at least the minimal set heart rate.
- Patient's heart and lungs maintain adequate function to sustain life.
- Patient does not experience injury.

IMPLEMENTATION

ACTION	RATIONALE
1. Verify the order for a transcutaneous pacemaker in the patient's medical record.	This ensures that the correct intervention is performed on the correct patient.
2. Gather all equipment.	Assembling equipment provides for an organized approach to the task.
3. Perform hand hygiene and put on PPE, if indicated.	Hand hygiene and PPE prevent the transmission of microorganisms. PPE is required based on transmission precautions.

ACTION	RATIONALE
4. Identify the patient.	Verifying the patient's identity validates that the correct procedure is being done on the correct patient.
5. If the patient is responsive, explain the procedure to the patient. Explain that it involves some discomfort and that you will administer medication to keep him or her comfortable and help him or her to relax. Administer analgesia and sedation, as ordered, if not an emergency situation.	External pacemakers are typically used with unconscious patients because most alert patients cannot tolerate the uncomfortable sensations produced by the high energy levels needed to pace externally. If responsive, the patient will most likely be sedated.
6. Close the curtains around the bed and close the door to the room, if possible. Obtain vital signs.	This provides for patient privacy. Vital signs provide baseline for assessing pacing effectiveness (Del Monte, 2009).
7. If necessary, clip the hair over the areas of electrode placement. **Do not shave the area.**	Shaving can cause tiny nicks in the skin, causing skin irritation. Also, the current from the pulse generator could cause discomfort.
8. Attach cardiac monitoring electrodes to the patient in the lead I, II, and III position. Do this even if the patient is already on telemetry monitoring. If you select the lead II position, adjust the LL (left leg) electrode placement to accommodate the anterior pacing electrode and the patient's anatomy.	Connecting the telemetry electrodes to the pacemaker is required.
9. Attach the patient monitoring electrodes to the ECG cable and into the ECG input connection on the front of the pacing generator. Set the selector switch to the 'Monitor on' position.	These actions ensure that the equipment is functioning properly.

ACTION	RATIONALE
10. Note the ECG waveform on the monitor. Adjust the R-wave beeper volume to a suitable level and activate the alarm by pressing the 'Alarm on' button. Set the alarm for 10 to 20 beats lower and 20 to 30 beats higher than the intrinsic rate.	These actions ensure that the equipment is functioning properly.
11. Press the 'Start/Stop' button for a printout of the waveform.	A printout provides objective data.
12. Apply the two pacing electrodes. Make sure the patient's skin is clean and dry to ensure good skin contact. Pull the protective strip from the posterior electrode (marked 'Back') and apply the electrode on the left side of the thoracic spinal column, just below the scapula (Figure 1).	This placement ensures that the electrical stimulus will travel only a short distance to the heart.

Anterior pacing electrode

Posterior pacing electrode

FIGURE 1 Transcutaneous pacemaker pads in place.

| 13. Apply the anterior pacing electrode (marked 'Front'), which has two protective strips—one covering the gelled area and one covering the outer rim. Expose the | This placement ensures that the electrical stimulus will travel only a short distance to the heart. |

ACTION	RATIONALE

gelled area and apply it to the skin in the anterior position, to the left of the precordium in the V$_2$ to the V$_5$ position (see Figure 1). Move this electrode around to get the best waveform. Then expose the electrode's outer rim and firmly press it to the skin.

14. Prepare to pace the heart. After making sure the energy output in milliamperes (mA) is on 0, connect the electrode cable to the monitor output cable.

   This sets the pacing threshold.

15. Check the waveform, looking for a tall QRS complex in lead II.

16. Check the selector switch to 'Pacer on.' Select synchronous (demand) or asynchronous (fixed-rate or nondemand) mode, per medical orders. **Tell the patient he or she may feel a thumping or twitching sensation. Reassure the patient you will provide medication if the discomfort is intolerable.**

   Asynchronous pacing delivers a stimulus at a set (fixed) rate regardless of the occurrence of spontaneous myocardial depolarizations. Synchronous pacing delivers a stimulus only when the heart's intrinsic pacemaker fails to function at a predetermined rate. Analgesia and/or sedation may be administered, as ordered, for discomfort associated with pacing.

17. Set the pacing rate dial to 60 to 70 beats per minute. Look for pacer artifact or spikes, which will appear as you increase the rate.

   Setting the pacing rate dial higher than the intrinsic rhythm ensures adequate cardiac output.

18. Set the pacing current output (in milliamperes [mA]), if not automatically done by pacemaker. For patients with bradycardia, start with the minimal setting and **slowly increase the amount of energy delivered to the heart by adjusting the**

   Setting the pacing current output ensures adequate cardiac output.

ACTION	RATIONALE

'Output' mA dial. Do this until electrical capture is achieved: you will see a pacer spike followed by a widened QRS complex and a tall broad T wave that resembles a premature ventricular contraction.

19. Increase output by 2 mA or 10%. **Do not go higher because of the increased risk of discomfort to the patient.**

Increasing the output ensures consistent capture. With full capture, the patient's heart rate should be approximately the same as the pacemaker rate set on the machine. The usual pacing threshold is 40 to 80 mA. Thresholds may vary due to recent cardiothoracic surgery, pericardial effusions, cardiac tamponade, acidosis, and hypoxia. These conditions may require higher thresholds.

20. Assess for effectiveness of pacing and mechanical capture: observe for pacemaker spike with subsequent capture; assess heart rate and rhythm (using right carotid, brachial or femoral artery); assess blood pressure (using right arm); assess for signs of improved cardiac output (increased blood pressure, improved level of consciousness, improved body temperature).

Both electrical and mechanical capture must occur to benefit the patient (Del Monte, 2009). Use of patient's right side for pulse assessment avoids inaccuracy related to strong contractions from the pacemaker. Use of right arm for blood pressure measurement avoids interference from the pacemaker (Morton & Fontaine, 2013).

21. For patients with asystole, in certain circumstances in hospitalized patients, start with the full output. If capture occurs, slowly decrease the output until capture is lost, then add 2 mA or 10% more.

Although transcutaneous pacing is not recommended for all patients in asystole, there are circumstances when it should be used in hospitalized patients with sudden asystole (Link et al., 2010). Increasing the output ensures consistent capture. With full capture, the patient's heart rate should be approximately the

ACTION	RATIONALE
	same as the pacemaker rate set on the machine. The usual pacing threshold is 40 to 80 mA.
22. Secure the pacing leads and cable to the patient's body.	This prevents accidental displacement of the electrode, resulting in failure to pace or sense.
23. Monitor the patient's heart rate and rhythm to assess ventricular response to pacing. Assess the patient's vital signs, skin color, level of consciousness, and peripheral pulses. Take blood pressure in both arms.	Assessment helps determine the effectiveness of the paced rhythm. If the blood pressure reading is significantly higher in one arm, use that arm for measurements.
24. Assess the patient's pain and administer analgesia/sedation, as ordered, to ease the discomfort of chest wall muscle contractions (Craig, 2005).	Analgesia and sedation promote patient comfort.
25. Perform a 12-lead ECG and additional ECG daily or with clinical changes.	ECG monitoring provides a baseline for further evaluation.
26. Continually monitor the ECG readings, noting capture, sensing, rate, intrinsic beats, and competition of paced and intrinsic rhythms. If the pacemaker is sensing correctly, the sense indicator on the pulse generator should flash with each beat.	Continuous monitoring helps evaluate the patient's condition and determine the effectiveness of therapy.
27. Remove PPE, if used. Perform hand hygiene.	Removing PPE properly reduces the risk for infection transmission and contamination of other items. Hand hygiene and proper disposal of equipment reduces the transmission of microorganisms.

EVALUATION

• The external transcutaneous pacemaker is applied correctly without adverse effect to the patient.

- Patient regains signs of circulation, including the capture of at least the minimal set heart rate.
- Patient's heart and lungs maintain adequate function to sustain life.
- Patient does not experience injury.

DOCUMENTATION

- Document the reason for pacemaker use, time that pacing began, electrode locations, pacemaker settings, patient's response to the procedure and to temporary pacing, complications, and nursing actions taken. Document the patient's pain-intensity rating, analgesia or sedation administered, and the patient's response. If possible, obtain a rhythm strip before, during, and after pacemaker placement; anytime that pacemaker settings are changed; and whenever the patient receives treatment because of a complication due to the pacemaker.

SKILL 126 CARING FOR A PATIENT RECEIVING CONTINUOUS WOUND PERFUSION PAIN MANAGEMENT

Continuous wound perfusion pain management systems deliver a continuous infusion of local analgesia to surgical wound beds. These systems are used as an adjuvant in the management of postoperative pain in a wide range of surgical procedures, such as cardiothoracic and orthopedic procedures. The system consists of a balloon type pump filled with local anesthetic and a catheter placed near an incision, in a nerve close to a surgical site, or in a wound bed (Figure 1). The catheter delivers a consistent flow rate and uniform distribution to the surgical site. Continuous wound perfusion catheters decrease postoperative pain and opioid use and side effects, and have been associated with decreased postoperative nausea and vomiting (D'Arcy, 2012; Charous, 2008). The

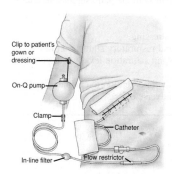

Clip to patient's gown or dressing

On-Q pump

Clamp

In-line filter

Catheter

Flow restrictor

FIGURE 1 Wound perfusion pain management system consists of a balloon (pump), filter, and catheter that delivers a specific amount of prescribed local anesthetic at the rate determined by the prescriber. (Redrawn from I-Flow, LLC, a Kimberly-Clark Health Care Company, with permission.)

catheter is placed during surgery and is not sutured into place; the site dressing holds it in place.

DELEGATION CONSIDERATIONS

Care related to continuous wound perfusion pain management systems is not delegated to nursing assistive personnel (NAP) or to unlicensed assistive personnel (UAP). Depending on the state's nurse practice act and the organization's policies and procedures, specific aspects of the care related to continuous wound perfusion pain management systems, such as monitoring the infusion and assessment of patient response, may be delegated to licensed practical/vocational nurses (LPN/LVNs). The decision to delegate must be based on careful analysis of the patient's needs and circumstances, as well as the qualifications of the person to whom the task is being delegated. Refer to the Delegation Guidelines in Appendix A.

EQUIPMENT

- Computerized medication administration record (CMAR) or medication administration record (MAR)
- Pain assessment tool and pain scale
- Gauze and tape, or other dressing, based on facility policy
- Gloves
- Additional PPE, as indicated

ASSESSMENT

- Review the patient's medical record and plan of care for specific instructions related to continuous wound perfusion pain management therapy, including the medical order for the drug and conditions indicating the need for therapy.
- Review the patient's history for allergy to the prescribed medication.
- Assess the patient's understanding of a continuous wound perfusion pain management system and the rationale for its use.
- Assess the patient's level of discomfort and pain using an appropriate assessment tool. Assess the characteristics of any pain. Assess for other symptoms that often occur with the pain, such as headache or restlessness.
- Assess the surgical site.
- Assess the catheter insertion site dressing.
- Assess the patient's vital signs and respiratory status, including rate, depth, and rhythm, and oxygen saturation level using pulse oximetry.
- Assess the patient's response to the intervention to evaluate its effectiveness and for the presence of adverse effects.

NURSING DIAGNOSIS

- Acute Pain
- Deficient Knowledge
- Risk for Infection

OUTCOME IDENTIFICATION AND PLANNING

- Patient reports increased comfort and/or decreased pain, without adverse effects.
- Patient displays decreased anxiety.
- Patient exhibits a dry, intact dressing with catheter in place.
- Patient remains free from infection.
- Patient verbalizes an understanding of the therapy and the reason for its use.

IMPLEMENTATION

ACTION	RATIONALE
1. Check the medication order against the original medical order, according to facility policy. Clarify any inconsistencies. Check the patient's medical record for allergies.	This comparison helps to identify errors that may have occurred when orders were transcribed. The medical order is the legal record-of-medication order for each agency.
2. Know the actions, special nursing considerations, safe dose ranges, purpose of administration, and adverse effects of the medications to be administered. Consider the appropriateness of the medication for this patient.	This knowledge aids the nurse in evaluating the therapeutic effect of the medication in relation to the patient's disorder and can also be used to educate the patient about the medication.
3. Perform hand hygiene and put on PPE, if indicated.	Hand hygiene and PPE prevent the spread of microorganisms. PPE is required based on transmission precautions.
4. Identify the patient.	Identifying the patient ensures that the right patient receives the intervention and helps prevent errors.
5. Close the door to the room or pull the bedside curtain.	Closing the door or curtain provides patient privacy.
6. Assess the patient's pain. Administer postoperative analgesic, as ordered.	Continuous wound perfusion pain management is an adjuvant therapy; patients will likely require postoperative pain medication, with reduced frequency.

ACTION	RATIONALE
7. Check the medication label attached to the pain management system balloon. Compare it with the medical order and MAR, per facility policy. Assess the patient for perioral numbness or tingling, numbness or tingling of fingers or toes, blurred vision, ringing in the ears, metallic taste in the mouth, confusion, seizures, drowsiness, nausea and/or vomiting. Assess the patient's vital signs.	Checking the medication label with the order and MAR ensures correct therapy for the patient. These symptoms may indicate local anesthetic toxicity (I-Flow, 2012; D'Arcy, 2007a). Changes in vital signs may indicate adverse effect. Cardiac dysrhythmias and hypertension are possible adverse effects (Layzell, 2008).
8. Put on gloves. Assess the wound perfusion system. Inspect tubing for kinks; check that the white tubing clamps are open. If tubing appears crimped, massage area on tubing to facilitate flow. Check filter in tubing, which should be unrestricted and free from tape.	Gloves prevent contact with blood and body fluids. Tubing must be unclamped and free of kinks and/or crimping to maintain consistent flow of analgesic. Tape over filter interferes with properly functioning system.
9. Check the flow restrictor to ensure it is in contact with the patient's skin. Tape in place, as necessary.	Checking the flow restrictor for adequate contact ensures accurate flow rate.
10. Check the insertion site dressing. Ensure that it is intact. Assess for leakage and dislodgement. Assess for redness, warmth, swelling, pain at site, and drainage.	Transparent dressing holds the catheter in place. Dressing must stay in place to prevent accidental dislodgement or removal. These symptoms may indicate infection.
11. Review the device with the patient. Review the function of the device and reason for its use. Reinforce the purpose and action of the medication to the patient.	Explanation encourages patient understanding and cooperation and reduces apprehension.

To Remove the Catheter

12. Check to ensure that infusion is complete. Infusion is complete when the delivery time	Depending on the size and volume of the balloon, the infusion typically lasts 2 to 5 days.

ACTION	RATIONALE
has passed and the balloon is no longer inflated.	Infusion time should be recorded in the operative note or postoperative instructions. The balloon will no longer appear full, the outside bag will be flat, and a hard tube can be felt in the middle of the balloon (I-Flow, 2010).

13. Perform hand hygiene. Identify the patient. Put on gloves. Remove the catheter site dressing. Loosen adhesive skin closure strips at the catheter site.

Hand hygiene and use of gloves reduces the risk of infection transmission. Identifying the patient ensures that the right patient receives the intervention and helps prevent errors. Loosening of materials allows the catheter to be free of constraints.

14. Grasp the catheter close to the patient's skin at the insertion site. Gently pull catheter to remove. Catheter should be easy to remove and not painful. Do not tug or quickly pull on the catheter during removal. Check the distal end of the catheter for the black marking.

Gentle removal prevents patient discomfort and accidental breakage of the catheter. Checking for the black mark at the distal end ensures the entire catheter was removed.

15. Cover puncture site with a dry dressing, according to facility policy.

Covering the wound prevents contamination.

16. Dispose of the balloon, tubing, and catheter according to facility policy.

Proper disposal reduces the risk for infection transmission and contamination of other items.

17. Remove gloves and additional PPE, if used. Perform hand hygiene.

Removing PPE properly reduces the risk for infection transmission and contamination of other items. Hand hygiene prevents transmission of microorganisms.

EVALUATION
- Patient verbalizes pain relief.
- Patient exhibits a dry, intact dressing, and the catheter exit site is free of signs and symptoms of complications, injury, or infection.

- Patient reports a decrease in anxiety and an increased ability to cope with pain.
- Patient verbalizes information related to the functioning of the system and the reasons for its use.

DOCUMENTATION

- Document system patency, the condition of the insertion site and dressing, vital signs and assessment information, analgesics administered, and the patient's response.

SKILL 127 | CARING FOR A PATIENT RECEIVING PATIENT-CONTROLLED ANALGESIA

Patient-controlled analgesia (PCA) allows patients to control the administration of their own medication within predetermined safety limits. This approach can be used with oral analgesic agents as well as with infusions of opioid analgesic agents by intravenous, subcutaneous, epidural, and perineural routes (Hinkle & Cheever, 2014; Cranwell-Bruce, 2009; D'Arcy, 2008a; Hicks et al., 2012). PCA provides effective individualized analgesia and comfort. This drug delivery system can be used to manage acute and chronic pain in a health care facility or the home.

The PCA pump permits the patient to self-administer medication (bolus doses) with episodes of increased pain or painful activities. A timing device electronically controls the PCA pump. The PCA system consists of a portable infusion pump containing a reservoir or chamber for a syringe or other reservoir that is prefilled with the prescribed medication, usually an opioid, or dilute anesthetic solutions in the case of epidural administration (Hinkle & Cheever, 2014; Cranwell-Bruce, 2009; D'Arcy, 2008a; Hicks et al., 2012). When pain occurs, the patient pushes a button that activates the PCA device to deliver a small, preset bolus dose of the analgesic. A lockout interval that is programmed into the PCA unit prevents reactivation of the pump and administration of another dose during that period of time. The pump mechanism can also be programmed to deliver only a specified amount of analgesic within a given time interval (basal rate; most commonly every hour or, occasionally, every 4 hours). These safeguards limit the risk for overmedication and allow the patient to evaluate the effect of the previous dose. PCA pumps also have a locked safety system that prohibits tampering with the device.

Nursing responsibilities for patients receiving medications via a PCA pump include patient/family teaching, initial device setup, monitoring the device to ensure proper functioning, and frequent assessment of the patient's response, including pain and discomfort control and presence of adverse effects. Additional information related to epidural infusions is discussed in Skill 68.

DELEGATION CONSIDERATIONS

The care related to patient-controlled analgesia is not delegated to nursing assistive personnel (NAP) or to unlicensed assistive personnel (UAP). Depending on the state's nurse practice act and the organization's policies and procedures, specific aspects of the care related to PCA, such as monitoring the infusion and assessment of patient response, may be delegated to licensed practical/vocational nurses (LPN/LVNs). The decision to delegate must be based on careful analysis of the patient's needs and circumstances, as well as the qualifications of the person to whom the task is being delegated. Refer to the Delegation Guidelines in Appendix A.

EQUIPMENT

- PCA system
- Syringe (or appropriate reservoir for device) filled with medication
- PCA system tubing
- Antimicrobial swabs
- Appropriate label for syringe and tubing, based on facility policy and procedure
- Second nurse to verify medication and programmed pump
- information, if necessary, according to facility policy
- Pain assessment tool and pain scale
- Computerized medication administration record (CMAR) or medication administration record (MAR)
- Gloves
- Additional PPE, as indicated

ASSESSMENT

- Review the patient's medical record and plan of care for specific instructions related to PCA therapy, including the primary care provider's orders and conditions indicating the need for therapy.
- Check the medical order for the prescribed drug, initial loading dose, dose for self-administration, and lockout interval.
- Check to ensure proper functioning of the unit.
- Assess the patient's level of consciousness and understanding of PCA therapy and the rationale for its use.
- Review the patient's history for conditions that might contraindicate therapy, such as respiratory limitations, history of substance abuse, or psychiatric disorder.
- Review the patient's medical record and assess for factors contributing to an increased risk for respiratory depression, such as the use of a basal infusion, the patient's age, obesity, upper abdominal or thoracic surgery, sleep apnea, history of smoking, concurrent CNS depressants, and impaired major organ functioning (The Joint Commission, 2012; Jarzyna et al., 2011).
- Determine the prescribed route for administration.
- Inspect the site to be used for the infusion for signs of infiltration or infection. If the route is via an IV infusion, ensure that the line is patent and the current solution is compatible with the drug ordered.
- Assess the patient's pain and level of discomfort using an appropriate assessment tool and pain scale. Assess the characteristics of any

pain, and for other symptoms that often occur with the pain, such as headache or restlessness. Ask the patient what interventions have and have not been successful in the past to promote comfort and relieve pain.
- Assess the patient's vital signs. Assess the patient's respiratory status, including rate, depth, and rhythm; oxygen saturation level using pulse oximetry; and level of carbon dioxide concentration using capnography. Assess the patient's sedation score.
- Determine the patient's response to the intervention to evaluate effectiveness and for the presence of adverse effects.

NURSING DIAGNOSIS
- Acute Pain
- Chronic Pain
- Deficient Knowledge

OUTCOME IDENTIFICATION AND PLANNING
- Patient reports increased comfort and/or decreased pain, without adverse effects, oversedation, and respiratory depression.
- Patient displays decreased anxiety, improved coping skills, and an understanding of the therapy and the reason for its use.

ACTION	RATIONALE

4. Perform hand hygiene and put on PPE, if indicated.

Hand hygiene and PPE prevent the spread of microorganisms. PPE is required based on transmission precautions.

5. Identify the patient.

Identifying the patient ensures that the right patient receives the intervention and helps prevent errors.

6. Show the patient the device, and explain its function and the reason for use. Explain the purpose and action of the medication to the patient.

Explanation encourages patient understanding and cooperation and reduces apprehension.

7. Plug the PCA device into the electrical outlet, if necessary. Check status of battery power, if appropriate.

The PCA device requires a power source (electricity or battery) to run. Most units will alarm to acknowledge a low battery state.

8. Close the door to the room or pull the bedside curtain.

Closing the door or pulling the curtain provides patient privacy.

9. Complete necessary assessments before administering medication. Check allergy bracelet or ask patient about allergies. Assess the patient's pain, using an appropriate assessment tool and measurement scale.

Assessment is a prerequisite to medication administration. Accurate assessment is necessary to guide treatment and relief interventions and to evaluate the effectiveness of pain control measures.

10. **Check the label on the prefilled drug syringe or reservoir with the medication record and patient identification.** Obtain verification of information from a second nurse, according to facility policy.

This action verifies that the correct drug and dosage will be administered to the correct patient. Confirmation of information by a second nurse helps prevent errors (D'Arcy, 2008a).

11. Scan the patient's barcode on the identification band, if required.

This provides an additional check to ensure that the medication is given to the right patient.

ACTION	RATIONALE
12. Connect tubing to prefilled syringe and place the syringe into the PCA device. **Prime the tubing.**	Doing so prepares the device to deliver the drug. Priming the tubing purges air from the tubing and reduces the risk for air embolism.
13. Set the PCA device to administer the loading dose, if ordered, and then program the device based on the medical order for medication dosage, dose interval, and lockout interval. Obtain verification of information from a second nurse, according to facility policy.	These actions ensure that the appropriate drug dosage will be administered. Confirmation of information by a second nurse helps prevent errors.
14. Put on gloves. Using an antimicrobial swab, clean connection port on IV infusion line or other site access, based on route of administration. Connect the PCA tubing to the patient's IV infusion line or appropriate access site, based on the specific site used. Secure the site per facility policy and procedure. Remove gloves. Initiate the therapy by activating the appropriate button on the pump. Lock the PCA device, per facility policy.	Gloves prevent contact with blood and body fluids. Cleaning the connection port reduces the risk of infection. Connection and initiation are necessary to allow drug delivery to the patient. Locking the device prevents tampering with the settings.
15. Remind the patient to press the button each time he or she needs relief from pain.	Instruction promotes correct use of the device.
16. Assess the patient's pain at least every 4 hours or more often, as needed, based on patient's individual risk factors. Monitor vital signs, especially respiratory status, including oxygen saturation at least every 4 hours or more often as needed, based on patient's individual risk factors.	Continued assessment at frequent intervals helps evaluate the effectiveness of the drug and reduce the risk for complications (Jarzyna et al., 2011; D'Arcy, 2008a; D'Arcy, 2007b).

ACTION	RATIONALE
17. Assess the patient's sedation score and end-tidal carbon dioxide level (capnography) at least every 4 hours or more often as needed, based on patient's individual risk factors.	Sedation occurs before clinically significant respiratory depression (D'Arcy, 2008). Respiratory depression can occur with the use of narcotic analgesics. Capnography is a more reliable indicator of respiratory depression (Capnography, 2012; Hicks et al., 2012; Jarzyna et al., 2011; Johnson et al., 2011).
18. Assess the infusion site periodically, according to facility policy and nursing judgment. Assess the patient's use of the medication, noting number of attempts and number of doses delivered. Replace the drug syringe when it is empty.	Continued assessment of the infusion site is necessary for early detection of problems. Continued assessment of the patient's use of medication and effect is necessary to ensure adequate pain control without adverse effect. Replacing the syringe ensures continued drug delivery.
19. Make sure the patient control (dosing button) is within the patient's reach.	Easy access to the control is essential for the patient to use the device.
20. Remove gloves and additional PPE, if used. Perform hand hygiene.	Removing PPE properly reduces the risk for infection transmission and contamination of other items. Hand hygiene prevents transmission of microorganisms.

EVALUATION

- Patient reports increased comfort and/or decreased pain, without adverse effects, oversedation, and respiratory depression.
- Patient displays decreased anxiety and improved coping skills.
- Patient verbalizes an understanding of the therapy and the reason for its use.

DOCUMENTATION

- Document the date and time PCA therapy was initiated, initial pain assessment, drug and loading dose administered, if appropriate, and individual dosing and time interval.
- Document continued pain, sedation level, vital signs and assessments, and patient's response to therapy.

SKILL 128

When a continuous IV is no longer necessary, the primary IV line (short peripheral venous catheter or CVAD) can be capped and converted to an intermittent infusion device. A capped line consists of the IV catheter connected to a short length of extension tubing sealed with a cap. Capping of a short peripheral venous catheter is commonly referred to as a medication or saline lock. Capping of a vascular access device provides venous access for intermittent infusions or emergency medications. This can be accomplished in different ways. Refer to facility policy for the procedure to convert an access for intermittent use. Vascular access devices used for intermittent infusions should be flushed with normal saline solution prior to each infusion as part of the assessment of catheter function. Flushing of the device is also required after each infusion to clear the infused medication or other solution from the catheter lumen. Vascular access devices should also be 'locked' after completion of the flush solution at each use to decrease the risk of occlusion. According to the guidelines from the INS (2011), short peripheral venous access devices are locked with normal saline solution after each intermittent use. If the device is not in use, periodic flushing according to facility policy is required to keep the catheter patent. Refer to facility policy for specific guidelines.

The following skill describes converting a primary line when extension tubing is present; the accompanying skill variation describes converting a primary line when the administration set is connected directly to the hub of the IV catheter, without extension tubing.

DELEGATION CONSIDERATIONS

Capping and flushing of a peripheral venous access device is not delegated to nursing assistive personnel (NAP) or to unlicensed assistive personnel (UAP). Depending on the state's nurse practice act and the organization's policies and procedures, these procedures may be delegated to licensed practical/vocational nurses (LPN/LVNs). The decision to delegate must be based on careful analysis of the patient's needs and circumstances, as well as the qualifications of the person to whom the task is being delegated. Refer to the Delegation Guidelines in Appendix A.

EQUIPMENT

- End cap device
- Clean gloves
- Additional PPE, as indicated
- 4 × 4 gauze pad
- Normal saline flush prepared in a syringe (1 to
- 3 mL) according to facility policy
- Alcohol or other disinfectant wipes
- Tape

ASSESSMENT

- Assess the insertion site for signs of any complications
- Verify the medical order for discontinuation of IV fluid infusion.

NURSING DIAGNOSIS

- Risk for Infection
- Risk for Injury

OUTCOME IDENTIFICATION AND PLANNING

- Patient will remain free of injury and any signs and symptoms of IV complications.
- Capped venous access device will remain patent.

IMPLEMENTATION

ACTION	RATIONALE
1. Determine the need for conversion to an intermittent access. Verify medical order. Check facility policy. Gather equipment.	Ensures correct intervention for correct patient. Preparation promotes efficient time management and an organized approach to the task.
2. Perform hand hygiene and put on PPE, if indicated.	Hand hygiene and PPE prevent the spread of microorganisms. PPE is required based on transmission precautions.
3. Identify the patient.	Identifying the patient ensures the right patient receives the intervention and helps prevent errors.
4. Close the curtains around the bed and close the door to the room, if possible. Explain what you are going to do and why you are going to do it to the patient. Ask the patient about allergies to tape and skin antiseptics.	This ensures the patient's privacy. Explanation relieves anxiety and facilitates cooperation. Possible allergies may exist related to tape or antiseptics.
5. Assess the IV site. Refer to Skill 92.	Complications, such as infiltration, phlebitis, or infection, necessitate discontinuation of the IV infusion at that site.

ACTION	RATIONALE
6. If using an electronic infusion device, stop the device. Close the roller clamp on the administration set. If using gravity infusion, close the roller clamp on the administration set.	The action of the infusion device needs to be stopped and clamps closed to prevent leaking of fluid when tubing is disconnected.
7. Put on gloves. Close the clamp on the short extension tubing connected to the IV catheter in the patient's arm.	Clamping the tubing on the extension set prevents introduction of air into the extension tubing.
8. Remove the administration set tubing from the extension set. Cleanse the end cap with an antimicrobial swab.	Removing the infusion tubing discontinues the infusion. Cleaning the cap reduces the risk for contamination.
9. Insert the saline flush syringe into the cap on the extension tubing. Pull back on the syringe to aspirate the catheter for positive blood return. If positive, instill the solution over 1 minute or flush the line according to facility policy. Remove syringe and reclamp the extension tubing.	Positive blood return confirms patency before administration of medications and solutions (INS, 2011, p. S60). Flushing maintains patency of the IV line. Action of positive pressure end cap is maintained with removal of syringe before clamp is engaged. Clamping prevents air from entering the extension set.
10. If necessary, loop the extension tubing near the entry site and anchor it with tape (nonallergenic) close to the site.	The weight of the tubing is sufficient to pull it out of the vein if it is not well anchored. Nonallergenic tape is less likely to tear fragile skin.
11. Remove equipment. Ensure patient's comfort. Remove gloves. Lower bed, if not in lowest position.	Promotes patient comfort and safety. Removing gloves properly reduces the risk for infection transmission and contamination of other items.
12. Remove additional PPE, if used. Perform hand hygiene.	Removing PPE properly reduces the risk for infection transmission and contamination of other items. Hand hygiene prevents transmission of microorganisms.

EVALUATION

- Peripheral venous access device flushes without resistance.
- Patient exhibits an access site that is intact, free of the signs and symptoms of infection, phlebitis, or infiltration.
- Site dressing is clean, dry, and intact.

DOCUMENTATION

- Document discontinuation of IV fluid infusion. Record the condition of the venous access site. Document the flushing of the venous access device. This is often done in the CMAR/MAR. Record the patient's reaction to the procedure and any patient teaching that has occurred.

SKILL VARIATION | **Capping a Primary Line When No Extension Tubing is in Place**

It is good practice to add a short extension tubing to decrease the risk of contact with blood, and for infection-control purposes if one was not placed during initiation of the peripheral venous access. After checking the medical order to convert the peripheral venous access, the nurse brings the end cap and the extension tubing to the bedside, as well as other required equipment.

1. Gather equipment and verify medical order.
2. Perform hand hygiene.

3. Put on PPE, as indicated.
4. Identify the patient.

5. Explain the procedure to the patient.
6. Fill the cap and extension tubing with normal saline.

7. Assess IV site.
8. Put on gloves.
9. Remove site dressing as outlined in Skill 55.
10. Put on sterile gloves. Place gauze 4 × 4-inch sponge underneath IV connection hub, between IV catheter and tubing.
11. **Stabilize hub of IV catheter with nondominant hand. Use dominant hand to quickly twist and disconnect IV tubing from the catheter. Discard it. Attach the primed extension tubing to the IV catheter hub using aseptic technique.**
12. Cleanse cap with an antimicrobial solution.
13. Insert the syringe into the cap and gently flush with saline per facility policy. Remove syringe. Engage slide clamp on extension tubing.
14. Redress site as outlined in Skill 55.
15. Remove gloves.

continued on page 684

Capping a Primary Line When No Extension Tubing is in Place *continued*	
16. Loop the extension tubing near the entry site and anchor with tape (nonallergenic) close to the site.	purpose of the device and the importance of safeguarding the site when using the extremity.
17. Apply an IV securement/stabilization device if not already in place as part of the dressing, as indicated, based on facility policy. Explain to patient the	18. Ensure that the patient is comfortable. Perform hand hygiene.
	19. Chart on IV administration record, MAR, or CMAR, per facility policy.

SKILL 129 INITIATING A PERIPHERAL VENOUS ACCESS IV INFUSION

Administering and monitoring IV fluids is an essential part of routine patient care. The primary care provider often orders IV therapy to prevent or correct problems in fluid and electrolyte balance. For IV fluid and other therapies to be administered, an intravenous access must be established.

The nurse must also verify the amount and type of solution to be administered, as well as the prescribed infusion rate. The nurse is responsible for critically evaluating all patient orders prior to administration. Any concerns regarding the type or amount of therapy prescribed should be immediately and clearly communicated to the prescribing practitioner. The nurse must understand the patient's need for IV therapy, the type of solution being used, its desired effect, and potential adverse reactions and effects. Follow the facility's policies and guidelines to determine if the infusion should be administered by electronic infusion device or by gravity.

DELEGATION CONSIDERATIONS

The initiation of a peripheral venous access IV infusion is not delegated to nursing assistive personnel (NAP) or to unlicensed assistive personnel (UAP). Depending on the state's nurse practice act and the organization's policies and procedures, initiation of a peripheral venous access IV infusion may be delegated to licensed practical/vocational nurses (LPN/LVNs). The decision to delegate must be based on careful analysis of the patient's needs and circumstances, as well as the qualifications of the person to whom the task is being delegated. Refer to the Delegation Guidelines in Appendix A.

EQUIPMENT

- IV solution, as prescribed
- Medication administration record (MAR) or computer-generated MAR (CMAR)
- Towel or disposable pad
- Nonallergenic tape
- IV administration set
- Label for infusion set (for next change date)
- Transparent site dressing
- Electronic infusion device (if appropriate)
- Tourniquet
- Time tape and/or label (for IV container)
- Cleansing swabs (chlorhexidine preferred; 70% alcohol,

iodine, or povidone-iodine are also acceptable)
- IV securement/stabilization device, as appropriate
- Clean gloves
- Additional PPE, as indicated
- IV pole
- Local anesthetic (if ordered)
- IV catheter
- Short extension tubing
- End cap for extension tubing
- Alcohol or other disinfectant wipes
- Skin protectant wipe (e.g., SkinPrep)
- Prefilled 2-mL syringe with sterile normal saline for injection

ASSESSMENT

- Review the patient's record for baseline data, such as vital signs, intake and output balance, and pertinent laboratory values, such as serum electrolytes.
- Assess the appropriateness of the solution for the patient.
- Review assessment and laboratory data that may influence solution administration.
- Assess arms and hands for potential sites for initiating the IV. Keep in mind the following guidelines related to peripheral venous catheters and access sites:
  - Determine the most desirable accessible vein. The dorsal and ventral surfaces of the upper extremities are appropriate sites for infusion (INS, 2011). The superficial veins on the dorsal aspect of the hand can also be used successfully for some people, but can be more painful (I.V. Rounds, 2008). Avoid the ventral surface of the wrist and the lateral surface of the wrist for approximately 4 to 5 inches because of the potential risk for nerve damage. Initiate venous access in the distal areas of the upper extremities, as this allows for future sites proximal to the previous insertion site (INS, 2011).
  - Generally, either arm may be used for IV therapy. Usually the nondominant arm is selected for patient comfort and to limit movement in the impacted extremity. For example, if the patient is right-handed, the IV is preferably placed on the left extremity to improve the patient's ability to complete activities of daily living. This is particularly important if the duration of infusion is expected to be prolonged.
  - Determine accessibility based on the patient's condition. The use of an extremity for IV therapy may be contraindicated in some circumstances. For example, patients with a history of breast cancer

with same side surgical axillary lymph node removal; patients with burns, infections or traumatic injury to the extremity; and patients with upper extremity arterial-venous fistulas or catheters for dialysis treatment will not be able to have an IV catheter placed on the impacted extremity.

- Do not use the antecubital veins if another vein is available. They are not a good choice for infusion because flexion of the patient's arm can displace the IV catheter over time. By avoiding the antecubital veins for peripheral venous catheters, a PICC line may be inserted at a later time, if needed.

- Do not use veins in the leg of an adult, unless other sites are inaccessible, because of the danger of stagnation of peripheral circulation and possible serious complications. The cannulation of the lower extremities is associated with risk of tissue damage, thrombophlebitis, and ulceration (INS, 2011). Some facilities require a medical order to insert an IV catheter in an adult patient's lower extremity.

NURSING DIAGNOSIS

- Deficient Fluid Volume
- Risk for Shock
- Risk for Deficient Fluid Volume

OUTCOME IDENTIFICATION AND PLANNING

- Access device is inserted using sterile technique on the first attempt.
- Patient experiences minimal trauma, and the IV solution infuses without difficulty.

IMPLEMENTATION

ACTION	RATIONALE
1. Verify the IV solution order on the MAR/CMAR with the medical order. Consider the appropriateness of the prescribed therapy in relation to the patient. Clarify any inconsistencies. Check the patient's chart for allergies. Check for color, leaking, and expiration date. Know techniques for IV insertion, precautions, purpose of the IV administration, and medications if ordered. Gather necessary supplies.	This ensures that the correct IV solution and rate of infusion, and/or medication will be administered. The nurse is responsible for critically evaluating all patient orders prior to administration. Any concerns regarding the type or amount of therapy prescribed should be immediately and clearly communicated to the prescribing practitioner. This knowledge and skill is essential for safe and accurate IV and medication administration. Preparation promotes efficient time management and an organized approach to the task.

ACTION	RATIONALE
2. Perform hand hygiene and put on PPE, if indicated.	Hand hygiene and PPE prevent the spread of microorganisms. PPE is required based on transmission precautions.
3. Identify the patient.	Identifying the patient ensures the right patient receives the intervention and helps prevent errors.
4. Close the curtains around the bed and close the door to the room, if possible. Explain what you are going to do and why you are going to do it to the patient. Ask the patient about allergies to medications, tape, or skin antiseptics, as appropriate. If considering using a local anesthetic, inquire about allergies for these substances as well.	This ensures the patient's privacy. Explanation relieves anxiety and facilitates cooperation. Possible allergies may exist related to medications, tape, or local anesthetic. Injectable anesthetic can result in allergic reactions and tissue damage.
5. If using a local anesthetic, explain the rationale and procedure to the patient. Apply the anesthetic to a few potential insertion sites. Allow sufficient time for the anesthetic to take effect.	Explanations provide reassurance and facilitate the patient's cooperation. Local anesthetic decreases the degree of pain felt at the insertion site. Some of the anesthetics take up to an hour to become effective.

Prepare the IV Solution and Administration Set

6. Compare the IV container label with the MAR/CMAR. Remove IV bag from outer wrapper, if indicated. Check expiration dates. Scan bar code on container, if necessary. Compare on patient identification band with the MAR/CMAR. Alternately, label the solution container with the patient's name, solution type, additives, date,	Checking the label with MAR/CMAR ensures the correct IV solution will be administered. Identifying the patient ensures the right patient receives the medications and helps prevent errors. Time strip allows for quick visual reference by the nurse to monitor infusion accuracy.

ACTION	RATIONALE

and time. Complete a time strip for the infusion and apply to IV container.

7. Maintain aseptic technique when opening sterile packages and IV solution. Remove administration set from package. Apply label to tubing reflecting the day/date for next set change, per facility guidelines.

Asepsis is essential for preventing the spread of microorganisms. Labeling tubing ensures adherence to facility policy regarding administration set changes and reduces the risk of spread of microorganisms.

8. Close the roller clamp or slide the clamp on the IV administration set. Invert the IV solution container and remove the cap on the entry site, taking care not to touch the exposed entry site. Remove the cap from the spike on the administration set. Using a twisting and pushing motion, insert the administration set spike into the entry site of the IV container. Alternately, follow the manufacturer's directions for insertion.

Clamping the IV tubing prevents air and fluid from entering the IV tubing at this time.

Inverting the container allows easy access to the entry site. Touching the opened entry site on the IV container and/or the spike on the administration set results in contamination and the container/administration set would have to be discarded. Inserting the spike punctures the seal in the IV container and allows access to the contents.

9. Hang the IV container on the IV pole. Squeeze the drip chamber and fill at least halfway.

Suction causes fluid to move into drip chamber. Fluid prevents air from moving down the tubing.

10. Open the IV tubing clamp, and allow fluid to move through tubing. Follow additional manufacturer's instructions for specific electronic infusion pump, as indicated. **Allow fluid to flow until all air bubbles have disappeared and the entire length of the tubing is primed (filled) with IV solution.** Close the clamp. Alternately, some brands of tubing may require removal

This technique prepares for IV fluid administration and removes air from the tubing. If not removed from the tubing, large amounts of air can act as an embolus. Touching the open end of the tubing results in contamination and the administration set would have to be discarded.

ACTION	RATIONALE
of the cap at the end of the IV tubing to allow fluid to flow. Maintain its sterility. After fluid has filled the tubing, recap the end of the tubing.	
11. If an electronic device is to be used, follow manufacturer's instructions for inserting tubing into the device.	This ensures proper use of equipment.

Initiate Peripheral Venous Access

ACTION	RATIONALE
12. Place patient in low-Fowler's position in bed. Place protective towel or pad under patient's arm.	The supine position permits either arm to be used and allows for good body alignment. Towel protects underlying surface from blood contamination.
13. Provide emotional support, as needed.	Patient may experience anxiety because he or she may, in general, fear needlestick or IV infusion.
14. Open the short extension tubing package. Attach end cap, if not in place. Clean end cap with alcohol wipe. Insert syringe with normal saline into extension tubing. Fill extension tubing with normal saline and apply slide clamp. Remove the syringe and place extension tubing and syringe back on package, within easy reach.	Priming the extension tubing removes air from the tubing and prevents administration of air when connected to venous access. Having tubing within easy reach facilitates accomplishment of procedure.
15. Select and palpate for an appropriate vein. Refer to guidelines in previous Assessment section. If the intended insertion site is visibly soiled, clean area with soap and water.	The use of an appropriate vein decreases discomfort for the patient and reduces the risk for damage to body tissues.
16. If the site is hairy and agency policy permits, clip a 2-inch area around the intended entry site.	Hair can harbor microorganisms and inhibit adhesion of site dressing. Shaving causes microabrasions and increases risk for infection (INS, 2011, p. S44).

ACTION	RATIONALE
17. Put on gloves.	Gloves prevent contact with blood and body fluids.
18. Apply a tourniquet 3 to 4 inches above the venipuncture site to obstruct venous blood flow and distend the vein. Direct the ends of the tourniquet away from the entry site. Make sure the radial pulse is still present.	Interrupting the blood flow to the heart causes the vein to distend. Distended veins are easy to see, palpate, and enter. The end of the tourniquet could contaminate the area of injection if directed toward the entry site.
	Tourniquet may be applied too tightly so assessment for radial pulse is important.
	Checking radial pulse ensures arterial supply is not compromised.
19. Instruct the patient to hold the arm lower than the heart.	Lowering the arm below the heart level helps distend the veins by filling them.
20. Ask the patient to open and close the fist. Observe and palpate for a suitable vein. Try the following techniques if a vein cannot be felt:	Contracting the muscles of the forearm forces blood into the veins, thereby distending them further.
a. Lightly stroke the vein downward.	Massaging and tapping the vein help distend veins by filling them with blood.
b. Remove tourniquet and place warm, dry compresses over intended vein for 10 to 15 minutes.	Warm compresses help dilate veins. The use of dry heat increases the likelihood of successful peripheral catheter insertion (INS, 2011).
21. **Cleanse site with an antiseptic solution such as chlorhexidine or according to facility policy. Press applicator against the skin and apply chlorhexidine using a gentle back and forth motion. Do not wipe or blot. Allow to dry completely.**	Cleansing is necessary because organisms on the skin can be introduced into the tissues or the bloodstream with the needle. Chlorhexidine is the preferred antiseptic solution, but iodine, povidone-iodine, and 70% alcohol are considered acceptable alternatives (INS, 2011). Scrubbing motion creates friction and lets the solution more effectively penetrate the epidermal layers (Hadaway, 2006).

ACTION	RATIONALE

22. Alternately, for patients who bruise easily, are at risk for bleeding, or have fragile skin, **apply the chlorhexidine without scrubbing for at least 30 seconds. Allow to dry completely. Do not wipe or blot.**

Cleansing is necessary because organisms on the skin can be introduced into the tissues or the bloodstream with the needle. Avoiding use of scrubbing decreases risk of injury. A minimum of 30 seconds is the length of time that is necessary for chlorhexidine to be effective (Hadaway, 2006).

23. Using the nondominant hand placed about 1 or 2 inches below the entry site, hold the skin taut against the vein. **Avoid touching the prepared site.** Ask the patient to remain still while performing the venipuncture.

Pressure on the vein and surrounding tissues helps prevent movement of the vein as the needle or catheter is being inserted. The planned IV insertion site is not palpated after skin cleansing unless sterile gloves are worn to prevent contamination (INS, 2011). Patient movement may prevent proper technique for IV insertion.

24. Enter the skin gently, holding the catheter by the hub in your dominant hand, bevel side up, at a 10- to 15-degree angle. Insert the catheter from directly over the vein or from the side of the vein. While following the course of the vein, advance the needle or catheter into the vein. A sensation of "give" can be felt when the needle enters the vein.

This allows the needle or catheter to enter the vein with minimal trauma and deters passage of the needle through the vein.

25. When blood returns through the lumen of the needle or the flashback chamber of the catheter, advance either device into the vein until the hub is at the venipuncture site. The exact technique depends on the type of device used.

The tourniquet causes increased venous pressure, resulting in automatic backflow. Placing the access device well into the vein helps to prevent dislodgement.

26. Release the tourniquet. Quickly remove the protective cap from the extension

Bleeding is minimized and the patency of the vein is maintained if the connection is made

ACTION	RATIONALE
tubing and attach it to the catheter or needle. Stabilize the catheter or needle with your nondominant hand.	smoothly between the catheter and tubing.
27. Continue to stabilize the catheter or needle and flush gently with the saline, observing the site for infiltration and leaking.	Infiltration and/or leaking and patient reports of pain and/or discomfort indicate that the insertion into the vein is not successful and should be discontinued.
28. Open the skin protectant wipe. Apply the skin protectant to the site, making sure to apply—at minimum—the area to be covered with the dressing. Place sterile transparent dressing or catheter securing/stabilization device over venipuncture site. Loop the tubing near the entry site, and anchor with tape (nonallergenic) close to the site.	Skin protectant aids in adhesion of the dressing and decreases the risk for skin trauma when the dressing is removed. Transparent dressing allows easy visualization and protects the site. Stabilization/securing devices preserve the integrity of the access device, minimize catheter movement at the hub, and prevent catheter dislodgement and loss of access (INS, 2011, p. S46). Some stabilization devices act as a site dressing also. The weight of the tubing is sufficient to pull it out of the vein if it is not well anchored. Nonallergenic tape is less likely to tear fragile skin.
29. Label the IV dressing with the date, time, site, and type and size of catheter or needle used for the infusion.	Other personnel working with the infusion will know the site, what type of device is being used, and when it was inserted. Peripheral venous catheter IV insertion sites are changed every 72 to 96 hours for an adult (O'Grady et al., 2011).
30. Using an antimicrobial swab, cleanse the access cap on the extension tubing. Remove the end cap from the administration set. Insert the end of the administration set into the end cap. Loop the administration set tubing near the entry site, and anchor with tape (nonallergenic) close to the site. Remove gloves.	Inserting the administration set allows initiation of the fluid infusion. The weight of the tubing is sufficient to pull it out of the vein if it is not well anchored. Nonallergenic tape is less likely to tear fragile skin. Removing gloves properly reduces the risk for infection transmission and contamination of other items.

ACTION	RATIONALE
31. Open the clamp on the administration set. Set the flow rate and begin the fluid infusion. Alternately, start the flow of solution by releasing the clamp on the tubing and counting the drops. Adjust until the correct drop rate is achieved. Assess the flow of the solution and function of the infusion device. Inspect the insertion site for signs of infiltration.	Verifying the rate and device settings ensures the patient receives the correct volume of solution. If the catheter slips out of the vein, the solution will accumulate (infiltrate) into the surrounding tissue.
32. Apply an IV securement/ stabilization device if not already in place as part of the dressing, as indicated, based on facility policy. Explain to the patient the purpose of the device and the importance of safeguarding the site when using the extremity.	These systems are recommended for use on all venous access sites, and particularly central venous access sites, to preserve the integrity of the access device, minimize catheter movement at the hub, and prevent catheter dislodgement and loss of access (INS, 2011, p. S46). Some devices act as a site dressing also and may already have been applied.
33. Remove equipment and return the patient to a position of comfort. Lower bed, if not in lowest position.	Promotes patient comfort and safety.
34. Remove additional PPE, if used. Perform hand hygiene.	Removing PPE properly reduces the risk for infection transmission and contamination of other items. Hand hygiene prevents transmission of microorganisms.
35. Return to check flow rate and observe IV site for infiltration and/or other complications 30 minutes after starting infusion, and at least hourly thereafter. Ask the patient if he or she is experiencing any pain or discomfort related to the IV infusion.	Continued monitoring is important to maintain correct flow rate. Early detection of problems ensures prompt intervention.

EVALUATION

- IV access is initiated on the first attempt.
- Fluid flows easily into the vein without any sign of infiltration.
- Patient verbalizes minimal discomfort related to insertion and demonstrates an understanding of the reasons for the IV.

DOCUMENTATION

- Document the location where the IV access was placed, as well as the size of the IV catheter or needle, the type of IV solution, and the rate of the IV infusion, as well as the use of a securing or stabilization device. Additionally, document the condition of the site. Record the patient's reaction to the procedure and pertinent patient teaching, such as alerting the nurse if the patient experiences any pain from the IV or notices any swelling at the site. Document the IV fluid solution on the intake and output record.

SKILL 130 CARING FOR A PERITONEAL DIALYSIS CATHETER

Peritoneal dialysis is a method of removing fluid and wastes from the body of a patient with kidney failure. A catheter inserted through the abdominal wall into the peritoneal cavity allows a special fluid (dialysate) to be infused and then drained from the body, removing waste products and excess fluid (Figure 1). The exit site should be protected and kept clean and dry to allow for healing, which will take approximately 2 to 3 weeks (Lee & Park, 2012). Exit site dressings are initially changed weekly, until the site is healed. Frequent dressing changes in the immediate postoperative period are not necessary unless there is excessive oozing, bleeding, or signs of infection, to decrease the risk of contamination and unnecessary movement of the catheter (Lee & Park). Once the exit site has healed, exit site care is an important part of patient care. The catheter insertion site is a site for potential infection, possibly leading to catheter tunnel infection and peritonitis, therefore, meticulous care is

FIGURE 1 Position of catheter in peritoneal space. Patient is set up for peritoneal dialysis.

needed. The incidence of exit site infections can be reduced through a cleansing regimen by the patient or caregiver. Chronic exit site care is performed daily or every other day (Hain & Chan, 2013). In the postoperative period, catheter care is performed using aseptic technique, to reduce the risk for a health care-acquired infection. At home, clean technique can be used by the patient and caregivers.

DELEGATION CONSIDERATIONS

The care of a peritoneal dialysis catheter is not delegated to nursing assistive personnel (NAP) or to unlicensed assistive personnel (UAP). Depending on the state's nurse practice act and the organization's policies and procedures, care of a peritoneal dialysis catheter may be delegated to licensed practical/vocational nurses (LPN/LVNs). The decision to delegate must be based on careful analysis of the patient's needs and circumstances, as well as the qualifications of the person to whom the task is being delegated. Refer to the Delegation Guidelines in Appendix A.

EQUIPMENT

- Face masks (2)
- Sterile gloves
- Nonsterile gloves
- Additional PPE, as indicated
- Antimicrobial cleansing agent, per facility policy
- Sterile gauze squares (4)
- Sterile basin
- Sterile drain sponge
- Transparent, occlusive site dressing
- Topical antibiotic, such as mupirocin or gentamicin, depending on order and policy
- Sterile applicator
- Plastic trash bag
- Bath blanket

ASSESSMENT

- Inspect the peritoneal dialysis catheter exit site for any erythema, drainage, bleeding, tenderness, swelling, skin irritation or breakdown, or leakage. These signs could indicate exit site or tunnel infection.
- Assess abdomen for tenderness, pain, and guarding.
- Assess the patient for nausea, vomiting, and fever, which could indicate peritonitis.
- Assess the patient's knowledge about measures used to care for the exit site.

NURSING DIAGNOSIS

- Risk for Impaired Skin Integrity
- Deficient Knowledge
- Risk for Infection

OUTCOME IDENTIFICATION AND PLANNING

- Peritoneal dialysis catheter dressing change is completed using aseptic technique without trauma to the site or patient.
- Site is clean, dry, and intact, without evidence of inflammation or infection.

• Patient exhibits fluid balance and participates in care, as appropriate.
• Patient verbalizes an understanding of, and participates in care, as appropriate.

IMPLEMENTATION

ACTION	RATIONALE
1. Review the patient's medical record for orders related to catheter site care. Gather equipment.	Ensures appropriate interventions for the patient. Assembling equipment provides for an organized approach to the task.
2. Perform hand hygiene and put on PPE, if indicated.	Hand hygiene and PPE prevent the spread of microorganisms. PPE is required based on transmission precautions.
3. Identify the patient.	Identifying the patient ensures the right patient receives the intervention and helps prevent errors.
4. Close the curtains around the bed and close the door to the room, if possible. Explain what you are going to do and why you are going to do it to the patient. Encourage the patient to observe or participate if possible.	This ensures the patient's privacy. Explanation relieves anxiety and facilitates cooperation. Discussion promotes cooperation and helps to minimize anxiety. Having the patient observe or assist encourages self-acceptance.
5. Assemble equipment on overbed table within reach.	Arranging items nearby is convenient, saves time, and avoids unnecessary stretching and twisting of muscles on the part of the nurse.
6. Adjust the bed to a comfortable working height, usually elbow height of the caregiver (VISN 8 Patient Safety Center, 2009). Assist the patient to a supine position. Expose the abdomen, draping the patient's chest with the bath blanket, exposing only the catheter site.	Having the bed at the proper height prevents back and muscle strain. The supine position is usually the best way to gain access to the peritoneal dialysis catheter. Use of bath blanket provides patient warmth and avoids unnecessary exposure.

ACTION	RATIONALE
7. Put on nonsterile gloves. Put on one of the facemasks; have patient put on the other mask.	Gloves protect the nurse from contact with blood and bodily fluids. Use of facemasks deters the spread of microorganisms.
8. Gently remove old dressing, noting odor, amount, and color of drainage; leakage; and condition of skin around the catheter. Discard dressing in appropriate container.	Drainage, leakage, and skin condition can indicate problems with the catheter, such as infection.
9. Remove gloves and discard. Set up sterile field. Open packages. Using aseptic technique, place two sterile gauze squares in basin with antimicrobial agent. Leave two sterile gauze squares opened on sterile field. Alternately (based on facility's policy), place sterile antimicrobial swabs on the sterile field. Place sterile applicator on field. Squeeze a small amount of the topical antibiotic on one of the gauze squares on the sterile field.	Until catheter site has healed, aseptic technique is necessary for site care to prevent infection.
10. Put on sterile gloves. Pick up dialysis catheter with nondominant hand. **With the antimicrobial-soaked gauze/ swab, cleanse the skin around the exit site using a circular motion, starting at the exit site and then slowly going outward 3 to 4 inches. Gently remove crusted scabs, if necessary.**	Aseptic technique is necessary to prevent infection. The antimicrobial agent cleanses the skin and removes any drainage or crust from the wound, reducing the risk for infection.
11. **Continue to hold the catheter with your nondominant hand. After skin has dried, clean the catheter with an antimicrobial-soaked gauze, beginning at the exit site, going around catheter, and then moving up to**	Antimicrobial agents cleanse the catheter and remove any drainage or crust from the tube, reducing the risk for infection.

ACTION	RATIONALE
end of the catheter. Gently remove crusted secretions on the tube, if necessary.	
12. Using the sterile applicator, apply the topical antibiotic to the catheter exit site, if prescribed.	Application of mupirocin or gentamicin at catheter exit site prevents exit site infection and peritonitis (Bernardini et al., 2005; The Joanna Briggs Institute, 2004).
13. Place sterile drain sponge around the exit site. Then place a 4 × 4 gauze over the exit site. Cover with transparent, occlusive dressing. Remove masks.	The drain sponge and 4 × 4 gauze are used to absorb any drainage from the exit site. Occlusion of the site with a dressing deters site contamination. Once the site is covered, masks are no longer necessary.
14. Label dressing with date, time of change, and initials.	Other personnel working with the catheter will know information related to site care.
15. Coil the exposed length of tubing and secure to the dressing or the patient's abdomen with tape.	Anchoring the catheter absorbs any tugging, preventing tension on and irritation to the skin or abdomen.
16. Assist the patient to a comfortable position. Cover the patient with bed linens. Place the bed in the lowest position.	Positioning and covering provide warmth and promote comfort. A bed in the low position promotes patient safety.
17. Put on clean gloves. Remove or discard equipment and assess the patient's response to the procedure.	These actions deter the spread of microorganisms. The patient's response may indicate acceptance of the catheter or the need for health teaching.
18. Remove gloves and additional PPE, if used. Perform hand hygiene.	Removing PPE properly reduces the risk for infection transmission and contamination of other items. Hand hygiene prevents the spread of microorganisms.

EVALUATION

• Peritoneal dialysis catheter dressing change is completed using aseptic technique without trauma to the site or the patient.

- Site is clean, dry, and intact, without evidence of redness, irritation, or excoriation.
- Patient's fluid balance is maintained.
- Patient verbalizes and demonstrates appropriate measures to care for the site.

DOCUMENTATION

- Document the dressing change, including condition of skin surrounding the exit site, drainage, or odor, as well as the patient's reaction to procedure, and any patient teaching provided.

SKILL 131   USING PERSONAL PROTECTIVE EQUIPMENT

Personal protective equipment refers to specialized clothing or equipment worn by an employee for protection against infectious materials. PPE is used in health care settings to improve personnel safety in the health care environment through the appropriate use of PPE (CDC, 2004). This equipment includes clean (nonsterile) and sterile gloves, impervious gowns/aprons, surgical and high-efficiency particulate air (HEPA) masks, N95 disposable masks, face shields, and protective eyewear/goggles.

Understanding the potential contamination hazards related to the patient's diagnosis and condition and the institutional policies governing PPE is very important. The type of PPE used will vary based on the type of exposure anticipated and category of precautions: Standard Precautions and Transmission-Based Precautions, including Contact, Droplet, or Airborne Precautions. It is the nurse's responsibility to enforce the proper wearing of PPE during patient care for members of the health care team.

DELEGATION CONSIDERATIONS

The application and use of PPE is appropriate for all health care providers.

EQUIPMENT

- Gloves
- Mask (surgical or particulate respirator)
- Impervious gown
- Protective eyewear (does not include eyeglasses)

Note: Equipment for PPE may vary depending on facility policy.

ASSESSMENT

- Assess the situation to determine the necessity for PPE.
- Check the patient's chart for information about a suspected or diagnosed infection or communicable disease.

- Determine the possibility of exposure to blood and body fluids and identify the necessary equipment to prevent exposure. Refer to the infection control manual provided by your facility.

NURSING DIAGNOSIS

- Risk for Infection
- Ineffective Protection
- Diarrhea

OUTCOME IDENTIFICATION AND PLANNING

- The prevention of microorganism transmission.
- The patient and staff remain free of exposure to potentially infectious microorganisms.
- The patient verbalizes information about the rationale for use of PPE.

IMPLEMENTATION

ACTION	RATIONALE
1. Check medical record and nursing plan of care for type of precautions and review precautions in infection control manual.	Mode of transmission of organism determines type of precautions required.
2. Plan nursing activities before entering patient's room.	Organization facilitates performance of task and adherence to precautions.
3. Perform hand hygiene.	Hand hygiene prevents the spread of microorganisms.
4. Provide instruction about precautions to patient, family members, and visitors.	Explanation encourages cooperation of patient and family and reduces apprehension about precaution procedures.
5. Put on gown, mask, protective eyewear, and gloves based on the type of exposure anticipated and category of isolation precautions.	Use of PPE interrupts chain of infection and protects patient and nurse. Gown should protect entire uniform. Gloves protect hands and wrists from microorganisms. Masks protect nurse or patient from droplet nuclei and large-particle aerosols. Eyewear protects mucous membranes in the eye from splashes.

ACTION	RATIONALE
a. Put on the gown, with the opening in the back. Tie gown securely at neck and waist.	Gown should fully cover the torso from the neck to knees, arms to the end of wrists, and wrap around the back.
b. Put on the mask or respirator over your nose, mouth, and chin. Secure ties or elastic bands at the middle of the head and neck. If respirator is used, perform a fit check. Inhale; the respirator should collapse. Exhale; air should not leak out.	Masks protect nurse or patient from droplet nuclei and large-particle aerosols. A mask must fit securely to provide protection.
c. Put on goggles. Place over eyes and adjust to fit. Alternately, a face shield could be used to take the place of the mask and goggles.	Eyewear protects mucous membranes in the eye from splashes. Must fit securely to provide protection.
d. Put on clean disposable gloves. Extend gloves to cover the cuffs of the gown.	Gloves protect hands and wrists from microorganisms.
6. Identify the patient. Explain the procedure to the patient. Continue with patient care as appropriate.	Patient identification validates the correct patient and correct procedure. Discussion and explanation help allay anxiety and prepare the patient for what to expect.

Remove PPE

7. Remove PPE: Except for respirator, remove PPE at the doorway or in an anteroom. **Remove respirator after leaving the patient's room and closing the door.**	Proper removal prevents contact with and the spread of microorganisms. Removing respirator outside the patient's room prevents contact with airborne microorganisms.
a. If impervious gown has been tied in front of the body at the waistline, untie waist strings before removing gloves.	Outside front of equipment is considered contaminated. The inside, outside back, ties on head and back, are considered clean, which are areas of PPE that are not likely to have been in contact with infectious organisms. Front of gown, including waist strings, are contaminated. If tied in front

ACTION	RATIONALE
	of body, the ties must be untied before removing gloves.
b. Grasp the outside of one glove with the opposite gloved hand and peel off, turning the glove inside out as you pull it off. Hold the removed glove in the remaining gloved hand.	Outside of gloves are contaminated.
c. Slide fingers of ungloved hand under the remaining glove at the wrist, **taking care not to touch the outer surface of the glove.**	Ungloved hand is clean and should not touch contaminated areas.
d. Peel off the glove over the first glove, containing the one glove inside the other. Discard in appropriate container.	Proper disposal prevents transmission of microorganisms.
e. To remove the goggles or face shield: Handle by the headband or earpieces. Lift away from the face. Place in designated receptacle for reprocessing or in an appropriate waste container.	Outside of goggles or face shield is contaminated. **Do not touch.** Handling by headband or earpieces and lifting away from face prevents transmission of microorganisms. Proper disposal prevents transmission of microorganisms.
f. To remove gown: Unfasten ties, if at the neck and back. Allow the gown to fall away from shoulders. **Touching only the inside of the gown,** pull away from the torso. Keeping hands on the inner surface of the gown, pull gown from arms. Turn gown inside out. Fold or roll into a bundle and discard.	Gown front and sleeves are contaminated. Touching only the inside of the gown and pulling it away from the torso prevents transmission of microorganisms. Proper disposal prevents transmission of microorganisms.
g. To remove mask or respirator: Grasp the neck ties or elastic, then top ties or elastic and remove. **Take care to avoid touching**	Front of mask or respirator is contaminated. **Do not touch.** Not touching the front and proper disposal prevent transmission of microorganisms.

ACTION	RATIONALE

front of mask or respira-
tor. Discard in waste container. If using a respirator,
save for future use in the
designated area.

8. Perform hand hygiene
immediately after
removing all PPE.

Hand hygiene prevents spread of
microorganisms.

EVALUATION

- The transmission of microorganisms is prevented.
- Patient and staff remain free from exposure to potentially infectious microorganisms.
- Patient verbalizes an understanding about the rationale for use of PPE.

DOCUMENTATION

- It is not usually necessary to document the use of specific articles of PPE or each application of PPE. However, document the implementation and continuation of specific transmission-based precautions as part of the patient's care.

SKILL 132   APPLYING PNEUMATIC COMPRESSION DEVICES

Pneumatic compression devices (PCD) consist of fabric sleeves containing air bladders that apply brief pressure to the legs. Intermittent compression pushes blood from the smaller blood vessels into the deeper vessels and into the femoral veins. This action enhances blood flow and venous return and promotes fibrinolysis, deterring venous thrombosis. The sleeves are attached by tubing to an air pump. The sleeve may cover the entire leg or may extend from the foot to the knee.

Pneumatic compression devices may be used in combination with graduated compression stockings (antiembolism stockings) and anticoagulant therapy to prevent thrombosis formation. They can be used preoperatively and postoperatively with patients at risk for blood clot formation. They are also prescribed for patients with other risk factors for clot formation, including inactivity or immobilization, chronic venous disease, and malignancies.

DELEGATION CONSIDERATIONS

The application and removal of pneumatic compression devices may be delegated to nursing assistive personnel (NAP) or to unlicensed assistive personnel (UAP), as well as to licensed practical/vocational nurses (LPN/LVNs). The decision to delegate must be based on careful analysis of the patient's needs and circumstances, as well as the qualifications of the person to whom the task is being delegated. Refer to the Delegation Guidelines in Appendix A.

EQUIPMENT

- Compression sleeves of appropriate size based on the manufacturer's guidelines
- Inflation pump with connection tubing
- PPE, as indicated

ASSESSMENT

- Assess the patient's history, medical record, and current condition and status to identify risk for development of deep-vein thrombosis (DVT).
- Assess the lower extremity skin integrity.
- Identify any leg conditions that would be exacerbated by the use of the compression device or would contraindicate its use.

NURSING DIAGNOSIS

- Impaired Physical Mobility
- Risk for Peripheral Neurovascular Dysfunction
- Delayed Surgical Recovery

OUTCOME IDENTIFICATION AND PLANNING

- Patient maintains adequate circulation in extremities.
- Patient is free from symptoms of neurovascular compromise.

ACTION	RATIONALE
3. Identify the patient. Explain the procedure to the patient.	Patient identification validates the correct patient and correct procedure. Discussion and explanation help allay anxiety and prepare the patient for what to expect.
4. Close the curtains around the bed and close the door to the room, if possible. Place the bed at an appropriate and comfortable working height, usually elbow height of the caregiver (VISN 8 Patient Safety Center, 2009).	Closing the door or curtains provides privacy. Proper bed height helps reduce back strain.
5. Hang the compression pump on the foot of the bed and plug it into an electrical outlet. Attach the connecting tubing to the pump.	Equipment preparation promotes efficient time management and provides an organized approach to the task.
6. Remove the compression sleeves from the package and unfold them. Lay the unfolded sleeves on the bed with the cotton lining facing up. **Note the markings indicating the correct placement for the ankle and popliteal areas.**	Proper placement of the sleeves prevents injury.
7. Apply graduated compression stockings, if ordered. Place a sleeve under the patient's leg with the tubing toward the heel. Each one fits either leg. **For total leg sleeves, place the behind-the-knee opening at the popliteal space to prevent pressure there. For knee-high sleeves, make sure the back of the ankle is over the ankle marking.**	Proper placement prevents injury.
8. Wrap the sleeve snugly around the patient's leg so that two fingers fit between the leg and the sleeve. Secure the sleeve with the	Correct placement ensures appropriate, but not excessive, compression of the extremity.

ACTION	RATIONALE
fasteners. Repeat for the second leg, if bilateral therapy is ordered. Connect each sleeve to the tubing, following manufacturer's recommendations.	
9. Set the pump to the pre-scribed maximal pressure (usually 35 to 55 mm Hg). Make sure the tubing is free from kinks. Check that the patient can move about without interrupting the airflow. Turn on the pump. Initiate cooling setting, if available.	Proper pressure setting ensures patient safety and prevents injury. Some devices have a cooling setting available to increase patient comfort.
10. **Observe the patient and the device during the first cycle. Check the audible alarms. Check the sleeves and pump at least once per shift or per facility policy.**	Observation and frequent check-ing ensure proper fit and inflation and reduce the risk for injury from the device.
11. Place the bed in the lowest position. Make sure the call bell and other essential items are within easy reach.	Returning the bed to the lowest position and having the call bell and other essential items readily available promote patient safety.
12. Remove PPE, if used. Perform hand hygiene.	Removing PPE properly reduces the risk for infection transmission and contamination of other items. Hand hygiene prevents the spread of microorganisms.
13. Assess the extremities for peripheral pulses, edema, changes in sensation, and movement. Remove the sleeves and assess and document skin integrity every 8 hours.	Assessment provides for early detection and prompt interven-tion for possible complications, including skin irritation.

EVALUATION

- Patient exhibits adequate circulation in extremities without symptoms of neurovascular compromise.

DOCUMENTATION

- Document the time and date of application of the PCD, the patient's response to the therapy, and the patient's understanding of the therapy. Document the status of the alarms and pressure settings. Note the use of the cooling setting, if appropriate.

SKILL 133 | PROVIDING POSTOPERATIVE CARE WHEN PATIENT RETURNS TO ROOM

Postoperative care facilitates recovery from surgery and supports the patient in coping with physical changes or alterations. Nursing interventions promote physical and psychological health, prevent complications, and teach self-care skills for the patient to use after the hospital stay. After surgery, patients spend time on the postanesthesia care unit (PACU). From the PACU, they are transferred back to their rooms. At this time, nursing care focuses on accurate assessments and associated interventions. Ongoing assessments are crucial for early identification of postoperative complications.

DELEGATION CONSIDERATIONS

Postoperative measurement of vital signs may be delegated to nursing assistive personnel (NAP) or to unlicensed assistive personnel (UAP), as well as to licensed practical/vocational nurses (LPN/LVNs). Postoperative assessment and teaching is not delegated to nursing assistive personnel (NAP) or to unlicensed assistive personnel (UAP). Depending on the state's nurse practice act and the organization's policies and procedures, postoperative teaching may be delegated to licensed practical/vocational nurses (LPN/LVNs) after an assessment of education needs by the registered nurse. The decision to delegate must be based on careful analysis of the patient's needs and circumstances, as well as the qualifications of the person to whom the task is being delegated. Refer to the Delegation Guidelines in Appendix A.

EQUIPMENT (VARIES, DEPENDING ON THE SURGERY)

- Electronic blood pressure monitor
- Blood pressure cuff
- Electronic thermometer
- Pulse oximeter
- Stethoscope
- IV pump, IV solutions
- Graduated compression stockings
- Pneumatic compression devices
- Tubes, drains, vascular access tubing
- Incentive spirometer
- PPE, as indicated
- Blankets, as needed

ASSESSMENT

- Assess the patient's mental status, positioning, and vital signs.
- Assess the patient's oxygen saturation level, skin color, respiratory status, and cardiovascular status.
- Assess the patient's neurovascular status, depending on the type of surgery.
- Assess the operative site, drains/tubes, and intravenous site(s).
- Perform a pain assessment.
- A wide variety of factors increase the risk for postoperative complications. Ongoing postoperative assessments and interventions are used to decrease the risk for postoperative complications.
- Assess the learning needs of the patient and family.

NURSING DIAGNOSIS

- Acute Pain
- Risk for Imbalanced Fluid Volume
- Impaired Gas Exchange
- Hypothermia
- Impaired Skin Integrity
- Risk for Aspiration

OUTCOME IDENTIFICATION AND PLANNING

- Patient will recover from the surgery.
- Patient is free from anxiety.
- Patient's temperature remains between 97.7°F and 99.5°F (36.5°C and 37.5°C).
- Patient's vital signs remain stable.
- Patient will remain free from infection.
- Patient will not experience any skin breakdown.
- Patient will regain mobility.
- Patient will have pain managed appropriately.
- Patient is comfortable with body image.
- Specific expected outcomes are individualized based on risk factors, the surgical procedure, and the patient's unique needs.

ACTION	RATIONALE
2. Perform hand hygiene and put on PPE, if indicated.	Hand hygiene and PPE prevent the spread of microorganisms. PPE is required based on transmission precautions.
3. Identify the patient.	Identifying the patient ensures the right patient receives the intervention and helps prevent errors.
4. Close the curtains around the bed and close the door to the room, if possible. Explain what you are going to do and why you are going to do it to the patient or significant other. Place necessary supplies on the bedside stand or overbed table, within easy reach.	This ensures the patient's privacy. Explanation relieves anxiety and facilitates cooperation. Bringing everything to the bedside conserves time and energy. Arranging items nearby is convenient, saves time, and avoids unnecessary stretching and twisting of muscles on the part of the nurse.
5. **Place patient in safe position (semi- or high Fowler's or side-lying). Note level of consciousness.**	A sitting position (head of bed [HOB] elevated) facilitates deep breathing; the side-lying position with neck slightly extended prevents aspiration and airway obstruction. Alternate positions may be appropriate based on the type of surgery.
6. **Obtain vital signs. Monitor and record vital signs frequently.** Assessment order may vary, but usual frequency includes taking vital signs every 15 minutes the first hour, every 30 minutes the next 2 hours, every hour for 4 hours, and finally every 4 hours.	Comparison with baseline preoperative vital signs may indicate impending shock or hemorrhage. Some institutions use a paper or computer flow sheet to record initial postoperative data.
7. Assess the patient's respiratory status. Measure the patient's oxygen saturation level.	Comparison with baseline preoperative respiratory assessment may indicate impending respiratory complications.

ACTION	RATIONALE
8. Assess the patient's cardiovascular status.	Comparison with baseline preoperative cardiovascular assessment may indicate impending cardiovascular complications.
9. Assess the patient's neurovascular status, based on the type of surgery performed.	Comparison with baseline preoperative neurovascular assessment may indicate impending neurovascular complications.
10. Provide for warmth, using heated or extra blankets, as necessary. Refer to Skill 183. Assess skin color and condition.	The operating room is a cold environment. Hypothermia is uncomfortable and may lead to cardiac arrhythmias and impaired wound healing.
11. Check dressings for color, odor, presence of drains, and amount of drainage. Mark the drainage on the dressing by circling the amount, and include the time. Turn the patient to assess visually under the patient for bleeding from the surgical site.	Hemorrhage and shock are life-threatening complications of surgery and early recognition is essential.
12. Verify that all tubes and drains are patent and the equipment is working; note amount of drainage in collection device. If an indwelling urinary (Foley) catheter is in place, note urinary output.	This ensures function of drainage devices.
13. Verify and maintain IV infusion at prescribed rate.	This replaces fluid loss and prevents dehydration and electrolyte imbalances.
14. Assess for pain and relieve it by administering medications ordered by the primary care provider. If the patient has been instructed in the use of PCA for pain management, review its use. Check record to verify if analgesic medication was administered in the PACU.	Use a facility-approved pain scale. Observe for nonverbal behavior that may indicate pain, such as grimacing, crying, and restlessness. Analgesics and other nonpharmacologic pain strategies are used for relief of postoperative pain.

ACTION	RATIONALE
15. Provide for a safe environment. Keep bed in low position with side rails up, based on facility policy. Have call bell within patient's reach.	This prevents accidental injury. Easy access to call bell permits patient to call for nurse when necessary.
16. Remove PPE, if used. Perform hand hygiene.	Removing PPE properly reduces the risk for infection transmission and contamination of other items. Hand hygiene prevents transmission of microorganisms.

Ongoing Care

ACTION	RATIONALE
17. Promote optimal respiratory function.	Anesthetic agents may depress respiratory function. Patients who have existing respiratory or cardiovascular disease, have abdominal or chest incisions, who are obese, older (Shippee-Rice et al., 2012), or in a poor state of nutrition are at greater risk for respiratory complications.
a. Assess respiratory rate, depth, quality, color, and capillary refill. Ask if the patient is experiencing any difficulty breathing.	Postoperative analgesic medication can reduce the rate and quality of the respiratory effort.
b. Assist with coughing and deep breathing exercises (refer to Skill 46).	
c. Assist with incentive spirometry (refer to Skill 84).	
d. Assist with early ambulation.	
e. Provide frequent position changes.	
f. Administer oxygen as ordered.	
g. Monitor pulse oximetry (refer to Skill 137).	

ACTION	RATIONALE

18. Promote optimal cardiovascular function:

Preventive measures can improve venous return and circulatory status.

   a. Assess apical rate, rhythm, and quality and compare with peripheral pulses, color, and blood pressure. Ask if the patient has any chest pains or shortness of breath.

   b. Provide frequent position changes.

   c. Assist with early ambulation.

   d. Apply graduated compression stockings or pneumatic compression devices, if ordered and not in place. If in place, assess for integrity.

   e. Provide leg and range-of-motion exercises if not contraindicated (refer to Skill 93).

19. Promote optimal neurologic function:

   a. Assess level of consciousness, movement, and sensation.

Anesthetic and pain management agents can alter neurologic function.

   b. Determine the level of orientation to person, place, and time.

Older patients may take longer to return to their level of orientation before surgery. Drug and anesthetics will delay this return (Shippee-Rice et al., 2012).

   c. Test motor ability by asking the patient to move each extremity.

Anesthesia alters motor and sensory function.

   d. Evaluate sensation by asking the patient if he or she can feel your touch on an extremity.

ACTION	RATIONALE
20. Promote optimal renal and urinary function and fluid and electrolyte status. Assess intake and output, evaluate for urinary retention and monitor serum electrolyte levels.	Anesthetic agents and surgical manipulation in the area may temporarily depress bladder tone and response causing urinary retention.
a. Promote voiding by offering bedpan at regular intervals, noting the frequency, amount, and if any burning or urgency symptoms.	Frequency, burning, or urgency may indicate possible urinary tract abnormality.
b. Monitor urinary catheter drainage if present.	The primary care provider needs to be notified if the urinary output is less than 30 mL/hour or 240 mL/8-hour period.
c. Measure intake and output.	Intake and output are good indicators of fluid balance.
21. Promote optimal gastrointestinal function and meet nutritional needs:	Anesthetic agents and narcotics depress peristalsis and normal functioning of the gastrointestinal tract. Flatus indicates return of peristalsis.
a. Assess abdomen for distention and firmness. Ask if patient feels nauseated, any vomiting, and if passing flatus.	
b. Auscultate for bowel sounds.	Presence of bowel sounds indicates return of peristalsis.
c. Assist with diet progression; encourage fluid intake; monitor intake.	Patients may experience nausea after surgery and are encouraged to resume diet slowly, starting with clear liquids and advancing as tolerated.
d. Medicate for nausea and vomiting, as ordered.	Antiemetics are frequently ordered to alleviate postoperative nausea.
22. Promote optimal wound healing.	Alterations in nutritional, circulatory, and metabolic status may predispose the patient to infection and delayed healing.
a. Assess condition of wound for presence of drains and any drainage.	

ACTION	RATIONALE
b. Use surgical asepsis for dressing changes and drain care. Refer to Skills 51, 52, 53, 56, and 57.	Surgical asepsis reduces the risk of infection.
c. Inspect all skin surfaces for beginning signs of pressure ulcer development and use pressure-relieving supports to minimize potential skin breakdown.	Lying on the operating room table in the same position can predispose some patients to pressure ulcer formation, especially in patients who have undergone lengthy procedures.
23. Promote optimal comfort and relief from pain.	This shortens recovery period and facilitates return to normal function.
a. Assess of pain (location and intensity using pain scale).	Control of postoperative pain promotes patient comfort and recovery.
b. Provide for rest and comfort; provide extra blankets, as needed, for warmth.	Patients may experience chills in the postoperative period.
c. Administer pain medications, as needed, and/or initiate nonpharmacologic methods, as appropriate.	
24. Promote optimal meeting of psychosocial needs:	This facilitates individualized care, anxiety reduction, and patient's return to normal health.
a. Provide emotional support to patient and family, as needed.	
b. Explain procedures and offer explanations regarding postoperative recovery, as needed, to both patient and family members.	

EVALUATION

- Patient recovers from surgery.
- Patient is free from anxiety.
- Patient's temperature remains between 36.5°C and 37.5°C (97.7°F and 99.5°F).

- Patient's vital signs remain stable.
- Patient remains free from infection.
- Patient does not experience skin breakdown.
- Patient regains mobility.
- Patient experiences adequate pain control.
- Patient is comfortable with body image.
- Specific expected outcomes are individualized based on risk factors, the surgical procedure, and the patient's unique needs.

DOCUMENTATION

- Document the time that the patient returns from PACU to the surgical unit. Record the patient's level of consciousness, vital signs, all assessments, and condition of dressing. If patient has oxygen running, an IV, or any other equipment, record this information. Document pain assessment, interventions that were instituted to alleviate pain, and the patient's response to the interventions. Document any patient teaching that is reviewed with the patient, such as use of incentive spirometer.

SKILL 134 | ASSESSING THE APICAL PULSE BY AUSCULTATION

An apical pulse is auscultated (listened to) over the apex of the heart, as the heart beats. The heart is a cone-shaped, muscular pump, divided into four hollow chambers. The upper chambers, the atria (singular, atrium), receive blood from the veins (the superior and inferior vena cava and the left and right pulmonary veins). The lower chambers, the ventricles, force blood out of the heart through the arteries (the left and right pulmonary arteries and the aorta). One-way valves that direct blood flow through the heart are located at the entrance (tricuspid and mitral valves) and exit (pulmonic and aortic valves) of each ventricle. Heart sounds, which are produced by closure of the valves of the heart, are characterized as "lub-dub." The apical pulse is the result of closure of the mitral and tricuspid valves ("lub") and the aortic and pulmonic valves ("dub"). The combination of the two sounds is counted as one beat. Pulse rates are measured in beats per minute. The normal pulse rate for adolescents and adults ranges from 60 to 100 beats per minute. Pulse rhythm is also assessed. Pulse rhythm is the pattern of the beats and the pauses between them. Pulse rhythm is normally regular; the beats and the pauses between occur at regular intervals. An irregular pulse rhythm occurs when the beats and pauses between beats occur at unequal intervals.

An apical pulse is assessed when giving medications that alter heart rate and rhythm. In addition, if a peripheral pulse is difficult to assess accurately because it is irregular, feeble, or extremely rapid, assess the apical rate. In adults, the apical rate is counted for 1 full minute by listening with a stethoscope over the apex of the heart. Apical pulse measurement is also the preferred method of pulse assessment in children less than 10 years of age (Jarvis, 2012).

DELEGATION CONSIDERATIONS

The assessment of an apical pulse is not delegated to nursing assistive personnel (NAP) or to unlicensed assistive personnel (UAP). The assessment of an apical pulse may be delegated to licensed practical/vocational nurses (LPN/LVNs). The decision to delegate must be based on careful analysis of the patient's needs and circumstances, as well as the qualifications of the person to whom the task is being delegated. Refer to the Delegation Guidelines in Appendix A.

EQUIPMENT

- Watch with second hand or digital readout
- Stethoscope
- Alcohol swab
- Pencil or pen, paper or flow sheet, computerized record
- Nonsterile gloves, if appropriate; additional PPE, as indicated

ASSESSMENT

- Assess for factors that could affect apical pulse rate and rhythm, such as the patient's age, amount of exercise, fluid balance, and medications.
- Note baseline or previous apical pulse measurements.

NURSING DIAGNOSIS

- Decreased Cardiac Output
- Deficient Fluid Volume

OUTCOME IDENTIFICATION AND PLANNING

- Patient's pulse is assessed accurately without injury.
- Patient experiences minimal discomfort.

IMPLEMENTATION

ACTION	RATIONALE
1. Check medical order or nursing care plan for frequency of pulse assessment. More frequent pulse measurement may be appropriate based on nursing judgment. Identify the need to obtain an apical pulse measurement.	Provides for patient safety and appropriate care.

ACTION	RATIONALE
2. Perform hand hygiene and put on PPE, if indicated.	Hand hygiene and PPE prevent the spread of microorganisms. PPE is required based on transmission precautions.
3. Identify the patient.	Identifying the patient ensures the right patient receives the intervention and helps prevent errors.
4. Close the curtains around the bed and close the door to the room, if possible. Discuss the procedure with the patient and assess the patient's ability to assist with the procedure.	This ensures the patient's privacy. Explanation relieves anxiety and facilitates cooperation.
5. Put on gloves, if indicated.	Gloves are not usually worn to obtain a pulse measurement unless contact with blood or body fluids is anticipated. Gloves prevent contact with blood and body fluids.
6. Use an alcohol swab to clean the diaphragm of the stethoscope. Use another swab to clean the earpieces, if necessary.	Cleaning with alcohol deters transmission of microorganisms.
7. Assist the patient to a sitting or reclining position and expose the chest area.	This position facilitates identification of the site for stethoscope placement.
8. Move the patient's clothing to expose only the apical site.	The site must be exposed for pulse assessment. Exposing only the apical site keeps the patient warm and maintains his or her dignity.
9. Hold the stethoscope diaphragm against the palm of your hand for a few seconds.	Warming the diaphragm promotes patient comfort.
10. **Palpate the space between the fifth and sixth ribs (fifth intercostal space), and move to the left midclavicular line.** Place the	Position the stethoscope over the apex of the heart, where the heartbeat is best heard.

ACTION	RATIONALE

stethoscope diaphragm over the apex of the heart (Figures 1 and 2).

Midsternum Midclavicular line

FIGURE 1 Locating the apical pulse: apex area.

FIGURE 2 The apical pulse is usually found at (**A**) the fifth intercostal space just inside the midclavicular line and can be heard (**B**) over the apex of the heart.

11. Listen for heart sounds ("lub-dub"). Each "lub-dub" counts as one beat.

These sounds occur as the heart valves close.

12. Using a watch with a second hand, count the heartbeat for 1 minute.

Counting for a full minute increases the accuracy of assessment.

13. When measurement is completed, cover the patient and help him or her to a position of comfort.

Ensures patient comfort.

14. Clean the diaphragm of the stethoscope with an alcohol swab.

Cleaning with alcohol deters transmission of microorganisms.

15. Remove gloves and additional PPE, if used. Perform hand hygiene.

Removing PPE properly reduces the risk for infection transmission and contamination of other items. Hand hygiene prevents the spread of microorganisms.

EVALUATION

• The expected outcomes are met when the patient's apical pulse is assessed accurately without injury and the patient experiences minimal discomfort.

DOCUMENTATION

• Record pulse rate and rhythm on paper, flow sheet, or computerized record. Report abnormal findings to the appropriate person. Identify site of assessment.

SKILL 135 | ASSESSING A PERIPHERAL PULSE BY PALPATION

The pulse is a throbbing sensation that can be palpated over a peripheral artery, such as the radial artery or the carotid artery. Peripheral pulses result from a wave of blood being pumped into the arterial circulation by the contraction of the left ventricle. Each time the left ventricle contracts to eject blood into an already full aorta, the arterial walls in the cardiovascular system expand to compensate for the increase in pressure of the blood. Characteristics of the pulse, including rate, quality or amplitude, and rhythm provide information about the effectiveness of the heart as a pump and the adequacy of peripheral blood flow.

Pulse rates are measured in beats per minute. The normal pulse rate for adolescents and adults ranges from 60 to 100 beats per minute. Pulse quality (amplitude) describes the quality of the pulse in terms of its fullness—strong or weak. It is assessed by the feel of the blood flow through the vessel. Pulse rhythm is the pattern of the pulsations and the pauses between them. Pulse rhythm is normally regular; the pulsations and the pauses between occur at regular intervals. An irregular pulse rhythm occurs when the pulsations and pauses between beats occur at unequal intervals.

Assess the pulse by palpating peripheral arteries, by auscultating the apical pulse with a stethoscope, or by using a portable Doppler ultrasound (see Skill 136). To assess the pulse accurately, you need to know which site to choose and what method is most appropriate for the patient. Place your fingers over the artery so that the ends of your fingers are flat against the patient's skin when palpating peripheral pulses. Do not press with the tip of the fingers only.

DELEGATION CONSIDERATIONS

The assessment of the radial and brachial peripheral pulses may be delegated to nursing assistive personnel (NAP) or unlicensed assistive personnel (UAP). The assessment of peripheral pulses may be delegated to licensed practical/vocational nurses (LPN/LVNs). The decision to delegate must be based on careful analysis of the patient's needs and circumstances, as well as the qualifications of the person to whom the task is being delegated. Refer to the Delegation Guidelines in Appendix A.

EQUIPMENT

- Watch with second hand or digital readout
- Pencil or pen, paper or flow sheet, computerized record
- Nonsterile gloves, if appropriate; additional PPE, as indicated

ASSESSMENT

- Choose a site to assess the pulse. For an adult patient, adolescent, and older child, the most common site for obtaining a peripheral pulse is the radial pulse. Apical pulse measurement is the preferred method of pulse assessment for infants and children less than 2 years of age (Jarvis, 2012).
- Assess for factors that could affect pulse characteristics, such as the patient's age, amount of exercise, fluid balance, and medications. Note baseline or previous pulse measurements.

NURSING DIAGNOSIS

- Decreased Cardiac Output
- Ineffective Peripheral Tissue Perfusion
- Acute Pain

OUTCOME IDENTIFICATION AND PLANNING

- Patient's pulse is assessed accurately without injury.
- Patient experiences minimal discomfort.

ACTION	RATIONALE
3. Identify the patient.	Identifying the patient ensures the right patient receives the intervention and helps prevent errors.
4. Close the curtains around the bed and close the door to the room, if possible. Discuss the procedure with the patient and assess the patient's ability to assist with the procedure.	This ensures the patient's privacy. Explanation relieves anxiety and facilitates cooperation.
5. Put on gloves, if indicated.	Gloves are not usually worn to obtain a pulse measurement unless contact with blood or body fluids is anticipated. Gloves prevent contact with blood and body fluids.
6. Select the appropriate peripheral site based on assessment data.	Ensures safety and accuracy of measurement.
7. Move the patient's clothing to expose only the site chosen.	The site must be exposed for pulse assessment. Exposing only the site keeps the patient warm and maintains his or her dignity.
8. Place your first, second, and third fingers over the artery (Figure 1). **Lightly compress the artery so pulsations can be felt and counted.**	The sensitive fingertips can feel the pulsation of the artery.

FIGURE 1 Palpating the radial pulse.

ACTION	RATIONALE
9. Using a watch with a second hand, count the number of pulsations felt for 30 seconds. Multiply this number by 2 to calculate the rate for 1 minute.	Ensures accuracy of measurement and assessment.

ACTION	RATIONALE
If the rate, rhythm, or amplitude of the pulse is abnormal in any way, palpate and count the pulse for 1 minute.	
10. Note the rhythm and amplitude of the pulse.	Provides additional assessment data regarding the patient's cardiovascular status.
11. When measurement is completed, remove gloves, if worn. Cover the patient and help him or her to a position of comfort.	Removing PPE properly reduces the risk for infection transmission and contamination of other items. Ensures patient comfort.
12. Remove additional PPE, if used. Perform hand hygiene.	Removing PPE properly reduces the risk for infection transmission and contamination of other items. Hand hygiene prevents the spread of microorganisms.

EVALUATION

- Patient's pulse is assessed accurately without injury.
- Patient experiences minimal discomfort.

DOCUMENTATION

- Record pulse rate, amplitude, and rhythm on paper, flow sheet, or computerized record. Identify site of assessment. Report abnormal findings to the primary care provider.

SKILL 136 | ASSESSING PERIPHERAL PULSE USING A PORTABLE DOPPLER ULTRASOUND

Pulse rates are measured in beats per minute. The normal pulse rate for adolescents and adults ranges from 60 to 100 beats per minute. Pulse rhythm is the pattern of the pulsations and the pauses between them. Pulse rhythm is normally regular; the pulsations and the pauses between occur at regular intervals. An irregular pulse rhythm occurs when the pulsations and pauses between beats occur at unequal intervals.

Assess the pulse by palpating peripheral arteries (Skill 135), by auscultating the apical pulse with a stethoscope, or by using a portable Doppler ultrasound. An ultrasound or Doppler device amplifies sound. It is especially useful if the pulse is weak, or to assess the circulatory status of a surgical or injury site. Doppler ultrasound is used to assess peripheral pulses. To assess the pulse accurately, you need to know which site to choose and what method is most appropriate for the patient.

DELEGATION CONSIDERATIONS

The assessment of the radial and brachial peripheral pulses may be delegated to nursing assistive personnel (NAP) or to unlicensed assistive personnel (UAP). The assessment of peripheral pulses may be delegated to licensed practical/vocational nurses (LPN/LVNs). The decision to delegate must be based on careful analysis of the patient's needs and circumstances, as well as the qualifications of the person to whom the task is being delegated. Refer to the Delegation Guidelines in Appendix A.

EQUIPMENT

- Watch with second hand or digital readout
- Portable Doppler Ultrasound
- Conducting gel
- Pencil or pen, paper or flow sheet, computerized record
- Nonsterile gloves, if appropriate; additional PPE, as indicated

ASSESSMENT

- Choose a site to assess the pulse. For an adult patient, adolescent, and older child, the most common site for obtaining a peripheral pulse is the radial pulse. Apical pulse measurement is the preferred method of pulse assessment for infants and children less than 2 years of age (Jarvis, 2012). The site may be determined by other patient health problems, such as recent arteriovenous surgery or injury.
- Assess for factors that could affect pulse characteristics, such as the patient's age, amount of exercise, fluid balance, and medications. Note baseline or previous pulse measurements.

NURSING DIAGNOSIS

- Decreased Cardiac Output
- Ineffective Peripheral Tissue Perfusion
- Acute Pain

OUTCOME IDENTIFICATION AND PLANNING

- Patient's pulse is assessed accurately without injury.
- Patient experiences minimal discomfort.

IMPLEMENTATION

ACTION	RATIONALE
1. Check medical order or nursing care plan for frequency	Assessment and measurement of vital signs at appropriate

ACTION	RATIONALE
of pulse assessment. More frequent pulse measurement may be appropriate based on nursing judgment. Determine the need to use a Doppler ultrasound device for pulse assessment.	intervals provide important data about the patient's health status.
2. Bring necessary equipment to the bedside stand or overbed table.	Provides an organized approach.
3. Perform hand hygiene and put on PPE, if indicated.	Hand hygiene and PPE prevent the spread of microorganisms. PPE is required based on transmission precautions.
4. Identify the patient.	Identifying the patient ensures the right patient receives the intervention and helps prevent errors.
5. Close the curtains around the bed and close the door to the room, if possible. Discuss the procedure with the patient and assess the patient's ability to assist with the procedure.	This ensures the patient's privacy. Explanation relieves anxiety and facilitates cooperation.
6. Put on gloves, if indicated.	Gloves are not usually worn to obtain a pulse measurement unless contact with blood or body fluids is anticipated. Gloves prevent contact with blood and body fluids.
7. Select the appropriate peripheral site based on assessment data.	Ensures safety and accuracy of measurement.
8. Move the patient's clothing to expose only the site chosen.	The site must be exposed for pulse assessment. Exposing only the site keeps the patient warm and maintains his or her dignity.
9. Remove Doppler from charger and turn it on. Make sure that volume is set at low.	Removing from charger and turning on prepare the device for use. Low volume setting prevents unnecessary loud noise.

ACTION	RATIONALE
10. Apply conducting gel to the site where you are auscultating the pulse.	Conducting gel facilitates transmission of sound from artery to Doppler.
11. Hold the Doppler base in your nondominant hand. With your dominant hand, place the Doppler probe tip in the gel. Adjust the volume, as needed. Move the Doppler tip around until the pulse is heard (Figure 1). **Using a watch with a second hand, count the heartbeat for 1 minute.**	Locates arterial pulse for reading. Ensures accuracy of measurement and assessment.

FIGURE 1 Moving the Doppler tip until pulse is heard.

ACTION	RATIONALE
12. Note the rhythm of the pulse.	Provides additional assessment data regarding patient's cardiovascular status.
13. Remove the Doppler tip and turn the Doppler off. Wipe excess gel off of the patient's skin with a tissue. Place a small X over the spot where the pulse is located with an indelible pen, depending on facility policy.	Removing gel from the patient's skin promotes patient comfort. Marking the site allows for easier future assessment. It can also make palpating the pulse easier since the exact location of the pulse is known.
14. Wipe any gel remaining on the Doppler probe off with a tissue. Clean the Doppler probe per facility policy or manufacturer's recommendations.	Appropriate cleaning deters the spread of microorganisms. Equipment should be left ready for use.
15. Remove gloves, if worn. Cover the patient and help him or her to a position of comfort.	Removing PPE properly reduces the risk for infection transmission and contamination of other items. Ensures patient comfort.

ACTION	RATIONALE
16. Remove additional PPE, if used. Perform hand hygiene.	Removing PPE properly reduces the risk for infection transmission and contamination of other items. Hand hygiene prevents the spread of microorganisms.
17. Return Doppler ultrasound device to the charge base.	Equipment should be left ready for use.
18. Record pulse rate, rhythm, and site, and that it was obtained with a Doppler ultrasound device.	

EVALUATION

- Patient's pulse is assessed accurately without injury.
- Patient experiences minimal discomfort.

DOCUMENTATION

- Record pulse rate and rhythm on paper, flow sheet, or computerized record. Identify assessment site and that it was obtained with a Doppler. Report abnormal findings to the primary care provider.

SKILL 137 USING A PULSE OXIMETER

Pulse oximetry is a noninvasive technique that measures the arterial oxyhemoglobin saturation (SaO_2 or SpO_2) of arterial blood. The reported result is a ratio, expressed as a percentage, between the actual oxygen content of the hemoglobin and the potential maximum oxygen-carrying capacity of the hemoglobin (Van Leeuwen et al., 2011). A sensor, or probe, uses a beam of red and infrared light that travels through tissue and blood vessels. One part of the sensor emits the light and another part receives the light. The oximeter then calculates the amount of light that has been absorbed by arterial blood. Oxygen saturation is determined by the amount of each light absorbed; nonoxygenated hemoglobin absorbs more red light and oxygenated hemoglobin absorbs more infrared light.

Sensors are available for use on a finger, a toe, a foot (infants), an earlobe, forehead, and the bridge of the nose. It is important to use the appropriate sensor for the intended site; use of a sensor on a site other than what it is intended can result in inaccurate or unreliable readings (Johnson et al., 2012). Circulation to the sensor site must be adequate to ensure accurate readings. Pulse oximeters also display a measured pulse rate.

It is important to know the patient's hemoglobin level before evaluating oxygen saturation because the test measures only the percentage of oxygen carried by the available hemoglobin. Thus, even a patient with a low hemoglobin level could appear to have a normal SpO_2 because most of that hemoglobin is saturated. However, the patient may not have enough oxygen to meet body needs. Also, take into consideration the presence of preexisting health conditions, such as COPD. Parameters for acceptable oxygen saturation readings may be different for these patients. Be aware of any medical orders regarding acceptable ranges and/or check with the patient's physician. A range of 95% to 100% is considered normal SpO_2. Values ≤90% are abnormal, indicating that oxygenation to the tissues is inadequate. It is important to investigate these low values for potential hypoxia or technical error.

Pulse oximetry is useful for monitoring patients receiving oxygen therapy, titrating oxygen therapy, monitoring those at risk for hypoxia, monitoring those at risk of hypoventilation (opioids use, neurologic compromise), and postoperative patients. Pulse oximetry does not replace arterial blood gas analysis. Desaturation (decreased level of SpO_2) indicates gas exchange abnormalities. Oxygen desaturation is considered a late sign of respiratory compromise in patients with reduced rate and depth of breathing (Johnson et al., 2011).

DELEGATION CONSIDERATIONS

The measurement of oxygen saturation using a pulse oximeter may be delegated to nursing assistive personnel (NAP) or to unlicensed assistive personnel (UAP), as well as to licensed practical/vocational nurses (LPN/LVNs). The decision to delegate must be based on careful analysis of the patient's needs and circumstances, as well as the qualifications of the person to whom the task is being delegated. Refer to the Delegation Guidelines in Appendix A.

EQUIPMENT

- Pulse oximeter with an appropriate sensor or probe
- Alcohol wipe(s) or disposable cleansing cloth
- Nail polish remover (if necessary)
- PPE, as indicated

ASSESSMENT

- Assess the patient's skin temperature and color, including the color of the nail beds. Temperature is a good indicator of blood flow. Warm skin indicates adequate circulation. In a well-oxygenated patient, the skin and nail beds are usually pink. Skin that is bluish or dusky indicates hypoxia (inadequate amount of oxygen available to the cells). Check capillary refill; prolonged capillary refill indicates a reduction in blood flow. Assess the quality of the pulse proximal to the sensor application site. Assess for edema of the sensor site. Avoid placing a sensor on edematous tissue; the presence of edema can interfere with readings.

- Auscultate the lungs. Note the amount of oxygen and delivery method if the patient is receiving supplemental oxygen.

NURSING DIAGNOSIS
- Impaired Gas Exchange
- Ineffective Airway Clearance
- Activity Intolerance

OUTCOME IDENTIFICATION AND PLANNING
- Patient will exhibit oxygen saturation within acceptable parameters, or greater than 95%.

IMPLEMENTATION

ACTION	RATIONALE
1. Review health record for any health problems that would affect the patient's oxygenation status.	Identifying influencing factors aids in interpretation of results.
2. Bring necessary equipment to the bedside stand or overbed table.	Bringing everything to the bedside conserves time and energy. Arranging items nearby is convenient, saves time, and avoids unnecessary stretching and twisting of muscles on the part of the nurse.
3. Perform hand hygiene and put on PPE, if indicated.	Hand hygiene and PPE prevent the spread of microorganisms. PPE is required based on transmission precautions.
4. Identify the patient.	Identifying the patient ensures the right patient receives the intervention and helps prevent errors.
5. Close the curtains around the bed and close the door to the room, if possible. Explain what you are going to do and why you are going to do it to the patient.	This ensures the patient's privacy. Explanation relieves anxiety and facilitates cooperation.
6. Select an adequate site for application of the sensor.	Inadequate circulation can interfere with the oxygen saturation (SpO_2) reading.

ACTION	RATIONALE
a. Use the patient's index, middle, or ring finger.	Fingers are easily accessible.
b. Check the proximal pulse and capillary refill at the pulse closest to the site.	Brisk capillary refill and a strong pulse indicate adequate circulation to the site.
c. If circulation to the site is inadequate, consider using the earlobe, forehead, or bridge of nose. Use the appropriate oximetry sensor for the chosen site.	These alternate sites are highly vascular alternatives. Correct use of appropriate equipment is vital for accurate results. The appropriate ear oximetry sensor should be used to obtain measurements from a patient's ear. The use of a finger sensor should be limited to use on the finger (Johnson et al., 2012).
d. Use a toe only if lower extremity circulation is not compromised.	Peripheral vascular disease is common in lower extremities.
7. Select proper equipment:	
a. If one finger is too large for the probe, use a smaller finger.	Inaccurate readings can result if probe or sensor is not attached correctly.
b. Use probes appropriate for patient's age and size. Use a pediatric probe for a small adult, if necessary.	Probes come in adult, pediatric, and infant sizes.
c. Check if patient is allergic to adhesive. A nonadhesive finger clip or reflectance sensor is available.	A reaction may occur if the patient is allergic to an adhesive substance.
8. Prepare the monitoring site. Cleanse the selected area with the alcohol wipe or disposable cleansing cloth. Allow the area to dry. If necessary, remove nail polish and artificial nails after checking pulse oximeter's manufacturer's instructions.	Skin oils, dirt, or grime on the site can interfere with the passage of light waves. Research is conflicting regarding the effect of dark color nail polish and artificial nails. It is prudent to remove nail polish (Hess et al., 2012). Refer to facility policy and pulse oximeter's manufacturer's instructions regarding nail polish and artificial nails for additional information (Collins & Andersen, 2007; DeMeulenaere, 2007).

ACTION	RATIONALE
9. **Attach probe securely to skin. Make sure that the light-emitting sensor and the light-receiving sensor are aligned opposite each other (not necessary to check if placed on forehead or bridge of nose).**	Secure attachment and proper alignment promote satisfactory operation of the equipment and accurate recording of the SpO_2.
10. Connect the sensor probe to the pulse oximeter, turn the oximeter on, and check operation of the equipment (audible beep, fluctuation of bar of light or waveform on face of oximeter).	Audible beep represents the arterial pulse, and fluctuating waveform or light bar indicates the strength of the pulse. A weak signal will produce an inaccurate recording of the SpO_2. Tone of beep reflects SpO_2 reading. If SpO_2 drops, tone becomes lower in pitch.
11. Set alarms on pulse oximeter. Check manufacturer's alarm limits for high and low pulse rate.	Alarm provides additional safeguard and signals when high or low limits have been surpassed.
12. Check oxygen saturation at regular intervals, as ordered by primary care provider, nursing assessment, and signaled by alarms. Monitor hemoglobin level.	Monitoring SpO_2 provides ongoing assessment of patient's condition. A low hemoglobin level may be satisfactorily saturated yet inadequate to meet a patient's oxygen needs.
13. Remove sensor on a regular basis and check for skin irritation or signs of pressure (every 2 hours for spring-tension sensor or every 4 hours for adhesive finger or toe sensor).	Prolonged pressure may lead to tissue necrosis. Adhesive sensor may cause skin irritation.
14. Clean nondisposable sensors according to the manufacturer's directions. Remove PPE, if used. Perform hand hygiene.	Cleaning equipment between patient use reduces the spread of microorganisms. Removing PPE properly reduces the risk for infection transmission and contamination of other items. Hand hygiene prevents the spread of microorganisms.

EVALUATION

- Patient exhibits an oxygen saturation level within acceptable parameters, or greater than 95%, and a heart rate that correlates with the pulse measurement.

DOCUMENTATION

- Documentation should include the type of sensor and location used; assessment of the proximal pulse and capillary refill; pulse oximeter reading; the amount of oxygen and delivery method if the patient is receiving supplemental oxygen; lung assessment, if relevant; and any other relevant interventions required as a result of the reading.

SKILL 138 PROVIDING RANGE-OF-MOTION EXERCISES

Range of motion (ROM) is the complete extent of movement of which a joint is normally capable. When a person performs routine activities of daily living (ADLs), he or she is using muscle groups that help to keep many joints in an effective range of motion. When all or some of the normal ADLs are impossible due to illness or injury, it is important to give attention to the joints not being used or to those that have limited use. When the patient does the exercise for him- or herself, it is referred to as *active range of motion*. Exercises performed by the nurse without participation by the patient are referred to as *passive range of motion*. Exercises should be as active as the patient's physical condition permits. Allow the patient to do as much individual activity as his or her condition permits. Initiate ROM exercises as soon as possible because body changes can occur after only 3 days of impaired mobility.

DELEGATION CONSIDERATIONS

Patient teaching regarding range-of-motion exercises cannot be delegated to nursing assistive personnel (NAP) or to unlicensed assistive personnel (UAP). Reinforcement or implementation of ROM exercises may be delegated to NAP or UAP, as well as to licensed practical/vocational nurses (LPN/LVNs). The decision to delegate must be based on careful analysis of the patient's needs and circumstances, as well as the qualifications of the person to whom the task is being delegated. Refer to the Delegation Guidelines in Appendix A.

EQUIPMENT

No special equipment or supplies are necessary to perform ROM exercises. Wear nonsterile gloves and/or other PPE, as appropriate.

ASSESSMENT

- Review the medical record and nursing plan of care for any conditions or orders that will limit mobility.
- Perform a pain assessment before the time for the exercises. If the patient reports pain, administer the prescribed medication in sufficient time to allow for the full effect of the analgesic.
- Assess the patient's ability to perform ROM exercises.
- Inspect and palpate joints for redness, tenderness, pain, swelling, or deformities.

NURSING DIAGNOSIS

- Impaired Physical Mobility
- Fatigue
- Deficient Knowledge

OUTCOME IDENTIFICATION AND PLANNING

- Patient maintains joint mobility.
- Patient improves or maintains muscle strength.
- Prevention of muscle atrophy and contractures.

ACTION	RATIONALE
caregiver (VISN 8 Patient Safety Center, 2009). Adjust the head of the bed to a flat position or as low as the patient can tolerate.	
5. Stand on the side of the bed where the joints are to be exercised. Lower side rail on that side, if in place. Uncover only the limb to be used during the exercise.	Standing on the side to be exercised and lowering the side rail prevent strain on the nurse's back. Proper draping provides for privacy and warmth.
6. Perform the exercises slowly and gently, providing support by holding the areas proximal and distal to the joint. Repeat each exercise two to five times, moving each joint in a smooth and rhythmic manner. **Stop movement if the patient complains of pain or if you meet resistance.**	Slow, gentle movements with support prevent discomfort and muscle spasms resulting from jerky movements. Repeated movement of muscles and joints improves flexibility and increases circulation to the body part. Pain may indicate the exercises are causing damage.
7. While performing the exercises, begin at the head and move down one side of the body at a time. **Encourage the patient to do as many of these exercises independently as possible.**	Proceeding from head to toe one side at a time promotes efficient time management and an organized approach to the task. Both active and passive exercises improve joint mobility and increase circulation to the affected part, but only active exercise increases muscle mass, tone, and strength and improves cardiac and respiratory functioning.
8. Move the chin down to rest on the chest. Return the head to a normal upright position. Tilt the head as far as possible toward each shoulder.	These movements provide for flexion, extension, and lateral flexion of the head and neck.
9. Move the head from side to side, bringing the chin toward each shoulder.	These movements provide for rotation of neck.
10. Start with the arm at the patient's side and lift the arm forward to above the head.	These movements provide for flexion and extension of the shoulder.

ACTION	RATIONALE
Return the arm to the starting position at the side of the body.	
11. With the arm back at the patient's side, move the arm laterally to an upright position above the head, and then return it to the original position. Move the arm across the body as far as possible.	These movements provide for abduction and adduction of the shoulder.
12. Raise the arm at the side until the upper arm is in line with the shoulder. Bend the elbow at a 90-degree angle and move the forearm upward and downward, then return the arm to the side.	These movements provide for internal and external rotation of the shoulder.
13. Bend the elbow and move the lower arm and hand upward toward the shoulder. Return the lower arm and hand to the original position while straightening the elbow.	These movements provide for flexion and extension of the elbow.
14. Rotate the lower arm and hand so the palm is up. Rotate the lower arm and hand so the palm of the hand is down.	These movements provide for supination and pronation of the forearm.
15. Move the hand downward toward the inner aspect of the forearm. Return the hand to a neutral position even with the forearm. Then move the dorsal portion of the hand backward as far as possible.	These movements provide for flexion, extension, and hyperextension of the wrist.
16. Bend the fingers to make a fist, and then straighten them out. Spread the fingers apart and return them back together. Touch the thumb to each finger on the hand.	These movements provide for flexion, extension, abduction, and adduction of the fingers.

ACTION	RATIONALE
17. Extend the leg and lift it upward. Return the leg to the original position beside the other leg.	These movements provide for flexion and extension of the hip.
18. Lift the leg laterally away from the patient's body. Return the leg back toward the other leg and try to extend it beyond the midline.	These movements provide for abduction and adduction of the hip.
19. Turn the foot and leg toward the opposite leg to rotate it internally. Turn the foot and leg outward away from the opposite leg to rotate it externally.	These movements provide for internal and external rotation of the hip.
20. Bend the leg and bring the heel toward the back of the leg. Return the leg to a straight position.	These movements provide for flexion and extension of the knee.
21. At the ankle, move the foot up and back until the toes are upright. Move the foot with the toes pointing downward.	These movements provide for dorsiflexion and plantar flexion of the ankle.
22. Turn the sole of the foot toward the midline. Turn the sole of the foot outward.	These movements provide for inversion and eversion of the ankle.
23. Curl the toes downward, and then straighten them out. Spread the toes apart and bring them together.	These movements provide for flexion, extension, abduction, and adduction of the toes.
24. Repeat these exercises on the other side of the body. Encourage the patient to do as many of these exercises independently as possible.	Repeating motions on the other side provides exercise for the entire body. Self-esteem, self-care, and independence are encouraged through the patient performing the exercises on his or her own.
25. When finished, make sure the patient is comfortable, with the side rails up and the bed in the lowest position. Place call bell and other essential items within reach.	Proper positioning with raised side rails and proper bed height provides for patient comfort and safety. Having the call bell and other essential items within reach promotes safety.

ACTION	RATIONALE
26. Remove gloves and any other PPE, if used. Perform hand hygiene.	Removing PPE properly reduces the risk for infection transmission and contamination of other items. Hand hygiene prevents the spread of micro-organisms.

EVALUATION

• Patient maintains or improves joint mobility and muscle strength, and muscle atrophy and contractures are prevented.

DOCUMENTATION

• Document the exercises performed, any significant observations, and the patient's reaction to the activities.

SKILL 139 ADMINISTERING A RECTAL SUPPOSITORY

Rectal suppositories are used primarily for their local action, such as laxatives and fecal softeners. Systemic effects are also achieved with rectal suppositories. It is important to ensure the suppository is placed past the internal anal sphincter and against the rectal mucosa.

DELEGATION CONSIDERATIONS

The administration of medication as a rectal suppository is not delegated to nursing assistive personnel (NAP) or to unlicensed assistive personnel (UAP). Depending on the state's nurse practice act and the organization's policies and procedures, administration of a vaginal cream may be delegated to licensed practical/vocational nurses (LPN/LVNs). The decision to delegate must be based on careful analysis of the patient's needs and circumstances, as well as the qualifications of the person to whom the task is being delegated. Refer to the Delegation Guidelines in Appendix A.

EQUIPMENT

• Suppository (rectal)
• Water-soluble lubricant
• Non-latex, disposable gloves
• Computer-generated Medica-tion Administration Record

(CMAR) or Medication Administration Record (MAR)
• Additional PPE, as indicated

ASSESSMENT

- Assess the rectal area for any alterations in integrity. Do not administer suppositories to patients who have had recent rectal or prostate surgery.
- Assess recent laboratory values, particularly the patient's white blood cell and platelet counts. Patients who are thrombocytopenic or neutropenic should not receive rectal suppositories.
- Do not administer rectal suppositories to patients at risk for cardiac arrhythmias.
- Assess relevant body systems for the particular medication being administered.
- Assess the patient for allergies.
- Verify patient name, dose, route, and time of administration.
- Assess the patient's knowledge of the medication and procedure. If the patient has a knowledge deficit about the medication, this may be an appropriate time to begin education about the medication.
- Assess the patient's ability to cooperate with the procedure.

NURSING DIAGNOSIS

- Anxiety
- Risk for Injury
- Constipation

OUTCOME IDENTIFICATION AND PLANNING

- Medication is administered successfully into the rectum.
- Patient understands the rationale for the rectal instillation.
- Patient experiences no allergy response.
- Patient's mucosa and skin remain intact.
- Patient experiences no, or minimal, pain.
- Patient experiences minimal anxiety.

IMPLEMENTATION

ACTION	RATIONALE
1. Gather equipment. Check medication order against the original order in the medical record, according to facility policy. Clarify any inconsistencies. Check the patient's chart for allergies.	This comparison helps to identify errors that may have occurred when orders were transcribed. The primary care provider's order is the legal record of medication orders for each facility.
2. Know the actions, special nursing considerations, safe dose ranges, purpose of administration, and adverse	This knowledge aids the nurse in evaluating the therapeutic effect of the medication in relation to the patient's disorder and

ACTION	RATIONALE

effects of the medication to be administered. Consider the appropriateness of the medication for this patient.

3. Perform hand hygiene.

Hand hygiene prevents the spread of microorganisms.

4. Move the medication cart to the outside of the patient's room or prepare for administration in the medication area.

Organization facilitates error-free administration and saves time.

5. Unlock the medication cart or drawer. Enter pass code and scan employee identification, if required.

Locking the cart or drawer safeguards each patient's medication supply. Hospital accrediting organizations require medication carts to be locked when not in use. Entering pass code and scanning ID allows only authorized users into the system and identifies the user for documentation by the computer.

6. **Prepare medications for one patient at a time.**

This prevents errors in medication administration.

7. Read the CMAR/MAR and select the proper medication from unit stock or the patient's medication drawer.

This is the *first* check of the label.

8. Compare the label with the CMAR/MAR. Check expiration dates and perform calculations, if necessary. Scan the bar code on the package, if required.

This is the *second* check of the label. Verify calculations with another nurse to ensure safety, if necessary.

9. **Depending on facility policy, the third check of the label may occur at this point. If so, when all medications for one patient have been prepared, recheck the labels with the CMAR/ MAR before taking the medications to the patient.**

This *third* check ensures accuracy and helps to prevent errors. *Note:* Many facilities require the *third* check to occur at the bedside, after identifying the patient and before administration.

ACTION	RATIONALE
10. Lock the medication cart before leaving it.	Locking the cart or drawer safeguards the patient's medication supply. Hospital accrediting organizations require medication carts to be locked when not in use.
11. Transport medications to the patient's bedside carefully, and keep the medications in sight at all times.	Careful handling and close observation prevent accidental or deliberate disarrangement of medications.
12. **Ensure that the patient receives the medications at the correct time.**	Check agency policy, which may allow for administration within a period of 30 minutes before or 30 minutes after the designated time.
13. Perform hand hygiene and put on PPE, if indicated.	Hand hygiene and PPE prevent the spread of microorganisms. PPE is required based on transmission precautions.
14. **Identify the patient. Compare the information with the CMAR/MAR. The patient should be identified using at least two methods** (The Joint Commission, 2013):	Identifying the patient ensures the right patient receives the medications and helps prevent errors. The patient's room number or physical location is not used as an identifier (The Joint Commission, 2013). Replace the identification band if it is missing or inaccurate in any way.
a. Check the name on the patient's identification band.	
b. Check the identification number on the patient's identification band.	
c. Check the birth date on the patient's identification band.	
d. Ask the patient to state his or her name and birth date, based on facility policy.	This requires a response from the patient, but illness and strange surroundings often cause patients to be confused.

ACTION	RATIONALE
15. **Complete necessary assessments before administering medications. Check the patient's allergy bracelet or ask the patient about allergies. Explain the purpose and action of each medication to the patient.**	Assessment is a prerequisite to administration of medications.
16. Scan the patient's bar code on the identification band, if required.	Provides an additional check to ensure that the medication is given to the right patient.
17. **Based on facility policy, the third check of the label may occur at this point. If so, recheck the labels with the CMAR/MAR before administering the medications to the patient.**	Many facilities require the *third* check to occur at the bedside, after identifying the patient and before administration. If facility policy directs the *third* check at this time, this *third* check ensures accuracy and helps to prevent errors.
18. Put on gloves.	Gloves protect the nurse from potential contact with contaminants and body fluids.
19. Assist the patient to his or her left side in a Sims' position. Drape accordingly to expose only the buttocks.	Sims' positioning allows for easy access to the anal area. Left side decreases chance of expulsion of the suppository. Proper draping maintains privacy.
20. Remove the suppository from its wrapper. Apply lubricant to the rounded end. Lubricate the index finger of your dominant hand.	Lubricant reduces friction on administration and increases patient comfort.
21. Separate the buttocks with your nondominant hand and instruct the patient to breathe slowly and deeply through his or her mouth while the suppository is being inserted.	Slow, deep breaths help to relax the anal sphincter and reduce discomfort.
22. Using your index finger, insert the suppository, round end first, along the rectal wall. Insert about 3 to 4 inches (adult).	Suppository must make contact with the rectal mucosa for absorption to occur.

ACTION	RATIONALE
23. Use toilet tissue to clean any stool or lubricant from around the anus. Release the buttocks. Encourage the patient to remain on his or her side for at least 5 minutes and retain the suppository for the appropriate amount of time for the specific medication.	Prevents skin irritation. Prevents accidental expulsion of suppository and ensures absorption of the medication.
24. Remove additional PPE, if used. Perform hand hygiene.	Removing PPE properly reduces the risk for infection transmission and contamination of other items. Hand hygiene prevents the spread of microorganisms.
25. Document the administration of the medication immediately after administration. See Documentation section below.	Timely documentation helps to ensure patient safety.
26. Evaluate the patient's response to the medication within an appropriate time frame.	The patient needs to be evaluated for therapeutic and adverse effects from the medication.

EVALUATION

- Medication is administered successfully into the rectum.
- Patient understood the rationale for the rectal instillation.
- Patient did not experience adverse effects.
- Patient's mucosa and skin remain intact.
- Patient experiences minimal anxiety.

DOCUMENTATION

- Document the administration of the medication immediately after administration, including date, time, dose, and route of administration on the CMAR/MAR or record using the required format. If using a bar-code system, medication administration is automatically recorded when the bar code is scanned. PRN medications require documentation of the reason for administration. Prompt recording avoids the possibility of accidentally repeating the administration of the drug. Document your assessments, and the patient's response to the treatment, if appropriate. If the drug was refused or omitted, record this in the appropriate area on the medication record and notify the primary care provider. This verifies the reason medication was omitted and ensures that the primary care provider is aware of the patient's condition.

SKILL 140 ASSESSING RESPIRATION

Under normal conditions, healthy adults breathe about 12 to 20 times per minute. Infants and children breathe more rapidly. The depth of respirations varies normally from shallow to deep. The rhythm of respirations is normally regular, with each inhalation/exhalation and the pauses between occurring at regular intervals. An irregular respiratory rhythm occurs when the inhalation/exhalation cycle and the pauses between occur at unequal intervals.

Assess respiratory rate, depth, and rhythm by inspection (observing and listening) or by listening with the stethoscope. Determine the rate by counting the number of breaths per minute. If respirations are very shallow and difficult to detect, observe the sternal notch, where respiration is more apparent. With an infant or young child, assess respirations before taking the temperature so that the child is not crying, which would alter the respiratory status.

Move immediately from the pulse assessment to counting the respiratory rate to avoid letting the patient know you are counting respirations. Patients should be unaware of the respiratory assessment because, if they are conscious of the procedure, they might alter their breathing patterns or rate.

DELEGATION CONSIDERATIONS

The assessment of respiration may be delegated to nursing assistive personnel (NAP) or to unlicensed assistive personnel (UAP), as well as to licensed practical/vocational nurses (LPN/LVNs). The decision to delegate must be based on careful analysis of the patient's needs and circumstances, as well as the qualifications of the person to whom the task is being delegated. Refer to the Delegation Guidelines in Appendix A.

EQUIPMENT

- Watch with second hand or digital readout
- Pencil or pen, paper or flow sheet, computerized record
- PPE, as indicated

ASSESSMENT

- Assess the patient for factors that could affect respirations, such as exercise, medications, smoking, chronic illness or conditions, neurologic injury, pain, and anxiety.
- Note baseline or previous respiratory measurements.
- Assess patient for any signs of respiratory distress, which include retractions, nasal flaring, grunting, orthopnea (breathing more easily in an upright position), or tachypnea (rapid respirations).

NURSING DIAGNOSIS

- Ineffective Breathing Pattern
- Impaired Gas Exchange

- Risk for Activity Intolerance
- Ineffective Airway Clearance

OUTCOME IDENTIFICATION AND PLANNING

- Patient's respirations are assessed accurately without injury.
- Patient experiences minimal discomfort.

IMPLEMENTATION

ACTION	RATIONALE
1. **While your fingers are still in place for the pulse measurement, after counting the pulse rate, observe the patient's respirations.**	The patient may alter the rate of respirations if he or she is aware they are being counted.
2. Note the rise and fall of the patient's chest.	A complete cycle of an inspiration and an expiration composes one respiration.
3. Using a watch with a second hand, count the number of respirations for 30 seconds. Multiply this number by 2 to calculate the respiratory rate per minute.	Sufficient time is necessary to observe the rate, depth, and other characteristics.
4. **If respirations are abnormal in any way, count the respirations for at least 1 full minute.**	Increased time allows the detection of unequal timing between respirations.
5. Note the depth and rhythm of the respirations.	Provides additional assessment data regarding the patient's respiratory status.
6. When measurement is completed, remove gloves, if worn. Cover the patient and help him or her to a position of comfort.	Removing gloves properly reduces the risk for infection transmission and contamination of other items. Ensures patient comfort.
7. Remove additional PPE, if used. Perform hand hygiene.	Removing PPE properly reduces the risk for infection transmission and contamination of other items. Hand hygiene deters the spread of microorganisms.

EVALUATION

- Patient's respirations are assessed accurately without injury.
- Patient experiences minimal discomfort.

DOCUMENTATION

- Document respiratory rate, depth, and rhythm on paper, flow sheet, or computerized record. Report any abnormal findings to the appropriate person.

SKILL 141 APPLYING AN ELBOW RESTRAINT

Elbow restraints are generally used on infants and children, but may be used with adults. They prevent the patient from bending the elbows and reaching incisions or therapeutic devices. The patient can move all joints and extremities except the elbow. **Restraints should be used only after less-restrictive methods have failed.** Refer to Skill 145. Ensure compliance with ordering, assessment, and maintenance procedures.

DELEGATION CONSIDERATIONS

After assessment of the patient by the RN, the application of an elbow restraint may be delegated to nursing assistive personnel (NAP) or unlicensed assistive personnel (UAP), as well as to licensed practical/vocational nurses (LPN/LVNs). The decision to delegate must be based on careful analysis of the patient's needs and circumstances, as well as the qualifications of the person to whom the task is being delegated. Refer to the Delegation Guidelines in Appendix A.

EQUIPMENT

- Elbow restraint
- Padding, as necessary
- PPE, as indicated

ASSESSMENT

- Assess the patient's physical condition and for the potential for injury to self or others. Assess the patient's behavior, including the presence of confusion, agitation, combativeness, and ability to understand and follow directions. A confused patient who might remove devices needed to sustain life is considered at risk for injury to self and may require the use of restraints.
- Evaluate the appropriateness of the least restrictive restraint device.
- Inspect the arm where the restraint will be applied. Baseline skin condition should be established for comparison at future assessments while the restraint is in place. Consider using another form of restraint if the restraint may cause further injury at the site.

Assess capillary refill and proximal pulses in the arm to which the restraint is to be applied. This helps to determine the circulation in the extremity before applying the restraint. The restraint should not interfere with circulation.

• Measure the distance from the patient's shoulder to wrist to determine the appropriate size of elbow restraint to apply.

NURSING DIAGNOSIS

• Risk for Injury
• Acute Confusion
• Risk for Impaired Skin Integrity

OUTCOME IDENTIFICATION AND PLANNING

• Patient is constrained by the restraint, remains free from injury, and the restraint does not interfere with therapeutic devices.
• Patient does not experience impaired skin integrity.
• Patient does not injure himself or herself due to the restraint.
• Patient and the patient's family demonstrate an understanding about the use of the restraint and its role in the patient's care.

IMPLEMENTATION

ACTION	RATIONALE
1. Determine need for restraints. Assess the patient's physical condition, behavior, and mental status.	Restraints should be used only as a last resort when alternative measures have failed and the patient is at increased risk for harming self or others.
2. Confirm agency policy for application of restraints. **Secure an order from the primary care provider, or validate that the order has been obtained within the required time frame.**	Policy protects the patient and the nurse and specifies guidelines for application as well as type of restraint and duration of use. **Each order for restraint or seclusion used for the management of violent or self-destructive behavior that jeopardizes the immediate physical safety of the patient, a staff member, or others may only be renewed in accordance with the following limits for up to a total of 24 hours: (A) 4 hours for adults 18 years of age or older; (B) 2 hours for children and adolescents 9 to 17 years of age; or (C) 1 hour for children**

ACTION	RATIONALE
	under 9 years of age. After 24 hours, before writing a new order for the use of restraint or seclusion for the management of violent or self-destructive behavior, a physician or other licensed independent practitioner who is responsible for the care of the patient must see and assess the patient (CMS, 2006).
3. Perform hand hygiene and put on PPE, if indicated.	Hand hygiene and PPE prevent the spread of microorganisms. PPE is required based on transmission precautions.
4. Identify the patient.	Identifying the patient ensures the right patient receives the intervention and helps prevent errors.
5. Explain the reason for use to the patient and family. Clarify how care will be given and how needs will be met. Explain that restraint is a temporary measure.	Explanation to patient and family may lessen confusion and anger and provide reassurance. A clearly stated agency policy on application of restraints should be available for patient and family to read. In a long-term care facility, the family must give consent before a restraint is applied.
6. Apply restraint according to manufacturer's directions:	Proper application prevents injury. Proper application ensures that there is no interference with patient's circulation.
a. Choose the correct size of the least restrictive type of device that allows the greatest possible degree of mobility.	This provides minimal restriction.
b. Pad bony prominences that may be affected by the restraint.	Padding helps prevent injury.

ACTION	RATIONALE
c. Spread elbow restraint out flat. Place middle of elbow restraint behind patient's elbow. **The restraint should not extend below the wrist or place pressure on the axilla.**	Elbow restraint should be placed in the middle of the arm to ensure that the patient cannot bend the elbow. Patient should be able to move the wrist. Pressure on the axilla may lead to skin impairment.
d. **Wrap restraint snugly around patient's arm, but make sure that two fingers can easily fit under the restraint.**	Wrapping snugly ensures that the patient will not be able to remove the device. Being able to insert two fingers helps to prevent impaired circulation and potential alterations in neurovascular status.
e. Secure Velcro straps around the restraint.	Velcro straps will hold the restraint in place and prevent removal of the restraint.
f. Apply the restraint to the opposite arm if the patient can move arm.	Bilateral elbow restraints are needed if the patient can move both arms.
g. Thread Velcro strap from one elbow restraint across the back and into the loop on the opposite elbow restraint.	Strap across the back prevents the patient from wiggling out of elbow restraints.
7. **Assess circulation to fingers and hand.**	Circulation should not be impaired by the elbow restraint.
8. Remove PPE, if used. Perform hand hygiene.	Removing PPE properly reduces the risk for infection transmission and contamination of other items. Hand hygiene prevents transmission of microorganisms.
9. Assess the patient at least every hour or according to facility policy. An assessment should include the placement of the restraint, neurovascular assessment, and skin integrity. Assess for signs of sensory deprivation, such as increased sleeping, daydreaming, anxiety, inconsolable crying, and panic.	Improperly applied restraints may cause alterations in circulation, skin tears, abrasions, or bruises. Decreased circulation may result in impaired skin integrity. Use of restraints may decrease environmental stimulation and result in sensory deprivation.

ACTION	RATIONALE
10. **Remove restraint at least every 2 hours or according to agency policy and patient need. Remove restraint at least every 2 hours for children ages 9 to 17 years and at least every 1 hour for children under age 9, or according to agency policy and patient need.** Perform ROM exercises.	Removal allows you to assess patient and reevaluate need for restraint. Allows interventions for toileting; provision of nutrition and liquids, and exercise; and change of position. Exercise increases circulation in restrained extremity.
11. Evaluate patient for continued need of restraint. Reapply restraint only if continued need is evident.	Continued need must be documented for reapplication.
12. Reassure patient at regular intervals. **Keep call bell within easy reach of patient.**	Reassurance demonstrates caring and provides opportunity for sensory situation as well as ongoing assessment and evaluation. Parent or child old enough to use call bell can use it to summon assistance quickly.

EVALUATION

- Restraint prevents injury to patient or others.
- Patient cannot bend the elbow.
- Skin integrity is maintained under the restraint.
- Patient and family demonstrate an understanding of the rationale for the elbow restraint.

DOCUMENTATION

- Document alternative measures attempted before applying restraint. Document patient assessment before application. Record patient and family education regarding restraint use and their understanding. Document family consent, if necessary, according to facility policy. Document reason for restraining patient, date and time of application, type of restraint, times when removed, and result and frequency of nursing assessment.

SKILL 142 | APPLYING AN EXTREMITY RESTRAINT

Cloth extremity restraints immobilize one or more extremities. They may be indicated after other measures have failed to prevent a patient from removing therapeutic devices, such as intravenous (IV) access devices, endotracheal tubes, oxygen, or other treatment interventions. **Restraints should be used only after less-restrictive methods have failed. Ensure compliance with ordering, assessment, and maintenance procedures.** Restraints can be applied to the hands, wrists, or ankles. Refer to Skill 145.

DELEGATION CONSIDERATIONS

After assessment of the patient by the RN, the application of an extremity restraint may be delegated to nursing assistive personnel (NAP) or unlicensed assistive personnel (UAP), as well as to licensed practical/vocational nurses (LPN/LVNs). The decision to delegate must be based on careful analysis of the patient's needs and circumstances, as well as the qualifications of the person to whom the task is being delegated. Refer to the Delegation Guidelines in Appendix A.

EQUIPMENT

- Appropriate cloth restraint for the extremity that is to be immobilized
- Padding, if necessary, for bony prominences
- PPE, as indicated

ASSESSMENT

- Assess both the patient's physical condition and the potential for injury to self or others. Assess the patient's behavior, including the presence of confusion, agitation, and combativeness, as well as the patient's ability to understand and follow directions. A confused patient who might remove devices needed to sustain life is considered at risk for injury to self and may require the use of restraints.
- Evaluate the appropriateness of the least restrictive restraint device. For example, if the patient has had a stroke and cannot move the left arm, a restraint may be needed only on the right arm.
- Inspect the extremity where the restraint will be applied. Establish baseline skin condition for comparison at future assessments while the restraint is in place. Consider using another form of restraint if the restraint may cause further injury at the site. Before application, assess for adequate circulation in the extremity to which the restraint is to be applied, including capillary refill and proximal pulses.

NURSING DIAGNOSIS

- Risk for Injury
- Risk for Impaired Skin Integrity
- Acute Confusion

OUTCOME IDENTIFICATION AND PLANNING

- Patient is constrained by the restraint, remains free from injury, and the restraint does not interfere with therapeutic devices.
- Patient does not experience impaired skin integrity.
- Patient does not injure himself or herself due to the restraints.
- Patient's family will demonstrate an understanding about the use of the restraint and their role in the patient's care.

ACTION	RATIONALE
3. Perform hand hygiene and put on PPE, if indicated.	Hand hygiene and PPE prevent the spread of microorganisms. PPE is required based on transmission precautions.
4. Identify the patient.	Identifying the patient ensures the right patient receives the intervention and helps prevent errors.
5. Explain the reason for restraint use to patient and family. Clarify how care will be given and how needs will be met. Explain that restraint is a temporary measure.	Explanation to patient and family may lessen confusion and anger and provide reassurance. A clearly stated agency policy on application of restraints should be available for patient and family to read. In a long-term care facility, the family must give consent before a restraint is applied.
6. Include the patient's family and/or significant others in the plan of care.	This promotes continuity of care and cooperation.
7. Apply restraint according to manufacturer's directions:	Proper application prevents injury.
a. Choose the least restrictive type of device that allows the greatest possible degree of mobility.	This provides minimal restriction.
b. Pad bony prominences.	Padding helps prevent skin injury.
c. Wrap the restraint around the extremity with the soft part in contact with the skin. If a hand mitt is being used, pull over the hand with cushion to the palmar aspect of hand.	This prevents excess pressure on the extremity.
8. Secure in place with the Velcro straps or other mechanism, depending on specific restraint device. Depending on characteristics of specific restraint, it may	Proper application secures restraint and ensures that there is no interference with patient's circulation and potential alteration in neurovascular status.

ACTION	RATIONALE

be necessary to tie a knot in the restraint ties, to ensure the restraint remains secure on the extremity.

9. **Ensure that two fingers can be inserted between the restraint and patient's extremity.**

Proper application ensures that nothing interferes with patient's circulation and potential alteration in neurovascular status.

10. Maintain restrained extremity in normal anatomic position. **Use a quick-release knot to tie the restraint to the bed frame, not side rail.** The restraint may also be attached to a chair frame. The site should not be readily accessible to the patient.

Maintaining a normal position lessens possibility of injury. A quick-release knot ensures that the restraint will not tighten when pulled and can be removed quickly in an emergency. Securing the restraint to a side rail may injure the patient when the side rail is lowered. Tying the restraint out of the patient's reach promotes security.

11. Remove PPE, if used. Perform hand hygiene.

Removing PPE properly reduces the risk for infection transmission and contamination of other items. Hand hygiene prevents transmission of microorganisms.

12. Assess the patient at least every hour or according to facility policy. Assessment should include the placement of the restraint, neurovascular assessment of the affected extremity, and skin integrity. In addition, assess for signs of sensory deprivation, such as increased sleeping, daydreaming, anxiety, panic, and hallucinations.

Improperly applied restraints may cause skin tears, abrasions, or bruises. Decreased circulation may result in paleness, coolness, decreased sensation, tingling, numbness, or pain in extremity. Use of restraints may decrease environmental stimulation and result in sensory deprivation.

13. **Remove restraint at least every 2 hours, or according to agency policy and patient need.** Perform range-of-motion (ROM) exercises.

Removal allows you to assess the patient and re-evaluate need for restraint. It also allows interventions for toileting, provision of nutrition and liquids, exercise, and change of position. Exercise increases circulation in the restrained extremity.

ACTION	RATIONALE
14. Evaluate patient for continued need of restraint. Reapply restraint only if continued need is evident and order is still valid.	Continued need must be documented for reapplication.
15. Reassure patient at regular intervals. Provide continued explanation of rationale for interventions, reorientation if necessary, and plan of care. **Keep call bell within patient's easy reach.**	Reassurance demonstrates caring and provides an opportunity for sensory stimulation as well as ongoing assessment and evaluation. Patient can use call bell to summon assistance quickly.

EVALUATION

- Patient remains free of injury to self or others.
- Circulation to extremity remains adequate.
- Skin integrity is not impaired under the restraint.
- Patient and family are aware of rationale for restraints.

DOCUMENTATION

- Document alternative measures attempted before applying restraint. Document patient assessment before application. Record patient and family education and understanding regarding restraint use. Document family consent, if necessary, according to facility policy. Document reason for restraining patient, date and time of application, type of restraint, times when removed, and result and frequency of nursing assessment.

SKILL 143 APPLYING A MUMMY RESTRAINT

A mummy restraint is appropriate for short-term restraint of an infant or small child to control the child's movements during examination or to provide care for the head and neck. **Restraints should be used only after less-restrictive methods have failed.** Refer to Skill 145. Ensure compliance with ordering, assessment, and maintenance procedures.

DELEGATION CONSIDERATIONS

After assessment of the patient by the RN, the application of a mummy restraint may be delegated to nursing assistive personnel (NAP) or unlicensed assistive personnel (UAP), as well as to licensed practical/vocational nurses (LPN/LVNs). The decision to delegate must be based on careful analysis of the patient's needs and circumstances, as well as the qualifications of the person to whom the task is being delegated. Refer to the Delegation Guidelines in Appendix A.

EQUIPMENT

- Small blanket or sheet
- PPE, as indicated

ASSESSMENT

- Assess patient's behavior and need for restraint.
- Assess for wounds or therapeutic devices that may be affected by the restraint.
- Evaluate the appropriateness of the least restrictive restraint device. Another form of restraint may be more appropriate to prevent injury.

NURSING DIAGNOSIS

- Risk for Injury
- Anxiety
- Impaired Physical Mobility

OUTCOME IDENTIFICATION AND PLANNING

- Patient is constrained by the restraint, remains free from injury, and the restraint does not interfere with therapeutic devices.
- Examination and/or treatment is provided without incident.
- Patient's family will demonstrate an understanding about the use of the restraint and its role in the patient's care.

ACTION	RATIONALE
	the patient, a staff member, or others may only be renewed in accordance with the following limits for up to a total of 24 hours: (A) 4 hours for adults 18 years of age or older; (B) 2 hours for children and adolescents 9 to 17 years of age; or (C) 1 hour for children under 9 years of age. After 24 hours, before writing a new order for the use of restraint or seclusion for the management of violent or self-destructive behavior, a physician or other licensed independent practitioner who is responsible for the care of the patient must see and assess the patient (CMS, 2006).
3. Perform hand hygiene and put on PPE, if indicated.	Hand hygiene and PPE prevent the spread of microorganisms. PPE is required based on transmission precautions.
4. Identify the patient.	Identifying the patient ensures the right patient receives the intervention and helps prevent errors.
5. Explain the reason for use to the patient and family. Clarify how care will be given and how needs will be met. Explain that restraint is a temporary measure.	Explanation to patient and family may lessen confusion and anger and provide reassurance. A clearly stated agency policy on application of restraints should be available for patient and family to read. In a long-term care facility, the family must give consent before a restraint is applied.
6. Open the blanket or sheet. Place the child on the blanket, with the edge of blanket at or above neck level.	This positions the child correctly on the blanket.

ACTION	RATIONALE
7. Position the child's right arm alongside the child's body. Left arm should not be constrained at this time. Pull the right side of the blanket tightly over the child's right shoulder and chest. Secure under the left side of the child's body (Figure 1).	Wrapping snugly ensures that child will not be able to wiggle out.
8. Position the left arm alongside the child's body. Pull the left side of the blanket tightly over the child's left shoulder and chest. Secure under the right side of the child's body (Figure 2).	Wrapping snugly ensures that child will not be able to wiggle out.

FIGURE 1 Pulling blanket over right shoulder and chest and securing under patient's left side.

FIGURE 2 Securing blanket under right side of body.

9. Fold the lower part of blanket up and pull over the child's body. Secure under the child's body on each side or with safety pins (Figure 3).	This ensures that child will not be able to wiggle out.

ACTION	RATIONALE

FIGURE 3 Securing lower corner of blanket under each side of patient's body.

ACTION	RATIONALE
10. Stay with the child while the mummy wrap is in place. Reassure the child and parents at regular intervals. Once examination or treatment is completed, unwrap the child.	Remaining with the child prevents injury. Reassurance demonstrates caring and provides opportunity for ongoing assessment and evaluation.
11. Remove PPE, if used. Perform hand hygiene.	Removing PPE properly reduces the risk for infection transmission and contamination of other items. Hand hygiene prevents transmission of microorganisms.

EVALUATION

• Restraint prevents injury to patient or others.
• Examination or treatment is provided without incident.
• The family demonstrate an understanding of the rationale for the mummy restraint.

DOCUMENTATION

• Document alternative measures attempted before applying restraint. Document patient assessment before application. Record patient and family education and understanding regarding restraint use. Document family consent, if necessary, according to facility policy. Document reason for restraining patient, date and time of application, type of restraint, times when removed, and result and frequency of nursing assessment.

Waist restraints are a form of restraint that is applied to the patient's torso. It is applied over the patient's clothes, gown, or pajamas. When using a waist restraint, patients can move their extremities, but cannot get out of the chair or bed. **Restraints should be used only after less-restrictive methods have failed. Refer to Skill 145. Ensure compliance with ordering, assessment, and maintenance procedures. Historically, vest or jacket restraints were used to prevent similar patient movement, but their use has significantly decreased due to concerns for the potential risk for asphyxiation with these devices. However, research suggests that waist restraints pose the same potential risk for asphyxial death as vest restraints (Capezuti et al., 2008).** Health care providers need to be aware of the potential outcome of using this device and weigh it against possible benefit from its use.

DELEGATION CONSIDERATIONS

After assessment of the patient by the RN, the application of a waist restraint may be delegated to nursing assistive personnel (NAP) or unlicensed assistive personnel (UAP), as well as to licensed practical/vocational nurses (LPN/LVNs). The decision to delegate must be based on careful analysis of the patient's needs and circumstances, as well as the qualifications of the person to whom the task is being delegated. Refer to the Delegation Guidelines in Appendix A.

EQUIPMENT

- Waist restraint
- Additional padding as needed
- PPE, as indicated

ASSESSMENT

- Assess the patient's physical condition and for the potential for injury to self or others. Assess the patient's behavior, including the presence of confusion, agitation, combativeness, and ability to understand and follow directions. A confused patient who is being treated with devices needed to sustain life, such as pulmonary intubation, might attempt to ambulate and is considered at risk for injury to self, and may require the use of restraints.
- Assess the patient's behavior, including the presence of confusion, agitation, combativeness, and ability to understand and follow directions.
- Evaluate the appropriateness of the least restrictive restraint device.
- Inspect patient's torso for any wounds or therapeutic devices that may be affected by the waist restraint. Consider using another form of restraint if the restraint may cause further injury at the site.
- Assess the patient's respiratory effort. If applied incorrectly, the waist restraint can restrict the patient's ability to breathe.

NURSING DIAGNOSIS

- Risk for Injury
- Wandering
- Acute Confusion

OUTCOME IDENTIFICATION AND PLANNING

- Patient is constrained by the restraint, remains free from injury, and the restraint does not interfere with therapeutic devices.
- Patient does not experience impaired skin integrity.
- Patient does not injure himself or herself due to the restraints.
- Patient and the patient's family demonstrate an understanding about the use of the restraint and its role in the patient's care.

IMPLEMENTATION

ACTION	RATIONALE
1. Determine need for restraints. Assess patient's physical condition, behavior, and mental status.	Restraints should be used only as a last resort when alternative measures have failed and the patient is at increased risk for harming self or others.
2. Confirm agency policy for application of restraints. **Secure an order from the primary care provider, or validate that the order has been obtained within the required time frame.**	Policy protects the patient and the nurse and specifies guidelines for application as well as type of restraint and duration. **Each order for restraint or seclusion used for the management of violent or self-destructive behavior that jeopardizes the immediate physical safety of the patient, a staff member, or others may only be renewed in accordance with the following limits for up to a total of 24 hours: (A) 4 hours for adults 18 years of age or older; (B) 2 hours for children and adolescents 9 to 17 years of age; or (C) 1 hour for children under 9 years of age. After 24 hours, before writing a new order for the use of restraint or seclusion for the management of violent or self-destructive behavior, a physician or other**

ACTION	RATIONALE
	licensed independent practitioner who is responsible for the care of the patient must see and assess the patient (CMS, 2006).
3. Perform hand hygiene and put on PPE, if indicated.	Hand hygiene and PPE prevent the spread of microorganisms. PPE is required based on transmission precautions.
4. Identify the patient.	Identifying the patient ensures the right patient receives the intervention and helps prevent errors.
5. Explain reason for use of restraint to patient and family. Clarify how care will be given and how needs will be met. Explain that restraint is a temporary measure.	Explanation to patient and family may lessen confusion and anger and provide reassurance. A clearly stated agency policy on application of restraints should be available for patient and family to read. In a long-term care facility, the family must give consent before a restraint is applied.
6. Include the patient's family and/or significant others in the plan of care.	This promotes continuity of care and cooperation.
7. Apply restraint according to manufacturer's directions:	Proper application prevents injury. Proper application ensures that there is no interference with patient's respiration.
a. Choose the correct size of the least restrictive type of device that allows the greatest possible degree of mobility.	This provides minimal restriction.
b. Pad bony prominences that may be affected by the waist restraint.	Padding helps prevent injury.
c. Assist patient to a sitting position, if not contraindicated.	This will assist you in helping the patient into the waist restraint.

ACTION	RATIONALE
d. Place waist restraint on patient over gown. Bring ties through slots in restraint. Position slots at patient's back.	Placing the waist restraint over the gown protects the patient's skin. Positioning the slots with the ties at the back keeps them out of the patient's vision.
e. Pull the ties secure. **Ensure that the restraint is not too tight and has no wrinkles.**	Securing too tightly could impede breathing. Wrinkles in the restraint may lead to skin impairment.
f. **Insert fist between restraint and patient to ensure that breathing is not constricted.** Assess respirations after restraint is applied.	This prevents impaired respirations.
8. **Use a quick-release knot to tie the restraint to the bed frame, not side rail.** If patient is in a wheelchair, lock the wheels and place the ties under the arm rests and tie behind the chair. Site should not be readily accessible to the patient.	A quick-release knot ensures that the restraint will not tighten when pulled and can be removed quickly in an emergency. Securing the restraint to a side rail may injure the patient when the side rail is lowered. Tying the restraint out of patient's reach promotes security.
9. Remove PPE, if used. Perform hand hygiene.	Removing PPE properly reduces the risk for infection transmission and contamination of other items. Hand hygiene prevents transmission of microorganisms.
10. Assess the patient at least every hour or according to facility policy. An assessment should include the placement of the restraint, respiration, and skin integrity. Assess for signs of sensory deprivation, such as increased sleeping, daydreaming, anxiety, panic, and hallucinations.	Improperly applied restraints may cause difficulty breathing, skin tears, abrasions, or bruises. Decreased circulation can result in impaired skin integrity. Use of restraints may decrease environmental stimulation and result in sensory deprivation.
11. **Remove restraint at least every 2 hours or according to agency policy and patient need.** Perform ROM exercises.	Removal allows you to assess patient and reevaluate need for restraint. Allows interventions for toileting, provision of nutrition and liquids, exercise, and

ACTION	RATIONALE
	change of position. Exercise increases circulation in restrained extremity.
12. Evaluate patient for continued need of restraint. Reapply restraint only if continued need is evident and order is still valid.	Continued need must be documented for reapplication.
13. Reassure patient at regular intervals. Provide continued explanation of rationale for interventions, reorientation if necessary, and plan of care. **Keep call bell within easy reach of patient.**	Reassurance demonstrates caring and provides an opportunity for sensory situation as well as ongoing assessment and evaluation. Patient can use call bell to summon assistance quickly.

EVALUATION

- Patient remains free of injury.
- Restraint prevents injury to the patient or others.
- Respirations are easy and effortless.
- Skin integrity is maintained under the restraint.
- Patient and family demonstrate understanding of the rationale for using the restraints.

DOCUMENTATION

- Document alternative measures attempted before applying restraint. Document patient assessment before application. Record patient and family education and understanding regarding restraint use. Document family consent, if necessary, according to facility policy. Document reason for restraining patient, date and time of application, type of restraint, times when removed, and result and frequency of nursing assessment.

Physical restraints increase the possibility of serious injury due to a fall. They do not prevent falls. The adverse health consequences associated with restraint use actually result in the need for additional staff because the condition of residents in long-term care facilities can deteriorate when restraints are employed. Additional negative outcomes of restraint use include skin breakdown and contractures, incontinence, depression, delirium, anxiety, aspiration and respiratory difficulties, and even death (Taylor et al., 2015). The following skill outlines possible alternatives to restraint use. Restraints should be used only after less-restrictive methods have failed.

DELEGATION CONSIDERATIONS

After assessment by the RN, activities related to the use of alternatives to restraints may be delegated to nursing assistive personnel (NAP) or unlicensed assistive personnel (UAP), as well as to licensed practical/vocational nurses (LPN/LVNs). The decision to delegate must be based on careful analysis of the patient's needs and circumstances, as well as the qualifications of the person to whom the task is being delegated. Refer to the Delegation Guidelines in Appendix A.

EQUIPMENT

- PPE, as indicated
- Additional intervention tools, as appropriate (refer to sample

intervention equipment in this skill)

ASSESSMENT

- Assess the patient's status. Determine whether the patient's pattern of behavior (wandering, fall risk, interfering with medical devices, resistive to care, danger to self or others) exists that increases the need for restraint use. Assess to determine the meaning of the behavior and its cause.
- Assess for pain. Assess respiratory status, vital signs, blood glucose level, fluid and electrolyte issues, and medications.
- Assess the patient's functional, mental, and psychological status.
- Evaluate the patient's environment, including noise level, lighting, floor surfaces, design/suitability of equipment and furniture, visual cues, barriers to mobility, space for privacy, and clothing.
- Assess and evaluate the effectiveness of restraint alternatives.

NURSING DIAGNOSIS

- Acute Confusion
- Risk for Injury
- Risk for Other-Directed Violence

OUTCOME IDENTIFICATION AND PLANNING

The expected outcomes may include:
- Use of restraints is avoided.
- Patient and others remain free from harm.

IMPLEMENTATION

ACTION	RATIONALE
1. Perform hand hygiene and put on PPE, if indicated.	Hand hygiene and PPE prevent the spread of microorganisms. PPE is required based on transmission precautions.
2. Identify the patient.	Identifying the patient ensures the right patient receives the intervention and helps prevent errors.
3. Explain the rationale for interventions to the patient and family/significant others.	Explanation helps reduce anxiety and promotes compliance and understanding.
4. Include the patient's family and/or significant others in the plan of care.	This promotes continuity of care and cooperation.
5. Identify behavior(s) that place the patient at risk for restraint use. Assess the patient's status and environment, as outlined above.	Behaviors such as interference with therapy or treatment, risk for falls, agitation/restlessness, resistance to care, wandering, and/or cognitive impairment put the patient at risk for restraint use. Assessment and interpretation of patient behavior identifies unmet physiologic or psychosocial needs, acute changes in mental or physical status, provides for appropriate environments and individualized care, and respects patient's needs and rights.
6. Identify triggers or contributing factors to patient behaviors. Evaluate medication usage for medications that can contribute to cognitive and movement dysfunction and to increased risk for falls.	Removal of contributing factors and/or triggers can decrease need for restraint use. Possible changes in prescribed medications can be addressed to decrease adverse effects and decrease the need for restraint use.

ACTION	RATIONALE
7. Assess the patient's functional, mental, and psychological status and the environment, as outlined above.	Assessment provides a better understanding of the reason for the behavior, leading to individualized interventions that can eliminate restraint use and provide for patient safety.
8. Provide adequate lighting. Use a night light during sleeping hours.	Appropriate lighting can reduce disruptive behavior related to fear in an unfamiliar environment.
9. Consult with primary care provider and other appropriate health care providers regarding the continued need for treatments/therapies and the use of the least invasive method to deliver care.	Exploring the possibility of administering treatment in a less intrusive manner or discontinuing treatment no longer needed can remove the stimulus for behavior that increases risk for use of restraints.
10. Assess the patient for pain and discomfort. Provide appropriate pharmacologic and nonpharmacologic interventions.	Unrelieved pain can contribute to behaviors that increase the risk for the use of restraints.
11. Ask a family member or significant other to stay with the patient.	Having someone stay with the patient provides companionship and familiarity.
12. Reduce unnecessary environmental stimulation and noise.	Increased stimulation can contribute to behaviors that increase the risk for use of restraints.
13. Provide simple, clear, and direct explanations for treatments and care. Repeat to reinforce as needed.	Explanation helps reduce anxiety and promotes compliance and understanding.
14. Distract and redirect using a calm voice.	Distraction and redirection can reduce or remove behaviors that increase risk for use of restraints.
15. Increase the frequency of patient observation and surveillance; 1- or 2-hour nursing rounds, including pain assessment, toileting assistance, patient comfort, keeping personal items in reach, and meeting patient needs.	Patient care rounds/nursing rounds improve identification of unmet needs, which can decrease behaviors that increase risk for use of restraints.

ACTION	RATIONALE
16. Implement fall precaution interventions. Refer to Skill 72.	Behaviors that increase risk for use of restraints also increase risk for falls.
17. Camouflage tube and other treatment sites with clothing, elastic sleeves, or bandaging.	Camouflaging tubes and other treatment sites removes stimulus that can trigger behaviors that increase risk for use of restraints.
18. Ensure the use of glasses and hearing aids, if necessary.	Glasses and hearing aids allow for correct interpretation of the environment and activities to reduce confusion.
19. Consider relocation to a room close to the nursing station.	Relocation close to the nursing station provides the opportunity for increased frequency of observation.
20. Encourage daily exercise/ provide exercise and activities or relaxation techniques.	Activity provides an outlet for energy and stimulation, decreasing behaviors associated with increased risk for use of restraints.
21. Make the environment as homelike as possible; provide familiar objects.	Familiarity provides reassurance and comfort, decreasing apprehension and reducing behaviors associated with increased risk for use of restraints.
22. Allow restless patient to walk after ensuring that environment is safe. Use a large plant or piece of furniture as a barrier to limit wandering from the designated area.	Activity provides an outlet for energy and stimulation, decreasing behaviors associated with increased risk for use of restraints.
23. Consider the use of patient attendant or sitter.	An attendant or sitter provides companionship and supervision.
24. Remove PPE, if used. Perform hand hygiene.	Removing PPE properly reduces the risk for infection transmission and contamination of other items. Hand hygiene prevents transmission of microorganisms.

EVALUATION

- Use of restraints is avoided.
- Patient and others remain free from harm.

DOCUMENTATION

- Document patient assessment. Include appropriate interventions to reduce need for restraints in nursing plan of care. Document patient and family teaching relative to use of interventions. Document interventions included in care.

SKILL 146 | USING A MANUAL RESUSCITATION BAG AND MASK

If the patient is not breathing with an adequate rate and depth, or if the patient has lost the respiratory drive, a bag and mask may be used to deliver oxygen until the patient is resuscitated or can be intubated with an endotracheal tube. Bag and mask devices are frequently referred to as Ambu bags ("air mask bag unit") or BVM ("bag-valve-mask" device). The bags come in infant, pediatric, and adult sizes. The bag consists of an oxygen reservoir (commonly referred to as the tail), oxygen tubing, the bag itself, a one-way valve to prevent secretions from entering the bag, an exhalation port, an elbow so that the bag can lie across the patient's chest, and a mask.

DELEGATION CONSIDERATIONS

The use of a BVM may be delegated to nursing assistive personnel (NAP) or to unlicensed assistive personnel (UAP) in an emergency situation. The use of a BVM may be delegated to licensed practical/vocational nurses (LPN/LVNs). The decision to delegate must be based on careful analysis of the patient's needs and circumstances, as well as the qualifications of the person to whom the task is being delegated. Refer to the Delegation Guidelines in Appendix A.

EQUIPMENT

- Handheld resuscitation device with a mask
- Oxygen source
- Disposable gloves
- Face shield or goggles and mask
- Additional PPE, as indicated

ASSESSMENT

- Assess the patient's respiratory effort and drive. If the patient is breathing less than 10 breaths per minute, is breathing too shallowly, or is not breathing at all, assistance with a BVM may be needed.
- Assess the oxygen saturation level. Patients who have decreased respiratory effort and drive may also have a decreased oxygen saturation level.
- Assess heart rate and rhythm. Bradycardia may occur with a decreased oxygen saturation level, leading to a cardiac dysrhythmia.
- Many times, a BVM is used in a crisis situation. Manual ventilation is also used during airway suctioning.

NURSING DIAGNOSIS
- Ineffective Breathing Pattern
- Impaired Gas Exchange

OUTCOME IDENTIFICATION AND PLANNING
- Patient will exhibit signs and symptoms of adequate oxygen saturation.
- Patient will receive adequate volume of respirations with the BVM.
- Patient will maintain normal sinus rhythm.

IMPLEMENTATION

ACTION	RATIONALE
1. If not a crisis situation, perform hand hygiene.	Hand hygiene prevents the spread of microorganisms.
2. Put on PPE, as indicated.	PPE prevents the spread of microorganisms. PPE is required based on transmission precautions.
3. If not a crisis situation, identify the patient.	Identifying the patient ensures the right patient receives the intervention and helps prevent errors.
4. Explain what you are going to do and the reason for doing it to the patient, even if the patient does not appear to be alert.	Explanation alleviates fears. Even if the patient appears unconscious, the nurse should explain what is happening.
5. Put on disposable gloves. Put on face shield or goggles and mask.	Using gloves deters the spread of microorganisms. PPE protects the nurse from pathogens.
6. **Ensure that the mask is connected to the bag device, the oxygen tubing is connected to the oxygen source, and the oxygen is turned on, at a flow rate of 10 to 15 L per minute.** This may be done visualizing or by listening to the open end of the reservoir or tail: if air is heard flowing, the oxygen tubing is attached and on.	Expected results might **not** be accomplished if the oxygen tubing is not attached and on.

ACTION	RATIONALE

7. Initiate CPR, if indicated.

Start CPR in any situation in which either breathing alone or breathing and a heartbeat are absent. The brain is sensitive to hypoxia and will sustain irreversible damage after 4 to 6 minutes of no oxygen. The faster CPR is initiated, the greater the chance of survival.

8. If possible, get behind head of bed and remove headboard. **Slightly hyperextend the patient's neck (unless contraindicated). If unable to hyperextend, use jaw thrust maneuver to open airway.**

Standing at head of bed makes positioning easier when obtaining seal of mask to face. Hyperextending the neck opens the airway.

9. Place mask over the patient's face with opening over oral cavity. If mask is teardrop-shaped, the narrow portion should be placed over the bridge of the nose.

This helps ensure an adequate seal so that oxygen can be forced into the lungs.

10. **With dominant hand, place three fingers on the mandible, keeping head slightly hyperextended. Place thumb and one finger in C position around the mask, pressing hard enough to form a seal around the patient's face (Figure 1).**

This helps ensure that an adequate seal is formed so that oxygen can be forced into the lungs.

FIGURE 1 Creating a seal between mask and patient's face.

11. Using nondominant hand, gently and slowly (over 2 to 3 seconds) squeeze the bag,

Volume of air needed is based on patient's size. Enough has been delivered if the chest is rising. If

ACTION	RATIONALE
watching the chest for symmetric rise. If two health care providers are available, one person should maintain a seal on the mask with two hands while the other squeezes the bag to deliver the ventilation and oxygenation.	air is introduced rapidly, it may enter the stomach.
12. Deliver the breaths with the patient's own inspiratory effort, if present. Avoid delivering breaths when the patient exhales. Deliver one breath every 5 seconds, if patient's own respiratory drive is absent. Continue delivering breaths until the patient's drive returns or until the patient is intubated and attached to mechanical ventilation.	Once patient's airway has been stabilized or patient is breathing on own, bag-mask delivery can be stopped.
13. Dispose of equipment appropriately.	Reduces the risk for transmission of microorganisms and contamination of other items.
14. Remove face shield or goggles and mask. Remove gloves and additional PPE, if used. Perform hand hygiene.	Removing PPE properly reduces the risk for infection transmission and contamination of other items. Hand hygiene prevents the spread of microorganisms.

EVALUATION

• Patient demonstrates improved skin color and nail beds without evidence of cyanosis, the oxygen saturation level is within acceptable parameters, and normal sinus rhythm is evident.
• Patient maintains a patent airway and exhibits spontaneous respirations.

DOCUMENTATION

• Document the incident, including patient's respiratory effort before initiation of bag-mask breaths, lung sounds, oxygen saturation, chest symmetry, and resolution of incident (i.e., intubation or patient's respiratory drive returns).

SKILL 147 | EMPLOYING SEIZURE PRECAUTIONS AND SEIZURE MANAGEMENT

Seizures occur when the electrical system of the brain malfunctions. Sudden abnormal and excessive discharge from cerebral neurons results in episodes of abnormal motor, sensory, autonomic, or psychic activity, or a combination of these (Hickey, 2014; Hinkle & Cheever, 2014). A seizure manifests as an alteration in sensation, behavior, movement, perception, or consciousness (Barker, 2008). During a seizure, patients are at risk for hypoxia, vomiting, and pulmonary aspiration. Patients who are at risk for seizures and those who have had a seizure(s) are often placed under seizure precautions to minimize the risk of physical injury. Causes of seizures include cerebrovascular disease, hypoxemia, head injury, hypertension, central nervous system infections, metabolic and toxic conditions, brain tumor, drug and alcohol withdrawal, allergies, and a history of epilepsy (seizure disorder) (Hinkle & Cheever, 2014). Seizure management includes interventions by the nurse to prevent aspiration, protect the patient from injury, provide care after the seizure, and observe and document the details of the event (Hinkle & Cheever, 2014; Hickey).

DELEGATION CONSIDERATIONS

The implementation of seizure precautions may be delegated to nursing assistive personnel (NAP) or to unlicensed assistive personnel (UAP). The implementation of seizure management may not be delegated to nursing assistive personnel (NAP) or to unlicensed assistive personnel (UAP). Implementation of seizure precautions as well as seizure management may be delegated to licensed practical/vocational nurses (LPN/LVNs). The decision to delegate must be based on careful analysis of the patient's needs and circumstances, as well as the qualifications of the person to whom the task is being delegated. Refer to the Delegation Guidelines in Appendix A.

EQUIPMENT

- PPE, as indicated
- Portable or wall suction unit with tubing
- A commercially prepared suction kit with an appropriate size catheter or:
  - Sterile suction catheter with Y-port in the appropriate size (adult: 10F to 16F)
- Sterile disposable container
- Sterile gloves
- Oral airway
- Bed rail padding
- Oxygen apparatus
- Nasal cannula or mask to deliver oxygen
- Handheld bag valve/resuscitation bag

ASSESSMENT

- Assess for preexisting conditions that increase the patient's risk for seizure activity. For example, assess for a history of seizure disorder or epilepsy, cerebrovascular disease, hypoxemia, head injury, hypertension, central nervous system infections, metabolic conditions (e.g., renal failure, hypocalcemia, hypoglycemia), brain tumor, drug/alcohol withdrawal, or allergies.

- Assess circumstances before the seizure, such as visual, auditory, or olfactory stimuli, tactile stimuli, emotional or psychological disturbances, sleep, or hyperventilation. Assess for the occurrence of an aura.
- Note where the movements or stiffness begin; and the gaze position and position of the head when the seizure begins. Assess the body part(s) and the type of movement(s) involved in the seizure.
- Assess pupil sizes; if eyes remained open during seizure; and whether eyes or head turned to one side.
- Assess for the presence or absence of repeated involuntary motor activity (e.g., repeated swallowing); incontinence of urine or stool; duration of seizure; presence of unconsciousness and duration; obvious paralysis or weakness of arms or legs after seizure; and inability to speak, movements, sleeping, and/or confusion after seizure.
- Assess the patient's neurologic status and for injury after the seizure is over.

NURSING DIAGNOSIS
- Risk for Injury
- Risk for Aspiration
- Deficient Knowledge

OUTCOME IDENTIFICATION AND PLANNING
- Patient remains free from injury.
- Other specific outcomes will be formulated depending on the identified nursing diagnosis.

IMPLEMENTATION

ACTION	RATIONALE
1. Review the medical record and nursing plan of care for conditions that would place the patient at risk for seizures. Review the medical orders and the nursing plan of care for orders for seizure precautions.	Reviewing the order and plan of care validates the correct patient and correct procedure.

Seizure Precautions

2. Gather the necessary supplies.	Preparation promotes efficient time management and an organized approach to the task.

ACTION	RATIONALE
3. Perform hand hygiene and put on PPE, if indicated.	Hand hygiene and PPE prevent the spread of microorganisms. PPE is required based on transmission precautions.
4. Identify the patient.	Identifying the patient ensures the right patient receives the intervention and helps prevent errors.
5. Close curtains around the bed and close the door to the room, if possible. Explain what you are going to do and why you are going to do it to the patient.	This ensures the patient's privacy. Explanation relieves anxiety and facilitates cooperation.
6. Assemble equipment on overbed table within reach.	Arranging items nearby is convenient, saves time, and avoids unnecessary stretching and twisting of muscles on the part of the nurse.
7. Place the bed in the lowest position with two to three side rails elevated. Apply padding to the side rails.	Bed in lowest position promotes safety and decreases risk of injury. Rail padding decreases the risk of injury.
8. Attach oxygen apparatus to oxygen access in the wall at the head of the bed. Place nasal cannula or mask equipment in a location where it can be easily reached if needed.	During a seizure, patients are at risk for hypoxia, vomiting, and pulmonary aspiration. Ready access ensures availability of oxygen in the event of a seizure.
9. Attach suction apparatus to vacuum access in the wall at the head of the bed. Place suction catheter, oral airway, and resuscitation bag in a location where they are easily reached if needed.	During a seizure, patients are at risk for hypoxia, vomiting, and pulmonary aspiration. Ready access ensures availability of suction in the event of a seizure. Oral airway and resuscitation bag ensure availability of emergency ventilation in the event of respiratory arrest.

ACTION	RATIONALE

10. Remove PPE, if used. Perform hand hygiene.

Removing PPE properly reduces the risk for infection transmission and contamination of other items. Hand hygiene prevents the spread of micro-organisms.

Seizure Management

11. For patients with known seizures, be alert for the occurrence of an aura, if known. If the patient reports experiencing an aura, have the patient lie down.

Some patients report a warning or premonition before seizures occur; an aura can be a visual, auditory, or olfactory sensation that indicates a seizure is going to occur. Lying down prevents injury that might occur if the patient falls to the floor.

12. Once a seizure begins, close the curtains around the bed and close the door to the room, if possible.

Closing the door or curtain provides for patient privacy.

13. If the patient is seated, ease the patient to the floor.

Getting the patient to the floor prevents injury that might occur if the patient falls to the floor.

14. Remove patient's eyeglasses. Loosen any constricting clothing. Place something flat and soft, such as a folded blanket, under the head. Push aside furniture or other objects in area.

Removing objects and loosening clothing prevents possible injury. Blanket prevents injury from striking a hard surface (floor).

15. If the patient is in bed, remove the pillow, place bed in lowest position, and raise side rails.

Prevents injury.

16. Do not restrain patient. Guide movements, if necessary. Do not try to insert anything in the patient's mouth or open jaws.

Guiding movements prevents injury. Restraint can injure the patient. Attempting to open the mouth and/or insert anything into the mouth can result in broken teeth, and injury to mouth, lips, or tongue.

17. If possible, place patient on the side with the head flexed forward, head of bed

During a seizure, patients are at risk for hypoxia, vomiting, and pulmonary aspiration. This

ACTION	RATIONALE
elevated 30 degrees. Begin administration of oxygen, based on facility policy. Clear airway using suction, as appropriate. (Refer to Skill 160.)	position allows the tongue to fall forward, and facilitates drainage of saliva and mucus and minimizes risk for aspiration. Oxygen supports the increased metabolism associated with neurologic and muscular hyperactivity. Patent airway is necessary to support ventilation.
18. Provide supervision throughout the seizure and time the length of the seizure.	Supervision of the patient ensures safety. Timing of event contributes to accurate information and documentation.
19. Establish/maintain intravenous access, as necessary. Administer medications, as appropriate, based on medical order and facility policy.	Pharmacologic therapy may be appropriate, based on patient history and medical diagnoses. Intravenous access is necessary to administer emergency medications.
20. After the seizure, place the patient in a side-lying position. Clear airway using suction, as appropriate.	Side-lying position facilitates drainage of secretions. Patent airway is necessary to support ventilation.
21. Monitor vital signs, oxygen saturation, response to medications administered, and capillary glucose, as appropriate.	Monitoring of parameters provides information for accurate assessment of patient status.
22. Place the bed in the lowest position. Make sure the call bell is in reach.	Bed in lowest position and access to call bell contribute to patient safety.
23. Reassess the patient's neurologic status and comfort level.	Reassessment helps to evaluate the effects of the event on the patient.
24. Allow the patient to sleep after the seizure. On awakening, orient and reassure the patient. Reassess as indicated.	The patient will probably experience an inability to recall the seizure; patients may also experience confusion, anxiety, embarrassment, and/or fatigue after a seizure. Reassessment helps to evaluate the effects of the event on the patient.

ACTION	RATIONALE
25. Remove PPE, if used. Perform hand hygiene.	Removing PPE properly reduces the risk for infection transmission and contamination of other items. Hand hygiene prevents the spread of microorganisms.

EVALUATION

• Patient remains free from injury.

DOCUMENTATION

• Document initiation of seizure precautions, including specific interventions put in place. Document if the beginning of the seizure was witnessed. If so, record noted circumstances before the seizure, such as visual, auditory, or olfactory stimuli, tactile stimuli, emotional or psychological disturbances, sleep, or hyperventilation. Note the occurrence of an aura; where the movements or stiffness began; gaze position and position of the head when the seizure began. Record the body part(s) and the type of movement(s) involved in the seizure. Document pupil sizes; if eyes remained open during seizure; whether eyes or head turned to one side; presence or absence of repeated involuntary motor activity (e.g., repeated swallowing); incontinence of urine or stool; duration of seizure; presence of unconsciousness and duration; obvious paralysis or weakness of arms or legs after seizure; and inability to speak, movements, sleeping, and/or confusion after seizure. Document oxygen administration, airway suction, safety measures, and medication administration, if used. If the patient was injured during the seizure, document assessment of injury.

SKILL 148 | SHAMPOOING A PATIENT'S HAIR IN BED

The easiest way to wash a patient's hair is to assist him or her in the shower, but not all patients can take showers. If the patient's hair needs to be washed but the patient is unable or not allowed to get out of bed, a bed shampoo can be performed. Shampoo caps are available, and are being used with increasing frequency. These commercially prepared, disposable caps contain a rinseless shampoo product. See the accompanying Skill Variation.

DELEGATION CONSIDERATIONS

The shampooing of a patient's hair may be delegated to nursing assistive personnel (NAP) or to unlicensed assistive personnel (UAP), as well as to licensed practical/vocational nurses (LPN/LVNs). The decision to delegate must be based on careful analysis of the patient's needs and circumstances, as well as the qualifications of the person to whom the task is being delegated. Refer to the Delegation Guidelines in Appendix A.

EQUIPMENT

- Water pitcher
- Warm water
- Shampoo
- Conditioner (optional)
- Disposable gloves
- Additional PPE, as indicated
- Protective pad for bed
- Shampoo board
- Bucket
- Towels
- Gown
- Comb or brush
- Blow dryer (optional)

ASSESSMENT

- Assess the patient's hygiene preferences: frequency, time of day, and type of hygiene products.
- Assess for any physical activity limitations.
- Assess the patient's ability to get out of bed to have his or her hair washed. If the medical orders allow it and patient is physically able to wash his or her hair in the shower, the patient may prefer to do so. If the patient cannot tolerate being out of bed or is not allowed to do so, perform a bed shampoo.
- Assess for any activity or positioning limitations.
- Inspect the patient's scalp for any cuts, lesions, or bumps. Note any flaking, drying, or excessive oiliness, or evidence of problems, such as pediculosis.

NURSING DIAGNOSIS

- Bathing Self-Care Deficit
- Impaired Physical Mobility
- Impaired Transfer Ability

OUTCOME IDENTIFICATION AND PLANNING

- Patient's hair will be clean.
- Patient will tolerate the shampoo with little to no difficulty.
- Patient will demonstrate an improved body image.
- Patient will verbalize an increase in comfort.

IMPLEMENTATION

ACTION	RATIONALE
1. Review health record for any limitations in physical activity, or contraindications to the	Identifying limitations prevents patient discomfort and injury. In some settings, a medical order

ACTION	RATIONALE
procedure. Confirm presence of medical order for shampooing the patient's hair, if required by facility policy.	is required for shampooing a patient's hair.
2. Perform hand hygiene. Put on PPE, as indicated.	Hand hygiene and PPE prevent the spread of microorganisms. PPE is required based on transmission precautions.
3. Identify the patient. Explain the procedure to the patient.	Patient identification validates the correct patient and correct procedure. Discussion and explanation help allay anxiety and prepare the patient for what to expect.
4. Assemble equipment on overbed table within reach.	Organization facilitates performance of task.
5. Close the curtains around the bed and close the door to the room, if possible.	Provides for patient privacy.
6. Lower the head of the bed. Raise bed to a comfortable working position, usually elbow height of the caregiver (VISN 8 Patient Safety Center, 2009). Lower side rail. Remove pillow and place protective pad under patient's head and shoulders.	Proper bed height helps reduce back strain while performing the procedure. A protective pad keeps the sheets from getting wet.
7. **Fill the pitcher with comfortably warm water (100°F to less than 120°F to 125°F).** Position the patient at the top of the bed, in a supine position. Have the patient lift his or her head and place the shampoo board underneath patient's head. If necessary, pad the edge of the board with a small towel.	Warm water is comfortable and relaxing for the patient. It also stimulates circulation and provides for more effective cleaning. Adjusting the water temperature to 100°F to less than 120°F to 125°F decreases risk of burns and drying of the skin. The lower temperature is recommended for children and adults over 65 years of age (Burn Foundation, 2012). Padding the edge of the shampoo board may help increase patient comfort.
8. Place a drain container underneath the drain of the shampoo board.	The container will catch the runoff water, preventing a mess on the floor.

ACTION	RATIONALE
9. Put on gloves. If the patient is able, have him or her hold a folded washcloth at the forehead. Pour a pitcher of warm water slowly over the patient's head, making sure that all hair is saturated. Refill pitcher, if needed.	Gloves prevent the spread of microorganisms. A washcloth prevents water from running into the patient's eyes. By pouring slowly, more hair will become wet, and it is more soothing for the patient.
10. Apply a small amount of shampoo to patient's hair. Lather shampoo. Massage deep into the scalp, avoiding any cuts, lesions, or sore spots.	Shampoo will help to remove dirt or oil.
11. Rinse with comfortably warm water until all shampoo is out of hair. Repeat shampoo, if necessary.	Shampoo left in hair may cause pruritus. If hair is still dirty, another shampoo treatment may be needed.
12. If patient has thick hair or requests it, apply a small amount of conditioner to hair and massage throughout. Avoid any cuts, lesions, or sore spots.	Conditioner eases tangles and moisturizes hair and scalp.
13. If drain container is small, empty before rinsing hair. Rinse with comfortably warm water until all conditioner is out of hair.	Container may overflow if not emptied. Conditioner left in hair may cause pruritus.
14. Remove shampoo board. Place towel around patient's hair.	This prevents the patient from getting cold.
15. Pat hair dry, avoiding any cuts, lesions, or sore spots. Remove protective padding, but keep one dry protective pad under patient's hair.	Patting dry removes any excess water without damaging hair or scalp.
16. Gently brush hair, removing tangles, as needed.	Removing tangles helps hair to dry faster. Brushing hair improves patient's self-image.
17. Blow-dry hair on a cool setting, if allowed and if patient wishes. If not,	Blow-drying hair helps hair to dry faster and prevents patient from becoming chilled. Keeping

ACTION	RATIONALE
consider covering the patient's head with a dry towel, until hair is dry.	the head covered prevents chilling while hair is drying.
18. Change patient's gown and remove protective pad. Replace pillow.	If patient's gown is damp, patient will become chilled. Protective pad is no longer needed once hair is dry.
19. Remove equipment and return patient to a position of comfort. Remove your gloves. Raise side rail and lower bed.	Promotes patient comfort and safety. Removing gloves properly reduces the risk for infection transmission and contamination of other items.
20. Remove additional PPE, if used. Perform hand hygiene.	Removing PPE properly reduces the risk for infection transmission and contamination of other items. Hand hygiene deters spread of microorganisms.

EVALUATION

• Patient's hair is clean.
• Patient verbalizes a positive body image.
• Patient reports an increase in comfort level.

DOCUMENTATION

• Record your assessment, significant observations, and unusual findings, such as bleeding or inflammation. Document any teaching done. Document procedure and patient response.

SKILL VARIATION	Shampooing a Patient's Hair with a Shampoo Cap

Shampoo caps are available and are being used with increasing frequency. These commercially prepared, disposable caps contain a rinseless shampoo product. The cap is warmed in the microwave or stored in a warmer until use. After shampooing for the manufacturer's suggested length of time, the cap is removed and discarded.

1. Review chart for any limitations in physical activity, or contraindications to the procedure. Confirm presence of medical order for shampooing patient's hair, if required by facility policy.
2. Warm the cap in the microwave, according to the manufacturer's directions,

Shampooing a Patient's Hair with a Shampoo Cap   *continued*

or remove it from the storage warmer.

3. Perform hand hygiene and put on PPE, if indicated.

4. Identify the patient.

5. Explain what you are going to do and the reason for doing it to the patient.

6. Assemble necessary equipment on the bedside stand or overbed table.

7. Close the curtains around the bed and close the door to the room, if possible.

8. Put on gloves. Raise bed to a comfortable working position, usually elbow height of the caregiver (VISN 8 Patient Safety Center, 2009). Place a towel across the patient's chest. Place the shampoo cap on the patient's head.

9. Massage the scalp and hair through the cap to lather the shampoo. Continue to massage according to the time frame specified by the manufacturer's directions.

10. Remove and discard the shampoo cap.

11. Dry the patient's hair with a towel.

12. Remove the towel from the patient's chest.

13. Comb and style the hair.

14. Remove gloves. Lower bed. Assist the patient to a comfortable position.

15. Remove additional PPE, if used. Perform hand hygiene.

SKILL 149   ASSISTING THE PATIENT TO SHAVE

For many patients shaving is a daily hygiene ritual. They may feel disheveled and unclean without shaving. Some patients may need help with shaving when using a regular blade or may require that the nurse perform the shaving procedure for them completely. Patients with beards or mustaches may require nursing assistance to keep the beard and mustache clean. However, never trim or shave a patient's beard or mustache without the patient's consent. Female patients may require assistance with shaving underarm and leg hair, depending on the patient's personal preference and abilities. If available and permitted by the facility, electric shavers are usually recommended when the patient is receiving anticoagulant therapy or has a bleeding disorder. Electric shavers are especially convenient for ill and bedridden patients.

DELEGATION CONSIDERATIONS

The shaving of a patient's hair may be delegated to nursing assistive personnel (NAP) or to unlicensed assistive personnel (UAP) after assessment by the registered nurse, as well as to licensed practical/ vocational nurses (LPN/LVNs). The decision to delegate must be based on careful analysis of the patient's needs and circumstances, as well as the qualifications of the person to whom the task is being delegated. Refer to the Delegation Guidelines Appendix A.

EQUIPMENT

- Shaving cream
- Safety razor
- Towel
- Washcloth
- Bath basin
- Disposable gloves
- Additional PPE, as indicated
- Waterproof pad
- Aftershave or lotion (optional)

ASSESSMENT

- Assess the patient's shaving preferences: frequency, time of day, and type of shaving products.
- Assess for any physical activity limitations.
- Assess patient for any bleeding problems. If patient is receiving any anticoagulant, such as heparin or warfarin (Coumadin), has received an antithrombolytic agent, or has a low platelet count, consider using an electric razor.
- Inspect the area to be shaved for any lesions or weeping areas.
- Assess the patient's ability to shave himself or assist with the procedure.

NURSING DIAGNOSIS

- Risk for Injury
- Bathing Self-Care Deficit
- Impaired Physical Mobility

OUTCOME IDENTIFICATION AND PLANNING

- Patient will be clean, without evidence of hair growth or trauma to the skin.
- Patient tolerates shaving with minimal to no difficulty.
- Patient verbalizes feelings of improved self-esteem.

IMPLEMENTATION

ACTION	RATIONALE
1. Review health record for any limitations in physical activity, or contraindications to the procedure. Confirm	Identifying limitations prevents patient discomfort and injury. In some settings, a medical order is required for shaving a patient

ACTION	RATIONALE
presence of medical order for shaving the patient, if required by facility policy.	with certain health problems or taking medications that affect coagulation.
2. Perform hand hygiene. Put on PPE, as indicated.	Hand hygiene and PPE prevent the spread of microorganisms. PPE is required based on transmission precautions.
3. Identify patient. Explain the procedure to the patient.	Identifying the patient ensures the right patient receives the intervention and helps prevent errors. Explanation facilitates cooperation.
4. Assemble equipment on overbed table within reach.	Organization facilitates performance of task.
5. Close the curtains around the bed and close the door to the room, if possible.	Provides for patient privacy.
6. Raise bed to a comfortable working position, usually elbow height of the caregiver (VISN 8 Patient Safety Center, 2009). Lower side rail. Cover patient's chest with a towel or waterproof pad. Fill bath basin with comfortably warm (100°F to less than 120°F to125°F) water. Put on gloves. Press a warm washcloth on the area to be shaved.	Proper bed height helps reduce back strain while performing the procedure. Adjusting the water temperature to 100°F to less than 120°F to 125°F decreases risk of burns and drying of the skin. The lower temperature is recommended for children and adults over 65 years of age (Burn Foundation, 2012). Warm water is comfortable and relaxing for the patient. Moistens skin and softens hair. Gloves prevent the spread of microorganisms. Warm water softens the hair, making the process easier.
7. Dispense shaving cream into palm of hand. Apply cream to area to be shaved in a layer about 0.5 inch thick.	Using shaving cream helps to prevent skin irritation and prevents hair from pulling.
8. With one hand, pull the skin taut at the area to be shaved. Using a smooth stroke, begin shaving. *If shaving the face,*	The skin on the face is more sensitive and needs to be shaved with the direction of hair growth to prevent discomfort.

ACTION	RATIONALE

shave with the direction of hair growth in short strokes (Figure 1). *If shaving a leg,* shave against the hair in upward, short strokes. *If shaving an underarm,* pull skin taut and use short, upward strokes.

FIGURE 1 Shaving the face.

ACTION	RATIONALE
9. Remove residual shaving cream with wet washcloth.	Shaving cream can lead to irritation if left on the skin.
10. If patient requests, apply aftershave or lotion to area shaved.	Aftershave and lotion can reduce skin irritation.
11. Remove equipment and return patient to a position of comfort. Remove your gloves. Raise side rail and lower bed.	Promotes patient comfort and safety. Removing gloves properly reduces the risk for infection transmission and contamination of other items.
12. Remove additional PPE, if used. Perform hand hygiene.	Removing PPE properly reduces the risk for infection transmission and contamination of other items. Hand hygiene deters spread of microorganisms.

EVALUATION

- Patient is clean-shaven without evidence of trauma, irritation, or redness.
- Patient verbalizes feeling refreshed and demonstrates improved self-esteem.

DOCUMENTATION

- Shaving a patient does not usually require documentation. However, if your skin assessment reveals any unusual findings, document your assessment and the procedure. If the patient or nurse breaks the skin while shaving, document the occurrence and your assessment of the patient.

SKILL 150   APPLYING A SLING

A sling is a bandage that can provide support for an arm or immobilize an injured arm, wrist, or hand. Slings can be used to restrict movement of a fracture or dislocation and to support a muscle sprain. They may also be used to support a splint or secure dressings. Health care agencies usually use commercial slings. The sling should distribute the supported weight over a large area, not the back of the neck, to prevent pressure on the cervical spinal nerves.

DELEGATION CONSIDERATIONS

The application of a sling may not be delegated to nursing assistive personnel (NAP) or to unlicensed assistive personnel (UAP). The application of a sling may be delegated to licensed practical/vocational nurses (LPN/LVNs). The decision to delegate must be based on careful analysis of the patient's needs and circumstances, as well as the qualifications of the person to whom the task is being delegated. Refer to the Delegation Guidelines in Appendix A.

EQUIPMENT

- Commercial arm sling
- ABD gauze pad
- Nonsterile gloves and/or other PPE, as indicated

ASSESSMENT

- Assess the situation to determine the need for a sling.
- Assess the affected limb for pain and edema.
- Perform a neurovascular assessment of the affected extremity.
- Assess body parts distal to the site for cyanosis, pallor, coolness, numbness, tingling, swelling, and absent or diminished pulses.

NURSING DIAGNOSIS

- Impaired Physical Mobility
- Risk for Impaired Skin Integrity
- Risk for Peripheral Neurovascular Dysfunction

OUTCOME IDENTIFICATION AND PLANNING

• Arm is immobilized, and the patient maintains muscle strength and joint range of motion.
• Patient shows no evidence of contractures, venous stasis, thrombus formation, or skin breakdown.

IMPLEMENTATION

ACTION	RATIONALE
1. Review the medical record and nursing plan of care to determine the need for the use of a sling.	Reviewing the medical record and plan of care validates the correct patient and correct procedure and prevents injury.
2. Perform hand hygiene. Put on PPE, as indicated.	Hand hygiene and PPE prevent the spread of microorganisms. PPE is required based on transmission precautions.
3. Identify the patient. Explain the procedure to the patient.	Patient identification validates the correct patient and correct procedure. Discussion and explanation help allay anxiety and prepare the patient for what to expect.
4. Close the curtains around the bed and close the door to the room, if possible. Place the bed at an appropriate and comfortable working height, usually elbow height of the caregiver (VISN 8 Patient Safety Center, 2009).	Closing the door or curtain provides privacy. Proper bed height helps reduce back strain.
5. Assist the patient to a sitting position. Place the patient's forearm across the chest with the elbow flexed and the palm against the chest. Measure the sleeve length, if indicated.	Proper positioning facilitates sling application. Measurement ensures proper sizing of the sling and proper placement of the arm.
6. Enclose the arm in the sling, making sure the elbow fits into the corner of the fabric. Run the strap up the patient's back and across the shoulder opposite the injury, then down the chest to the fastener on the end of the sling.	This position ensures adequate support and keeps the arm out of a dependent position, preventing edema.

ACTION	RATIONALE
7. Place the ABD pad under the strap, between the strap and the patient's neck. **Ensure that the sling and forearm are slightly elevated and at a right angle to the body (Figure 1).**	Padding prevents skin irritation and reduces pressure on the neck. Proper positioning ensures alignment, provides support, and prevents edema.

FIGURE 1 Patient with sling in place.

ACTION	RATIONALE
8. Place the bed in the lowest position, with the side rails up. Make sure the call bell and other essential items are within easy reach.	Having the bed at proper height and leaving the call bell and other items within reach ensure patient safety.
9. Remove PPE, if used. Perform hand hygiene.	Removing PPE properly reduces the risk for infection transmission and contamination of other items. Hand hygiene prevents the spread of microorganisms.
10. Check the patient's level of comfort, arm positioning, and neurovascular status of the affected limb every 4 hours or according to facility policy. Assess the axillary and cervical skin frequently for irritation or breakdown.	Frequent assessment ensures patient safety, prevents injury, and provides early intervention for skin irritation and other complications.

EVALUATION

- Patient demonstrates the extremity in proper alignment with adequate muscle strength and joint range of motion.

- Patient demonstrates proper use of the sling and remains free of complications, including contractures, venous stasis, thrombus formation, or skin breakdown.

DOCUMENTATION

- Document the time and date the sling was applied. Document the patient's response to the sling and the neurovascular status of the extremity.

SKILL 151 | COLLECTING A SPUTUM SPECIMEN FOR CULTURE

Sputum production is the result of the reaction of the lungs to any constant recurring irritant (Hinkle & Cheever, 2014). A sputum specimen comes from deep within the bronchi, not from the postnasal region. Sputum analysis is used to diagnose disease, test for drug sensitivity, and guide patient treatment. Sputum may be obtained to identify pathogenic organisms, determine if malignant cells are present, and assess for hypersensitivity states. A sputum specimen may be ordered if a bacterial, viral, or fungal infection of the pulmonary system is suspected. A sputum specimen can be collected by patient expectoration into a sterile container, by endotracheal suctioning, during bronchoscopy, and via transtracheal aspiration. Because secretions have accumulated during the night, it is desirable to collect an expectorated sputum specimen first thing in the morning when the patient rises, which aids in the collection process (Hinkle & Cheever, 2014). The following procedure describes collecting an expectorated sample. Collecting a sputum specimen by suctioning via an endotracheal tube is discussed in the Skill Variation at the end of this skill.

DELEGATION CONSIDERATIONS

Obtaining a sputum specimen is not delegated to nursing assistive personnel (NAP) or to unlicensed assistive personnel (UAP). Obtaining a sputum specimen may be delegated to licensed practical/vocational nurses (LPN/LVNs). The decision to delegate must be based on careful analysis of the patient's needs and circumstances, as well as the qualifications of the person to whom the task is being delegated. Refer to the Delegation Guidelines in Appendix A.

EQUIPMENT

- Sterile sputum specimen container
- Nonsterile gloves
- Goggles or safety glasses
- Additional PPE, as indicated
- Biohazard bag
- Appropriate label for specimen, based on facility policy and procedure

ASSESSMENT

- Assess the patient's lung sounds. Patients with a productive cough may have crackles, rhonchi, wheezing, or diminished lung sounds.
- Monitor oxygen saturation levels, because patients with excessive pulmonary secretions may have decreased oxygen saturation.
- Assess the patient's level of pain. Consider administering pain medication before obtaining the sample, because the patient will have to cough.
- Assess the characteristics of the sputum: color, quantity, presence of blood, and viscosity.

NURSING DIAGNOSIS

- Acute Pain
- Ineffective Airway Clearance
- Impaired Gas Exchange

OUTCOME IDENTIFICATION AND PLANNING

- Patient produces an adequate sample (based on facility policy) from the lungs.
- Airway patency is maintained.
- Oxygen saturation increases.
- Patient demonstrates an understanding about the need for specimen collection.
- Patient demonstrates improved respiratory status.

IMPLEMENTATION

ACTION	RATIONALE
1. Verify the order for a sputum specimen collection in the medical record. Gather equipment.	Verifying the medical order is crucial to ensuring that the proper procedure is administered to the right patient. Assembling equipment provides for an organized approach to the task.
2. Perform hand hygiene and put on PPE, if indicated.	Hand hygiene and PPE prevent the transmission of microorganisms. PPE is required based on transmission precautions.
3. Identify the patient.	Identifying the patient ensures the right patient receives the intervention and helps prevent errors.

ACTION	RATIONALE
4. Explain the procedure to the patient. Administer pain medication (if ordered) if the patient might have pain with coughing. If the patient can perform the task without assistance after instruction, leave the container at bedside with instructions to call the nurse as soon as a specimen is produced.	Explanation provides reassurance and promotes cooperation. Pain relief facilitates compliance.
5. Check specimen label with the patient's identification bracelet. Label should include the patient's name and identification number, time specimen was collected, route of collection, identification of the person obtaining the sample, and any other information required by facility policy.	Confirmation of patient identification information ensures the specimen is labeled correctly for the right patient.
6. Assemble equipment on overbed table within reach.	Arranging items nearby is convenient, saves time, and avoids unnecessary stretching and twisting of muscles on the part of the nurse.
7. Close curtains around the bed and close the door to the room, if possible.	Closing the curtain or door provides for patient privacy.
8. Put on disposable gloves and goggles.	The gloves and goggles prevent contact with blood and body fluids.
9. Adjust the bed to a comfortable working height, usually elbow height of the caregiver (VISN 8 Patient Safety Center, 2009). Lower side rail closest to you. Place patient in semi-Fowler's position. **Have patient clear nose and throat and rinse mouth with water before beginning procedure.**	Having the bed at the proper height prevents back and muscle strain. The semi-Fowler's position will help the patient to cough and expectorate the sputum specimen. Water will rinse the oral cavity of saliva and any food particles.

ACTION	RATIONALE
10. Caution the patient to avoid spitting saliva secretion in to the sterile container. **Instruct the patient to inhale deeply two or three times and cough with exhalation.** If the patient has had abdominal surgery, assist the patient to splint the abdomen.	Saliva can contaminate the sputum specimen. The specimen will need to come from the lungs; saliva is not acceptable. Splinting helps to reduce the pain in the abdominal incision.
11. If the patient produces sputum, open the lid to the container and have the patient expectorate the specimen into the container. Caution the patient to avoid touching the edge or the inside of the collection container.	The specimen needs to come from the lungs; saliva is not acceptable. Touching the edge or inside of the sterile collection container contaminates the specimen.
12. If patient believes he or she can produce more sputum for the specimen, have the patient repeat the procedure. Collect a volume of sputum based on facility policy.	This ensures an adequate amount of sputum specimen is obtained for analysis.
13. Close the container lid. Offer oral hygiene to the patient.	Closing the container prevents contamination of the specimen and possible infection transmission. Oral hygiene helps to remove pathogens from the oral cavity.
14. Remove equipment and return the patient to a position of comfort. Raise side rail and lower bed.	Repositioning promotes patient comfort. Raising rails promotes safety.
15. Remove gloves and goggles. Perform hand hygiene.	Removing gloves and goggles properly reduces the risk for infection transmission and con- tamination of other items. Hand hygiene reduces the transmission of microorganisms.
16. Place label on the container per facility policy. Place container in plastic, sealable biohazard bag.	Proper labeling of the specimen ensures the specimen is for the right patient. Packaging the specimen in a biohazard bag

ACTION	RATIONALE
	prevents the person transporting the container from coming in contact with the specimen.
17. Remove other PPE, if used. Perform hand hygiene.	Removing PPE properly reduces the risk for infection transmission and contamination of other items. Hand hygiene reduces the transmission of microorganisms.
18. Transport the specimen to the laboratory immediately. If immediate transport is not possible, check with laboratory personnel or policy manual whether refrigeration is contraindicated.	Timely transport ensures accurate results.

EVALUATION

- Patient expectorates sputum, and it is collected in a sterile container and sent to the laboratory as soon as possible.
- Patient maintains a patent airway and oxygen saturation level is within expected parameters.
- Patient demonstrates understanding about the rationale for the specimen collection.

DOCUMENTATION

- Record the time the sputum specimen was collected and sent to the laboratory, and the characteristics and amount of secretions. Document the tests for which the specimen was collected. Note the respiratory assessment pre- and post-collection. Note antibiotics administered in the past 24 hours on the laboratory request form, if required by the facility.

SKILL VARIATION | **Collecting Sputum Specimen via Endotracheal Suctioning**

1. Sputum specimens can be collected by suctioning an endotracheal tube or tracheostomy tube. A sterile collection receptacle is attached between the suction catheter and the suction tubing to trap sputum as it is removed from the patient's airway, before reaching the suction collection canister.

2. Refer to Skills 63, 64, and 166 for the procedure for endotracheal suctioning.

Collecting Sputum Specimen via Endotracheal Suctioning *continued*

3. After checking suction pressure (Step 8, Skill 63; Step 9, Skill 64; Step 9, Skill 166), attach a sterile specimen trap to the suction tubing, taking care to avoid contaminating the open ends (Figure A).

FIGURE A Suction trap for sputum collection.

4. Continue with Step 9, Skill 63; Step 10, Skill 64, Step 10, Skill 166 taking care to handle the suction tubing and sputum trap with your nondominant hand. Proceed with suction procedure.

5. After first suction pass, if 5 to 10 mL of sputum has been obtained, disconnect the specimen container, and set aside (LeFever Kee, 2013). If less than this amount has been collected, re-suction the patient, after

waiting the appropriate amount of time for the patient to recover.

6. If secretions are extremely thick or tenacious, flush the catheter with a small amount (1 to 2 mL) of sterile normal saline to aid in moving the secretions into the trap.

7. Once the sputum trap is removed, connect suction tubing to the suction catheter. The catheter may then be flushed with normal saline before suctioning again. Continue with the suctioning procedure, if necessary, based on remaining steps in Skill 63, Skill 64, or Skill 166.

8. When suctioning is completed, check the specimen label with the patient's identification bracelet. Label should include the patient's name and identification number, time specimen was collected, route of collection, identification of person obtaining the sample, and any other information required by facility policy. Place label on the container per facility policy. Place container in plastic, sealable biohazard bag and send to the laboratory immediately.

Skin staples made of stainless steel are used to hold tissue and skin together. Staples decrease the risk of infection and allow for faster wound closure. Surgical staples are removed when enough tensile strength has developed to hold the wound edges together during healing. The time frame for removal varies depending on the patient's age, nutritional status, and wound location. After skin staples are removed, adhesive wound closure strips are applied across the wound to keep the skin edges approximated as it continues to heal. The removal of surgical staples may be done by the primary care provider or by the nurse with a medical order.

DELEGATION CONSIDERATIONS

The removal of surgical staples is not delegated to nursing assistive personnel (NAP) or to unlicensed assistive personnel (UAP). Depending on the state's nurse practice act and the organization's policies and procedures, the removal of surgical staples may be delegated to licensed practical/vocational nurses (LPN/LVNs). The decision to delegate must be based on careful analysis of the patient's needs and circumstances, as well as the qualifications of the person to whom the task is being delegated. Refer to the Delegation Guidelines in Appendix A.

EQUIPMENT

- Staple remover
- Gauze
- Wound cleansing agent, according to facility policy

- Clean, disposable gloves
- Additional PPE, as indicated
- Adhesive wound closure strips
- Skin protectant wipes

ASSESSMENT

- Inspect the surgical incision and the surrounding tissue.
- Assess the appearance of the wound for the approximation of wound edges, the color of the wound and surrounding area, and signs of dehiscence. Note the stage of the healing process and the characteristics of any drainage.
- Assess the surrounding skin for color, temperature, and the presence of edema or ecchymosis.

NURSING DIAGNOSIS

- Impaired Skin Integrity
- Acute Pain
- Delayed Surgical Recovery

OUTCOME IDENTIFICATION AND PLANNING

- Staples are removed without contaminating the incisional area, causing trauma to the wound, and/or causing the patient to experience pain or discomfort.

- Patient remains free of complications that would delay recovery.
- Patient verbalizes an understanding of the procedure.

IMPLEMENTATION

ACTION	RATIONALE
1. Review the medical order for staple removal. Gather necessary supplies.	Reviewing the order and plan of care validates the correct patient and correct procedure. Preparation promotes efficient time management and an organized approach to the task.
2. Perform hand hygiene and put on PPE, if indicated.	Hand hygiene and PPE prevent the spread of microorganisms. PPE is required based on transmission precautions.
3. Identify the patient.	Identifying the patient ensures the right patient receives the intervention and helps prevent errors.
4. Assemble equipment on overbed table within reach.	Organization facilitates performance of task.
5. Close the curtains around the bed and close the door to the room, if possible. Explain what you are going to do and why you are going to do it to the patient. Describe the sensation of staple removal as a pulling experience.	This ensures the patient's privacy. Explanation relieves anxiety and facilitates cooperation.
6. Assess the patient for possible need for nonpharmacologic pain-reducing interventions or analgesic medication before beginning the procedure. Administer appropriate prescribed analgesic. Allow enough time for the analgesic to achieve its effectiveness before beginning procedure.	Pain is a subjective experience influenced by past experience. Wound care and dressing changes may cause pain for some patients.

ACTION	RATIONALE
7. Place a waste receptacle at a convenient location for use during the procedure.	Having a waste container handy means that the soiled dressing may be discarded easily, without the spread of microorganisms.
8. Adjust bed to comfortable working height, usually elbow height of the caregiver (VISN 8, 2009).	Having the bed at the proper height prevents back and muscle strain.
9. Assist the patient to a comfortable position that provides easy access to the incision area. Use a bath blanket to cover any exposed area other than the incision. Place a waterproof pad under the incision site.	Patient positioning and use of a bath blanket provide for comfort and warmth. Waterproof pad protects underlying surfaces.
10. Put on clean gloves. Carefully and gently remove the soiled dressings. If there is resistance, use a silicone-based adhesive remover to help remove the tape. If any part of the dressing sticks to the underlying skin, use small amounts of sterile saline to help loosen and remove it. Inspect the incision area.	Gloves protect the nurse from handling contaminated dressings. Cautious removal of the dressing is more comfortable for the patient and ensures that any drain present is not removed. A silicone-based adhesive remover allows for the easy, rapid, and painless removal without the associated problems of skin stripping (Denyer, 2011; Benbow, 2011). Sterile saline moistens the dressing for easier removal and minimizes damage and pain.
11. Clean the incision using the wound cleanser and gauze, according to facility policies and procedures.	Incision cleaning prevents the spread of microorganisms and contamination of the wound.
12. Grasp the staple remover. **Position the staple remover under the staple to be removed. Firmly close the staple remover.** The staple will bend in the middle and the edges will pull up out of the skin.	Correct use of the staple remover prevents accidental injury to the wound and contamination of the incision area and resulting infection.

ACTION	RATIONALE
13. Remove every other staple to be sure the wound edges are healed. If they are, remove the remaining staples as ordered. Dispose of staples in the sharps container.	Removing every other staple allows for inspection of the wound, while leaving an adequate number of staples in place to promote continued healing if the edges are not totally approximated.
14. If wound closure strips are to be used, apply skin protectant to skin around incision. **Do not apply to incision.** Apply adhesive closure strips. Take care to handle the strips by the paper backing.	Skin protectant helps adherence of closure strips and prevents skin irritation. Adhesive wound closure strips provide additional support to the wound as it continues to heal. Handling by the paper backing avoids contamination.
15. Reapply the dressing, depending on the medical orders and facility policy.	A new dressing protects the wound. Some policies advise leaving the area uncovered.
16. Remove gloves and discard. Remove all remaining equipment; place the patient in a comfortable position, with side rails up and bed in the lowest position.	Proper removal of gloves prevents spread of microorganisms. Proper patient and bed positioning promotes safety and comfort.
17. Remove additional PPE, if used. Perform hand hygiene.	Removing PPE properly reduces the risk for infection transmission and contamination of other items. Hand hygiene prevents the spread of microorganisms.
18. Assess all wounds every shift. More frequent checks may be needed if the wound is more complex.	Checking wound and dressings ensures the assessment of changes in patient condition and timely intervention to prevent complications.

EVALUATION

- Patient exhibits an incision area that is clean, dry, and intact without staples.
- Incision area is free of trauma and infection.
- Patient verbalizes little to no pain or discomfort during the removal.
- Patient verbalizes an understanding of the procedure.

DOCUMENTATION

- Document the location of the incision and the assessment of the site. Include the appearance of the surrounding skin. Document cleansing of the site and staple removal. Record any skin care and the dressing applied, if appropriate. Note pertinent patient and family education and any patient reaction to this procedure, including patient's pain level and effectiveness of nonpharmacologic interventions or analgesia if administered.

SKILL 153 ADDING STERILE ITEMS TO A STERILE FIELD

A sterile field is created to provide a surgically aseptic workspace. It should be considered a restricted area. After establishing the sterile field, add other sterile items, including solutions, as needed. Items can be wrapped and sterilized within the agency or commercially prepared. Take care to ensure that nothing unsterile touches the field or other items in the field, including hands or clothes.

DELEGATION CONSIDERATIONS

Procedures requiring the use of a sterile field and other sterile items are not delegated to nursing assistive personnel (NAP) or unlicensed assistive personnel (UAP). Depending on the state's nurse practice act and the organization's policies and procedures, these procedures may be delegated to licensed practical/vocational nurses (LPN/LVNs). The decision to delegate must be based on careful analysis of the patient's needs and circumstances, as well as the qualifications of the person to whom the task is being delegated. Refer to the Delegation Guidelines in Appendix A.

EQUIPMENT

- Sterile field
- Sterile gauze, forceps, dressings, containers, solutions,
- or other sterile supplies, as needed
- PPE, as indicated

ASSESSMENT

- Assess the situation to determine the necessity for creating a sterile field.
- Assess the area in which the sterile field is to be prepared. Move any unnecessary equipment out of the immediate vicinity.
- Identify additional supplies needed for the procedure.

NURSING DIAGNOSIS

- Risk for Infection
- Ineffective Protection

OUTCOME IDENTIFICATION AND PLANNING

- The sterile field is created without contamination and the sterile supplies are not contaminated.
- Patient remains free of exposure to potential infection-causing microorganisms.

IMPLEMENTATION

ACTION	RATIONALE
1. Perform hand hygiene and put on PPE, if indicated.	Hand hygiene and PPE prevent the spread of microorganisms. PPE is required based on transmission precautions.
2. Identify the patient. Explain the procedure to the patient.	Patient identification validates the correct patient and correct procedure. Discussion and explanation help allay anxiety and prepare the patient for what to expect.
3. Check that the sterile, packaged drape and supplies are dry and unopened. Also note expiration date, making sure that the date is still valid.	Moisture contaminates a sterile package. Expiration date indicates period that package remains sterile.
4. Select a work area that is waist level or higher.	Work area is within sight. Bacteria tend to settle, so there is less contamination above the waist.
5. Prepare sterile field as described in Skill 154 or Skill 155.	Proper technique maintains sterility.
6. Add sterile item: **To Add an Agency-Wrapped and Sterilized Item**	
a. Hold agency-wrapped item in the dominant hand, with top flap opening away from the body. With other hand, reach around the package and unfold top flap and both sides.	Only sterile surface and item are exposed before dropping onto sterile field.

ACTION	RATIONALE
b. Keep a secure hold on the item through the wrapper with the dominant hand. Grasp the remaining flap of the wrapper closest to the body, taking care not to touch the inner surface of the wrapper or the item. Pull the flap back toward the wrist, so the wrapper covers the hand and wrist.	Only sterile surface and item are exposed before dropping onto sterile field.
c. Grasp all the corners of the wrapper together with the nondominant hand and pull back toward wrist, covering hand and wrist. Hold in place.	Only sterile surface and item are exposed before dropping onto sterile field.
d. Hold the item 6 inches above the surface of the sterile field and drop onto the field. Be careful to avoid touching the surface or other items or dropping any item onto the 1-inch border.	This prevents contamination of the field and inadvertent dropping of the sterile item too close to the edge or off the field. Any items landing on the 1-inch border are considered contaminated.

To Add a Commercially Wrapped and Sterilized Item

ACTION	RATIONALE
a. Hold package in one hand. Pull back top cover with other hand. Alternately, carefully peel the edges apart using both hands.	Contents remain uncontaminated by hands.
b. After top cover or edges are partially separated, hold the item 6 inches above the surface of the sterile field. Continue opening the package and drop the item onto the field. **Be careful to avoid touching the surface or other items or dropping an item onto the 1-inch border.**	This prevents contamination of the field and inadvertent dropping of the sterile item too close to the edge or off the field. Any items landing on the 1-inch border are considered contaminated.

ACTION	RATIONALE
c. Discard wrapper.	A neat work area promotes proper technique and avoids inadvertent contamination of the field.

To Add a Sterile Solution

ACTION	RATIONALE
a. Obtain appropriate solution and check expiration date.	Once opened, label any bottles with date and time. Solution remains sterile for 24 hours once opened.
b. Open solution container according to directions and **place cap on table away from the field with edges up.**	Sterility of inside cap is maintained.
c. Hold bottle outside the edge of the sterile field with the label side facing the palm of your hand and prepare to pour from a height of 4 to 6 inches (10 to 15 cm). **Never touch the tip of the bottle to the sterile container or field.**	Label remains dry, and solution may be poured without reaching across sterile field. Minimal splashing occurs from that height. Accidentally touching the tip of the bottle to a container or dressing contaminates them both.
d. Pour required amount of solution steadily into sterile container previously added to the sterile field and positioned at side of sterile field or onto dressings. **Avoid splashing any liquid.**	A steady stream minimizes the risk of splashing; moisture contaminates sterile field.
e. Touch only the outside of the lid when recapping. Label solution with date and time of opening.	Solution remains uncontaminated and available for future use.
7. Continue with procedure as indicated.	
8. When procedure is completed, remove PPE, if used. Perform hand hygiene.	Removing PPE properly reduces the risk for infection transmission and contamination of other items. Hand hygiene prevents the spread of microorganisms.

EVALUATION
- Sterile field is created without contamination.
- Sterile supplies are not contaminated.
- Patient remains free of exposure to potential infection-causing microorganisms.

DOCUMENTATION
- It is not usually necessary to document the addition of sterile items to a sterile field. However, document the use of performing sterile technique for any procedure.

SKILL 154   PREPARING A STERILE FIELD USING A COMMERCIALLY PREPARED STERILE KIT OR TRAY

A sterile field is created to provide a surgically aseptic workspace. Consider it a restricted area. Commercially prepared sterile kits and trays are wrapped in a sterile wrapper that, once opened, becomes the sterile field. Sterile items and sterile gloved hands are the only objects allowed in the sterile field. If the area is breached, the entire sterile field is considered contaminated.

DELEGATION CONSIDERATIONS

Procedures requiring the use of a sterile field and other sterile items are not delegated to nursing assistive personnel (NAP) or to unlicensed assistive personnel (UAP). Depending on the state's nurse practice act and the organization's policies and procedures, these procedures may be delegated to licensed practical/vocational nurses (LPN/LVNs). The decision to delegate must be based on careful analysis of the patient's needs and circumstances, as well as the qualifications of the person to whom the task is being delegated. Refer to the Delegation Guidelines in Appendix A.

EQUIPMENT
- Commercially prepared sterile package
- Additional sterile supplies, such as dressings, containers, or solution, as needed
- PPE, as indicated

ASSESSMENT
- Assess the situation to determine the necessity for creating a sterile field.
- Assess the area in which the sterile field is to be prepared. Move any unnecessary equipment out of the immediate vicinity.

NURSING DIAGNOSIS

- Risk for Infection
- Ineffective Protection

OUTCOME IDENTIFICATION AND PLANNING

- A sterile field is created without contamination and the contents of the package remain sterile.
- Patient remains free of exposure to potential infection-causing microorganisms.

IMPLEMENTATION

ACTION	RATIONALE
1. Perform hand hygiene and put on PPE, if indicated.	Hand hygiene and PPE prevent the spread of microorganisms. PPE is required based on transmission precautions.
2. Identify the patient. Explain the procedure to the patient.	Patient identification validates the correct patient and correct procedure. Discussion and explanation help allay anxiety and prepare the patient for what to expect.
3. Check that the packaged kit or tray is dry and unopened. Also note expiration date, making sure that the date is still valid.	Moisture contaminates a sterile package. Expiration date indicates period that package remains sterile.
4. Select a work area that is waist level or higher.	Work area is within sight. Bacteria tend to settle, so there is less contamination above the waist.
5. Open the outside cover of the package and remove the kit or tray. Place in the center of the work surface, with the topmost flap positioned on the far side of the package. Discard outside cover.	This allows sufficient room for sterile field.
6. Reach around the package and grasp the outer surface of the end of the topmost flap, holding no more than	This maintains sterility of inside of wrapper, which is to become the sterile field. Outer surface of the wrapper is considered

1 inch from the border of the flap. Pull open away from the body, keeping the arm outstretched and away from the inside of the wrapper (Figure 1). Allow the wrapper to lie flat on the work surface.

unsterile. Outer 1-inch border of the wrapper is considered contaminated.

FIGURE 1 Pulling top flap open, away from body.

7. Reach around the package and grasp the outer surface of the first side flap, holding no more than 1 inch from the border of the flap. Pull open to the side of the package, keeping the arm outstretched and away from the inside of the wrapper (Figure 2). Allow the wrapper to lie flat on the work surface.

This maintains sterility of inside of wrapper, which is to become the sterile field. Outer surface of the wrapper is considered unsterile. Outer 1-inch border of the wrapper is considered contaminated.

FIGURE 2 Pulling open the first side flap.

8. Reach around the package and grasp the outer surface of the remaining side flap, holding no more than 1 inch from the border of the flap.

This maintains sterility of inside of wrapper, which is to become the sterile field. Outer surface of the wrapper is considered unsterile. Outer 1 inch of border

ACTION	RATIONALE

Pull open to the side of the package, keeping the arm outstretched and away from the inside of the wrapper (Figure 3). Allow the wrapper to lie flat on the work surface.

of the wrapper is considered contaminated.

9. Stand away from the package and work surface. Grasp the outer surface of the remaining flap closest to the body, holding not more than 1 inch from the border of the flap. Pull the flap back toward the body, keeping arm outstretched and away from the inside of the wrapper (Figure 4). Keep this hand in place. Use other hand to grasp the wrapper on the underside (the side that is down to the work surface). Position the wrapper so that when flat, edges are on the work surface, and do not hang down over sides of work surface. Allow the wrapper to lie flat on the work surface.

This maintains sterility of the inside of the wrapper, which is to become the sterile field. Outer surface of the wrapper is considered unsterile. Outer 1-inch border of the wrapper is considered contaminated.

FIGURE 3 Pulling open the remaining side flap.

FIGURE 4 Pulling open flap closest to body.

10. The outer wrapper of the package has become a sterile field with the packaged supplies in the center. Do not touch or reach over the sterile field. Place additional

Sterility of the field and contents are maintained.

ACTION	RATIONALE
sterile items on field as needed. Refer to Skill 153. Continue with the procedure as indicated.	
11. When procedure is completed, remove PPE, if used. Perform hand hygiene.	Removing PPE properly reduces the risk for infection transmission and contamination of other items. Hand hygiene prevents the spread of microorganisms.

EVALUATION

- The sterile field is prepared without contamination.
- The contents of the package remain sterile.
- Patient remains free of exposure to potential infection-causing microorganisms.

DOCUMENTATION

- It is not usually necessary to document the preparation of a sterile field. However, do document the use of sterile technique for any procedure performed using sterile technique.

SKILL 155 PREPARING A STERILE FIELD USING A PACKAGED STERILE DRAPE

A sterile field is created to provide a surgically aseptic workspace. It should be considered a restricted area. A sterile drape may be used to establish a sterile field or to extend the sterile working area. The sterile drape should be waterproof on one side, with that side placed down on the work surface. After establishing the sterile field, add other sterile items as needed, including solutions. Sterile items and sterile gloved hands are the only objects allowed in the sterile field.

DELEGATION CONSIDERATIONS

Procedures requiring the use of a sterile field and other sterile items are not delegated to nursing assistive personnel (NAP) or unlicensed assistive personnel (UAP). Depending on the state's nurse practice act and the organization's policies and procedures, these procedures may be delegated to licensed practical/vocational nurses (LPN/LVNs). The decision to delegate must be based on careful analysis of the patient's needs and circumstances, as well as the qualifications of the person to

whom the task is being delegated. Refer to the Delegation Guidelines in Appendix A.

EQUIPMENT

- Sterile wrapped drape
- Additional sterile supplies, such as dressings,
- containers, or solution, as needed
- PPE, as indicated

ASSESSMENT

- Assess the situation to determine the necessity for creating a sterile field.
- Assess the area in which the sterile field is to be prepared. Move any unnecessary equipment out of the immediate vicinity.

NURSING DIAGNOSIS

- Risk for Infection
- Ineffective Protection

OUTCOME IDENTIFICATION AND PLANNING

- The sterile field is created without contamination.
- Patient remains free of exposure to potential infection-causing microorganisms.

IMPLEMENTATION

ACTION	RATIONALE
1. Perform hand hygiene and put on PPE, if indicated.	Hand hygiene and PPE prevent the spread of microorganisms. PPE is required based on transmission precautions.
2. Identify the patient. Explain the procedure to the patient.	Patient identification validates the correct patient and correct procedure. Discussion and explanation help allay anxiety and prepare the patient for what to expect.
3. Check that packaged sterile drape is dry and unopened. Also note expiration date, making sure that the date is still valid.	Moisture contaminates a sterile package. Expiration date indicates period that package remains sterile.
4. Select a work area that is waist level or higher.	Work area is within sight. Bacteria tend to settle, so there is less contamination above the waist.

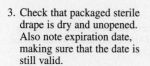

ACTION	RATIONALE
5. Open the outer covering of the drape. Remove sterile drape, lifting it carefully by its corners. Hold away from body and above the waist and work surface.	Outer 1 inch (2.5 cm) of drape is considered contaminated. Any item touching this area is also considered contaminated.
6. Continue to hold only by the corners. Allow the drape to unfold, away from your body and any other surface.	Touching the outer side of the wrapper maintains the sterile field. Contact with any surface would contaminate the field.
7. Position the drape on the work surface with the moisture-proof side down. This would be the shiny or blue side. Avoid touching any other surface or object with the drape. If any portion of the drape hangs off the work surface, that part of the drape is considered contaminated.	Moisture-proof side prevents contamination of the field if it becomes wet. The moisture penetrates the sterile cloth or paper and carries organisms by capillary action to contaminate the field. A wet field is considered contaminated if the surface immediately below it is not sterile.
8. Place additional sterile items on field as needed. Refer to Skill 153. Continue with the procedure as indicated.	Sterility of the field is maintained.
9. When procedure is completed, remove PPE, if used. Perform hand hygiene.	Removing PPE properly reduces the risk for infection transmission and contamination of other items. Hand hygiene prevents the spread of microorganisms.

EVALUATION
• The sterile field is prepared without contamination.
• Patient has remained free of exposure to potentially infectious microorganisms.

DOCUMENTATION
• It is not usually necessary to document the preparation of a sterile field. However, document the use of sterile technique for any procedure performed using sterile technique.

SKILL 156 EMPTYING AND CHANGING A STOMA APPLIANCE ON AN ILEAL CONDUIT

An ileal conduit is a cutaneous urinary diversion. An ileal conduit involves a surgical resection of the small intestine, with transplantation of the ureters to the isolated segment of small bowel. This separated section of the small intestine is then brought to the abdominal wall, where urine is excreted through a stoma, a surgically created opening on the body surface. Such diversions are usually permanent, and the patient wears an external appliance to collect the urine because urine elimination from the stoma cannot be controlled voluntarily. Appliances are available in a one-piece (barrier backing already attached to the pouch) or two-piece (separate pouch that fastens to the barrier backing) system; they are usually changed every 3 to 7 days, although they could be changed more often. Proper application minimizes the risk for skin breakdown around the stoma. This skill addresses changing a one-piece appliance. A one-piece appliance consists of a pouch with an integral adhesive section that adheres to the patient's skin. The adhesive flange is generally made from hydrocolloid. The accompanying Skill Variation addresses changing a two-piece appliance.

The appliance usually is changed after a time of low fluid intake, such as in the early morning. Urine production is less at this time, making changing the appliance easier. Proper application minimizes the risk for skin breakdown around the stoma.

DELEGATION CONSIDERATIONS

The empting of a stoma appliance on an ileal conduit may be delegated to nursing assistive personnel (NAP) or to unlicensed assistive personnel (UAP), as well as to licensed practical/vocational nurses (LPN/LVNs). The changing of a stoma appliance on an ileal conduit may be delegated to LPN/LVNs. The decision to delegate must be based on careful analysis of the patient's needs and circumstances, as well as the qualifications of the person to whom the task is being delegated. Refer to the Delegation Guidelines in Appendix A.

EQUIPMENT

- Basin with warm water
- Skin cleanser, towel, washcloth
- Silicone-based adhesive remover
- Gauze squares
- Skin protectant, such as SkinPrep
- Ostomy appliance
- Stoma measuring guide
- Graduated container
- Ostomy belt (optional)
- Disposable gloves
- Additional PPE, as indicated
- Waterproof, disposable pad
- Small plastic trash bag

ASSESSMENT

- Assess current ileal conduit appliance, observing product style, condition of appliance, and stoma (if bag is clear). Note length of time the appliance has been in place.
- Determine the patient's knowledge of ileal conduit care, including level of self-care and ability to manipulate the equipment.
- After the appliance is removed, assess the skin surrounding the ileal conduit.
- Assess the condition of any abdominal scars or incisional areas, if surgery to create the urinary diversion was recent.

NURSING DIAGNOSIS

- Disturbed Body Image
- Risk for Impaired Skin Integrity
- Deficient Knowledge

OUTCOME IDENTIFICATION AND PLANNING

- Stoma appliance is applied correctly to the skin to allow urine to drain freely.
- Patient exhibits a moist red stoma with intact skin surrounding the stoma.
- Patient demonstrates knowledge of how to apply the appliance.
- Patient verbalizes positive self-image.

IMPLEMENTATION

ACTION	RATIONALE
1. Gather equipment.	Assembling equipment provides for an organized approach to task.
2. Perform hand hygiene and put on PPE, if indicated.	Hand hygiene and PPE prevent the spread of microorganisms. PPE is required based on transmission precautions.
3. Identify the patient.	Identifying the patient ensures the right patient receives the intervention and helps prevent errors.
4. Close the curtains around the bed and close the door to the room, if possible. Explain what you are going to do and	This ensures the patient's privacy. Explanation relieves anxiety and facilitates cooperation. Discussion promotes cooperation and helps

ACTION	RATIONALE
why you are going to do it to the patient. Encourage the patient to observe or participate, if possible.	to minimize anxiety. Having the patient observe or assist encourages self-acceptance.
5. Assemble equipment on overbed table within reach.	Arranging items nearby is convenient, saves time, and avoids unnecessary stretching and twisting of muscles on the part of the nurse.
6. Assist the patient to a comfortable sitting or lying position in bed or a standing or sitting position in the bathroom. If the patient is in bed, adjust the bed to a comfortable working height, usually elbow height of the caregiver (VISN 8 Patient Safety Center, 2009). Place waterproof pad under the patient at the stoma site.	Either position should allow the patient to view the procedure in preparation for learning to perform it independently. Lying flat or sitting upright facilitates smooth application of the appliance. Having the bed at the proper height prevents back and muscle strain. A waterproof pad protects linens and the patient from moisture.

Emptying the Appliance

ACTION	RATIONALE
7. Put on gloves. Hold end of appliance over a bedpan, toilet, or measuring device. Remove the end cap from the spout. Open spout and empty the contents into the bedpan, toilet, or measuring device.	Gloves protect the nurse from exposure to blood and body fluids. Emptying the pouch before handling it reduces the likelihood of spilling the excretions.
8. Close the spout. Wipe the spout with toilet tissue. Replace the cap.	Drying the spout removes any urine.
9. Remove equipment. Remove gloves. Assist the patient to a comfortable position.	Proper removal of PPE prevents the transmission of microorganisms. Ensures patient comfort.
10. If appliance is not to be changed, place bed in lowest position. Remove additional PPE, if used. Perform hand hygiene.	Lowering the bed promotes patient safety. Removing PPE properly reduces the risk for infection transmission and contamination of other items. Hand hygiene prevents the spread of microorganisms.

ACTION	RATIONALE

Changing the Appliance

11. Place a disposable water-proof pad on the overbed table or other work area. Set up the washbasin with warm water and the rest of the supplies. Place a trash bag within reach.

The pad protects the surface. Organization facilitates performance of the procedure.

12. Put on clean gloves. Place waterproof pad under the patient at the stoma site. Empty the appliance if necessary as described in steps 6–8.

Waterproof pad protects linens and patient from moisture. Emptying the contents before removal prevents accidental spillage of fecal material.

13. Gently remove the appliance faceplate, starting at the top and keeping the abdominal skin taut. Remove appliance faceplate from skin by pushing skin from appliance rather than pulling appliance from skin. Apply a silicone-based adhesive remover by spraying or wiping with the remover wipe as needed.

The seal between the surface of the faceplate and the skin must be broken before the faceplate can be removed. Harsh handling of the appliance can damage the skin and impair the development of a secure seal in the future. Silicone-based adhesive remover allows for the rapid and painless removal of adhesives and prevents skin stripping (Rudoni, 2008; Stephen-Haynes, 2008).

14. Place the appliance in the trash bag, if disposable. If reusable, set aside to wash in lukewarm soap and water and allow to air dry after the new appliance is in place.

Thorough cleaning and airing of the appliance reduce odor and deterioration of appliance. For aesthetic and infection-control purposes, used appliances should be discarded appropriately.

15. Clean skin around stoma with mild skin cleanser and water or a cleansing agent and a washcloth. Remove all old adhesive from the skin; additional adhesive remover may be used. Do not apply lotion to the peristomal area.

Cleaning the skin removes excretions and old adhesive and skin protectant. Excretions or a buildup of other substances can irritate and damage the skin. Lotion will prevent a tight adhesive seal.

16. Gently pat area dry. **Make sure skin around stoma is thoroughly dry.** Assess

Careful drying prevents trauma to skin and stoma. An intact, properly applied urinary

ACTION	RATIONALE
stoma and condition of surrounding skin.	collection device protects skin integrity. Any change in color and size of the stoma may indicate circulatory problems.
17. Place one or two gauze squares over the stoma opening.	Continuous drainage must be absorbed to keep skin dry during appliance change.
18. Apply skin protectant to a 2-inch (5-cm) radius around the stoma, and allow it to dry completely, which takes about 30 seconds.	The skin needs protection from the potentially excoriating effect of the appliance adhesive. The skin must be perfectly dry before the appliance is placed to get good adherence and to prevent leaks.
19. Lift the gauze squares for a moment and measure the stoma opening, using the measurement guide. Replace the gauze. Trace the same size opening on the back center of the appliance. Cut the opening 1/8 inch larger than the stoma size. Use a finger to gently smooth the wafer edges after cutting. Check that the spout is closed and the end cap is in place.	The appliance should fit snugly around the stoma, with only 1/8 inch of skin visible around the opening. A faceplate opening that is too small can cause trauma to the stoma. If the opening is too large, exposed skin will be irritated by urine. Wafer edges may be uneven after cutting and could cause irritation to and/or pressure on the stoma. A closed spout and secured end cap prevent urine from leaking from the appliance.
20. Remove the paper backing from the appliance faceplate. Quickly remove the gauze squares and discard appropriately; ease the appliance over the stoma. Gently press onto the skin while smoothing over the surface. Apply gentle, even pressure to the appliance for approximately 30 seconds.	The appliance is effective only if it is properly positioned and adhered securely. Pressure on faceplate allows the faceplate to mold to the patient's skin and improves the seal.
21. Secure optional belt to appliance and around patient.	An elasticized belt helps support the appliance for some people.
22. Remove gloves. Assist the patient to a comfortable position. Cover the patient with bed linens. Place the bed in the lowest position.	Removing gloves reduces risk of transmission of microorganisms. Positioning and covering provide warmth and promote comfort. Bed in lowest position promotes patient safety.

ACTION	RATIONALE
23. Put on clean gloves. Remove or discard any remaining equipment and assess the patient's response to the procedure.	The patient's response may indicate acceptance of the ostomy as well as the need for health teaching.
24. Remove gloves and additional PPE, if used. Perform hand hygiene.	Removing PPE properly reduces the risk for infection transmission and contamination of other items. Hand hygiene prevents the spread of microorganisms.

EVALUATION
- Ileal conduit appliance is changed without trauma to the stoma or peristomal skin, or leaking.
- Urine is draining freely into the appliance.
- Skin surrounding the stoma is clean, dry, and intact.
- Patient shows an interest in learning to perform the appliance change and verbalizes positive self-image.

DOCUMENTATION
- Document the procedure, including the appearance of the stoma, condition of the peristomal skin, characteristics of the urine, the patient's response to the procedure, and pertinent patient teaching.

SKILL VARIATION | **Applying a Two-Piece Appliance**

A two-piece colostomy appliance is composed of a pouch and a separate adhesive faceplate that 'click' together. The faceplate is left in place for a period of time, usually 3 to 7 days. During this period, when the appliance requires changing, only the bag needs to be replaced.

1. Gather necessary equipment.
2. Perform hand hygiene and put on PPE, if indicated.

3. Identify the patient.

4. Close the curtains around the bed and close the door to room, if possible. Explain what you are going to do and why you are going to do it to the patient. Encourage the patient to observe or participate, if possible.
5. Assemble equipment on overbed table within reach.

6. Assist the patient to a comfortable sitting or lying position in bed or a standing or sitting position in the bathroom.

7. Place a disposable pad on the work surface. Set up the washbasin with warm water and the rest of the supplies. Place a trash bag within reach.

8. Put on gloves. Place waterproof pad under the patient at the stoma site. Empty the appliance as described previously in Skill 156 above.

9. Gently remove pouch faceplate from skin by pushing skin from appliance rather than pulling appliance from skin. Start at the top of the appliance, while keeping the abdominal skin taut. Apply a silicone-based adhesive remover by spraying or wiping with the remover wipe. Push the skin from the appliance rather than pulling the appliance from the skin.

10. Place the appliance in the trash bag, if disposable. If reusable, set aside to wash in lukewarm soap and water and allow to air dry after the new appliance is in place.

11. Clean skin around the stoma with a mild skin cleanser and water or a cleansing agent and a washcloth. Remove all old adhesive from skin; additional adhesive remover may be used. Do not apply lotion to peristomal area.

12. Gently pat area dry. Make sure skin around the stoma is thoroughly dry. Assess stoma and condition of surrounding skin. Place one or two gauze squares over stoma opening.

13. Apply skin protectant to a 2-inch (5 cm) radius around the stoma, and allow it to dry completely, which takes about 30 seconds.

14. Lift the gauze squares for a moment and measure the stoma opening, using the measurement guide. Replace the gauze. Trace the same-size opening on the back center of the appliance faceplate. Cut the opening 1/8 inch larger than the stoma size. Use a finger to gently smooth the wafer edges after cutting.

15. Remove the backing from the faceplate. Quickly remove the gauze squares and ease the faceplate over the stoma. Gently press onto the skin while smoothing over the surface. Apply gentle pressure to the faceplate for approximately 30 seconds.

16. Apply the appliance pouch to the faceplate following manufacturer's directions. Check that the spout is closed and the end cap is in place. If using a 'click' system, lay the ring on the

continued on page 816

pouch over the ring on the faceplate. Ask the patient to tighten stomach muscles, if possible. Beginning at one edge of the ring, push the pouch ring onto the faceplate ring. A 'click' should be heard when the pouch is secured onto the faceplate.

17. Remove gloves. Assist the patient to a comfortable position. Cover the patient with bed linens. Place the bed in the lowest position.

18. Put on clean gloves. Remove or discard equipment and assess the patient's response to the procedure.

19. Remove gloves and additional PPE, if used. Perform hand hygiene.

SKILL 157 COLLECTING A STOOL SPECIMEN FOR CULTURE

A stool specimen may be ordered to screen for pathogenic organisms, such as *Clostridium difficile* or ova and parasites, electrolytes, fat, and leukocytes. The nurse is responsible for obtaining the specimen according to facility procedure, labeling the specimen, and ensuring that the specimen is transported to the laboratory in a timely manner. The facility's policy and procedure manual or laboratory manual identifies specific information about the amount of stool needed, the time frame during which stool is to be collected, and the type of specimen container to use.

Usually, 1 inch (2.5 cm) of formed stool or 15 to 30 mL of liquid stool is sufficient. If portions of the stool include visible blood, mucus, or pus, include these with the specimen. Also be sure that the specimen is free of any barium or enema solution. Because a fresh specimen produces the most accurate results, send the specimen to the laboratory immediately. If this is not possible, refrigerate it unless contraindicated, such as when testing for ova and parasites. Refrigeration will affect parasites. Ova and parasites are best detected in warm stool. Some institutions require ova and parasite specimens to be placed in a container filled with preservatives; consult facility policy.

DELEGATION CONSIDERATIONS

Obtaining a stool specimen may be delegated to nursing assistive personnel (NAP) or to unlicensed assistive personnel (UAP), as well as to licensed practical/vocational nurses (LPN/LVNs). The decision to delegate must be based on careful analysis of the patient's needs and circumstances, as well as the qualifications of the person to whom the task is being delegated. Refer to the Delegation Guidelines in Appendix A.

EQUIPMENT

- Tongue blade (2)
- Clean specimen container (or container with preservatives for ova and parasites)
- Biohazard bag
- Nonsterile gloves
- Additional PPE, as indicated
- Appropriate label for specimen, based on facility policy and procedure

ASSESSMENT

- Assess the patient's understanding of the need for the test and the requirements of the test.
- Assess the patient's understanding of the collection procedure and ability to cooperate.
- Ask the patient when his or her last bowel movement was, and check the patient's medical record for this information.

NURSING DIAGNOSIS

- Deficient Knowledge
- Diarrhea
- Anxiety

OUTCOME IDENTIFICATION AND PLANNING

- Uncontaminated specimen is obtained and sent to the laboratory promptly.
- Patient demonstrates the ability to collect a stool specimen and verbalizes a decrease in anxiety related to stool collection.

IMPLEMENTATION

ACTION	RATIONALE
1. Verify the order for a stool specimen collection in the medical record. Gather equipment.	Verifying the medical order is crucial to ensuring that the proper procedure is administered to the right patient. Assembling equipment provides for an organized approach to the task.
2. Perform hand hygiene and put on PPE, if indicated.	Hand hygiene and PPE prevent the transmission of microorganisms. PPE is required based on transmission precautions.
3. Identify the patient.	Identifying the patient ensures the right patient receives the intervention and helps prevent errors.

ACTION	RATIONALE
4. Discuss with the patient the need for a stool sample. Explain to the patient the process by which the stool will be collected, either from a bedpan, commode, or plastic receptacle in the toilet to catch stool without urine. Instruct the patient to void first and not to discard toilet paper with stool. Tell the patient to call you as soon as a bowel movement is completed.	Discussion and explanation help to allay some of the patient's anxiety and prepare the patient for what to expect. The patient should void first because the laboratory study may be inaccurate if the stool contains urine. Placing a container in the toilet or bedside commode aids in obtaining a clean stool specimen uncontaminated by urine.
5. Check specimen label with the patient's identification bracelet. Label should include the patient's name and identification number, time specimen was collected, route of collection, identification of the person obtaining the sample, and any other information required by facility policy.	Confirmation of patient identification information ensures the specimen is labeled correctly for the right patient.
6. Assemble equipment on overbed table within reach.	Arranging items nearby is convenient, saves time, and avoids unnecessary stretching and twisting of muscles on the part of the nurse.
7. After the patient has passed a stool, put on gloves. Use the tongue blades to obtain a sample, free of blood or urine, and place it in the designated clean container.	The container does not have to be sterile, because stool is not sterile. To ensure accurate results, the stool should be free of urine or menstrual blood.
8. Collect as much of the stool as possible to send to the laboratory.	Different tests and laboratories require different amounts of stool. Collecting as much as possible helps to ensure that the laboratory has an adequate amount of specimen for testing.

ACTION	RATIONALE
9. Place lid on container. Dispose of used equipment per facility policy. Remove gloves and perform hand hygiene.	Proper disposal of equipment reduces the transmission of microorganisms. Removing gloves properly reduces the risk for infection transmission and contamination of other items. Hand hygiene deters the spread of microorganisms.
10. Place label on the container per facility policy. Place container in plastic, sealable biohazard bag.	Correct labeling is necessary to ensure accurate results. Packaging the specimen in a biohazard bag prevents the person transporting the container from coming in contact with stool.
11. Remove other PPE, if used. Perform hand hygiene.	Removing PPE properly reduces the risk for infection transmission and contamination of other items. Hand hygiene reduces the transmission of microorganisms.
12. Transport the specimen to the laboratory while stool is still warm. If immediate transport is impossible, check with laboratory personnel or policy manual whether refrigeration is contraindicated.	Most tests have better results with fresh stool. Different tests may require different preparation if the test is not immediately completed. Some tests will be compromised if the stool is refrigerated.

EVALUATION

• Patient passes a stool that is not contaminated by urine or menstrual blood and is placed in a clean container.
• Specimen is transported appropriately to the laboratory.
• Patient participates in stool collection and verbalizes feelings of diminished anxiety related to the procedure.

DOCUMENTATION

• Document amount, color, and consistency of stool obtained, time of collection, specific test for which the specimen was collected, and transport to laboratory.

When a patient develops a fecal impaction (prolonged retention or an accumulation of fecal material that forms a hardened mass in the rectum), the stool must sometimes be broken up manually. However, before digital removal of feces is considered, dietary interventions, adequate fluids, and medication adjustment should be included in the patient's plan of care (Ness et al., 2012; Kyle et al., 2004). Digital removal of stool is very uncomfortable and may cause great discomfort to the patient as well as irritation of the rectal mucosa and bleeding. The primary care provider may order an oil-retention enema to be given before the procedure to soften stool. In addition, many patients find that a sitz bath or tub bath after this procedure soothes the irritated perineal area.

DELEGATION CONSIDERATIONS

Digital removal of stool is not delegated to nursing assistive personnel (NAP) or to unlicensed assistive personnel (UAP). Depending on the state's nurse practice act and the organization's policies and procedures, the administration of a small-volume cleansing enema may be delegated to licensed practical/vocational nurses (LPN/LVNs). The decision to delegate must be based on careful analysis of the patient's needs and circumstances, as well as the qualifications of the person to whom the task is being delegated. Refer to the Delegation Guidelines in Appendix A.

EQUIPMENT

- Disposable gloves
- Additional PPE, as indicated
- Water-soluble lubricant
- Waterproof pad
- Bath blanket
- Bedpan
- Toilet paper, washcloth, skin cleanser, and towel
- Sitz bath (optional)

ASSESSMENT

- Verify the time of the patient's last bowel movement by asking the patient and checking the patient's medical record.
- Assess the abdomen, including auscultating for bowel sounds, and palpating for tenderness and/or firmness.
- Inspect the rectal area for any fissures, hemorrhoids, sores, or rectal tears. If any of these are noted, consult the prescriber for the appropriateness of the intervention.
- Assess the results of the patient's laboratory work, specifically the platelet count and WBC count. Digital removal of stool is contraindicated for patients with a low platelet count or low WBC count. Digital removal of stool may irritate or traumatize the GI mucosa, causing bleeding, bowel perforation, or infection. Do not perform any unnecessary procedures that would place the patient at risk for bleeding or infection.

- Assess for dizziness, light-headedness, diaphoresis, and clammy skin.
- Assess pulse rate and blood pressure before and after the procedure. The procedure may stimulate a vagal response, which increases parasympathetic stimulation, causing a decrease in heart rate and blood pressure.
- Do not perform digital removal of stool on patients who have bowel inflammation or bowel infection, or after rectal, prostate, and colon surgery.

NURSING DIAGNOSIS

- Constipation
- Acute Pain
- Risk for Injury

OUTCOME IDENTIFICATION AND PLANNING

- Patient will expel feces with assistance.
- Patient verbalizes decreased discomfort.
- Abdominal distention is absent.
- Patient remains free of any evidence of trauma to the rectal mucosa or other adverse effect.

IMPLEMENTATION

ACTION	RATIONALE
1. Verify the order for digital removal of stool. Gather equipment.	Digital removal of stool is considered an invasive procedure and requires a medical order. Verifying the medical order is crucial to ensuring that the proper procedure is administered to the right patient. Assembling equipment provides for an organized approach to the task.
2. Perform hand hygiene and put on PPE, if indicated.	Hand hygiene and PPE prevent the spread of microorganisms. PPE is required based on transmission precautions.
3. Identify the patient.	Identifying the patient ensures the right patient receives the intervention and helps prevent errors.

ACTION	RATIONALE
4. Explain the procedure to the patient and provide the rationale why the procedure is needed. Discuss the associated discomforts that may be experienced. Discuss signs and symptoms of a slow heart rate. Instruct the patient to alert you if any of these symptoms are felt during the procedure. Have a bedpan ready for use.	Explanation relieves anxiety and facilitates cooperation. The patient is better able to relax and cooperate if he or she is familiar with the procedure.
5. Assemble equipment on overbed table within reach.	Arranging items nearby is convenient, saves time, and avoids unnecessary stretching and twisting of muscles on the part of the nurse.
6. Close the curtains around the bed and close the door to the room, if possible. Discuss where the patient will defecate, if necessary. Have a bedpan, commode, or nearby bathroom ready for use.	This ensures the patient's privacy. Explanation relieves anxiety and facilitates cooperation. The patient is better able to relax and cooperate if he or she is familiar with the procedure and knows everything is in readiness if the urge to defecate is felt.
7. Adjust the bed to a comfortable working height, usually elbow height of the caregiver (VISN 8 Patient Safety Center, 2009). Position the patient on the left side (Sims' position), as dictated by patient comfort and condition. Fold top linen back just enough to allow access to the patient's rectal area. Drape the patient with the bath blanket, as necessary, to maintain privacy and provide warmth. Place a waterproof pad under the patient's hip.	Having the bed at the proper height prevents back and muscle strain. Sims' position facilitates access into the rectum and colon. Folding back the linen in this manner minimizes unnecessary exposure and promotes the patient's comfort and warmth. The waterproof pad will protect the bed.
8. Put on nonsterile gloves.	Gloves prevent contact with blood and body fluids, as well as feces.
9. Generously lubricate index finger of dominant hand with	Lubrication reduces irritation of the rectum. The presence of the

ACTION	RATIONALE
water-soluble lubricant and insert finger gently into anal canal, pointing toward the umbilicus.	finger added to the mass tends to cause discomfort for the patient if the work is not done slowly and gently.
10. Gently work the finger around and into the hardened mass to break it up and then remove pieces of it. Instruct patient to bear down, if possible, while extracting feces to ease in removal. Place extracted stool in bedpan.	Fecal mass may be large and may need to be removed in smaller pieces.
11. Remove impaction at intervals if it is severe. **Instruct the patient to alert you if he or she begins to feel light-headed or nauseated. If patient reports either symptom, stop removal and assess the patient.**	Removal of stool in intervals helps to prevent discomfort and irritation, and vagal nerve stimulation. Assessment allows for detection of a vagal response. The enema may stimulate a vagal response, which increases parasympathetic stimulation, causing a decrease in heart rate.
12. When the procedure is completed, put on clean gloves. Assist the patient, if necessary, with cleaning of anal area. Offer washcloth, skin cleanser, and water for handwashing. If the patient is able, offer sitz bath.	Cleaning deters the transmission of microorganisms and promotes hygiene. Sitz bath may relieve the irritated perianal area.
13. Remove gloves. Return the patient to a comfortable position. Make sure the linens under the patient are dry. Ensure that the patient is covered.	Removing contaminated gloves prevents spread of microorganisms. The other actions promote patient comfort.
14. Raise side rail. Lower bed height and adjust head of bed to a comfortable position.	These promote patient safety.
15. Remove additional PPE, if used. Perform hand hygiene.	Removing PPE properly reduces the risk for infection transmission and contamination of other items. Hand hygiene prevents the spread of microorganisms.

EVALUATION

- Fecal impaction is removed and the patient expels feces with assistance.
- Patient verbalizes decreased discomfort.
- Abdominal distention is absent.
- Patient remains free of any evidence of trauma to the rectal mucosa or other adverse effect.

DOCUMENTATION

- Document the following: abdominal assessment; color, consistency, and amount of stool removed; condition of perianal area after the procedure; pain assessment rating; and the patient's reaction to the procedure.

SKILL 159 | TESTING STOOL FOR OCCULT BLOOD

Fecal occult blood testing (FOBT) is used to detect occult blood in the stool. It is used for initial screening for disorders such as cancer and for gastrointestinal bleeding in conditions such as ulcer disease, inflammatory bowel disorders, and intestinal polyps. Three consecutive stool samples should be collected over several days to provide the most effective screening for colon cancer (AACC, 2013). FOBT may be performed within an institution, collected at the bedside and sent to the laboratory for analysis. They may also be collected by the patient at home and delivered or mailed to the health care provider's office or to the laboratory for analysis.

The *guaiac fecal occult blood test* (gFOBT) is a chemical test that detects the enzyme peroxidase in hemoglobin molecules when blood is present in the stool sample. A positive gFOBT result indicates that abnormal bleeding is occurring somewhere in the digestive tract. Ingestion of certain substances before the specimen collection can result in false–positive results. These substances include red meat, salmon, tuna, mackerel, sardines, tomatoes, broccoli, turnips, cauliflower, horseradish, apples, oranges, mushrooms, melon, bananas, and soybeans. Certain medications, such as a salicylate intake of more than 325 mg daily, other nonsteroidal anti-inflammatory drugs, steroids, iron preparations, and anticoagulants, also may lead to false–positive readings (AACC, 2013; Fischbach & Dunning, 2009). Vitamin C ingestion can produce false–negative results even if bleeding is present. Avoid the foods (for 3 days) and drugs (for 7 days) that may alter test results (if clinically possible).

The *immunochemical fecal occult blood test* (iFOBT or FIT) uses antibodies directed against human hemoglobin to detect blood in the stool. A positive iFOBT test indicates abnormal bleeding in the lower digestive tract. It cannot detect hemoglobin that came from bleeding sites in the upper gastrointestinal tract or small intestine. Because this test detects only human hemoglobin, other sources of blood, such as from the diet, do not cause a positive result. No dietary or drug restrictions are related to the iFOBT.

DELEGATION CONSIDERATIONS

Obtaining a stool specimen for FOBT may be delegated to nursing assistive personnel (NAP) or to unlicensed assistive personnel (UAP), as well as to licensed practical/vocational nurses (LPN/LVNs). Developing the FOBT at the point-of-care is not delegated to nursing assistive personnel (NAP) or to unlicensed assistive personnel (UAP). Developing the FOBT at the point-of-care may be delegated to LPN/LVNs. The decision to delegate must be based on careful analysis of the patient's needs and circumstances, as well as the qualifications of the person to whom the task is being delegated. Refer to the Delegation Guidelines in Appendix A.

EQUIPMENT

- Nonsterile gloves; other PPE as indicated
- Wooden applicator
- gFOBT: Wooden applicator, testing card, and developer (if processing is being done at point-of-care)
- iFOBT: Applicator stick or brush, depending on collection kit in use

- Bedpan, or plastic collection receptacle for commode or toilet
- Biohazard bag
- Appropriate label for specimen, based on facility policy and procedure

ASSESSMENT

- Assess the patient's understanding of the collection procedure and ability to cooperate.
- Assess the patient for a history of gastrointestinal bleeding. Review prescribed restrictions for medications and diet, and evaluate patient compliance with required restrictions.
- Assess patient for any blood in the perineal area, including hemorrhoids, menstruation, urinary tract infection, or vaginal or rectal tears. Blood may be from a source other than the gastrointestinal tract.

NURSING DIAGNOSIS

- Deficient Knowledge
- Anxiety

OUTCOME IDENTIFICATION AND PLANNING

- Uncontaminated stool sample is obtained, following collection guidelines, and then transported to the laboratory within the recommended time frame, without adverse effect.

- Patient demonstrates accurate understanding of testing instructions.
- Specimen is obtained with minimal discomfort or embarrassment.

IMPLEMENTATION

ACTION	RATIONALE
1. Verify the order for a stool specimen collection in the medical record. Gather equipment.	Verifying the medical order is crucial to ensuring that the proper procedure is administered to the right patient. Assembling equipment provides for an organized approach to the task.
2. Perform hand hygiene and put on PPE, if indicated.	Hand hygiene and PPE prevent the transmission of microorganisms. PPE is required based on transmission precautions.
3. Identify the patient.	Identifying the patient ensures the right patient receives the intervention and helps prevent errors.
4. Discuss with the patient the need for a stool sample. Explain to the patient the process by which the stool will be collected, either from a bedpan, commode, or plastic receptacle in the toilet.	Discussion and explanation help to allay some of the patient's anxiety and prepare the patient for what to expect.
5. If sending the specimen to the laboratory, check the specimen label with patient identification bracelet. Label should include the patient's name and identification number, time specimen was collected, route of collection, identification of the person obtaining the sample, and any other information required by facility policy.	Facilities may allow point-of-service testing (at bedside or on unit) or the specimen may have to be sent to the laboratory for testing. Confirmation of patient identification information ensures the specimen is labeled correctly for the right patient.
6. Assemble equipment on overbed table within reach.	Arranging items nearby is convenient, saves time, and avoids unnecessary stretching and twisting of muscles on the part of the nurse.

ACTION	RATIONALE
7. Close curtains around the bed or close the door to the room, if possible.	Closing the door or curtain provides for patient privacy.
8. Place the plastic collection receptacle in the toilet, if applicable. Assist the patient to the bathroom or onto the bedside commode or onto the bedpan. Instruct the patient not to urinate or discard toilet paper with the stool.	Proper collection into an appropriate receptacle for stool prevents inaccurate results. Urine or toilet paper can contaminate the specimen, interfering with accurate results.
9. After the patient defecates, assist the patient out of the bathroom, off the commode, or remove the bedpan. Perform hand hygiene and put on disposable gloves.	Hand hygiene deters the spread of microorganisms. Gloves protect the nurse from microorganisms in feces.

If using gFOBT:

ACTION	RATIONALE
10. Open flap on sample side of card. **With wooden applicator, apply a small amount of stool from the center of the bowel movement onto one window of the testing card. With the opposite end of the wooden applicator, obtain another sample of stool from another area and apply a small amount of stool onto second window of testing card.**	Two separate areas of the same stool sample are tested to ensure accuracy. By using opposite ends of the wooden applicator, cross-contamination is avoided.
11. Close flap over stool samples.	Closing the flap prevents contamination of the samples.
12. If sending stool to the laboratory, label the specimen card per facility policy. Place in a sealable plastic biohazard bag and send to the laboratory immediately.	Facilities may allow point-of-service testing (at bedside or on unit) or the specimen may have to be sent to the laboratory for testing. Correct labeling is necessary to ensure accurate results. Packaging the specimen in a biohazard bag prevents the person transporting the container from coming in contact with the specimen.

ACTION	RATIONALE
13. If testing at the point-of-care, wait 3 to 5 minutes before developing. Open flap on opposite side of card and **place two drops of developer over each window and wait the time stated in the manufacturer's instructions.**	If immediate testing is required, waiting 3 to 5 minutes before developing allows adequate time for the sample to penetrate the test paper (Beckman Coulter, 2009a). The developer will react with any blood in the stool. Following the manufacturer's instructions promotes accuracy of results.
14. Observe card for any blue areas.	Any blue coloring on the card indicates a positive test result for blood.

If using iFOBT:

ACTION	RATIONALE
15. Open flap on sample side of card. **With applicator, brush, or sampling probe, apply a small amount of stool from the center of the bowel movement onto the top half of window of the testing card. With the opposite end of the device, obtain another sample of stool from another area and apply a small amount of stool onto the bottom half of window of testing card.**	Two separate areas of the same stool sample are tested to ensure accuracy. By using opposite ends of the wooden applicator, cross-contamination is avoided.
16. Spread samples over entire window by pressing gently with device while mixing thoroughly. Close flap over sample (Beckman Coulter, 2009c). Allow card to dry.	Drying of sample stabilizes hemoglobin, if present.
17. If sending to the laboratory, label the specimen card per facility policy. Place in a sealable plastic biohazard bag and send to the laboratory immediately.	Facilities may allow point-of-service testing (at bedside or on unit) or the specimen may have to be sent to the laboratory for testing. Correct labeling is necessary to ensure accurate results. Packaging the specimen in a biohazard bag prevents the person transporting the container from coming in contact with the specimen.

ACTION	RATIONALE
18. If testing at the point-of-care, open collection card according to manufacturer's instructions. Add three drops of developer to center of sample on Sample Pad. Developer should flow through the test (T) line and through the control (C) line. Snap Test Device closed (Beckman Coulter, 2009b).	The developer will react with any blood in the stool. Following the manufacturer's instructions promotes accuracy of results.
19. Wait 5 minutes, or time specified by manufacturer. Observe card for pink color on the test (T) line. The control (C) line must also turn pink within 5 minutes. If the control (C) line turns pink, read and report the result.	The developer will react with any blood in the stool. Following the manufacturer's instructions promotes accuracy of results. Any pink color on the test (T) line indicates a positive result.
20. After reading results, discard testing slide appropriately, according to facility policy. Remove gloves and any other PPE, if used. Perform hand hygiene.	Removing PPE properly reduces the risk for infection transmission and contamination of other items. Hand hygiene and proper disposal of equipment reduces the transmission of microorganisms.

EVALUATION

- Stool sample is obtained following collection guidelines and transported to the laboratory within the recommended time frame, without adverse effect.
- Patient demonstrates accurate understanding of testing instructions.
- Specimen is obtained with minimal discomfort and embarrassment.
- If the patient is to obtain the stool sample on his or her own, another outcome is met when the patient is able to collect the stool, place it correctly on the collection device, and deliver it to the testing site.

DOCUMENTATION

- Document the method used to obtain the specimen and transport it to the laboratory. If testing is done by the nurse, document results and communication of results to the health care provider. Document significant assessment findings and stool characteristics.

Suctioning of the pharynx is indicated to maintain a patent airway and to remove saliva, pulmonary secretions, blood, vomitus, or foreign material from the pharynx. Suctioning helps a patient who cannot successfully clear his or her airway by coughing and expectorating (Sole, et al., 2011). When performing suctioning, position yourself on the appropriate side of the patient. If you are right-handed, stand on the patient's right side; if left-handed, stand on the patient's left side. This allows for comfortable use of the dominant hand to manipulate the suction catheter. The following skill describes suctioning of the oropharyngeal airway. See the accompanying Skill Variation for a description of suctioning of the nasopharyngeal airway.

DELEGATION CONSIDERATIONS

The suctioning of the oropharyngeal airway may be delegated to nursing assistive personnel (NAP) or to unlicensed assistive personnel (UAP) who have received appropriate training. Depending on the state's nurse practice act and the organization's policies and procedures, the suctioning of the oropharyngeal and nasopharyngeal airways may be delegated to licensed practical/vocational nurses (LPN/LVNs). The decision to delegate must be based on careful analysis of the patient's needs and circumstances, as well as the qualifications of the person to whom the task is being delegated. Refer to the Delegation Guidelines in Appendix A.

EQUIPMENT

- Portable or wall suction unit with tubing
- A commercially prepared suction kit with an appropriate size catheter or sterile suction catheter with Y-port in the appropriate size (Adult: 10F to 16F)
- Sterile disposable container
- Sterile gloves
- Sterile water or saline
- Towel or waterproof pad
- Goggles and mask or face shield
- Disposable, clean gloves
- Water-soluble lubricant
- Additional PPE, as indicated

ASSESSMENT

- Assess lung sounds. Patients who need to be suctioned may have wheezes, crackles, or gurgling present.
- Assess oxygen saturation level. Oxygen saturation usually decreases when a patient needs to be suctioned.
- Assess respiratory status, including respiratory rate, rhythm, and depth. Patients may become tachypneic when they need to be suctioned. Assess the patient for signs of respiratory distress, such as nasal flaring, retractions, or grunting.

- Assess effectiveness of coughing and expectoration. Suctioning of the airway may be necessary for patients with an ineffective cough who are unable to expectorate secretions.
- Assess for history of deviated septum, nasal polyps, nasal obstruction, nasal injury, epistaxis (nasal bleeding), or nasal swelling.
- Assess for pain.
- Assess the characteristics and amount of secretions while suctioning.

NURSING DIAGNOSIS
- Ineffective Airway Clearance
- Impaired Gas Exchange
- Ineffective Breathing Pattern
- Risk for Aspiration

OUTCOME IDENTIFICATION AND PLANNING
- Patient will exhibit improved breath sounds and a clear, patent airway.
- Patient will exhibit an oxygen saturation level within acceptable parameters.
- Patient will demonstrate a respiratory rate and depth within an age-acceptable range.
- Patient will remain free of any signs of respiratory distress, including retractions, nasal flaring, or grunting.

IMPLEMENTATION

ACTION	RATIONALE
1. Bring necessary equipment to the bedside stand or overbed table.	Bringing everything to the bedside conserves time and energy. Arranging items nearby is convenient, saves time, and avoids unnecessary stretching and twisting of muscles on the part of the nurse.
2. Perform hand hygiene and put on PPE, if indicated.	Hand hygiene and PPE prevent the spread of microorganisms. PPE is required based on transmission precautions.
3. Identify the patient.	Identifying the patient ensures the right patient receives the intervention and helps prevent errors.
4. Close the curtains around the bed and close the door to the room, if possible.	This ensures the patient's privacy.

ACTION	RATIONALE
5. Determine the need for suctioning. Verify the suction order in the patient's medical record, if necessary. **Assess for pain or the potential to cause pain. Administer pain medication, as prescribed, before suctioning.**	To minimize trauma to airway mucosa, suctioning should be done only when secretions have accumulated or adventitious breath sounds are audible. Some facilities require an order for naso- and oropharyngeal suctioning. Suctioning stimulates coughing, which is painful for patients with surgical incisions and other conditions.
6. Explain what you are going to do and the reason for suctioning to the patient, even if the patient does not appear to be alert. Reassure the patient you will interrupt the procedure if he or she indicates respiratory difficulty.	Explanation alleviates fears. Even if the patient appears unconscious, explain what is happening. Any procedure that compromises respiration is frightening for the patient.
7. Adjust the bed to a comfortable working height, usually elbow height of the caregiver (VISN 8 Patient Safety Center, 2009). Lower side rail closest to you. **If patient is conscious, place the patient in a semi-Fowler's position. If unconscious, place the patient in the lateral position, facing you.** Move the bedside table close to your work area and raise it to waist height.	Having the bed at the proper height prevents back and muscle strain. A sitting position helps the patient to cough and makes breathing easier. Gravity also facilitates catheter insertion. The lateral position prevents the airway from becoming obstructed and promotes drainage of secretions. The bedside table provides a work surface and helps maintain sterility of objects on the work surface.
8. Place towel or waterproof pad across the patient's chest.	This protects bed linens.
9. **Adjust suction to appropriate pressure.** For a wall unit for an adult: 100–150 mm Hg; neonates: 60–80 mm Hg; infants: 80–125 mm Hg; children: 80–125 mm Hg; adolescents: 80–150 mm Hg (Hess et al., 2012).	Higher pressures can cause excessive trauma, hypoxemia, and atelectasis.

ACTION	RATIONALE

For a portable unit for an adult: 10–15 cm Hg; neonates: 6–8 cm Hg; infants: 8–10 cm Hg; children: 8–10 cm Hg; adolescents: 8–15 cm Hg.

Put on a disposable, clean glove and occlude the end of the connecting tubing to check suction pressure. Place the connecting tubing in a convenient location.

10. Open sterile suction package using aseptic technique. The open wrapper or container becomes a sterile field to hold other supplies. Carefully remove the sterile container, touching only the outside surface. Set it up on the work surface and pour sterile saline into it.

Sterile normal saline or water is used to lubricate the outside of the catheter, minimizing irritation of mucosa during introduction. It is also used to clear the catheter between suction attempts.

11. Place a small amount of water-soluble lubricant on the sterile field, taking care to avoid touching the sterile field with the lubricant package.

Lubricant facilitates passage of the catheter and reduces trauma to mucous membranes.

12. Increase the patient's supplemental oxygen level or apply supplemental oxygen per facility policy or primary care provider order.

Suctioning removes air from the patient's airway and can cause hypoxemia. Hyperoxygenation can help prevent suction-induced hypoxemia.

13. Put on face shield or goggles and mask. Put on sterile gloves. **The dominant hand will manipulate the catheter and must remain sterile. The nondominant hand is considered clean rather than sterile and will control the suction valve (Y-port) on the catheter.** In the home setting and other

Gloves and other PPE protect the nurse from microorganisms. Handling the sterile catheter using a sterile glove helps prevent introducing organisms into the respiratory tract. In the home setting and other community-based settings, clean (instead of sterile) technique is used because the patient is not exposed to disease-causing organisms that

ACTION	RATIONALE
community-based settings, maintenance of sterility is not necessary.	may be found in health care settings, such as hospitals.
14. With dominant gloved hand, pick up sterile catheter. Pick up the connecting tubing with the nondominant hand and connect the tubing and suction catheter.	Sterility of the suction catheter is maintained.
15. Moisten the catheter by dipping it into the container of sterile saline. Occlude Y-tube to check suction.	Lubricating the inside of the catheter with saline helps move secretions in the catheter. Checking suction ensures equipment is working properly.
16. Encourage the patient to take several deep breaths.	Hyperventilation can help prevent suction-induced hypoxemia.
17. Apply lubricant to the first 2 to 3 inches of the catheter, using the lubricant that was placed on the sterile field.	Lubricant facilitates passage of the catheter and reduces trauma to mucous membranes.
18. Remove the oxygen delivery device, if appropriate. Do not apply suction as the catheter is inserted. Hold the catheter between your thumb and forefinger.	Suctioning removes air from the patient's airway and can cause hypoxemia. Using suction while inserting the catheter can cause trauma to the mucosa and remove excessive oxygen from the respiratory tract.
19. Insert the catheter:	Correct distance for insertion ensures proper placement of the catheter. The general guideline for determining insertion distance for nasopharyngeal suctioning for an individual patient is to estimate the distance from the patient's earlobe to the nose.
a. **For nasopharyngeal suctioning,** gently insert catheter through the naris and along the floor of the nostril toward the trachea. Roll the catheter between your fingers to help advance it. Advance the catheter approximately 5 to 6 inches to reach the pharynx.	
b. **For oropharyngeal suctioning,** insert catheter through the mouth, along the side of the mouth toward the trachea. Advance	

ACTION	RATIONALE

the catheter 3 to 4 inches to reach the pharynx. (For nasotracheal suctioning, see the accompanying Skill Variation display.)

20. **Apply suction by intermittently occluding the Y-port on the catheter with the thumb of your nondominant hand and gently rotating the catheter as it is being withdrawn. Do not suction for more than 10 to 15 seconds at a time.**

Turning the catheter as it is withdrawn minimizes trauma to the mucosa. Suctioning for longer than 10 to 15 seconds robs the respiratory tract of oxygen, which may result in hypoxemia. Suctioning too quickly may be ineffective at clearing all secretions.

21. Replace the oxygen delivery device using your nondominant hand, if appropriate, and have the patient take several deep breaths.

Suctioning removes air from the patient's airway and can cause hypoxemia. Hyperventilation can help prevent suction-induced hypoxemia.

22. Flush catheter with saline. Assess effectiveness of suctioning and repeat, as needed, and according to patient's tolerance. Wrap the suction catheter around your dominant hand between attempts.

Flushing clears the catheter and lubricates it for next insertion. Reassessment determines the need for additional suctioning. Wrapping prevents inadvertent contamination of the catheter.

23. **Allow at least a 30-second to 1-minute interval if additional suctioning is needed. No more than three suction passes should be made per suctioning episode. Alternate the nares, unless contraindicated, if repeated suctioning is required.** Do not force the catheter through the nares. Encourage the patient to cough and deep breathe between suctioning. **Suction the oropharynx after suctioning the nasopharynx.**

The interval allows for reventilation and reoxygenation of airways. Excessive suction passes contribute to complications. Alternating nares reduces trauma. Suctioning the oropharynx after the nasopharynx clears the mouth of secretions. More microorganisms are usually present in the mouth, so it is suctioned last to prevent transmission of contaminants.

24. When suctioning is completed, remove gloves from

This technique reduces transmission of microorganisms. Proper

ACTION	RATIONALE
dominant hand over the coiled catheter, pulling them off inside out. Remove glove from nondominant hand and dispose of gloves, catheter, and container with solution in the appropriate receptacle. Assist the patient to a comfortable position. Raise bed rail and place bed in the lowest position.	positioning with raised side rails and proper bed height provide for patient comfort and safety.
25. Turn off suction. Remove supplemental oxygen placed for suctioning, if appropriate. Remove face shield or goggles and mask. Perform hand hygiene.	Proper removal of PPE and hand hygiene reduces risk of transmission of microorganisms.
26. Offer oral hygiene after suctioning.	Respiratory secretions that are allowed to accumulate in the mouth are irritating to mucous membranes and unpleasant for the patient.
27. Reassess the patient's respiratory status, including respiratory rate, effort, oxygen saturation, and lung sounds.	This assesses effectiveness of suctioning and the presence of complications.
28. Remove additional PPE, if used. Perform hand hygiene.	Removing PPE properly reduces the risk for infection transmission and contamination of other items. Hand hygiene prevents the spread of microorganisms.

EVALUATION
- Patient exhibits improved breath sounds and a clear and patent airway.
- Oxygen saturation level is within acceptable parameters.
- Patient does not exhibit signs or symptoms of respiratory distress or complications.

DOCUMENTATION
- Document the time of suctioning, your assessments before and after intervention, reason for suctioning, route used, and the characteristics and amount of secretions.

SKILL VARIATION Nasotracheal Suctioning

Nasotracheal suctioning is indicated to maintain a patent airway and remove saliva, pulmonary secretions, blood, vomitus, or foreign material from the trachea. Tracheal suctioning can lead to hypoxemia, cardiac dysrhythmias, trauma, atelectasis, infection, bleeding, and pain. It is imperative to be diligent in maintaining aseptic technique and following facility guidelines and procedures to prevent potential hazards. In the home setting and other community-based settings, clean technique is used because the patient is not exposed to disease-causing organisms that may be found in health care settings, such as hospitals. When performing suctioning, position yourself on the appropriate side of the patient. If you are right-handed, stand on the patient's right side; if left-handed, stand on the patient's left side. This allows for comfortable use of the dominant hand to manipulate the suction catheter. To perform nasotracheal suctioning:

1. Perform hand hygiene. Put on PPE, as indicated.

2. Identify the patient.

3. Determine the need for suctioning. **Assess for pain or the potential to cause pain. Administer pain medication, as prescribed, before suctioning.**

4. Explain to the patient what you are going to do and the reason for doing it, even if the patient does not appear to be alert.

5. Adjust bed to a comfortable working position. Lower the side rail closest to you. **If the patient is conscious, place him or her in a semi-Fowler's position. If the patient is unconscious, place him or her in the lateral position, facing you.** Move the overbed table close to your work area and raise to waist height.

6. Place a towel or waterproof pad across the patient's chest.

7. **Turn suction to appropriate pressure. Put on a disposable, clean glove and occlude the end of the connecting tubing to check suction pressure.** Place the connecting tubing in a convenient location.

8. Open sterile suction package using aseptic technique. The open wrapper becomes a sterile field to hold other supplies. Carefully remove the sterile container, touching only the outside surface. Set it up on the work surface and pour sterile saline into it.

9. Place a small amount of water-soluble lubricant on the sterile field, taking care

continued on page 838

to avoid touching the sterile field with the lubricant package.

10. Increase the patient's supplemental oxygen level or apply supplemental oxygen per facility policy or medical order.

11. Put on face shield or goggles and mask. Put on sterile gloves. **The dominant hand will manipulate the catheter and must remain sterile.** The nondominant hand is considered clean rather than sterile and will control the suction valve.

12. With dominant gloved hand, pick up the sterile catheter. Pick up the connecting tubing with the nondominant hand and connect the tubing and suction catheter.

13. Moisten the catheter by dipping it into the container of sterile saline. Occlude the Y-tube to check suction.

14. Encourage the patient to take several deep breaths.

15. Apply lubricant to the first 2 to 3 inches of the catheter, using the lubricant that was placed on the sterile field.

16. Remove the oxygen-delivery device, if appropriate. Do not apply suction as the catheter is inserted. Hold the catheter in your thumb and forefinger. Gently insert the catheter through the naris and along the floor of the nostril toward the trachea. Roll the catheter between your fingers to help advance it. Advance the catheter

approximately 8 to 9 inches to reach the trachea. Resistance should not be met. If resistance is met, the carina or tracheal mucosa has been hit. Withdraw the catheter at least 12 inches before applying suction.

17. Apply suction by intermittently occluding the Y-port on the catheter with the thumb of your nondominant hand, and gently rotating the catheter as it is being withdrawn. **Do not suction for more than 10 to 15 seconds at a time.**

18. Replace the oxygen-delivery device using your nondominant hand and have the patient take several deep breaths.

19. Flush the catheter with saline. Assess effectiveness of suctioning and repeat, as needed, and according to patient's tolerance. Wrap the suction catheter around your dominant hand between attempts.

20. **Allow at least a 30-second to 1-minute interval if additional suctioning is needed. No more than three suction passes should be made per suctioning episode.** Alternate the nares, unless contraindicated, if repeated suctioning is required. Do not force catheter through the nares. Encourage the patient to cough and deep breathe between suctioning. Suction the oropharynx after suctioning the trachea.

21. When suctioning is completed, remove glove from dominant hand over the coiled catheter, pulling it off inside-out. Remove glove from nondominant hand and dispose of gloves, catheter, and container with solution in the appropriate receptacle. Remove face shield or goggles and mask. Perform hand hygiene.

22. Turn off suction. Remove supplemental oxygen placed for suctioning, if appropriate. Assist the patient to a comfortable position.

23. Offer oral hygiene after suctioning.

24. Reassess the patient's respiratory status, including respiratory rate, effort, oxygen saturation, and lung sounds.

25. Remove additional PPE, if used. Perform hand hygiene.

26. Document the time of suctioning, your assessments before and after intervention, the reason for suctioning, route used, and the characteristics and amount of secretions.

SKILL 161 REMOVING SUTURES

Skin sutures are used to hold tissue and skin together. Sutures may be black silk, synthetic material, or fine wire. Surgical sutures are removed when enough tensile strength has developed to hold the wound edges together during healing. The time frame varies depending on the patient's age, nutritional status, and wound location. Frequently, after skin sutures are removed, adhesive wound closure strips are applied across the wound to give additional support as it continues to heal. The removal of sutures may be done by the primary care provider or by the nurse with a medical order.

DELEGATION CONSIDERATIONS

The removal of surgical sutures is not delegated to nursing assistive personnel (NAP) or to unlicensed assistive personnel (UAP). Depending on the state's nurse practice act and the organization's policies and procedures, the removal of surgical sutures may be delegated to licensed practical/vocational nurses (LPN/LVNs). The decision to delegate must be based on careful analysis of the patient's needs and circumstances, as well as the qualifications of the person to whom the task is being delegated. Refer to the Delegation Guidelines in Appendix A.

EQUIPMENT

- Suture removal kit or forceps and scissors
- Gauze
- Wound cleansing agent, according to facility policy
- Clean, disposable gloves
- Additional PPE, as indicated
- Adhesive wound closure strips
- Skin protectant wipes

ASSESSMENT

- Inspect the surgical incision and the surrounding tissue. Assess the appearance of the wound for the approximation of wound edges, the color of the wound and surrounding area, presence of wound drainage noting color, volume, and odor, and for signs of dehiscence. Note the stage of the healing process and characteristics of any drainage.
- Assess the surrounding skin for color, temperature, and the presence of edema, maceration, or ecchymosis.

NURSING DIAGNOSIS

- Deficient Knowledge
- Risk for Infection
- Impaired Skin Integrity

OUTCOME IDENTIFICATION AND PLANNING

- Sutures are removed without contaminating the incisional area, causing trauma to the wound, and/or causing the patient to experience pain or discomfort.
- Patient remains free of complications that would delay recovery.
- Patient verbalizes an understanding of the procedure.

IMPLEMENTATION

ACTION	RATIONALE
1. Review the medical orders for suture removal. Gather necessary supplies.	Reviewing the order and plan of care validates the correct patient and correct procedure. Preparation promotes efficient time management and an organized approach to the task.
2. Perform hand hygiene and put on PPE, if indicated.	Hand hygiene and PPE prevent the spread of microorganisms. PPE is required based on transmission precautions.

ACTION	RATIONALE
3. Identify the patient.	Identifying the patient ensures the right patient receives the intervention and helps prevent errors.
4. Assemble equipment on overbed table within reach.	Organization facilitates performance of task.
5. Close the curtains around the bed and close the door to the room if possible. Explain what you are going to do and why you are going to do it to the patient. Describe the sensation of suture removal as a pulling or slightly uncomfortable experience.	This ensures the patient's privacy. Explanation relieves anxiety and facilitates cooperation.
6. Assess the patient for possible need for nonpharmacologic pain-reducing interventions or analgesic medication before beginning the procedure. Administer appropriate prescribed analgesic. Allow enough time for the analgesic to achieve its effectiveness before beginning the procedure.	Pain is a subjective experience influenced by past experience. Wound care and dressing changes may cause pain for some patients.
7. Place a waste receptacle at a convenient location for use during the procedure.	Having a waste container handy means that the soiled dressing may be discarded easily, without the spread of microorganisms.
8. Adjust bed to comfortable working height, usually elbow height of the caregiver (VISN 8, 2009).	Having the bed at the proper height prevents back and muscle strain.
9. Assist the patient to a comfortable position that provides easy access to the incision area. Use a bath blanket to cover any exposed area other than the incision. Place a waterproof pad under the incision site.	Patient positioning and use of a bath blanket provide for comfort and warmth. Waterproof pad protects underlying surfaces.

ACTION	RATIONALE
10. Put on clean gloves. Carefully and gently remove the soiled dressings. If there is resistance, use a silicone-based adhesive remover to help remove the tape. If any part of the dressing sticks to the underlying skin, use small amounts of sterile saline to help loosen and remove it. Inspect the incision area.	Gloves protect the nurse from handling contaminated dressings. Cautious removal of the dressing is more comfortable for the patient and ensures that any drain present is not removed. A silicone-based adhesive remover allows for the easy, rapid, and painless removal without the associated problems of skin stripping (Denyer, 2011; Benbow, 2011). Sterile saline moistens the dressing for easier removal and minimizes damage and pain.
11. Clean the incision using the wound cleanser and gauze, according to facility policies and procedures.	Incision cleaning prevents the spread of microorganisms and contamination of the wound.
12. Using the forceps, grasp the knot of the first suture and gently lift the knot up off the skin.	Raising the suture knot prevents accidental injury to the wound or skin when cutting.
13. Using the scissors, cut one side of the suture below the knot, close to the skin. Grasp the knot with the forceps and pull the cut suture through the skin. **Avoid pulling the visible portion of the suture through the underlying tissue.**	Pulling the cut suture through the skin helps reduce the risk for contamination of the incision area and resulting infection.
14. Remove every other suture to be sure the wound edges are healed. If they are, remove the remaining sutures as ordered. Dispose of sutures according to facility policy.	Removing every other suture allows for inspection of the wound, while leaving adequate suture in place to promote continued healing if the edges are not totally approximated. Follow *Standard Precautions* in disposing of sutures.
15. If wound closure strips are to be used, apply skin protectant to skin around incision. **Do not apply to incision.** Apply adhesive closure	Skin protectant helps adherence of closure strips and prevents skin irritation. Adhesive wound closure strips provide additional support to the wound as it

ACTION	RATIONALE
strips. Take care to handle the strips by the paper backing.	continues to heal. Handling by the paper backing avoids contamination.
16. Reapply the dressing, depending on the medical orders and facility policy.	A new dressing protects the wound. Some policies advise leaving the area uncovered.
17. Remove gloves and discard. Remove all remaining equipment; place the patient in a comfortable position, with side rails up and bed in the lowest position.	Proper removal of gloves prevents spread of microorganisms. Proper patient and bed positioning promotes safety and comfort.
18. Remove additional PPE, if used. Perform hand hygiene.	Removing PPE properly reduces the risk for infection transmission and contamination of other items. Hand hygiene prevents the spread of microorganisms.
19. Assess all wounds every shift. More frequent checks may be needed if the wound is more complex.	Checking wound and dressings ensures the assessment of changes in patient condition and timely intervention to prevent complications.

EVALUATION

- Patient exhibits an incision area that is clean, dry, and intact without sutures.
- Incision area is free of trauma and infection.
- Patient verbalizes little to no pain or discomfort during the removal.
- Patient verbalizes an understanding of the procedure.

DOCUMENTATION

- Document the location of the incision and the assessment of the site. Include the appearance of the surrounding skin. Document cleansing of the site and suture removal. Record any skin care, application of wound closure strips, and the dressing applied, if appropriate. Note pertinent patient and family education and any patient reaction to this procedure, including patient's pain level and effectiveness of nonpharmacologic interventions or analgesia if administered.

Body temperature is the difference between the amount of heat produced by the body and the amount of heat lost to the environment measured in degrees. Normal body temperature is 35.9°C to 38°C (96.7°F to 100.5°F), depending on the route used for measurement (Jensen, 2011). To obtain an accurate measurement, choose an appropriate site, the correct equipment, and the appropriate tool based on the patient's condition. If a temperature reading is obtained from a site other than the oral route, document the site used along with the measurement. If no site is listed with the documentation, it is generally assumed to be the oral route.

DELEGATION CONSIDERATIONS

Assessment of body temperature may be delegated to nursing assistive personnel (NAP) or to unlicensed assistive personnel (UAP), as well as to licensed practical/vocational nurses (LPN/LVNs). The decision to delegate must be based on careful analysis of the patient's needs and circumstances, as well as the qualifications of the person to whom the task is being delegated. Refer to the Delegation Guidelines in Appendix A.

EQUIPMENT

- Digital, glass, or electronic thermometer, appropriate for site to be used
- Disposable probe covers
- Water-soluble lubricant for rectal temperature measurement
- Nonsterile gloves, if appropriate
- Additional PPE, as indicated
- Toilet tissue, if needed
- Pencil or pen, paper or flow sheet, computerized record

ASSESSMENT

- Note baseline or previous temperature measurements.
- Assess the patient to ensure that his or her cognitive functioning is intact.
- Assess whether the patient can close his or her lips around the thermometer. Determine if the patient has a disease of the oral cavity; earache; significant ear drainage or a scarred tympanic membrane.
- Determine if the patient has had surgery of the nose, mouth, or rectum; has diarrhea or diseases of the rectum; or scar tissue, open lesions, or abrasions in the temporal areas.
- Determine if the patient is neutropenic or thrombocytopenic.
- Ask the patient if he or she has recently smoked, has been chewing gum, or was eating and drinking.

When taking a temporal artery temperature, assess for head coverings. Anything covering the area, such as a hat, hair, wigs, or bandages, would insulate the area, resulting in falsely high readings. If a patient is lying on his or her side, measure only the side of the head exposed to the environment. Do not measure temporal artery temperature over scar tissue, open lesions, or abrasions.

NURSING DIAGNOSIS

- Hyperthermia
- Hypothermia
- Risk for Imbalanced Body Temperature
- Ineffective Thermoregulation

OUTCOME IDENTIFICATION AND PLANNING

- Patient's temperature is assessed accurately without injury.
- Patient experiences minimal discomfort.

IMPLEMENTATION

ACTION	RATIONALE
1. Check medical order or nursing care plan for frequency of measurement and route. More frequent temperature measurement may be appropriate based on nursing judgment.	Assessment and measurement of vital signs at appropriate intervals provide important data about the patient's health status.
2. Perform hand hygiene and put on PPE, if indicated.	Hand hygiene and PPE prevent the spread of microorganisms. PPE is required based on transmission precautions.
3. Identify the patient.	Identifying the patient ensures that the right patient receives the intervention and helps prevent errors.
4. Close the curtains around the bed and close the door to the room, if possible. Discuss the procedure with the patient and assess the patient's ability to assist with the procedure.	This ensures the patient's privacy. Explanation relieves anxiety and facilitates cooperation. Dialogue encourages patient participation and allows for individualized nursing care.
5. Assemble equipment on the overbed table within reach.	Organization facilitates performance of task.
6. Ensure that the electronic or digital thermometer is in working condition.	Improperly functioning thermometer may not give an accurate reading.

ACTION	RATIONALE
7. Put on gloves, if indicated.	Gloves prevent contact with blood and body fluids. Gloves are usually not required for an oral, axillary, or tympanic temperature measurement, unless contact with blood or body fluids is anticipated. Gloves should be worn for rectal temperature measurement.
8. Select the appropriate site based on previous assessment data.	This ensures safety and accuracy of measurement.
9. Follow the steps as outlined below for the appropriate type of thermometer.	
10. When measurement is completed, remove gloves, if worn. Remove additional PPE, if used. Perform hand hygiene.	Removing PPE properly reduces the risk for infection transmission and contamination of other items. Hand hygiene prevents the spread of microorganisms.

Measuring an Oral Temperature

11. Remove the electronic unit from the charging unit, and remove the probe from within the recording unit.	Electronic unit must be taken into the patient's room to assess the patient's temperature. On some models, by removing the probe the machine is already turned on.
12. Cover thermometer probe with disposable probe cover and slide it on until it snaps into place.	Using a cover prevents contamination of the thermometer probe.
13. **Place the probe beneath the patient's tongue in the posterior sublingual pocket. Ask the patient to close his or her lips around the probe.**	When the probe rests deep in the posterior sublingual pocket, it is in contact with blood vessels lying close to the surface.
14. Continue to hold the probe until you hear a beep. Note the temperature reading.	If left unsupported, the weight of the probe tends to pull it away from the correct location. The signal indicates that the

ACTION	RATIONALE
	measurement is completed. The electronic thermometer provides a digital display of the measured temperature.
15. Remove the probe from the patient's mouth. Dispose of the probe cover by holding the probe over an appropriate receptacle and pressing the probe release button.	Disposing of the probe cover ensures that it will not be reused accidentally on another patient. Proper disposal prevents spread of microorganisms.
16. Return the thermometer probe to the storage place within the unit. Return the electronic unit to the charging unit, if appropriate.	The thermometer needs to be recharged for future use. If necessary, the thermometer should stay on the charger so that it is ready to use at all times.

Measuring a Tympanic Membrane Temperature

ACTION	RATIONALE
17. If necessary, push the "ON" button and wait for the "ready" signal on the unit.	For proper function, the thermometer must be turned on and warmed up.
18. Slide the disposable cover onto the tympanic probe.	Use of a disposable cover deters the spread of microorganisms.
19. **Insert the probe snugly into the external ear using gentle but firm pressure, angling the thermometer toward the patient's jaw line. Pull the pinna up and back to straighten the ear canal in an adult.**	If the probe is not inserted correctly, the patient's temperature may be noted as lower than normal.
20. Activate the unit by pushing the trigger button. The reading is immediate (usually within 2 seconds). Note the reading.	The digital thermometer must be activated to record the temperature.
21. Discard the probe cover in an appropriate receptacle by pushing the probe-release button or use the rim of cover to remove it from the probe. Replace the thermometer in its charger, if necessary.	Discarding the probe cover ensures that it will not be reused accidentally on another patient. Proper disposal prevents the spread of microorganisms. If necessary, the thermometer should stay on the charger so that it is ready to use at all times.

ACTION	RATIONALE

Measuring Temporal Artery Temperature

22. Brush the patient's hair aside if it is covering the temporal artery area.

Anything covering the area—such as a hat, hair, wigs, or bandages—would insulate the area, resulting in falsely high readings. Measure only the side of the head exposed to the environment.

23. Apply a probe cover.

Using a cover prevents contamination of the thermometer probe.

24. Hold the thermometer like a remote control device, with your thumb on the red "ON" button. Place the probe flush on the center of the forehead, with the body of the instrument sideways (not straight up and down), so it is not in the patient's face.

Allows for easy use of the device and reading of the display. Holding the instrument straight up and down could be intimidating for the patient, particularly young patients and/or those with alterations in mental status.

25. Depress the "ON" button. Keep the button depressed throughout the measurement.

26. Slowly slide the probe straight across the forehead, midline, to the hairline. The thermometer will click; fast clicking indicates a rise to a higher temperature, slow clicking indicates that the instrument is still scanning, but not finding any higher temperature.

Midline on the forehead, the temporal artery is less than 2 mm below the skin; whereas at the side of the face, the temporal artery is much deeper. Measuring there would result in falsely low readings.

27. Brush hair aside if it is covering the ear, exposing the area of the neck under the ear lobe. Lift the probe from the forehead and touch on the neck just behind the ear lobe, in the depression just below the mastoid.

Sweat causes evaporative cooling of the skin on the forehead, possibly leading to a falsely low reading. During diaphoresis, the area on the head behind the ear lobe exhibits high blood flow necessary for the arterial measurement; it is a double check for the thermometer (Exergen, 2007).

28. Release the button and read the thermometer measurement.

ACTION	RATIONALE
29. Hold the thermometer over a waste receptacle. Gently push the probe cover with your thumb against the proximal edge to dispose of the probe cover.	Discarding the probe cover ensures that it will not be reused accidentally on another patient.
30. The instrument will automatically turn off in 30 seconds, or press and release the power button.	Turns thermometer off.

Measuring Axillary Temperature

ACTION	RATIONALE
31. Move the patient's clothing to expose only the axilla.	The axilla must be exposed for placement of the thermometer. Exposing only the axilla keeps the patient warm and maintains his or her dignity.
32. Remove the probe from the recording unit of the electronic thermometer. Place a disposable probe cover on by sliding it on and snapping it securely.	Using a cover prevents contamination of the thermometer probe.
33. **Place the end of the probe in the center of the axilla. Have the patient bring the arm down and close to the body.**	The deepest area of the axilla provides the most accurate measurement; surrounding the bulb with skin surface provides a more reliable measurement.
34. Hold the probe in place until you hear a beep, and then carefully remove the probe. Note the temperature reading.	Axillary thermometers must be held in place to obtain an accurate temperature.
35. Cover the patient and help him or her to a position of comfort.	Ensures patient comfort.
36. Dispose of the probe cover by holding the probe over an appropriate waste receptacle and pushing the release button.	Discarding the probe cover ensures that it will not be reused accidentally on another patient.
37. Place the bed in the lowest position and elevate rails, as needed. Leave the patient clean and comfortable.	Low bed position and elevated side rails provide for patient safety.

ACTION	RATIONALE
38. Return the electronic thermometer to the charging unit.	Thermometer needs to be recharged for future use.

Measuring Rectal Temperature

39. Adjust the bed to a comfortable working height, usually elbow height of the care giver (VISN 8 Patient Safety Center, 2009). Put on non-sterile gloves.	Having the bed at the proper height prevents back and muscle strain. Gloves prevent contact with contaminants and body fluids.
40. Assist the patient to a side-lying position. Pull back the covers sufficiently to expose only the buttocks.	The side-lying position allows the nurse to visualize the buttocks. Exposing only the buttocks keeps the patient warm and maintains his or her dignity.
41. Remove the rectal probe from within the recording unit of the electronic thermometer. Cover the probe with a disposable probe cover and slide it until it snaps in place.	Using a cover prevents contamination of the thermometer.
42. **Lubricate about 1 inch of the probe with a water-soluble lubricant.**	Lubrication reduces friction and facilitates insertion, minimizing the risk of irritation or injury to the rectal mucous membranes.
43. Reassure the patient. Separate the buttocks until the anal sphincter is clearly visible.	If not placed directly into the anal opening, the thermometer probe may injure adjacent tissue or cause discomfort.
44. **Insert the thermometer probe into the anus about 1.5 inches in an adult or no more than 1 inch in a child.**	Depth of insertion must be adjusted based on the patient's age. Rectal temperatures are not normally taken in an infant, but may be indicated.
45. Hold the probe in place until you hear a beep, then carefully remove the probe. Note the temperature reading on the display.	If left unsupported, movement of the probe in the rectum could cause injury and/or discomfort. The signal indicates that the measurement is completed. The electronic thermometer provides a digital display of the measured temperature.

ACTION	RATIONALE
46. Dispose of the probe cover by holding the probe over an appropriate waste receptacle and pressing the release button.	Proper probe cover disposal reduces risk of microorganism transmission.
47. Using toilet tissue, wipe the anus of any feces or excess lubricant. Dispose of the toilet tissue. Remove gloves and discard them.	Wiping promotes cleanliness. Disposing of the toilet tissue avoids transmission of microorganisms.
48. Cover the patient and help him or her to a position of comfort.	Ensures patient comfort.
49. Place the bed in the lowest position; elevate rails as needed.	These actions provide for the patient's safety.
50. Return the thermometer to the charging unit.	The thermometer needs to be recharged for future use.

EVALUATION

- Patient's temperature is assessed accurately without injury.
- Patient experiences minimal discomfort.

DOCUMENTATION

- Record temperature on paper, flow sheet, or computerized record. Report abnormal findings to the appropriate person. Identify the site of assessment if other than oral.

SKILL 163   REGULATING TEMPERATURE USING AN OVERHEAD RADIANT WARMER

Neonates, infants who are exposed to stressors or chilling (e.g., from undergoing numerous procedures), and infants who have an underlying condition that interferes with thermoregulation (e.g., prematurity) are highly susceptible to heat loss. Therefore, radiant warmers are used for infants who have trouble maintaining body temperature. In addition, use of a radiant warmer minimizes the oxygen and calories that the infant would expend to maintain body temperature, thereby minimizing the effects of body temperature changes on metabolic activity.

An overhead radiant warmer uses infrared light to warm the infant. The infant's skin is warmed, causing an increase in blood flow, which heats both the underlying blood and tissue surfaces. The warmed blood and tissue transfer this heat to the rest of the body (Dondelinger, 2010). The warmer is adjusted to maintain an anterior abdominal skin temperature of 36.5°C (97.7°F), but at least 36°C (96.8°F), using servo-control (automatic thermostat) (Dondelinger, 2010; Sinclair, 2002).

DELEGATION CONSIDERATIONS

The assessment of body temperature for an infant in a radiant warmer is not delegated to nursing assistive personnel (NAP) or to unlicensed assistive personnel (UAP). Depending on the state's nurse practice act and the organization's policies and procedures, the assessment of body temperature for an infant in a radiant warmer may be delegated to a licensed practical/vocational nurse (LPN/LVN). The decision to delegate must be based on careful analysis of the patient's needs and circumstances, as well as the qualifications of the person to whom the task is being delegated. Refer to the Delegation Guidelines in Appendix A.

EQUIPMENT

- Overhead warmer
- Temperature probe
- Aluminum foil probe cover
- Axillary or rectal thermometer, based on facility policy
- PPE, as indicated

ASSESSMENT

- Assess the patient's temperature using the route specified in facility policy, and assess the patient's fluid intake and output.

NURSING DIAGNOSIS

- Hyperthermia
- Hypothermia
- Risk for Imbalanced Body Temperature
- Ineffective Thermoregulation
- Risk for Deficient Fluid Volume

OUTCOME IDENTIFICATION AND PLANNING

- Infant's temperature is maintained within normal limits without injury.

IMPLEMENTATION

ACTION	RATIONALE
1. Check the medical order or nursing care plan for the use of a radiant warmer.	Provides for patient safety and appropriate care.

ACTION	RATIONALE
2. Perform hand hygiene and put on PPE, if indicated.	Hand hygiene and PPE prevent the spread of microorganisms. PPE is required based on transmission precautions.
3. Identify the patient.	Identifying the patient ensures the right patient receives the intervention and helps prevent errors.
4. Close curtains around the bed and close the door to the room, if possible. Discuss the procedure with the patient's family.	This ensures the patient's privacy. Explanation reduces the family's apprehension and encourages family cooperation.
5. Plug in the warmer. Turn the warmer to the manual setting. Allow the blankets to warm before placing the infant under the warmer.	By allowing the blankets to warm before placing the infant under the warmer, you are preventing heat loss through conduction. By placing the warmer on the manual setting, you are keeping the warmer at a set temperature no matter how warm the blankets become.
6. **Switch the warmer setting to automatic. Set the warmer to the desired abdominal skin temperature, usually 36.5°C (97.7°F).**	The automatic setting ensures that the warmer will regulate the amount of radiant heat, depending on the temperature of the infant's skin. The temperature should be adjusted so that the infant does not become too warm or too cold.
7. Place the infant under the warmer. Attach the probe to the infant's abdominal skin at mid-epigastrium, halfway between the xiphoid and the umbilicus. Cover with a foil patch.	The foil patch prevents direct warming of the probe, allowing the probe to read only the infant's temperature.
8. When the abdominal skin temperature reaches the desired set point, check the patient's temperature using the route specified in facility policy, to be sure it is within the normal range.	By monitoring the infant's temperature, you are watching for signs of hyperthermia or hypothermia.

ACTION	RATIONALE
9. Adjust the warmer's set point slightly, as needed, if the patient's temperature is abnormal. Do not change the set point if the temperature is normal.	By monitoring the infant's temperature, you are watching for signs of hyperthermia or hypothermia. This prevents the infant from becoming too warm or too cool.
10. Remove additional PPE, if used. Perform hand hygiene.	Removing PPE properly reduces the risk for infection transmission and contamination of other items. Hand hygiene deters the spread of microorganisms.
11. Check frequently to be sure the probe maintains contact with the patient's skin. Continue to monitor temperature measurement and other vital signs.	Poor contact will cause overheating. Entrapment of the probe under the arm or between the infant and mattress will cause under-heating. Monitoring of vital signs assesses patient status.

EVALUATION
- Infant is placed under the radiant warmer.
- Infant's temperature is well controlled.
- Infant experiences no injury.

DOCUMENTATION
- Document initial assessment of the infant, including body temperature; the placement of the infant under the radiant warmer; and the settings of the radiant warmer. Document incubator air temperatures, as well as subsequent skin and axillary or rectal temperatures, and other vital signs measurements.

SKILL 164   APPLYING AND CARING FOR A PATIENT USING A TENS UNIT

Transcutaneous electrical nerve stimulation (TENS) is a noninvasive technique for providing pain relief that involves the electrical stimulation of large-diameter fibers to inhibit the transmission of painful impulses carried over small-diameter fibers. The TENS unit consists of a battery-powered portable unit, lead wires, and cutaneous electrode pads that are applied to or around the painful area. It is most beneficial when used to treat pain that is localized, and it requires an order from the primary care provider. The TENS unit can be applied intermittently throughout the day or worn for extended periods.

DELEGATION CONSIDERATIONS

The application of and care for a TENS unit is not delegated to nursing assistive personnel (NAP) or unlicensed assistive personnel (UAP). Depending on the state's nurse practice act and the organization's policies and procedures, the application of, and care for, a TENS unit may be delegated to licensed practical/vocational nurses (LPN/LVNs). The decision to delegate must be based on careful analysis of the patient's needs and circumstances, as well as the qualifications of the person to whom the task is being delegated. Refer to the Delegation Guidelines in Appendix A.

EQUIPMENT

- TENS unit
- Electrodes
- Electrode gel (if electrodes are not pre-gelled)
- Tape (if electrodes are not self-adhesive)
- Pain assessment tool and pain scale
- Skin cleanser and water
- Towel and washcloth
- PPE, as indicated

ASSESSMENT

- Review the patient's medical record and plan of care for specific instructions related to TENS therapy, including the order and conditions indicating the need for therapy.
- Review the patient's history for conditions that might contraindicate therapy, such as pacemaker insertion, cardiac monitoring, or electrocardiography.
- Determine the location of electrode placement in consultation with the ordering practitioner and on the patient's report of pain.
- Assess the patient's understanding of TENS therapy and the rationale for its use.
- Inspect the skin of the area designated for electrode placement for irritation, redness, or breakdown.
- Assess the patient's pain and level of discomfort using an appropriate assessment tool. Assess the characteristics of any pain. Assess for other symptoms that often occur with the pain, such as headache or restlessness. Ask the patient what interventions have and have not been successful in the past to promote comfort and relieve pain.
- Assess the patient's vital signs.
- Check the patient's medication administration record for the time an analgesic was last administered. Assess the patient's response to a particular intervention to evaluate effectiveness and presence of any adverse effect.
- Check the unit to ensure proper functioning and review the manufacturer's instructions for use.

NURSING DIAGNOSIS
- Acute Pain
- Chronic Pain
- Deficient Knowledge

OUTCOME IDENTIFICATION AND PLANNING
- Patient verbalizes decreased discomfort and pain, without experiencing any injury or skin irritation or breakdown.
- Patient displays decreased anxiety, improved coping skills, and an understanding of the therapy and the reason for its use.

IMPLEMENTATION

ACTION	RATIONALE
1. Perform hand hygiene and put on PPE, if indicated.	Hand hygiene and PPE prevent the spread of microorganisms. PPE is required based on transmission precautions.
2. Identify the patient.	Identifying the patient ensures that the right patient receives the intervention and helps prevent errors.
3. Show the patient the device, and explain its function and the reason for its use.	Explanation encourages patient understanding and cooperation and reduces apprehension.
4. Assess the patient's pain, using an appropriate assessment tool and measurement scale.	Accurate assessment is necessary to guide treatment and relief interventions and evaluate the effectiveness of pain control measures.
5. Inspect the area where the electrodes are to be placed. Clean the patient's skin, using skin cleanser and water. Dry the area thoroughly.	Inspection ensures that the electrodes will be applied to intact skin. Cleaning and drying help ensure that the electrodes will adhere.
6. Remove the adhesive backing from the electrodes and apply them to the specified location. If the electrodes are not pre-gelled, apply a small amount of electrode gel to the bottom of each	Application to the proper location enhances the success of the therapy. Gel is necessary to promote conduction of the electrical current.

ACTION	RATIONALE

electrode. If the electrodes are not self-adhering, tape them in place.

7. **Check the placement of the electrodes; leave at least a 2-inch (5-cm) space (about the width of one electrode) between them.**

Proper spacing is necessary to reduce the risk of burns due to the proximity of the electrodes.

8. **Check the controls on the TENS unit to make sure that they are off.** Connect the wires to the electrodes (if not already attached) and plug them into the unit.

Having controls off prevents flow of electricity. This connection completes the electrical circuit necessary to stimulate the nerve fibers.

9. Turn on the unit and adjust the intensity setting to the lowest intensity and determine if the patient can feel a tingling, burning, or buzzing sensation. Then adjust the intensity to the prescribed amount or the setting most comfortable for the patient. Secure the unit to the patient.

Using the lowest setting at first introduces the patient to the sensations. Adjusting the intensity is necessary to provide the proper amount of stimulation.

10. Set the pulse width (duration of the each pulsation) as indicated or recommended.

The pulse width determines the depth and width of the stimulation.

11. Assess the patient's pain level during therapy.

Pain assessment helps evaluate the effectiveness of therapy.

a. If intermittent use is ordered, turn the unit off after the specified duration of treatment and remove the electrodes. Provide skin care to the area.

TENS therapy can be ordered for intermittent or continuous use. Skin care reduces the risk for irritation and breakdown.

b. If continuous therapy is ordered, periodically remove the electrodes from the skin (after turning off the unit) to inspect the area and clean the skin, according to facility policy. Reapply the electrodes and

Periodic removal of electrodes allows for skin assessment. Skin care reduces the risk for irritation and breakdown. Reapplication ensures continued therapy.

ACTION	RATIONALE
continue therapy. Change the electrodes according to manufacturer's directions.	
12. When therapy is discontinued, turn off the unit and remove the electrodes. Clean the patient's skin. Clean the unit and replace the batteries.	Turning off the unit and removing electrodes when therapy is discontinued reduces the risk of injury to the patient. Cleaning the unit and replacing the batteries ensures that the unit is ready for future use.
13. Remove PPE, if used. Perform hand hygiene.	Removing PPE properly reduces the risk for infection transmission and contamination of other items. Hand hygiene prevents transmission of microorganisms.

EVALUATION

• Patient verbalizes pain relief.
• Patient remains free of signs and symptoms of skin irritation and breakdown, and injury.
• Patient reports decreased anxiety and increased ability to cope with pain.
• Patient verbalizes information related to the functioning of the unit and the reasons for its use.

DOCUMENTATION

• Document the date and time of application; patient's initial pain assessment; skin assessment; electrode placement location; intensity and pulse width; duration of therapy; pain assessments during therapy and patient's response; and time of removal or discontinuation of therapy.

SKILL 165 PROVIDING CARE OF A TRACHEOSTOMY TUBE

The nurse is responsible for either replacing a disposable inner cannula or cleaning a nondisposable inner cannula. The inner cannula requires replacement or cleaning to prevent accumulation of secretions that can interfere with respiration and occlude the airway. Because soiled tracheostomy dressings place the patient at risk for the development of skin breakdown and infection, regularly change dressings and tracheostomy collar or ties. Use gauze dressings that are not filled with cotton to prevent aspiration of foreign bodies (e.g., lint or cotton fibers) into the trachea. Clean the skin around a tracheostomy to prevent buildup of dried secretions and skin breakdown. Exercise care when changing the tracheostomy collar or ties to prevent accidental decannulation or expulsion of the tube. Have an assistant hold the tube in place during the changing of a collar. When changing a tracheostomy tie, keep the soiled tie in place until a clean one is securely attached. Agency policy and patient condition determine specific procedures and schedules, but a newly inserted tracheostomy may require attention every 1 to 2 hours. Because the respiratory tract is sterile and the tracheostomy provides a direct opening, meticulous care is necessary when using aseptic technique. Once the tracheostomy site is healed, in the home setting and other community-based settings, clean technique is used, as the patient is not exposed to disease-causing organisms that may be found in health care settings, such as hospitals.

DELEGATION CONSIDERATIONS

Care of a tracheostomy tube is not delegated to nursing assistive personnel (NAP) or to unlicensed assistive personnel (UAP). Depending on the state's nurse practice act and the organization's policies and procedures, care of a tracheostomy tube in a stable situation, such as long-term care and other community-based care settings, may be delegated to licensed practical/vocational nurses (LPN/LVNs). The decision to delegate must be based on careful analysis of the patient's needs and circumstances, as well as the qualifications of the person to whom the task is being delegated. Refer to the Delegation Guidelines in Appendix A.

EQUIPMENT

- Disposable gloves
- Sterile gloves
- Goggles and mask or face shield
- Additional PPE, as indicated
- Sterile normal saline
- Sterile cup or basin
- Sterile cotton-tipped applicators
- Sterile gauze sponges
- Disposable inner tracheostomy cannula, appropriate size for patient
- Sterile suction catheter and glove set
- Commercially prepared tracheostomy or drain dressing
- Commercially prepared tracheostomy holder
- Plastic disposal bag
- Additional nurse

ASSESSMENT

- Assess for signs and symptoms of the need to perform tracheostomy care, which include soiled dressings and holder or ties, secretions in the tracheostomy tube, and diminished airflow through the tracheostomy, or in accordance with facility policy.
- Assess insertion site for any redness or purulent drainage; if present, these may signify an infection.
- Assess patient for pain. If the tracheostomy is new, pain medication may be needed before performing tracheostomy care.

- Assess lung sounds and oxygen saturation levels. Lung sounds should be equal in all lobes, with an oxygen saturation level above 93%. If tracheostomy is dislodged, lung sounds and oxygen saturation level will diminish.
- Inspect the area on the posterior portion of the neck for any skin breakdown that may result from irritation or pressure from tracheostomy holder or ties.

NURSING DIAGNOSIS

- Impaired Skin Integrity
- Risk for Infection
- Ineffective Airway Clearance
- Risk for Aspiration

OUTCOME IDENTIFICATION AND PLANNING

- Patient will exhibit a tracheostomy tube and site free from drainage, secretions, and skin irritation or breakdown.
- Oxygen saturation levels will be within acceptable parameters.
- Patient will have no evidence of respiratory distress.

IMPLEMENTATION

ACTION	RATIONALE
1. Bring necessary equipment to the bedside stand or overbed table.	Bringing everything to the bedside conserves time and energy. Arranging items nearby is convenient, saves time, and avoids unnecessary stretching and twisting of muscles on the part of the nurse.
2. Perform hand hygiene and put on PPE, if indicated.	Hand hygiene and PPE prevent the spread of microorganisms. PPE is required based on transmission precautions.
3. Identify the patient.	Identifying the patient ensures the right patient receives the intervention and helps prevent errors.
4. Close the curtains around the bed and close the door to the room, if possible.	This ensures the patient's privacy.
5. Determine the need for tracheostomy care. **Assess**	If tracheostomy is new, pain medication may be needed

ACTION	RATIONALE

patient's pain and administer pain medication, if indicated.

before performing tracheostomy care.

6. Explain what you are going to do and the reason for doing it to the patient, even if the patient does not appear to be alert. Reassure the patient you will interrupt the procedure if he or she indicates respiratory difficulty.

Explanation alleviates fears. Even if the patient appears unconscious, the nurse should explain what is happening. Any procedure that compromises respiration is frightening for the patient.

7. Adjust the bed to a comfortable working position, usually elbow height of the caregiver (VISN 8 Patient Safety Center, 2009). Lower side rail closest to you. **If conscious, place the patient in a semi-Fowler's position. If unconscious, place the patient in the lateral position, facing you.** Move the overbed table close to your work area and raise it to waist height. Place a trash receptacle within easy reach of the work area.

Having the bed at the proper height prevents back and muscle strain. A sitting position helps the patient to cough and makes breathing easier. Gravity also facilitates catheter insertion. The lateral position prevents the airway from becoming obstructed and promotes drainage of secretions. The overbed table provides a work surface and maintains sterility of objects on the work surface. Trash receptacle within reach prevents reaching over the sterile field or turning back to the field to dispose of trash.

8. Put on face shield or goggles and mask. Suction tracheostomy, if necessary. If tracheostomy has just been suctioned, remove soiled site dressing and discard before removal of gloves used to perform suctioning.

PPE prevents contact with contaminants. Suctioning removes secretions to prevent occluding the outer cannula while the inner cannula is removed.

Cleaning the Tracheostomy: Disposable Inner Cannula

(See the accompanying Skill Variation for steps for cleaning a nondisposable inner cannula.)

9. Carefully open the package with the new disposable inner cannula, taking care not to contaminate the cannula

Inner cannula must remain sterile. Saline and applicators will be used to clean the tracheostomy site. Plastic disposable bag will

ACTION	RATIONALE

or the inside of the package. Carefully open the package with the sterile cotton-tipped applicators, taking care not to contaminate them. Open sterile cup or basin and fill 0.5 inch deep with saline. Open the plastic disposable bag and place within reach on work surface.

be used to discard removed inner cannula.

10. Put on disposable gloves.

Gloves protect against exposure to blood and body fluids.

11. Remove the oxygen source if one is present. Stabilize the outer cannula and faceplate of the tracheostomy with your nondominant hand. Grasp the locking mechanism of the inner cannula with your dominant hand. Press the tabs and release lock (Figure 1). Gently remove inner cannula and place in disposal bag. If not already removed, remove site dressing and dispose of it in the trash.

Stabilizing the faceplate prevents trauma to, and pain from, the stoma. Releasing the lock permits removal of the inner cannula.

FIGURE 1 Releasing lock on inner cannula.

12. Discard gloves and put on sterile gloves. Pick up the new inner cannula with your dominant hand, stabilize the faceplate with your nondominant hand, and gently insert the new inner cannula into the outer cannula. Press the tabs to allow the lock to grab the

Sterile gloves are necessary to prevent contamination of the new inner cannula. Locking to outer cannula secures the inner cannula in place. Maintains oxygen supply to the patient.

ACTION

outer cannula (Figure 2).
Reapply oxygen source, if
needed.

FIGURE 2 Locking new inner
cannula in place.

**Applying Clean Dressing and
Holder**

(See accompanying Skill Variations for steps for an alternate
site dressing if a commercially
prepared sponge is not available
and to secure a tracheostomy
with tracheostomy ties/tape
instead of a collar.)

13. Remove oxygen source,
    if necessary. Dip cotton-
    tipped applicator or gauze
    sponge in cup or basin with
    sterile saline and clean stoma
    under faceplate. Use each
    applicator or sponge only
    once, moving from stoma
    site outward.

14. Pat skin gently with dry
    4 × 4 gauze sponge.

15. Slide commercially prepared
    tracheostomy dressing or
    prefolded non–cotton-filled
    4 × 4-inch dressing under the
    faceplate.

16. Change the tracheostomy
    holder:

RATIONALE

Saline is nonirritating to tissue.
Cleansing from stoma outward
and using each applicator only
once promotes aseptic technique.

Gauze removes excess moisture.

Lint or fiber from a cut cotton-
filled gauze pad can be aspirated
into the trachea, causing respiratory distress, or can embed in
the stoma and cause irritation or
infection.

Holding the tracheostomy tube
in place ensures that the tracheostomy will not inadvertently be
expelled if the patient coughs or
moves.

ACTION	RATIONALE
a. **Obtain the assistance of a second individual to hold the tracheostomy tube in place while the old collar is removed and the new collar is placed.**	Doing so provides attachment for one side of the faceplate.
b. Open the package for the new tracheostomy collar.	Allows access to the new collar.
c. Both nurses should put on clean gloves.	Gloves prevent contact with blood, body fluids, and contaminants.
d. One nurse holds the faceplate while the other pulls up the Velcro tabs. Gently remove the collar.	Holding the tracheostomy tube in place ensures that the tracheostomy will not inadvertently be expelled if the patient coughs or moves. Pulling up the Velcro tabs loosens the collar.
e. The first nurse continues to hold the tracheostomy faceplate.	Prevents accidental extubation.
f. The other nurse places the collar around the patient's neck and inserts first one tab, then the other, into the openings on the faceplate and secures the Velcro tabs on the tracheostomy holder (Figure 3).	Securing the Velcro tabs holds the tracheostomy in place and prevents accidental expulsion of the tracheostomy tube.

FIGURE 3 Securing tabs on tracheostomy holder.

g. Check the fit of the tracheostomy collar. You should be able to fit one finger between the neck and the collar. Check to make sure that the patient can flex neck comfortably. Reapply oxygen source, if necessary.	Allowing one fingerbreadth under the collar permits neck flexion that is comfortable and ensures that the collar will not compromise circulation to the area. Maintains oxygen supply to the patient.

ACTION	RATIONALE
17. Remove gloves. Remove face shield or goggles and mask. Assist the patient to a comfortable position. Raise the bed rail and place the bed in the lowest position.	Removing PPE properly reduces the risk for infection transmission and contamination of other items. Ensures patient comfort. Proper positioning with raised side rails and proper bed height provide for patient comfort and safety.
18. Reassess the patient's respiratory status, including respiratory rate, effort, oxygen saturation, and lung sounds.	Assessments determine the effectiveness of interventions and for the presence of complications.
19. Remove additional PPE, if used. Perform hand hygiene.	Removing PPE properly reduces the risk for infection transmission and contamination of other items. Hand hygiene prevents the spread of microorganisms.

EVALUATION

- Patient exhibits a tracheostomy tube and site that are free from drainage, secretions, and skin irritation or breakdown.
- Patient's oxygen saturation level is within acceptable parameters.
- Patient is without evidence of respiratory distress.
- Patient verbalizes that the site is free of pain and exhibits no evidence of skin breakdown on the posterior portion of the neck.

DOCUMENTATION

- Document your assessments before and after interventions, including site assessment, presence of pain, lung sounds, and oxygen saturation levels. Document presence of skin breakdown that may result from irritation or pressure from the tracheostomy collar. Document care given.

SKILL VARIATION | **Cleaning a Nondisposable Inner Cannula**

Some tracheostomies use nondisposable inner cannulas, requiring the nurse to clean the inner cannula. Aseptic technique is maintained during the proce- dure. Clean, rather than sterile, technique can be used in the home setting. Additional equip- ment includes the following: sterile tracheostomy cleaning

continued on page 866

Cleaning a Nondisposable Inner Cannula   *continued*

kit, if available, or three sterile basins; sterile brush/pipe cleaners; and sterile cleaning solutions (hydrogen peroxide and normal saline solution).

1. Bring necessary equipment to the bedside stand or overbed table.

2. Perform hand hygiene and put on PPE, if indicated.

3. Identify the patient.

4. Close the curtains around the bed and close the door to the room, if possible.

5. Determine the need for tracheostomy care. **Assess the patient's pain and administer pain medication, if indicated.** Explain what you are going to do and the reason for doing it to the patient, even if the patient does not appear to be alert. Reassure the patient that you will interrupt the procedure if he or she indicates respiratory difficulty.

6. Adjust the bed to a comfortable working position, usually elbow height of the caregiver (VISN 8 Patient Safety Center, 2009). Lower the side rail closest to you. **If conscious, place the patient in a semi-Fowler's position. If unconscious, place the patient in the lateral position, facing you.** Move the overbed table close to your work area and raise it to waist height. Place a trash receptacle within easy reach of the work area.

7. Put on face shield or goggles and mask. Suction tracheostomy, if necessary. If tracheostomy has just been suctioned, remove soiled site dressing and discard before removal of gloves used to perform suctioning.

8. Prepare supplies: Open the tracheostomy care kit and separate basins, touching only the edges. If kit is not available, open three sterile basins. Fill one basin 0.5 inch deep with hydrogen peroxide or half hydrogen peroxide and half saline, based on facility policy. Fill other two basins 0.5 inch with saline. Open sterile brush or pipe cleaners, cotton-tipped applicators, and gauze pads, if they are not already available in the cleaning kit.

9. Put on disposable gloves.

10. Remove the oxygen source if one is present. If not already removed, remove site dressing and dispose of it in the trash can. Stabilize the outer cannula and faceplate of the tracheostomy with your nondominant hand. Rotate the inner cannula in a counterclockwise motion with your dominant

Cleaning a Nondisposable Inner Cannula *continued*

hand to release the lock (Figure A).

FIGURE A Rotating inner cannula while stabilizing outer cannula.

11. Continue to hold the faceplate. Gently remove the inner cannula and carefully drop it in the basin with the hydrogen peroxide. Replace the oxygen source over the outer cannula.

12. Discard gloves and put on sterile gloves. Remove the inner cannula from the soaking solution. Moisten the brush or pipe cleaner in saline and insert into tube, using a back-and-forth motion to clean.

13. Agitate the cannula in saline solution. Remove and tap against the inner surface of the basin. Place on sterile gauze pad. If secretions have accumulated in outer cannula during cleaning of inner cannula, suction outer cannula using sterile technique.

14. Stabilize the outer cannula and faceplate with non-dominant hand. Replace inner cannula into outer cannula with dominant hand (Figure B). Turn clockwise and check that the inner cannula is secure. Reapply oxygen source, if needed.

FIGURE B Replacing inner cannula.

15. Continue with site care as detailed above.

SKILL VARIATION | **Using Alternate Site Dressing if Commercially Prepared Sponge is Not Available**

If a commercially prepared site dressing or drain sponge is not available, do not cut a gauze sponge to use at the tracheostomy site. Cutting the gauze can cause loose fibers, which can

continued on page 868

Using Alternate Site Dressing if Commercially Prepared Sponge is Not Available *continued*

become lodged in the stoma, causing irritation or infection. Loose fibers could also be inhaled into the trachea, causing respiratory distress.

1. Bring necessary equipment to the bedside stand or overbed table.

2. Perform hand hygiene and put on PPE, if indicated.

3. Identify the patient.

4. Close the curtains around the bed and close the door to the room, if possible.

5. Determine the need for tracheostomy care. **Assess the patient's pain and administer pain medication, if indicated.**

6. Explain what you are going to do and the reason for doing it to the patient, even if the patient does not appear to be alert. Reassure the patient that you will interrupt the procedure if he or she indicates respiratory difficulty.

7. Adjust bed to comfortable working position, usually elbow height of the caregiver (VISN 8 Patient Safety Center, 2009). Lower side rail closest to you. **If conscious, place the patient in a semi-Fowler's position. If unconscious, place the patient in the lateral position, facing you.** Move the overbed table close to your work area and raise it to waist height. Place a trash receptacle within easy reach of the work area.

8. Remove oxygen source. Dip cotton-tipped applicator or gauze sponge in second basin with sterile saline and clean stoma under faceplate. Use each applicator or sponge only once, moving from stoma site outward.

9. Pat skin gently with dry 4 × 4 gauze sponge.

10. Fold two gauze sponges on the diagonal, to form triangles. Slide one triangle under the faceplate on each side of the stoma, with the longest side of the triangle against the tracheostomy tube.

SKILL VARIATION | Securing a Tracheostomy With Ties/Tape

A tracheostomy may be secured in place using twill ties or tape. One nurse working alone should always place new

tracheostomy ties in place before removing old ties to prevent accidental extubation of tracheostomy. If it is necessary

Securing a Tracheostomy With Ties/Tape   *continued*

to remove old ties first, obtain the assistance of a second person to hold the tracheostomy tube in place while the old tie is removed and the new tie is replaced.

1. Bring necessary equipment to the bedside stand or overbed table.

2. Perform hand hygiene and put on PPE, if indicated.

3. Identify the patient.

4. Close the curtains around the bed and close the door to the room, if possible.

5. Determine the need for tracheostomy care. **Assess the patient's pain and administer pain medication, if indicated.** Explain what you are going to do and the reason for doing it to the patient, even if the patient does not appear to be alert. Reassure the patient that you will interrupt the procedure if he or she indicates respiratory difficulty.

6. Adjust the bed to a comfortable working position, usually elbow height of the caregiver (VISN 8 Patient Safety Center, 2009). Lower side rail closest to you. **If conscious, place the patient in a semi-Fowler's position. If unconscious, place the patient in the lateral position, facing you.** Move the overbed table close to your work area and raise to waist height. Place a trash receptacle within easy reach of the work area.

7. Put on clean gloves. If another nurse is assisting, both nurses should put on clean gloves.

8. Cut a piece of the tape twice the length of the neck circumference plus 4 inches. Trim ends of tape on the diagonal.

9. Insert one end of the tape through the faceplate opening alongside the old tie. Pull through until both ends are even length (Figure C).

FIGURE C Pulling tape through faceplate opening alongside old tie.

10. Slide both ends of the tape under the patient's neck and insert one end through the remaining opening on other side of the faceplate. Pull snugly and tie ends in double square knot to the

continued on page 870

Securing a Tracheostomy With Ties/Tape   *continued*

side of the patient's neck. You should be able to fit one finger between the neck and the ties. Avoid tying knot at the back of patient's neck, as this can cause excess pressure and skin breakdown. In addition, the ties could be confused with the patient's gown and mistakenly untied. Check to make sure the patient can flex his/her neck comfortably.

11. Carefully cut and remove old ties. Reapply oxygen supply, if necessary.

12. Continue with care as detailed above.

SKILL 166   SUCTIONING A TRACHEOSTOMY: OPEN SYSTEM

Suctioning through a tracheostomy is indicated to maintain a patent airway. However, tracheal suctioning can lead to hypoxemia, cardiac dysrhythmias, trauma, atelectasis, infection, bleeding, and pain. Therefore, it is imperative to be diligent in maintaining aseptic technique and following facility guidelines and procedures to prevent potential hazards. In the home setting and other community-based settings, clean technique is used, as the patient is not exposed to disease-causing organisms that may be found in health care settings, such as hospitals. Suctioning frequency is based on clinical assessment to determine the need for suctioning.

The purpose of suctioning is to remove secretions that are not accessible to bypassed cilia, so the recommendation is to insert the catheter only as far as the end of the tracheostomy tube. Catheter contact and suction cause tracheal mucosal damage, loss of cilia, edema, and fibrosis, and increase the risk of infection and bleeding for the patient. Insertion of the suction catheter to a predetermined distance, no more than 1 cm past the length of the tracheostomy tube, avoids contact with the trachea and carina, reducing the effects of tracheal mucosal damage (Hahn, 2011; Ireton, 2007; Pate, 2004; Pate & Zapata, 2002).

Note: In-line, closed suction systems are available to suction mechanically ventilated patients. The use of closed suction catheter systems may avoid some of the infection control issues and other complications associated with open suction techniques. The closed suctioning procedure is the same for patients with tracheostomy tubes and endotracheal tubes connected to mechanical ventilation. See Skill 63.

DELEGATION CONSIDERATIONS

Suctioning a tracheostomy is not delegated to nursing assistive personnel (NAP) or to unlicensed assistive personnel (UAP). Depending on the state's nurse practice act and the organization's policies and procedures, suctioning of a tracheostomy in a stable situation, such as long-term care and other community-based care settings, may be delegated to licensed practical/vocational nurses (LPN/LVNs). The decision to delegate must be based on careful analysis of the patient's needs and circumstances, as well as the qualifications of the person to whom the task is being delegated. Refer to the Delegation Guidelines in Appendix A.

EQUIPMENT

- Portable or wall suction unit with tubing
- A commercially prepared suction kit with an appropriate-size catheter or
- Sterile suction catheter with Y-port in the appropriate size
- Sterile, disposable container

- Sterile gloves
- Towel or waterproof pad
- Goggles and mask or face shield
- Additional PPE, as indicated
- Disposable, clean gloves
- Resuscitation bag connected to 100% oxygen

ASSESSMENT

- Assess lung sounds. Patients who need to be suctioned may have wheezes, crackles, or gurgling present.
- Assess oxygen saturation level. Oxygen saturation usually decreases when a patient needs to be suctioned.
- Assess respiratory status, including respiratory rate and depth. Patients may become tachypneic when they need to be suctioned. Additional indications for suctioning via a tracheostomy tube include secretions in the tube, acute respiratory distress, and frequent or sustained coughing.
- Assess for pain and the potential to cause pain during the intervention. Perform individualized pain management in response to the patient's needs (Arroyo-Novoa et al., 2008). Administer pain medication, as prescribed, before suctioning.
- Assess appropriate suction catheter depth.
- Assess the characteristics and amount of secretions while suctioning.

NURSING DIAGNOSIS

- Ineffective Airway Clearance
- Risk for Aspiration
- Impaired Gas Exchange

OUTCOME IDENTIFICATION AND PLANNING

- Patient will exhibit improved breath sounds and a clear, patent airway.
- Patient will exhibit an oxygen saturation level within acceptable parameters.
- Patient will demonstrate a respiratory rate and depth within an acceptable range.
- Patient will remain free of any signs of respiratory distress.

IMPLEMENTATION

ACTION	RATIONALE
1. Gather equipment.	Bringing everything to the bedside conserves time and energy. Arranging items nearby is convenient, saves time, and avoids unnecessary stretching and twisting of muscles on the part of the nurse.
2. Perform hand hygiene and put on PPE, if indicated.	Hand hygiene and PPE prevent the spread of microorganisms. PPE is required based on transmission precautions.
3. Identify the patient.	Identifying the patient ensures the right patient receives the intervention and helps prevent errors.
4. Close the curtains around the bed and close the door to the room, if possible.	This ensures the patient's privacy.
5. Determine the need for suctioning. Verify the suction order in the patient's medical record. **Assess for pain or the potential to cause pain. Administer pain medication, as prescribed, before suctioning.**	To minimize trauma to airway mucosa, suctioning should be done only when secretions have accumulated or adventitious breath sounds are audible. Suctioning can cause moderate to severe pain for patients. Individualized pain management is imperative (Arroyo-Novoa et al., 2008). Suctioning stimulates coughing, which is painful for patients with surgical incisions.
6. Explain to the patient what you are going to do and the reason or doing it, even if the patient does not appear to be alert. Reassure the patient you will interrupt the procedure if he or she indicates respiratory difficulty.	Explanation alleviates fears. Even if the patient appears unconscious, the nurse should explain what is happening. Any procedure that compromises respiration is frightening for the patient.

ACTION	RATIONALE

7. Adjust the bed to a comfortable working position, usually elbow height of the caregiver (VISN 8 Patient Safety Center, 2009). Lower side rail closest to you. **If conscious, place the patient in a semi-Fowler's position. If unconscious, place the patient in the lateral position, facing you.** Move the overbed table close to your work area and raise to waist height.

Having the bed at the proper height prevents back and muscle strain. A sitting position helps the patient to cough and makes breathing easier. Gravity also facilitates catheter insertion. The lateral position prevents the airway from becoming obstructed and promotes drainage of secretions. The overbed table provides a work surface and maintains sterility of objects on the work surface.

8. Place towel or waterproof pad across patient's chest.

This protects bed linens and the patient.

9. Turn suction to appropriate pressure.

Higher pressures can cause excessive trauma, hypoxemia, and atelectasis. Glove prevents contact with blood and body fluids. Checking pressure ensures equipment is working properly. Allows for an organized approach to the procedure.

- For a wall unit for an adult: 100–150 mm Hg; neonates: 60–80 mm Hg; infants: 80–125 mm Hg; children: 80–125 mm Hg; adolescents: 80–150 mm Hg (Hess et al., 2012).
- For a portable unit for an adult: 10–15 cm Hg; neonates: 6–8 cm Hg; infants: 8–10 cm Hg; children: 8–10 cm Hg; adolescents: 8–15 cm Hg.

Put on a disposable, clean glove and occlude the end of the connecting tubing to check suction pressure. Place the connecting tubing in a convenient location. If using, place resuscitation bag connected to oxygen within convenient reach.

10. Open sterile suction package using aseptic technique. The open wrapper or container becomes a sterile field to

Sterile normal saline or water is used to lubricate the outside of the catheter, minimizing irritation of mucosa during introduction. It

ACTION	RATIONALE
hold other supplies. Carefully remove the sterile container, touching only the outside surface. Set it up on the work surface and pour sterile saline into it.	is also used to clear the catheter between suction attempts.
11. Put on face shield or goggles and mask. Put on sterile gloves. **The dominant hand will manipulate the catheter and must remain sterile. The nondominant hand is considered clean rather than sterile and will control the suction valve (Y-port) on the catheter.**	Handling the sterile catheter using a sterile glove helps prevent introducing organisms into the respiratory tract; the clean glove protects the nurse from microorganisms.
12. With dominant gloved hand, pick up sterile catheter. Pick up the connecting tubing with the nondominant hand and connect the tubing and suction catheter.	Suction catheter sterility is maintained.
13. Moisten the catheter by dipping it into the container of sterile saline, unless it is a silicone catheter. Occlude Y-tube to check suction.	Lubricating the inside of the catheter with saline helps move secretions in the catheter. Silicone catheters do not require lubrication. Checking ensures equipment is working properly.
14. Using your nondominant hand and a manual resuscitation bag, hyperventilate the patient, delivering three to six breaths or use the sigh mechanism on a mechanical ventilator.	Hyperoxygenation and hyperventilation aid in preventing hypoxemia during suctioning.
15. Open the adapter on the mechanical ventilator tubing or remove oxygen delivery setup with your nondominant hand.	This exposes the tracheostomy tube without contaminating sterile gloved hand.
16. Using your dominant hand, gently and quickly insert catheter into trachea. **Advance the catheter to**	Catheter contact and suction cause tracheal mucosal damage, loss of cilia, edema, and fibrosis, and increase the risk of infection

ACTION	RATIONALE

the predetermined length. Do not occlude Y-port when inserting the catheter.

and bleeding for the patient. Insertion of the suction catheter to a predetermined distance, no more than 1 cm past the length of the endotracheal tube, avoids contact with the trachea and carina, reducing the effects of tracheal mucosal damage (Hahn, 2010; Ireton, 2007; Pate, 2004; Pate & Zapata, 2002). If resistance is met, the carina or tracheal mucosa has been hit. Withdraw the catheter at least 0.5 inch before applying suction. Suctioning when inserting the catheter increases the risk for trauma to airway mucosa and increases risk of hypoxemia.

17. Apply suction by intermittently occluding the Y-port on the catheter with the thumb of your nondominant hand, and gently rotate the catheter as it is being withdrawn (Figure 1). **Do not suction for more than 10 to 15 seconds at a time.**

Turning the catheter as it is withdrawn minimizes trauma to the mucosa. Suctioning for longer than 10 to 15 seconds robs the respiratory tract of oxygen, which may result in hypoxemia. Suctioning too quickly may be ineffective at clearing all secretions.

FIGURE 1 Applying intermittent suction while withdrawing catheter.

18. Hyperventilate the patient using your nondominant hand and a manual resuscitation bag, delivering three to six breaths. Replace the oxygen delivery device,

Suctioning removes air from the patient's airway and can cause hypoxemia. Hyperventilation can help prevent suction-induced hypoxemia.

ACTION	RATIONALE

if applicable, using your nondominant hand and have the patient take several deep breaths. If the patient is mechanically ventilated, close the adapter on the mechanical ventilator tubing and use the sigh mechanism on a mechanical ventilator.

19. Flush catheter with saline. Assess the effectiveness of suctioning and repeat, as needed, and according to patient's tolerance. Wrap the suction catheter around your dominant hand between attempts.

Flushing clears the catheter and lubricates it for next insertion. Reassessment determines the need for additional suctioning. Prevents inadvertent contamination of the catheter.

20. **Allow at least a 30-second to 1-minute interval if additional suctioning is needed. Do not make more than three suction passes per suctioning episode. Encourage the patient to cough and deep breathe between suctioning attempts.** Suction the oropharynx after suctioning the trachea. Do not reinsert in the tracheostomy after suctioning the mouth.

The interval allows for reventilation and reoxygenation of airways. Excessive suction passes contribute to complications. Clears the mouth of secretions. More microorganisms are usually present in the mouth, so it is suctioned last to prevent transmission of contaminants.

21. When suctioning is completed, remove gloves from dominant hand over the coiled catheter, pulling it off inside out. Remove glove from nondominant hand and dispose of gloves, catheter, and container with solution in the appropriate receptacle. Assist the patient to a comfortable position. Raise bed rail and place bed in the lowest position.

This technique reduces transmission of microorganisms. Ensures patient comfort. Proper positioning with raised side rails and proper bed height provide for patient comfort and safety.

ACTION	RATIONALE

22. Turn off suction. Remove supplemental oxygen placed for suctioning, if appropriate. Remove face shield or goggles and mask. Perform hand hygiene.

Removing PPE properly reduces the risk for infection transmission and contamination of other items. Hand hygiene prevents transmission of microorganisms.

23. Offer oral hygiene after suctioning.

Respiratory secretions that are allowed to accumulate in the mouth are irritating to mucous membranes and unpleasant for the patient.

24. Reassess the patient's respiratory status, including respiratory rate, effort, oxygen saturation, and lung sounds.

Assesses the effectiveness of suctioning and the presence of complications.

25. Remove additional PPE, if used. Perform hand hygiene.

Removing PPE properly reduces the risk for infection transmission and contamination of other items. Hand hygiene prevents the spread of microorganisms.

EVALUATION

- Patient exhibits improved breath sounds and a clear and patent airway.
- Patient's oxygen saturation level is within acceptable parameters.
- Patient does not exhibit signs or symptoms of respiratory distress or complications.

DOCUMENTATION

- Document the time of suctioning, your assessments before and after intervention, reason for suctioning, and the characteristics and amount of secretions.

SKILL 167 — CARING FOR A PATIENT IN HALO TRACTION

Halo traction provides immobilization to patients with spinal cord injury. Halo traction consists of a metal ring that fits over the patient's head, connected with skull pins into the skull, and metal bars that connect the ring to a vest that distributes the weight of the device around the chest. It immobilizes the head and neck after traumatic injury to the cervical vertebrae and allows early mobility. It is also used to apply spinal traction.

Nursing responsibilities include reassuring the patient, maintaining the device, monitoring neurovascular status, monitoring respiratory status, promoting exercise, preventing complications from the therapy, preventing infection by providing pin-site care, and providing teaching to ensure compliance and self-care. A growing evidence base supports effective management of pin sites, but there is no clear consensus (Walker, 2012; Lagerquist et al., 2012; Sarro et al., 2010). Pin-site care often varies based on primary care provider and facility policy. Dressings are often applied for the first 48 to 72 hours, and then sites may be left open to air. Pin-site care may be performed frequently in the first 48 to 72 hours after application, when drainage may be heavy; other evidence suggests pin care should begin after the first 48 to 72 hours. Routine pin-site care may then be done on a daily or weekly basis (Timms & Pugh, 2012; Lagerquist et al., 2012). Refer to specific patient medical orders and facility guidelines.

DELEGATION CONSIDERATIONS

The care of a patient with halo traction may not be delegated to nursing assistive personnel (NAP) or to unlicensed assistive personnel (UAP). Depending on the state's nurse practice act and the organization's policies and procedures, care for these patients may be delegated to licensed practical/vocational nurses (LPN/LVNs). The decision to delegate must be based on careful analysis of the patient's needs and circumstances, as well as the qualifications of the person to whom the task is being delegated. Refer to the Delegation Guidelines in Appendix A.

EQUIPMENT

- Basin of warm water
- Bath towels
- Skin cleanser, based on facility policy
- Antimicrobial ointment, per primary care provider order or facility policy
- Sterile applicators
- Cleansing solution, usually sterile normal saline or chlorhexidine, per primary care provider order or facility policy
- Sterile gauze or dressing per primary care provider order or facility policy
- Analgesic, per physician's order
- Clean gloves, if appropriate, for bathing under the vest
- Sterile gloves for performing pin care, depending on facility policy
- Additional PPE, as indicated

ASSESSMENT

- Review the patient's medical record, medical orders, and nursing plan of care to determine the type of device being used and the prescribed care.
- Assess the halo traction device to ensure proper function and position.
- Perform respiratory, neurologic, and skin assessments.
- Inspect the pin-insertion sites for inflammation and infection, including swelling, cloudy or offensive drainage, pain, or redness.
- Assess the patient's knowledge regarding the device and self-care activities and responsibilities, and his/her feelings related to treatment.

NURSING DIAGNOSIS

- Disturbed Body Image
- Self-Care Deficit (toileting, bathing, dressing)
- Disturbed Sleep Pattern
- Risk for Infection

OUTCOME IDENTIFICATION AND PLANNING

The expected outcomes may include:
- Patient maintains cervical alignment.
- Patient shows no evidence of infection.
- Patient is free from complications, such as respiratory impairment, orthostatic hypotension, and skin breakdown.
- Patient experiences relief from pain.
- Patient is free from injury.

IMPLEMENTATION

ACTION	RATIONALE
1. Review the medical record and the nursing plan of care to determine the type of device being used and prescribed care.	Reviewing the medical record and care plan validates the correct patient and correct procedure.
2. Gather the necessary equipment.	Preparation promotes efficient time management and an organized approach to the task.
3. Perform hand hygiene and put on PPE, if indicated.	Hand hygiene and PPE prevent the spread of microorganisms. PPE is required based on transmission precautions.

ACTION	RATIONALE
4. Identify the patient.	Identifying the patient ensures the right patient receives the intervention and helps prevent errors.
5. Close curtains around the bed and close the door to the room, if possible. Explain what you are going to do and why you are going to do it to the patient.	This ensures the patient's privacy. Explanation relieves anxiety and facilitates cooperation.
6. Assemble equipment on overbed table within reach.	Arranging items nearby is convenient, saves time, and avoids unnecessary stretching and twisting of muscles on the part of the nurse.
7. Assess the patient for possible need for nonpharmacologic, pain-reducing interventions or analgesic medication before beginning. Administer appropriate prescribed analgesic. Allow sufficient time for analgesic to achieve its effectiveness before beginning the procedure.	Pain is a subjective experience influenced by past experience. Pin care may cause pain for some patients.
8. Place a waste receptacle at a convenient location for use during the procedure.	Having a waste container handy means that the soiled dressing may be discarded easily, without the spread of microorganisms.
9. Adjust bed to comfortable working height, usually elbow height of the caregiver if the patient will remain in bed (VISN 8 Patient Safety Center, 2009). Alternatively, have the patient sit up, if appropriate.	Having the bed at the proper height prevents back and muscle strain.
10. Assist the patient to a comfortable position that provides easy access to the head. Place a waterproof pad under the head if the patient is lying down.	Patient positioning provides for comfort. Waterproof pad protects underlying surfaces.

ACTION	RATIONALE
11. Monitor vital signs and perform a neurologic assessment, including level of consciousness, motor function, and sensation, per facility policy. This is usually at least every 2 hours for 24 hours, or possibly every hour for 48 hours.	Changes in the neurologic assessment could indicate spinal cord trauma, which would require immediate intervention.
12. Examine the halo vest unit every 8 hours for stability, secure connections, and positioning. Make sure the patient's head is centered in the halo without neck flexion or extension. Check each bolt for loosening.	Assessment ensures correct function of the device and patient safety. Loose bolts require attention from an appropriate advanced practice professional to maintain correct positioning, proper alignment, and unit stability.
13. Check the fit of the vest. With the patient in a supine position, you should be able to insert one or two fingers under the jacket at the shoulder and chest.	Checking the fit prevents compression on the chest, which could interfere with respiratory status.
14. Put on nonsterile gloves, if appropriate. Remove patient's shirt or gown. Wash the patient's chest and back daily. Loosen the bottom Velcro straps. Protect the vest liner with a waterproof pad.	Gloves prevent contact with blood and body fluids. Removal of clothing from torso allows visualization of, and access to, appropriate areas. Daily cleaning prevents skin breakdown and allows assessment. Loosening the straps allows access to the chest and back. Waterproof pad keeps the vest liner dry and prevents skin irritation and breakdown.
15. Wring out a bath towel soaked in warm water (and skin cleanser, depending of facility policy). Pull the towel back and forth in a drying motion beneath the front.	Using an overly wet towel could lead to skin maceration and breakdown.
16. Thoroughly dry the skin in the same manner with a dry towel. Inspect the skin for	Drying prevents skin irritation and breakdown. Powders and lotions can cause skin irritation.

ACTION	RATIONALE
tender, reddened areas or pressure spots. Do not use powder or lotion under the vest.	
17. Turn the patient on his/her side, less than 45 degrees if lying supine, and repeat the process on the back. Remove waterproof pad from the vest liner. Close the Velcro straps. Assist the patient with putting on a new shirt, if desired.	Doing so prevents skin breakdown. Cleansers and lotions can cause skin irritation.
18. Perform a respiratory assessment. Check for respiratory impairment, such as absence of breath sounds, the presence of adventitious sounds, reduced inspiratory effort, or shortness of breath.	The halo vest limits chest expansion, which could lead to alterations in respiratory function. Pulmonary embolus is a common complication associated with spinal cord injury.
19. Assess the pin sites for redness, tenting of the skin: prolonged or purulent drainage; swelling; and bowing, bending, or loosening of the pins. Monitor body temperature.	Pin sites provide an entry for microorganisms. Assessment allows for early detection and prompt intervention should problems arise.
20. Perform pin-site care. (See Skill 69 and Skill 168.)	Pin-site care reduces the risk of infection and subsequent osteomyelitis.
21. Depending on medical order and facility policy, apply antimicrobial ointment to pin sites and a dressing.	Antimicrobial ointment helps prevent infection. Dressing provides protection and helps contain any drainage.
22. Remove gloves and dispose of them appropriately. Raise rails, as appropriate, and place the bed in the lowest position. Assist the patient to a comfortable position.	Disposing of gloves reduces the risk of microorganism transmission. Rails assist with patient positioning. Proper bed height ensures patient safety.
23. Remove additional PPE, if used. Perform hand hygiene.	Removing PPE properly reduces the risk for infection transmission and contamination of other items. Hand hygiene prevents the spread of microorganisms.

EVALUATION
- Patient maintains cervical alignment.
- Patient shows no evidence of infection.
- Patient is free from complications, such as respiratory impairment, orthostatic hypotension, and skin breakdown.
- Patient experiences relief from pain.
- Patient is free from injury.

DOCUMENTATION
- Document the time, date, and type of device in place. Include the skin assessment, pin-site assessment, personal hygiene, and pin-site care. Document the patient's response to the device and the neurologic assessment and respiratory assessment.

SKILL 168 | CARING FOR A PATIENT IN SKELETAL TRACTION

Skeletal traction provides pull to a body part by attaching weight directly to the bone, using pins, screws, wires, or tongs. It is used to immobilize a body part for prolonged periods. This method of traction is used to treat fractures of the femur, tibia, and cervical spine. Nursing responsibilities related to skeletal traction include maintaining the traction, maintaining body alignment, monitoring neurovascular status, promoting exercise, preventing complications from the therapy and immobility, and preventing infection by providing pin site care. A growing evidence base supports effective management of pin sites, but no clear consensus (Walker, 2012; Lagerquist et al., 2012). Pin-site care often varies based on primary care provider and facility policy. Dressings are often applied for the first 48 to 72 hours, and then sites may be left open to air. Pin-site care may be performed frequently in the first 48 to 72 hours after application, when drainage may be heavy; other evidence suggests pin care should begin after the first 48 to 72 hours. Pin-site care may be done daily or weekly (Timms & Pugh, 2012; Lagerquist et al.). Refer to specific patient medical orders and facility guidelines.

DELEGATION CONSIDERATIONS

The care of a patient with skeletal traction may not be delegated to nursing assistive personnel (NAP) or to unlicensed assistive personnel (UAP). Depending on the state's nurse practice act and the organization's policies and procedures, care for these patients may be delegated to licensed practical/vocational nurses (LPN/LVNs). The decision to delegate must be based on careful analysis of the patient's needs and circumstances, as well as the qualifications of the person to whom the task is being delegated. Refer to the Delegation Guidelines in Appendix A.

EQUIPMENT

- Sterile gloves
- Sterile applicators
- Cleansing agent for pin care, usually sterile normal saline or chlorhexidine, per primary care provider order or facility policy
- Sterile container
- Antimicrobial ointment, per primary care provider order or facility policy
- Sterile gauze or dressing, per primary care provider order or facility policy
- Analgesic, as ordered
- Sterile gloves for performing pin care, depending on facility policy
- Additional PPE, as indicated

ASSESSMENT

- Review the patient's medical record and nursing plan of care to determine the type of traction, traction weight, and line of pull.
- Assess the traction equipment to ensure proper function, including inspecting the ropes for fraying and proper positioning.
- Assess the patient's body alignment.
- Assess the patient's pain and need for analgesia before providing care.
- Perform skin and neurovascular assessments.
- Inspect the pin insertion sites for inflammation and infection, including swelling, cloudy or offensive drainage, pain, or redness.
- Assess for complications of immobility, including alterations in respiratory function, constipation, alterations in skin integrity, alterations in urinary elimination, and muscle weakness, contractures, thrombophlebitis, pulmonary embolism, and fatigue.

NURSING DIAGNOSIS

- Self-Care Deficit (toileting, bathing, or dressing)
- Anxiety
- Deficient Knowledge
- Risk for Infection

OUTCOME IDENTIFICATION AND PLANNING

- Traction is maintained appropriately.
- Patient is free from complications of immobility and infection.
- Patient maintains proper body alignment.
- Patient reports an increased level of comfort.
- Patient is free from injury.

IMPLEMENTATION

ACTION	RATIONALE
1. Review the medical record and the nursing plan of care to determine the type of	Reviewing the medical record and plan of care validates the correct patient and correct procedure.

ACTION	RATIONALE
traction being used and the prescribed care.	
2. Perform hand hygiene. Put on PPE, as indicated. 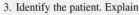	Hand hygiene and PPE prevent the spread of microorganisms. PPE is required based on transmission precautions.
3. Identify the patient. Explain the procedure to the patient, emphasizing the importance of maintaining counterbalance, alignment, and position.	Patient identification validates the correct patient and correct procedure. Discussion and explanation help allay anxiety and prepare the patient for what to expect.
4. Perform a pain assessment and assess for muscle spasm. Administer prescribed medications in sufficient time to allow for the full effect of the analgesic and/or muscle relaxant.	Assessing for pain and administering analgesics promote patient comfort.
5. Close the curtains around the bed and close the door to the room, if possible. Place the bed at an appropriate and comfortable working height, usually elbow height of the caregiver (VISN 8 Patient Safety Center, 2009).	Closing the door or curtains provides for privacy. Proper bed height prevents back and muscle strain.
6. Ensure the traction apparatus is attached securely to the bed. Assess the traction setup, including application of the ordered amount of weight. **Be sure that the weights hang freely, not touching the bed or the floor.**	Proper traction application reduces the risk of injury by promoting accurate counterbalance and traction function.
7. **Check that the ropes move freely through the pulleys. Check that all knots are tight and are positioned away from the pulleys. Pulleys should be free from the linens.**	Free ropes and pulleys ensure accurate counterbalance and traction function.

ACTION	RATIONALE
8. Check the alignment of the patient's body, as prescribed.	Proper alignment maintains an effective line of pull and prevents injury.
9. Perform a skin assessment. Pay attention to pressure points, including the ischial tuberosity, popliteal space, Achilles' tendon, sacrum, and heel.	Skin assessment provides early intervention for skin irritation, impaired tissue perfusion, and other complications.
10. Perform a neurovascular assessment. Assess the extremity distal to the traction for edema and peripheral pulses. Assess the temperature and color and compare with the unaffected limb. Check for pain, inability to move body parts distal to the traction, pallor, and abnormal sensations. Assess for indicators of deep-vein thrombosis (DVT), including calf tenderness, and swelling.	Neurovascular assessment aids in early identification and allows for prompt intervention should compromised circulation and oxygenation of tissues develop.
11. Assess the site at and around the pins for redness, edema, and odor. Assess for skin tenting, prolonged or purulent drainage, elevated body temperature, elevated pin site temperature, and bowing or bending of the pins.	Pin sites provide a possible entry for microorganisms. Skin inspection allows for early detection and prompt intervention should complications develop.
12. Provide pin-site care.	Performing pin-site care prevents crusting at the site that could lead to fluid buildup, infection, and osteomyelitis.
a. Using sterile technique, open the applicator package and pour the cleansing agent into the sterile container.	Using sterile technique reduces the risk for transmission of microorganisms.
b. Put on the sterile gloves.	Gloves prevent contact with blood and/or body fluids.
c. Place the applicators into the solution.	

ACTION	RATIONALE
d. **Clean the pin site starting at the insertion area and working outward, away from the pin site (Figure 1).**	Cleaning from the center outward ensures movement from the least to most contaminated area.

FIGURE 1 Cleaning around pin sites with normal saline on an applicator.

ACTION	RATIONALE
e. **Use each applicator once. Use a new applicator for each pin site.**	Using an applicator once reduces the risk of transmission of microorganisms.
13. Depending on medical order and facility policy, apply the antimicrobial ointment to pin sites and apply a dressing. Remove gloves and dispose of them appropriately.	Antimicrobial ointment helps reduce the risk of infection. A dressing aids in protecting the pin sites from contamination and containing any drainage. Disposing of gloves reduces the risk of microorganism transmission.
14. Perform range-of-motion (ROM) exercises on all joint areas, unless contraindicated. Encourage the patient to cough and deep breathe every 2 hours.	Range-of-motion exercises promote joint mobility. Coughing and deep breathing reduce the risk of respiratory complications related to immobility.
15. Place the bed in the lowest position that still allows the weight to hang freely. Make sure the call bell and other essential items are within easy reach.	Proper bed positioning ensures effective application of traction without patient injury. Having call bell and other items in easy reach contributes to patient safety.
16. Remove PPE, if used. Perform hand hygiene.	Removing PPE properly reduces the risk for infection transmission and contamination of other items. Hand hygiene prevents the spread of microorganisms.

EVALUATION

- Patient demonstrates maintenance of skeletal traction with pin sites free of infection.
- Patient maintains proper body alignment and joint function.
- Patient verbalizes pain relief.
- Patient states signs and symptoms to report.
- Patient remains free of injury.

DOCUMENTATION

- Document the time, date, type of traction, and the amount of weight used. Include skin and pin site assessments, and pin-site care. Document the patient's response to the traction and the neurovascular status of the extremity.

SKILL 169 | APPLYING SKIN TRACTION AND CARING FOR A PATIENT IN SKIN TRACTION

Traction is the application of a pulling force to a part of the body. It is used to reduce fractures, treat dislocations, correct or prevent deformities, improve or correct contractures, or decrease muscle spasms. It must be applied in the correct direction and magnitude to obtain the therapeutic effects desired.

With traction, the affected body part is immobilized by pulling with equal force on each end of the injured area, mixing traction and counter traction. Weights provide the pulling force or traction. The use of additional weights or positioning the patient's body weight against the traction pull provides the counter traction. Skin traction is applied directly to the skin, exerting indirect pull on the bone. The force may be applied using adhesive or nonadhesive traction tape or a boot, belt, or halter. Skin traction immobilizes a body part intermittently. Types of skin traction for adults include Buck's extension traction (lower leg), a cervical head halter, and the pelvic belt. Nursing care for skin traction includes setting the traction up, applying the traction, monitoring the application and patient response, and preventing complications from the therapy and immobility.

DELEGATION CONSIDERATIONS

The application of, and care for, a patient with skin traction may not be delegated to nursing assistive personnel (NAP) or to unlicensed assistive personnel (UAP). Depending on the state's nurse practice act and the organization's policies and procedures, this care may be delegated to licensed practical/vocational nurses (LPN/LVNs). The decision to delegate must be based on careful analysis of the patient's needs and circumstances, as well as the qualifications of the person to whom the task is being delegated. Refer to the Delegation Guidelines in Appendix A.

EQUIPMENT

- Bed with traction frame and trapeze
- Weights
- Velcro straps or other straps
- Rope and pulleys
- Boot with footplate
- Graduated compression stocking, as appropriate
- Nonsterile gloves and/or other PPE, as indicated
- Skin cleansing supplies

ASSESSMENT

- Assess the patient's medical record and the nursing plan of care to determine the type of traction, traction weight, and line of pull.
- Assess the traction equipment to ensure proper function, including inspecting the ropes for fraying and proper positioning.
- Assess the patient's body alignment.
- Perform skin and neurovascular assessments.
- Assess for complications of immobility, including alterations in respiratory function, skin integrity, urinary and bowel elimination, and muscle weakness, contractures, thrombophlebitis, pulmonary embolism, and fatigue.

NURSING DIAGNOSIS

- Risk for Injury
- Impaired Physical Mobility
- Self-Care Deficit (bathing, feeding, dressing, or toileting)
- Risk for Impaired Skin Integrity

OUTCOME IDENTIFICATION AND PLANNING

- Traction is maintained with the appropriate counterbalance and the patient is free from complications of immobility.
- Patient maintains proper body alignment.
- Patient reports an increased level of comfort.
- Patient is free from injury.

IMPLEMENTATION

ACTION	RATIONALE
1. Review the medical record and the nursing plan of care to determine the type of traction being used and care for the affected body part.	Reviewing the medical record and plan of care validates the correct patient and correct procedure.
2. Perform hand hygiene. Put on PPE, as indicated.	Hand hygiene and PPE prevent the spread of microorganisms. PPE is required based on transmission precautions.

ACTION	RATIONALE

3. Identify the patient. Explain the procedure to the patient, emphasizing the importance of maintaining counter-balance, alignment, and position.

Patient identification validates the correct patient and correct procedure. Discussion and explanation help allay anxiety and prepare the patient for what to expect.

4. Perform a pain assessment and assess for muscle spasm. Administer prescribed medications in sufficient time to allow for the full effect of the analgesic and/or muscle relaxant.

Assessing pain and administering analgesics promote patient comfort.

5. Close the curtains around the bed and close the door to the room, if possible. Place the bed at an appropriate and comfortable working height, usually elbow height of the caregiver (VISN 8 Patient Safety Center, 2009).

Closing the door or curtains provides for privacy. Proper bed height prevents back and muscle strain.

Applying Skin Traction

6. Ensure the traction apparatus is attached securely to the bed. Assess the traction setup.

Assessment of traction setup and weights promotes safety.

7. Check that the ropes move freely through the pulleys. Check that all knots are tight and are positioned away from the pulleys. Pulleys should be free from the linens.

Checking ropes and pulleys ensures that weight is being applied correctly, promoting accurate counterbalance and traction function.

8. Place the patient in a supine position with the foot of the bed elevated slightly. The patient's head should be near the head of the bed and in alignment.

Proper patient positioning maintains proper counterbalance and promotes safety.

9. Cleanse the affected area. Place the elastic stocking on the affected limb, as appropriate.

Skin care aids in preventing skin breakdown. Use of graduated compression stockings prevents edema and neurovascular complications.

ACTION	RATIONALE
10. Place the traction boot over the patient's leg. Be sure the patient's heel is in the heel of the boot. Secure the boot with the straps.	The boot provides a means for attaching traction; proper application ensures proper pull.
11. Attach the traction cord to the boot footplate. Pass the rope over the pulley fastened at the end of the bed. Attach the weight to the hook on the rope, usually 5 to 10 pounds for an adult. Gently let go of the weight. **The weight should hang freely, not touching the bed or the floor.**	Weight attachment applies the pull for the traction. Gently releasing the weight prevents a quick pull on the extremity and possible injury and pain. Properly hanging weights and correct patient positioning ensure accurate counterbalance and traction function.
12. **Check the patient's alignment with the traction.**	Proper alignment is necessary for proper counterbalance and ensures patient safety.
13. **Check the boot for placement and alignment. Make sure the line of pull is parallel to the bed and not angled downward.**	Misalignment causes ineffective traction and may interfere with healing. A properly positioned boot prevents pressure on the heel.
14. Place the bed in the lowest position that still allows the weight to hang freely. Make sure the call bell and other essential items are within easy reach.	Proper bed positioning ensures effective application of traction without patient injury. Having call bell and other items in easy reach contributes to patient safety.
15. Remove PPE, if used. Perform hand hygiene.	Removing PPE properly decreases the risk for infection transmission and contamination of other items. Hand hygiene prevents the spread of microorganisms.

Caring for a Patient With Skin Traction

16. Perform a skin-traction assessment per facility policy. This assessment includes checking the traction equipment, examining the affected body part, maintaining proper	Assessment provides information to determine proper application and alignment, thereby reducing the risk for injury. Misalignment causes ineffective traction and may interfere with healing.

ACTION	RATIONALE
body alignment, and performing skin and neurovascular assessments.	
17. Remove the straps every 4 hours per the physician's order or facility policy. Check bony prominences for skin breakdown, abrasions, and pressure areas. Remove the boot, per medical order or facility policy, every 8 hours. Put on gloves and wash, rinse, and thoroughly dry the skin.	Removing the straps provides assessment information for early detection and prompt intervention of potential complications should they arise. Washing the area enhances circulation to skin; thorough drying prevents skin breakdown. Using gloves prevents transfer of microorganisms.
18. Assess the extremity distal to the traction for edema, and assess peripheral pulses. Assess the temperature, color, and capillary refill, and compare with the unaffected limb. Check for pain, inability to move body parts distal to the traction, pallor, and abnormal sensations. Assess for indicators of DVT, including calf tenderness, and swelling.	Doing so helps detect signs of abnormal neurovascular function and allows for prompt intervention. Assessing neurovascular status determines the circulation and oxygenation of tissues. Pressure within the traction boot may increase with edema.
19. Replace the traction; remove gloves and dispose of them appropriately.	Replacing traction is necessary to provide immobilization and facilitate healing. Proper disposal of gloves prevents the transmission of microorganisms.
20. Check the boot for placement and alignment. **Make sure the line of pull is parallel to the bed and not angled downward.**	Misalignment causes ineffective traction and may interfere with healing. A properly positioned boot prevents pressure on the heel.
21. **Ensure the patient is positioned in the center of the bed, with the affected leg aligned with the trunk of the patient's body. Check overall alignment of the patient's body.**	Misalignment interferes with the effectiveness of traction and may lead to complications.

ACTION	RATIONALE
22. Examine the weights and pulley system. **Weights should hang freely, off the floor and bed. Knots should be secure. Ropes should move freely through the pulleys. The pulleys should not be constrained by knots.**	Checking the weights and pulley system ensures proper application and reduces the risk for patient injury from traction application.
23. Perform range-of-motion exercises on all unaffected joint areas, unless contra-indicated. Encourage the patient to cough and deep breathe every 2 hours.	ROM exercises maintain joint function. Coughing and deep breathing help to reduce the risk for respiratory complications related to immobility.
24. Raise the side rails. Place the bed in the lowest position that still allows the weight to hang freely. Make sure the call bell and other essential items are within easy reach.	Raising the side rails promotes patient safety. Proper bed positioning ensures effective application of traction without patient injury. Having call bell and other items in easy reach contributes to patient safety.
25. Remove PPE, if used. Perform hand hygiene.	Removing PPE properly decreases the risk for infection transmission and contamination of other items. Hand hygiene prevents the spread of micro-organisms.

EVALUATION

- Patient demonstrates proper body alignment with traction applied and maintained with appropriate counterbalance.
- Patient verbalizes pain relief, with pain rated at lower numbers.
- Patient remains free of injury.

DOCUMENTATION

- Document the time, date, type, amount of weight used, and the site where the traction was applied. Include the skin assessment and care provided before application. Document the patient's response to the traction and the neurovascular status of the extremity.

SKILL 170 | TRANSFERRING A PATIENT FROM THE BED TO A CHAIR

Often, moving a patient from the bed to a chair helps him or her begin engaging in physical activity. Also, changing a patient's position will help prevent complications related to immobility. Safety and comfort are key concerns when assisting the patient out of bed. Assessing the patient's response to activity is a major nursing responsibility. Before performing the transfer, identify any restrictions related to the patient's condition and determine how activity levels may be affected. Figure 1, Safe Patient Handling Algorithm 1, can assist in making decisions about safe patient handling and movement. Using assistance, appropriate lifting and repositioning devices, good body mechanics, and correct technique are important to avoid injuries to yourself and the patient. During any patient-handling task, if any caregiver is required to lift more than 35 pounds of a patient's weight, consider the patient to be fully dependent and use assistive devices (Waters, 2007).

DELEGATION CONSIDERATIONS

The transfer of a patient from bed to a chair may be delegated to nursing assistive personnel (NAP) or to unlicensed assistive personnel (UAP), as well as to licensed practical/vocational nurses (LPN/LVNs). The decision to delegate must be based on careful analysis of the patient's needs and circumstances, as well as the qualifications of the person to whom the task is being delegated. Refer to the Delegation Guidelines in Appendix A.

EQUIPMENT

- Chair or wheelchair
- Gait belt
- Stand-assist aid, if available
- Additional staff person to assist
- Blanket to cover the patient in the chair
- Nonsterile gloves and/or other PPE, as indicated

ASSESSMENT

- Assess the situation to determine the need to get the patient out of bed.
- Review the medical record and nursing plan of care for conditions that may influence the patient's ability to move or to be transferred.
- Check for tubes, IV lines, incisions, or equipment that may require modifying the transfer procedure.
- Assess the patient's level of consciousness, ability to understand and follow directions, and ability to assist with the transfer.
- Assess the patient's weight and your strength to determine if additional assistance is needed. Determine the need for bariatric equipment.
- Assess the patient's comfort level; if needed, medicate as ordered with analgesics.

Algorithm 1: Transfer to and From: Bed to Chair, Chair to Toilet, Chair to Chair, or Car to Chair

FIGURE 1 Step-by-step procedure or algorithm used to outline safe techniques for transferring a patient to and from bed to chair. (From VISN 8 Patient Safety Center. (2009). Safe patient handling and movement algorithms. Tampa, FL: Author. Available http://www.visn8.va.gov/visn8/patientsafetycenter/safePtHandling/default.asp.)

• If the patient is able to bear only partial weight, consider a second staff person to assist. If the patient is unable to bear even partial weight, or is uncooperative, use a full-body sling lift to move the patient.

NURSING DIAGNOSIS

• Activity Intolerance
• Risk for Falls
• Impaired Physical Mobility

OUTCOME IDENTIFICATION AND PLANNING

• Transfer is accomplished without injury to patient or nurse.
• Patient remains free of any complications of immobility.

IMPLEMENTATION

ACTION	RATIONALE
1. Review the medical record and nursing plan of care for conditions that may influence the patient's ability to move or to be positioned. Assess for tubes, IV lines, incisions, or equipment that may alter the positioning procedure. Identify any movement limitations. **Consult patient-handling algorithm, if available, to plan appropriate approach to moving the patient.**	Reviewing the medical record and plan of care validates the correct patient and correct procedure. Identification of limitations and ability and use of an algorithm help to prevent injury and aid in determining best plan for patient movement.
2. Perform hand hygiene and put on PPE, as indicated.	Hand hygiene and PPE prevent spread of microorganisms. PPE is required based on transmission precautions.
3. Identify the patient. Explain the procedure to the patient.	Patient identification validates the correct patient and correct procedure. Discussion and explanation help allay anxiety and prepare the patient for what to expect.
4. If needed, move equipment to make room for the chair. Close the curtains around the bed and close the door to the room, if possible.	A clear pathway from the bed to the chair facilitates the transfer. Closing the door or curtain provides for privacy.

ACTION	RATIONALE
5. Place the bed in the lowest position. Raise the head of the bed to a sitting position, or as high as the patient can tolerate.	Proper bed height and positioning facilitate the transfer. The amount of energy needed to move from a sitting position or elevated position to a sitting position is decreased.
6. **Make sure the bed brakes are locked. Put the chair next to the bed. If available, lock the brakes of the chair. If the chair does not have brakes, brace the chair against a secure object.**	Locking brakes or bracing the chair prevents movement during transfer and increases stability and patient safety.
7. Encourage the patient to make use of a stand-assist aid, either freestanding or attached to the side of the bed, if available, to move to the side of the bed and to a side-lying position, facing the side of the bed on which the patient will sit.	Encourages independence, reduces strain for staff, and decreases risk for patient injury.
8. Lower the side rail, if necessary, and stand near the patient's hips. Stand with your legs shoulder width apart with one foot near the head of the bed, slightly in front of the other foot.	The nurse's center of gravity is placed near the patient's greatest weight to assist the patient to a sitting position safely.
9. Encourage the patient to make use of the stand-assist device. Assist the patient to sit up on the side of the bed; ask the patient to swing his or her legs over the side of the bed. At the same time, pivot on your back leg to lift the patient's trunk and shoulders. Keep your back straight; avoid twisting.	Gravity lowers the patient's legs over the bed. The nurse transfers weight in the direction of motion and protects his or her back from injury.
10. **Stand in front of the patient, and assess for any balance problems or complaints of dizziness. Allow**	Standing in front of the patient prevents falls or injuries from orthostatic hypotension. The sitting position facilitates transfer to

ACTION	RATIONALE
the patient's legs to dangle a few minutes before continuing.	the chair and allows the circulatory system to adjust to a change in position.
11. Assist the patient to put on a robe, as necessary, and nonskid footwear.	Robe provides warmth and privacy. Nonskid soles reduce the risk for falling.
12. Wrap the gait belt around the patient's waist, based on assessed need and facility policy.	Gait belts improve the caregiver's grasp, reducing the risk of musculoskeletal injuries to staff and the patient. Provides firmer grasp for the caregiver if patient should lose his or her balance.
13. Stand facing the patient. Spread your feet about shoulder width apart and flex your hips and knees.	This position provides stability and allows for smooth movement using the legs' large muscle groups.
14. Ask the patient to slide his or her buttocks to the edge of the bed until the feet touch the floor. Position yourself as close as possible to the patient, with your foot positioned on the outside of the patient's foot. If a second staff person is assisting, have him or her assume a similar position. Grasp the gait belt (Figure 2).	Doing so provides balance and support.

FIGURE 2 Standing close to patient and grasping gait belt.

| 15. Encourage the patient to make use of the stand-assist device. If necessary, have second staff person grasp the gait belt on opposite side. Rock back and forth while counting to three. **On the** | Holding at the gait belt prevents injury to the patient. Bracing your knee against a weak extremity prevents a weak knee from buckling and the patient from falling. Assessing balance and strength helps to identify the |

ACTION	RATIONALE
count of three, using the gait belt and your legs (not your back), assist the patient to a standing position. If indicated, brace your front knee against the patient's weak extremity as he or she stands. Assess the patient's balance and leg strength. If the patient is weak or unsteady, return the patient to bed.	need for additional assistance to prevent falling.
16. Pivot on your back foot and assist the patient to turn until the patient feels the chair against his or her legs.	This action ensures proper positioning before sitting.
17. Ask the patient to use his arm to steady himself on the arm of the chair while slowly lowering to a sitting position. Continue to brace the patient's knees with your knees and hold the gait belt. Flex your hips and knees when helping the patient sit in the chair.	The patient uses his or her own arm for support and stability. Flexing hips and knees uses major muscle groups to aid in movement and reduce strain on the nurse's back.
18. Assess the patient's alignment in the chair. Remove gait belt, if desired. Depending on patient comfort, it could be left in place to use when returning to bed. Cover with a blanket, if needed. Make sure call bell and other essential items are within easy reach.	Assessment promotes comfort; blanket provides warmth and privacy; having the call bell and other essential items readily available helps promote safety.
19. Clean transfer aids, per facility policy, if not indicated for single patient use. Remove gloves and any other PPE, if used. Perform hand hygiene.	Proper cleaning of equipment between patient use prevents the spread of microorganisms. Removing PPE properly reduces the risk for infection transmission and contamination of other items. Hand hygiene prevents the spread of microorganisms.

EVALUATION
- Patient transfers from the bed to the chair without injury.
- Patient exhibits no signs and symptoms of problems or complications related to immobility.
- Nurse remains free of injury during the transfer.

DOCUMENTATION
- Document the activity, including the length of time the patient sat in the chair, any other pertinent observations, and the patient's tolerance of and reaction to the activity. Document the use of transfer aids and number of staff required for transfer.

SKILL 171 TRANSFERRING A PATIENT FROM THE BED TO A STRETCHER

While in the hospital, patients are often transported by stretcher to other areas for tests or procedures. Considerable care must be taken when moving someone from a bed to a stretcher or from a stretcher to a bed to prevent injury to the patient or staff. Refer to Figure 1, Safe Patient Handling Algorithm 2, to help in making decisions about safe patient handling and movement. Using assistance, appropriate lifting and repositioning devices, good body mechanics, and correct technique are important to avoid injuries to self and to the patient. During any patient-handling task, if any caregiver is required to lift more than 35 pounds of a patient's weight, consider the patient to be fully dependent and use assistive devices (Waters, 2007). Be familiar with the proper way to use lateral-assist devices, based on the manufacturer's directions.

DELEGATION CONSIDERATIONS
The transfer of a patient from bed to stretcher may be delegated to nursing assistive personnel (NAP) or to unlicensed assistive personnel (UAP), as well as to licensed practical/vocational nurses (LPN/LVNs). The decision to delegate must be based on careful analysis of the patient's needs and circumstances, as well as the qualifications of the person to whom the task is being delegated. Refer to the Delegation Guidelines in Appendix A.

EQUIPMENT
- Transport stretcher
- Friction-reducing sheet
- Lateral-assist device, such as a transfer board, roller board, or mechanical lateral-assist device, if available
- Bath blanket
- Regular blanket
- At least two assistants, depending on the patient's condition
- Nonsterile gloves and/or other PPE, as indicated

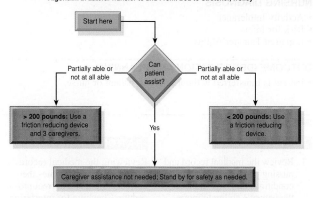

Algorithm 2: Lateral Transfer to and From: Bed to Stretcher, Trolley

General Notes:
- Surfaces should be even for all lateral patient moves.
- For patients with Stage 3 or 4 pressure ulcers, care must be taken to avoid shearing force.
- During any patient transferring task, if any caregiver is required to lift more than 35 pounds of a patient's weight, then the patient should be considered to be fully dependent and assistive devices should be used for the transfer.

FIGURE 1 Step-by-step procedure or algorithm used to outline safe technique for transferring a patient from bed to a stretcher. The first decision point in this algorithm is whether or not the patient can assist. If the patient is partially able or not at all able and weighs less than 200 pounds, use a friction-reducing device and three caregivers. If the patient can assist, caregiver assistance is not needed, but caregivers should stand by for safety. (From VISN 8 Patient Safety Center. (2009). *Safe patient handling and movement algorithms.* Tampa, FL: Author. Available. http://www.visn8.va.gov/visn8/patientsafetycenter/ safePtHandling/default.asp).

ASSESSMENT

- Review the medical record and nursing plan of care for conditions that may influence the patient's ability to move or to be transferred.
- Assess for tubes, IV lines, incisions, or equipment that may alter the transfer process.
- Assess the patient's level of consciousness, ability to understand and follow directions, and ability to assist with the transfer.
- Assess the patient's weight and your strength to determine if a fourth individual (or more) is required to assist with the activity. Determine a need for bariatric equipment.
- Assess the patient's comfort level; if needed, medicate, as ordered, with analgesics.

NURSING DIAGNOSIS

- Activity Intolerance
- Risk for Injury
- Impaired Transfer Ability

OUTCOME IDENTIFICATION AND PLANNING

- Patient is transferred without injury to patient or nurse.

IMPLEMENTATION

ACTION	RATIONALE
1. Review the medical record and nursing plan of care for any conditions that may influence the patient's ability to move or to be positioned. Assess for tubes, IV lines, incisions, or equipment that may alter the positioning procedure. Identify any movement limitations. **Consult patient handling algorithm, if available, to plan appropriate approach to moving the patient.**	Reviewing the medical record and plan of care validates the correct patient and correct procedure. Checking for interfering equipment helps reduce the risk for injury. Identification of limitations and ability along with use of an algorithm helps to prevent injury and aids in determining the best plan for patient movement.
2. Perform hand hygiene and put on PPE, if indicated.	Hand hygiene and PPE prevent the spread of microorganisms. PPE is required based on transmission precautions.
3. Identify the patient. Explain the procedure to the patient.	Patient identification validates the correct patient and correct procedure. Discussion and explanation help allay anxiety and prepare the patient for what to expect.
4. Close the curtains around the bed and close the door to the room, if possible. Adjust the head of the bed to a flat position or as low as the patient can tolerate. Raise the bed to a height that is even with the transport stretcher (VISN 8 Patient Safety Center, 2009). Lower the side rails, if in place.	Closing the door or curtain provides privacy. Proper bed height and lowering side rails make transfer easier and decrease the risk for injury.

ACTION	RATIONALE
5. Place the bath blanket over the patient and remove the top covers from underneath.	Bath blanket provides privacy and warmth.
6. If a friction-reducing transfer sheet is not in place under the patient, place one under the patient's midsection. Have patient fold arms against chest and move chin to chest. Use the friction-reducing sheet to move the patient to the side of the bed where the stretcher will be placed. Alternately, place a lateral-assist device under the patient. Follow manufacturer's directions for use.	A friction-reducing sheet supports the patient's weight, reduces friction during the lift, and provides for a secure hold. Positioning with chin to chest and arms folded provides assistance, reduces friction, and prevents hyperextension of the neck. A transfer board or other lateral-assist device makes it easier to move the patient and minimizes the risk for injury to the patient and nurses.
7. Position the stretcher next (and parallel) to the bed. **Lock the wheels on the stretcher and the bed.**	Positioning equipment makes the transfer easier and decreases the risk for injury. Locking the wheels keeps the bed and stretcher from moving.
8. Two nurses should stand on the stretcher side of the bed. A third nurse should stand on the side of the bed without the stretcher.	Team coordination provides for patient safety during transfer.
9. Use the friction-reducing sheet to roll the patient away from the stretcher. Place the transfer board across the space between the stretcher and the bed, partially under the patient (Figure 2). Roll the patient onto his or her	The transfer board or other lateral-assist device reduces friction, easing the workload to move patient.

FIGURE 2 Positioning transfer board under patient.

ACTION	RATIONALE

back, so that the patient is partially on the transfer board.

10. The nurse on the side of the bed without the stretcher should grasp the friction-reducing sheet at the head and chest areas of the patient. The nurse on the stretcher side of the bed should grasp the friction-reducing sheet at the head and chest, and the other nurse on that side should grasp the friction-reducing sheet at the chest and leg areas of the patient.

Grasping the friction-reducing sheet at these locations evenly supports the patient.

11. **At a signal given by one of the nurses, have the nurses standing on the stretcher side of the bed pull the friction-reducing sheet. At the same time, the nurse (or nurses) on the other side push, transferring the patient's weight toward the transfer board, and pushing the patient from the bed to the stretcher (Figure 3).**

Working in unison distributes the work of moving the patient and facilitates the transfer.

12. Once the patient is transferred to the stretcher, remove the transfer board, and secure the patient until the side rails are raised (Figure 4). Raise the side rails. To ensure the

Side rails promote safety. Blanket promotes comfort and warmth. Having the call bell and essential items readily available helps promote safety.

FIGURE 3 Transferring patient onto stretcher.

FIGURE 4 Securing the patient on the stretcher.

ACTION	RATIONALE
patient's comfort, cover the patient with blanket and remove the bath blanket from underneath. Leave the friction-reducing sheet in place for the return transfer. Make sure the call bell and other necessary items are within easy reach.	
13. Clean transfer aids per facility policy, if not indicated for single patient use. Remove gloves and any other PPE, if used. Perform hand hygiene.	Proper cleaning of equipment between patient use prevents the spread of microorganisms. Removing PPE properly reduces the risk for infection transmission and contamination of other items. Hand hygiene prevents the spread of microorganisms.

EVALUATION

The expected outcome is met when the patient is transferred to the stretcher without injury to patient or nurse.

DOCUMENTATION

Document the time and method of transport, and patient's destination, according to facility policy. Document the use of transfer aids and number of staff required for transfer.

SKILL 172 TRANSFERRING A PATIENT USING A POWERED FULL-BODY SLING LIFT

When it has been determined through the use of a transfer assessment and/or the patient cannot bear any weight, use a powered full-body sling lift device to move him or her up in or out of bed, into and out of a chair, and to a commode or stretcher. During any patient-handling task, if any caregiver is required to lift more than 35 pounds of a patient's weight, consider the patient to be fully dependent and use assistive devices (Waters, 2007). A full-body sling is placed under the patient's body, including head and torso, and then the sling is attached to the lift. The device slowly lifts the patient. Some devices can be lowered to the floor to pick up a patient who has fallen. These devices are available on portable bases and ceiling-mounted tracks. Each manufacturer's device is slightly different, so review the instructions for your particular device.

DELEGATION CONSIDERATIONS

The transfer of a patient from bed to a chair may be delegated to nursing assistive personnel (NAP) or to unlicensed assistive personnel (UAP), as well as to licensed practical/vocational nurses (LPN/LVNs). The decision to delegate must be based on careful analysis of the patient's needs and circumstances, as well as the qualifications of the person to whom the task is being delegated. Refer to the Delegation Guidelines in Appendix A.

EQUIPMENT

- Powered full-body sling lift
- Sheet or pad to cover the sling, if sling is not dedicated to only one patient
- Chair or wheelchair
- One or more caregivers for assistance, based on assessment
- Nonsterile gloves and/or other PPE, as indicated

ASSESSMENT

- Assess the situation to determine the need to use the lift.
- Review the medical record and nursing plan of care for conditions that may influence the patient's ability to move or to be transferred. Determine the need for bariatric equipment.
- Assess for tubes, IV lines, incisions, or equipment that may alter the transfer procedure.
- Assess the patient's level of consciousness and ability to understand and follow directions.
- Assess the patient's comfort level; if needed, medicate, as ordered, with analgesics.
- Assess the condition of the equipment to ensure proper functioning before using with the patient.

NURSING DIAGNOSIS

- Risk for Injury
- Impaired Transfer Ability
- Risk for Falls

OUTCOME IDENTIFICATION AND PLANNING

- Transfer is accomplished without injury to patient or nurse.
- Patient is free of any complications of immobility.

IMPLEMENTATION

ACTION	RATIONALE
1. Review the medical record and nursing plan of care for conditions that may influence the patient's ability to move	Reviewing the medical record and plan of care validates the correct patient and correct procedure. Checking for equipment and

ACTION	RATIONALE

or to be positioned. Assess for tubes, IV lines, incisions, or equipment that may alter the positioning procedure. Identify any movement limitations. **Consult patient-handling algorithm, if available, to plan appropriate approach to moving the patient.**

limitations reduces the risk for injury during the transfer.

2. Perform hand hygiene and put on PPE, if indicated.

Hand hygiene and PPE prevent the spread of microorganisms. PPE is required based on transmission precautions.

3. Identify the patient. Explain the procedure to the patient.

Patient identification validates the correct patient and correct procedure. Discussion and explanation allay anxiety and prepare the patient for what to expect.

4. If needed, move the equipment to make room for the chair. Close the curtains around the bed and close the door to the room, if possible.

Moving equipment out of the way provides a clear path and facilitates the transfer. Closing the door or curtain provides for privacy.

5. Adjust the bed to a comfortable working height, usually elbow height of the caregiver (VISN 8 Patient Safety Center, 2009). **Lock the bed brakes.**

Having the bed at the proper height prevents back and muscle strain. Locking the brakes prevents bed movement and ensures patient safety.

6. Lower the side rail, if in use, on the side of the bed you are working. If the sling is for use with more than one patient, place a cover or pad on the sling. Place the sling evenly under the patient. Roll the patient to one side and place half of the sling with the sheet or pad on it under the patient from shoulders to mid-thigh. Raise the rail and move to the other side. Lower the rail, if necessary. Roll

Lowering the side rail prevents strain on the nurse's back. Covering the sling prevents transmission of microorganisms. Some facilities, such as long-term care institutions, provide each patient with own transport sling. Rolling the patient positions the patient on the sling with minimal movement. Even distribution of the patient's weight in the sling provides for patient comfort and safety.

ACTION	RATIONALE

the patient to the other side and pull the sling under the patient. Raise the side rail.

7. Bring the chair to the side of the bed. **Lock the wheels, if present.**

Bringing the chair close to the bed minimizes the distance needed for transfer. Locking the wheels prevents chair movement and ensures patient safety.

8. Lower the side rail on the chair side of the bed. Roll the base of the lift under the side of the bed nearest to the chair. **Center the frame over the patient. Lock the wheels of the lift.**

Lowering the rail allows for ease of transfer. Doing so reduces the distance necessary for transfer. Centering the frame helps maintain the balance of the lift. Locking the lift's wheels prevents the lift from rolling.

9. **Using the base-adjustment lever, widen the stance of the base.**

A wider stance provides greater stability and prevents tipping.

10. Lower the arms close enough to attach the sling to the frame.

Lowering the arms is necessary to allow for the attachment of the sling's hooks.

11. Attach the straps on the sling to the hooks on the frame (Figure 1). Short straps attach behind the patient's back and long straps attach at the other end of the sling. Check the patient to make sure the straps are not pressing into the skin. Some lifts have straps or chains with hooks that attach to holes in the sling. Check the manufacturer's instructions for each lift.

Connecting the straps or chains permits attachment of the sling to the lift. Checking the patient's skin for pressure from the hooks prevents injury.

FIGURE 1 Connecting the straps to the lift.

ACTION	RATIONALE
12. Check all equipment, lines, and drains attached to the patient so that they are not interfering with the device. Have the patient fold his or her arms across the chest.	Ensuring that equipment and lines are free of the device prevents dislodgement and possible injury.
13. With a person standing on each side of the lift, tell the patient that he or she will be lifted from the bed. Support injured limbs as necessary. Engage the pump to raise the patient about 6 inches above the bed.	Having the necessary people available provides for safety. Supporting injured limbs helps maintain stability. Informing the patient about what will occur reassures the patient and reduces fear.
14. Unlock the wheels of the lift. **Carefully wheel the patient straight back and away from the bed. Support the patient's limbs, as needed.**	Moving in this manner promotes stability and safety.
15. Position the patient over the chair with the base of the lift straddling the chair (Figure 2). Lock the wheels of the lift.	Proper positioning of the patient and device promotes stability and safety.

FIGURE 2 Positioning the patient in the sling over the chair.

16. Gently lower the patient to the chair until the hooks or straps are slightly loosened from the sling or frame. Guide the patient into the chair with your hands as the sling lowers.	Gently lowering the patient in this manner places the patient fully in the chair and reduces the risk for injury.

ACTION	RATIONALE
17. Disconnect the hooks or strap from the frame. Keep the sling in place under the patient.	Disconnecting the hooks or straps allows the patient to be supported by the chair and promotes comfort. The sling will need to be reattached to the lift to move the patient back to bed.
18. Adjust the patient's position, using pillows, if necessary. Check the patient's alignment in the chair. Cover the patient with a blanket, if necessary. Make sure call bell and other essential items are within easy reach. When it is time for the patient to return to bed, reattach the hooks or straps and reverse the steps.	Pillows and proper alignment provide for patient safety and comfort. Having the call bell and other essential items readily available helps promote safety. Reattaching the hooks or straps allows the lift to support the patient for transfer back to bed.
19. Clean transfer aids per facility policy, if not indicated for single patient use. Remove gloves and any other PPE, if used. Perform hand hygiene.	Proper cleaning of equipment between patient use prevents the spread of microorganisms. Removing PPE properly reduces the risk for infection transmission and contamination of other items. Hand hygiene prevents the spread of microorganisms.

EVALUATION

• Transfer is accomplished without injury to patient or nurse.
• Patient exhibits no evidence of complications of immobility.

DOCUMENTATION

• Document the activity, transfer, any other pertinent observations, the patient's tolerance of the procedure, and the length of time in the chair. Document the use of transfer aids and number of staff required for transfer.

SKILL 173 ASSISTING A PATIENT WITH TURNING IN BED

People who are forced into inactivity by illness or injury are at high risk for serious health complications. One of the most common skills that you can use involves helping patients who cannot turn themselves in bed without assistance. You need to use your knowledge of correct body alignment and assistive devices to turn the patient in bed. Figure 1, Safe Patient Handling Algorithm 4, can help you make decisions about safe patient handling and movement. Mastering and using these techniques will help you maintain a turn schedule to prevent complications for a patient who is immobile. If a patient requires logrolling, please refer to Skill 94, Logrolling a Patient. During any patient-handling task, if any caregiver is required to lift more than 35 pounds of a patient's weight, consider the patient to be fully dependent and use assistive devices (Waters, 2007).

Algorithm 4: Reposition in Bed: From Side to Side or Up

Start here

Can patient assist?

Fully able → Caregiver assistance not needed: may or may not use positioning aid.

Partially able → Encourage patient to assist using positioning aid or cues

< 200 pounds: Use a friction-reducing device and 2 to 3 caregivers.

> 200 pounds: Use a friction-reducing device and at least 3 caregivers.

No → Use full-body sling lift and 2 or more caregivers.

General Notes:
- This is not a 1-person task; *do not pull from head of bed.*
- When pulling a patient up in bed, the bed should be flat or in a Trendelenburg position, with the side rail down.
- For patients with stage III or IV pressure ulcers, care must be taken to avoid shearing force.
- The height of the bed should be appropriate for staff safety (at the elbows).
- If the patient can assist when repositioning up in bed, ask him to flex the knees and push on the count of 3.
- During any patient-handling task, if the caregiver is required to lift more than 35 lbs. of a patient's weight, then the patient should be considered to be fully dependent and assistive devices should be used.

FIGURE 1 Step-by-step procedure or algorithm used to outline safe technique for repositioning a patient in bed. The first decision point is whether the patient can assist. (From VISN 8 Patient Safety Center. (2009). Safe patient handling and movement algorithms. Tampa, FL: Author. Available http://www.visn8.va.gov/visn8/patientsafetycenter/safePtHandling/default.asp.)

DELEGATION CONSIDERATIONS

Assisting a patient to turn in bed may be delegated to nursing assistive personnel (NAP) or to unlicensed assistive personnel (UAP), as well as to licensed practical/vocational nurses (LPN/LVNs). The decision to delegate must be based on careful analysis of the patient's needs and circumstances, as well as the qualifications of the person to whom the task is being delegated. Refer to the Delegation Guidelines in Appendix A.

EQUIPMENT

- Friction-reducing sheet or draw sheet
- Bed surface that inflates to aid in turning
- Pillows or other supports to help the patient maintain the desired position after turning
- and to maintain correct body alignment for the patient
- Additional caregivers and/or safe handling equipment to assist, based on assessment
- Nonsterile gloves, if indicated; other PPE as indicated

ASSESSMENT

- Before moving a patient, check the medical record for any conditions or orders that will limit mobility.
- Perform a pain assessment before the time for the activity. If the patient reports pain, administer the prescribed medication in sufficient time to allow for the full effect of the analgesic.
- Assess the patient's ability to assist with moving, the need for assistive devices, and the need for a second or third person to assist with the activity.
- Determine the need for bariatric equipment.
- Assess the patient's skin for signs of irritation, redness, edema, or blanching.

NURSING DIAGNOSIS

- Activity Intolerance
- Impaired Bed Mobility
- Acute Pain

OUTCOME IDENTIFICATION AND PLANNING

- Activity takes place without injury to patient or nurse.
- Patient is comfortable and in proper body alignment.

IMPLEMENTATION

ACTION	RATIONALE
1. Review the medical orders and nursing plan of care for patient activity. Identify any movement limitations and	Checking the medical orders and plan of care validates the correct patient and correct procedure. Identification of limitations and

ACTION	RATIONALE
the ability of the patient to assist with turning. **Consult patient handling algorithm, if available, to plan appropriate approach to moving the patient.**	ability along with use of an algorithm help to prevent injury and aids in determining best plan for patient movement.
2. Gather any positioning aids or supports, if necessary.	Having aids readily available promotes efficient time management.
3. Perform hand hygiene. Put on PPE, as indicated.	Hand hygiene and PPE prevent the spread of microorganisms. PPE is required based on transmission precautions.
4. Identify the patient. Explain the procedure to the patient.	Patient identification validates the correct patient and correct procedure. Discussion and explanation help allay anxiety and prepare the patient for what to expect.
5. Close the curtains around the bed and close the door to the room, if possible. Position at least one nurse on either side of the bed. Place pillows, wedges, or any other support to be used for positioning within easy reach. Place the bed at an appropriate and comfortable working height, usually elbow height of the caregiver (VISN 8 Patient Safety Center, 2009). Lower both side rails.	Closing the door or curtain provides privacy. Proper bed height helps reduce back strain while performing the procedure. Proper positioning and lowering of the side rails facilitates moving the patient and minimizes strain on the nurses.
6. If not already in place, position a friction-reducing sheet under the patient.	Friction-reducing sheets aid in preventing shearing and in reducing friction and the force required to move the patient.
7. Using the friction-reducing sheet, move the patient to the edge of the bed, opposite the side to which he or she will be turned. Raise the side rails.	With this placement, the patient will be on the center of the bed after turning is accomplished. Raising side rails ensures patient safety.

ACTION	RATIONALE
8. If the patient is able, have the patient grasp the side rail on the side of the bed toward which he or she is turning. Alternately, place the patient's arms across his or her chest and cross his or her far leg over the leg toward which they are turning.	This encourages the patient to assist as much as possible with the movement. This facilitates the turning motion and protects the patient's arms during the turn.
9. If available, activate the bed turn mechanism to inflate the side of the bed behind the patient's back.	Activating the turn mechanism inflates the side of the bed for approximately 10 seconds, aiding in propelling the patient to turn, and reducing the work required by the nurse. This helps avoid straining the nurse's lower back.
10. The nurse on the side of the bed toward which the patient is turning should stand opposite the patient's center with his or her feet spread about shoulder width and with one foot ahead of the other. Tighten your gluteal and abdominal muscles and flex your knees. Use your leg muscles to do the pulling. The other nurse should position his or her hands on the patient's shoulder and hip, assisting to roll the patient to the side. Instruct the patient to pull on the bed rail at the same time. Use the friction-reducing sheet to gently pull the patient over on his or her side (Figure 2).	Each nurse is in a stable position with good body alignment and prepared to use large muscle masses to turn the patient. These maneuvers support the patient's body and use the nurses' weight to assist with turning.

FIGURE 2 Using the friction-reducing sheet to pull the patient over on her side. (Photo by B. Proud.)

ACTION	RATIONALE
11. Use a pillow or other support behind the patient's back. Pull the shoulder blade forward and out from under the patient.	Pillow will provide support and help the patient maintain the desired position. Positioning the shoulder blade removes pressure from the bony prominence.
12. Make the patient comfortable and position in proper alignment, using pillows or other supports under the leg and arm, as needed. Readjust the pillow under the patient's head. Elevate the head of the bed as needed for comfort.	Positioning in proper alignment with supports ensures that the patient will be able to maintain the desired position and will be comfortable.
13. Place the bed in the lowest position, with the side rails up, as indicated. Make sure the call bell and other necessary items are within easy reach.	Adjusting the bed height ensures patient safety. Having the call bell and essential items readily available helps promote safety.
14. Clean transfer aids, per facility policy, if not indicated for single patient use. Remove gloves and other PPE, if used. Perform hand hygiene.	Proper cleaning of equipment between patient use prevents the spread of microorganisms. Removing PPE properly reduces the risk for infection transmission and contamination of other items. Hand hygiene prevents the spread of microorganisms.

EVALUATION

- Patient is turned and repositioned without injury to patient or nurse.
- Patient demonstrates proper body alignment and verbalizes comfort.

DOCUMENTATION

- Many facilities provide areas on the bedside flow sheet to document repositioning. Be sure to document the time the patient's position was changed, use of supports, and any pertinent observations, including skin assessment. Document the patient's tolerance of the position change. Document aids used to facilitate movement.

Male patients confined to bed usually prefer to use the urinal for voiding as a matter of convenience. Use of a urinal in the standing position facilitates emptying of the bladder. Patients who are unable to stand alone may benefit from assistance when voiding into a urinal. If the patient is unable to stand, the urinal may be used in bed. Patients may also use a urinal in the bathroom to facilitate measurement of urinary output. Many patients find it embarrassing to use the urinal. Promote comfort and normalcy as much as possible, while respecting the patient's privacy. Provide skin care, perineal hygiene, and hand hygiene after urinal use and maintain a professional manner.

DELEGATION CONSIDERATIONS

Assisting a patient with the use of a urinal may be delegated to nursing assistive personnel (NAP) or to unlicensed assistive personnel (UAP), as well as to licensed practical/vocational nurses (LPN/LVNs). The decision to delegate must be based on careful analysis of the patient's needs and circumstances, as well as the qualifications of the person to whom the task is being delegated. Refer to the Delegation Guidelines in Appendix A.

EQUIPMENT

- Urinal with end cover (usually attached)
- Toilet tissue
- Clean gloves
- Additional PPE, as indicated
- Disposable washcloths and skin cleanser
- Moist towelettes, skin cleanser and water, or hand sanitizer

ASSESSMENT

- Assess the patient's normal elimination habits. Determine why the patient needs to use a urinal (e.g., a medical order for strict bed rest or immobilization).
- Assess the patient's degree of limitation and ability to help with activity.
- Assess for activity limitations, such as hip surgery or spinal injury, which would contraindicate certain actions by the patient.
- Check for the presence of drains, dressings, intravenous fluid infusion sites/equipment, traction, or any other devices that could interfere with the patient's ability to help with the procedure or that could become dislodged.
- Assess the characteristics of the urine and the patient's skin.

NURSING DIAGNOSIS

- Impaired Physical Mobility
- Impaired Urinary Elimination
- Toileting Self-Care Deficit

OUTCOME IDENTIFICATION AND PLANNING

- Patient is able to void with assistance.
- Patient maintains continence.
- Patient demonstrates how to use the urinal.
- Patient maintains skin integrity.

IMPLEMENTATION

ACTION	RATIONALE
1. Review the patient's medical record for any limitations in physical activity. Gather equipment.	Activity limitations may contraindicate certain actions by the patient. Assembling equipment provides for an organized approach to the task.
2. Perform hand hygiene and put on PPE, if indicated.	Hand hygiene and PPE prevent the spread of microorganisms. PPE is required based on transmission precautions.
3. Identify the patient.	Identifying the patient ensures the right patient receives the intervention and helps prevent errors.
4. Assemble equipment on chair next to bed within reach.	Arranging items nearby is convenient, saves time, and avoids unnecessary stretching and twisting of muscles on the part of the nurse.
5. Close the curtains around the bed and close the door to the room, if possible. Discuss the procedure with the patient and assess the patient's ability to assist with the procedure, as well as personal hygiene preferences.	This ensures the patient's privacy. Discussion promotes reassurance and provides knowledge about the procedure. Dialogue encourages patient participation and allows for individualized nursing care.
6. Put on gloves.	Gloves prevent exposure to blood and body fluids.
7. Assist the patient to an appropriate position, as necessary: standing at the bedside, lying on one side or back, sitting in bed with the head elevated, or sitting on the side of the bed.	These positions facilitate voiding and emptying of the bladder.

ACTION	RATIONALE
8. If the patient remains in the bed, fold the linens just enough to allow for proper placement of the urinal.	Folding back the linen in this manner minimizes unnecessary exposure while still allowing the nurse to place the urinal.
9. If the patient is not standing, have him spread his legs slightly. **Hold the urinal close to the penis and position the penis completely within the urinal. Keep the bottom of the urinal lower than the penis. If necessary, assist the patient to hold the urinal in place.**	Slight spreading of the legs allows for proper positioning of the urinal. Placing penis completely within the urinal and keeping the bottom lower than the penis avoids urine spills.
10. Cover the patient with the bed linens.	Covering promotes warmth and privacy.
11. Place call bell and toilet tissue within easy reach. Have a receptacle, such as plastic trash bag, handy for discarding tissue. Ensure the bed is in the lowest position. Leave patient if it is safe to do so. Use side rails appropriately.	Falls can be prevented if the patient does not have to reach for items he needs. Placing the bed in the lowest position promotes patient safety. Leaving the patient alone, if possible, promotes self-esteem and shows respect for privacy. Side rails assist the patient in repositioning.
12. Remove gloves and additional PPE, if used. Perform hand hygiene.	Proper removal of PPE reduces transmission of microorganisms. Hand hygiene deters the spread of microorganisms.

Removing the Urinal

| 13. Perform hand hygiene. Put on gloves and additional PPE, as indicated. | Hand hygiene and PPE prevent the spread of microorganisms. Gloves prevent exposure to blood and body fluids. PPE is required based on transmission precautions. |
| 14. Pull back the patient's bed linens just enough to remove the urinal. Remove the urinal. Cover the open end of the urinal. Place on the bedside chair. If the patient | Covering the end of the urinal helps to prevent the spread of microorganisms. Cleaning the patient after he has used the urinal prevents offensive odors and skin irritation. |

ACTION	RATIONALE
needs assistance with hygiene, wrap tissue around the hand several times, and wipe patient dry. Place tissue in receptacle. Use warm, moist disposable washcloth and skin cleanser to clean perineal area, as necessary, and as per patient request.	
15. Return the patient to a comfortable position. Make sure the linens under the patient are dry. Remove your gloves and ensure that the patient is covered.	Proper positioning promotes patient comfort. Removing contaminated gloves prevents spread of microorganisms.
16. Ensure patient call bell is in reach.	Promotes patient safety.
17. Offer patient supplies to wash and dry his hands, assisting as necessary.	Washing hands after using the urinal helps prevent the spread of microorganisms.
18. Put on clean gloves. Empty and clean the urinal, measuring urine in graduated container, as necessary. Discard trash receptacle with used toilet paper per facility policy.	Measurement of urine volume is required for accurate intake and output records.
19. Remove gloves and additional PPE, if used, and perform hand hygiene.	Gloves prevent exposure to blood and body fluids. Removing PPE properly reduces the risk for infection transmission and contamination of other items. Hand hygiene prevents the spread of microorganisms.

EVALUATION
- Patient voids using the urinal.
- Patient remains dry.
- Patient does not experience episodes of incontinence.
- Patient demonstrates measures to assist with using the urinal.
- Patient does not experience impaired skin integrity.

DOCUMENTATION
• Document the patient's tolerance of the activity. Record the amount of urine voided on the intake and output record, if appropriate. Document any other assessments, such as unusual urine characteristics or alterations in the patient's skin.

SKILL 175 | CATHETERIZING THE FEMALE URINARY BLADDER

Urinary catheterization is the introduction of a catheter (tube) through the urethra into the bladder for the purpose of withdrawing urine. Catheter-associated urinary tract infections (UTIs) are the most common hospital-acquired infection in the United States and is one reason catheterization should be avoided whenever possible. When it is deemed necessary, it should be performed using strict aseptic technique and left in place for the shortest length of time possible (Hooton et al., 2010). The duration of catheterization is the most important risk factor for the development of a urinary tract infection (Bernard et al., 2012).

Intermittent urethral catheters, or straight catheters, are used to drain the bladder for shorter periods (5 to 10 minutes). If a catheter is to remain in place for continuous drainage, an indwelling urethral catheter is used. Indwelling catheters are also called *retention* or *Foley catheters.* The indwelling urethral catheter is designed so that it does not slip out of the bladder. A balloon is inflated to ensure that the catheter remains in the bladder once it is inserted. Intermittent catheterization should be considered as an alternative to short-term or long-term indwelling urethral catheterization to reduce catheter-associated UTIs (Hooton et al., 2012). Intermittent catheterization is becoming the gold standard for the management of bladder-emptying dysfunctions and following surgical interventions. Certain advantages to intermittent catheterization, including the lower risks of catheter-associated UTI and complications, may make it a more desirable and safer option than indwelling catheterization (Herter & Wallace Kazer, 2010, p. 343–344).

The following procedure reviews insertion of an indwelling catheter. The procedure for an intermittent catheter follows as a Skill Variation.

DELEGATION CONSIDERATIONS

The catheterization of the female urinary bladder is not delegated to nursing assistive personnel (NAP) or to unlicensed assistive personnel (UAP). Depending on the state's nurse practice act and the organization's policies and procedures, catheterization of the female urinary bladder may be delegated to licensed practical/vocational nurses (LPN/LVNs).The decision to delegate must be based on careful analysis of the patient's needs and circumstances, as well as the qualifications of the person to whom the task is being delegated. Refer to the Delegation Guidelines in Appendix A.

EQUIPMENT

- Sterile catheter kit that contains:
  - Sterile gloves
  - Sterile drapes (one of which is fenestrated)
  - Sterile catheter (Use the smallest appropriate-size catheter, usually a 14F to 16F catheter with a 5- to 10-mL balloon [Newman, 2008]).
- Antiseptic cleansing solution and cotton balls or gauze squares; antiseptic swabs
- Lubricant
- Forceps
- Prefilled syringe with sterile water (sufficient to inflate indwelling catheter balloon)

- Sterile basin (usually base of kit serves as this)
- Sterile specimen container (if specimen is required)
- Flashlight or lamp
- Waterproof, disposable pad
- Sterile, disposable urine collection bag and drainage tubing (may be connected to catheter in catheter kit)
- Velcro leg strap, catheter securing device, or tape
- Disposable gloves
- Additional PPE, as indicated
- Washcloth, skin cleanser, and warm water to perform perineal hygiene before and after catheterization

ASSESSMENT

- Assess the patient's normal elimination habits.
- Assess the patient's degree of limitations and ability to help with activity.
- Assess for activity limitations, such as hip surgery or spinal injury, which would contraindicate certain actions by the patient.
- Assess for the presence of any other conditions that may interfere with passage of the catheter or contraindicate insertion of the catheter, such as urethral strictures or bladder cancer.
- Check for the presence of drains, dressings, intravenous fluid infusion sites/equipment, traction, or any other devices that could interfere with the patient's ability to help with the procedure or that could become dislodged.
- Assess bladder fullness before performing the procedure, either by palpation or with a handheld bladder ultrasound device.
- Question patient about any allergies, especially to latex or iodine.
- Ask the patient if she has ever been catheterized. If she had an indwelling catheter previously, ask why and for how long it was used. The patient may have urethral strictures, which may make catheter insertion more difficult.
- Assess the characteristics of the urine and the patient's skin.

NURSING DIAGNOSIS

- Impaired Urinary Elimination
- Urinary Retention
- Risk for Infection

OUTCOME IDENTIFICATION AND PLANNING

- Patient's urinary elimination will be maintained, with a urine output of at least 30 mL/hour, and the patient's bladder will not be distended.
- Patient's skin remains clean, dry, and intact, without evidence of irritation or breakdown.
- Patient verbalizes an understanding of the purpose for, and care of, the catheter, as appropriate.

IMPLEMENTATION

ACTION	RATIONALE
1. Review the patient's chart for any limitations in physical activity. Confirm the medical order for indwelling catheter insertion.	Physical limitations may require adaptations in performing the skill. Verifying the medical order ensures that the correct intervention is administered to the right patient.
2. Gather equipment. Obtain assistance from another staff member, if necessary.	Assembling equipment provides for an organized approach to the task. Assistance from another person may be required to perform the intervention safely.
3. Perform hand hygiene and put on PPE, if indicated.	Hand hygiene and PPE prevent the spread of microorganisms. PPE is required based on transmission precautions.
4. Identify the patient.	Identifying the patient ensures the right patient receives the intervention and helps prevent errors.
5. Close the curtains around the bed and close the door to the room, if possible. Discuss the procedure with the patient and assess the patient's ability to assist with the procedure. Ask the patient if she has any allergies, especially to latex or iodine.	This ensures the patient's privacy. Discussion promotes reassurance and provides knowledge about the procedure. Dialogue encourages patient participation and allows for individualized nursing care. Some catheters and gloves in kits are made of latex. Some antiseptic solutions contain iodine.
6. Provide good lighting. Artificial light is recommended (use of a flashlight requires	Good lighting is necessary to see the meatus clearly. A readily available trash receptacle allows

ACTION	RATIONALE

an assistant to hold and position it). Place a trash receptacle within easy reach.

for prompt disposal of used supplies and reduces the risk of contaminating the sterile field.

7. Assemble equipment on overbed table within reach.

Arranging items nearby is convenient, saves time, and avoids unnecessary stretching and twisting of muscles on the part of the nurse.

8. Adjust the bed to a comfortable working height, usually elbow height of the caregiver (VISN 8 Patient Safety Center, 2009). Stand on the patient's right side if you are right-handed, patient's left side if you are left-handed.

Having the bed at the proper height prevents back and muscle strain. Positioning allows for ease of use of dominant hand for catheter insertion.

9. Assist the patient to a dorsal recumbent position with knees flexed, feet about 2 feet apart, with her legs abducted. Drape patient. Alternately, the Sims', or lateral, position can be used. Place the patient's buttocks near the edge of the bed with her shoulders at the opposite edge and her knees drawn toward her chest. Allow the patient to lie on either side, depending on which position is easiest for the nurse and best for the patient's comfort. Slide waterproof pad under patient.

Proper positioning allows adequate visualization of the urinary meatus. Embarrassment, chilliness, and tension can interfere with catheter insertion; draping the patient will promote comfort and relaxation. The Sims' position may allow better visualization and be more comfortable for the patient, especially if hip and knee movements are difficult. The smaller area of exposure is also less stressful for the patient. The waterproof pad will protect bed linens from moisture.

10. Put on clean gloves. Clean the perineal area with washcloth, skin cleanser, and warm water, using a different corner of the washcloth with each stroke. Wipe from above orifice downward toward sacrum (front to back). Rinse and dry. Remove gloves. Perform hand hygiene again.

Gloves reduce the risk of exposure to blood and body fluids. Cleaning reduces microorganisms near the urethral meatus and provides an opportunity to visualize the perineum and landmarks before the procedure. Hand hygiene reduces the spread of microorganisms.

ACTION	RATIONALE
11. Prepare urine drainage setup if a separate urine collection system is to be used. Secure to bed frame according to manufacturer's directions.	This facilitates connection of the catheter to the drainage system and provides for easy access.
12. Open sterile catheterization tray on a clean overbed table using sterile technique.	Placement of equipment near the worksite increases efficiency. Sterile technique protects the patient and prevents transmission of microorganisms.
13. Put on sterile gloves. Grasp upper corners of drape and unfold drape without touching nonsterile areas. Fold back a corner on each side to make a cuff over gloved hands. Ask the patient to lift her buttocks and slide sterile drape under her with gloves protected by cuff.	The drape provides a sterile field close to the meatus. Covering the gloved hands will help keep the gloves sterile while placing the drape.
14. Based on facility policy, position the fenestrated sterile drape. Place a fenestrated sterile drape over the perineal area, exposing the labia.	The drape expands the sterile field and protects against contamination. Use of a fenestrated drape may limit visualization and is considered optional by some practitioners and/or facility policies.
15. Place sterile tray on drape between the patient's thighs.	Provides easy access to supplies.
16. Open all the supplies. Open package of antiseptic swabs. Alternately, fluff cotton balls in tray before pouring antiseptic solution over them. Open specimen container if specimen is to be obtained.	It is necessary to open all supplies and prepare for the procedure while both hands are sterile.
17. Lubricate 1 to 2 inches of catheter tip.	Lubrication facilitates catheter insertion and reduces tissue trauma.

ACTION	RATIONALE
18. With thumb and one finger of nondominant hand, spread labia and identify meatus. **Be prepared to maintain separation of labia with one hand until catheter is inserted and urine is flowing well and continuously.** If the patient is in the side-lying position, lift the upper buttock and labia to expose the urinary meatus.	Smoothing the area immediately surrounding the meatus helps to make it visible. Allowing the labia to drop back into position may contaminate the area around the meatus, as well as the catheter. The nondominant hand is now contaminated.
19. Use the dominant hand to pick up an antiseptic swab or use forceps to pick up a cotton ball. **Clean one labial fold, top to bottom (from above the meatus down toward the rectum), then discard the cotton ball. Using a new cotton ball/swab for each stroke, continue to clean the other labial fold, then directly over the meatus.**	Moving from an area where there is likely to be less contamination to an area where there is more contamination helps prevent the spread of microorganisms. Cleaning the meatus last helps reduce the possibility of introducing microorganisms into the bladder.
20. With your noncontaminated, dominant hand, place the drainage end of the catheter in receptacle. If the catheter is pre-attached to sterile tubing and drainage container (closed drainage system), position catheter and setup within easy reach on sterile field. Ensure that the clamp on the drainage bag is closed.	This facilitates drainage of urine and minimizes risk of contaminating sterile equipment.
21. **Using your dominant hand, hold the catheter 2 to 3 inches from the tip and insert slowly into the urethra. Advance the catheter until there is a return of urine (approximately 2 to 3 inches [4.8 to 7.2 cm]). Once urine drains, advance catheter another 2 to**	The female urethra is about 1.5 to 2.5 inches (3.6 to 6.0 cm) long. Applying force on the catheter is likely to injure mucous membranes. The sphincter relaxes and the catheter can enter the bladder easily when the patient relaxes. Advancing an indwelling catheter an additional 2 to 3 inches

ACTION	RATIONALE

3 inches (4.8 to 7.2 cm). Do not force catheter through urethra into bladder. Ask patient to breathe deeply, and rotate catheter gently if slight resistance is met as catheter reaches external sphincter.

(4.8 to 7.2 cm) ensures placement in the bladder and facilitates inflation of the balloon without damaging the urethra.

22. Hold the catheter securely at the meatus with your nondominant hand. Use your dominant hand to inflate the catheter balloon. Inject entire volume of sterile water supplied in prefilled syringe.

Bladder or sphincter contraction could push the catheter out. The balloon anchors the catheter in place in the bladder. Manufacturer provides appropriate amount of sterile water for the size of catheter in the kit; as a result, use entire syringe provided in the kit.

23. Pull gently on catheter after balloon is inflated to feel resistance.

Improper inflation can cause patient discomfort and malpositioning of catheter.

24. Attach catheter to drainage system if not already preattached.

Closed drainage system minimizes the risk for microorganisms being introduced into the bladder.

25. Remove equipment and dispose of it according to facility policy. Discard syringe in sharps container. Wash and dry the perineal area, as needed.

Proper disposal prevents the spread of microorganisms. Placing syringe in sharps container prevents reuse. Cleaning promotes comfort and appropriate personal hygiene.

26. Remove gloves. **Secure catheter tubing to the patient's inner thigh with Velcro leg strap, catheter securing device, or tape.** Leave some slack in catheter for leg movement.

Proper attachment prevents trauma to the urethra and meatus from tension on the tubing. Whether to tape the drainage tubing over or under the leg depends on gravity flow, patient's mobility, and patient's comfort.

27. Assist the patient to a comfortable position. Cover the patient with bed linens. Place the bed in the lowest position.

Positioning and covering provides warmth and promotes comfort.

28. Secure drainage bag below the level of the bladder. Check that drainage tubing is not kinked and that movement of side rails does not interfere with catheter or drainage bag.

This facilitates drainage of urine and prevents the backflow of urine.

ACTION	RATIONALE
29. Put on clean gloves. Obtain urine specimen immediately, if needed, from drainage bag. Label specimen. Send urine specimen to the laboratory promptly or refrigerate it.	Catheter system is sterile. Obtaining specimen immediately allows access to sterile system. Keeping urine at room temperature may cause microorganisms, if present, to grow and distort laboratory findings.
30. Remove gloves and additional PPE, if used. Perform hand hygiene.	Removing PPE properly reduces the risk for infection transmission and contamination of other items. Hand hygiene prevents the spread of microorganisms.

EVALUATION

- Catheter is inserted using sterile technique, results in the immediate flow of urine, and the bladder is not distended.
- Patient does not experience trauma.
- Patient reports little to no pain on insertion.
- Patient's perineal area remains clean and dry.

DOCUMENTATION

- Document the type and size of catheter and balloon inserted, as well as the amount of fluid used to inflate the balloon. Document the patient's tolerance of the activity. Record the amount of urine obtained through the catheter and any specimen obtained. Document any other assessments, such as unusual urine characteristics or alterations in the patient's skin. Record urine amount on intake and output record, if appropriate.

SKILL VARIATION   **Intermittent Female Urethral Catheterization**

1. Check the medical record for the order for intermittent urethral catheterization. Review the patient's chart for any limitations in physical activity. Gather equipment. Obtain assistance from another staff member, if necessary.

2. Perform hand hygiene. Put on PPE, as indicated, based on transmission precautions.

3. Identify the patient. Discuss the procedure with the patient and assess the patient's ability to assist with

continued on page 928

Intermittent Female Urethral Catheterization   *continued*

the procedure. Ask the patient if she has any allergies, especially to latex or iodine.

4. Close the curtains around the bed and close the door to the room, if possible.

5. Provide good lighting. Artificial light is recommended (use of a flashlight requires an assistant to hold and position it). Place a trash receptacle within easy reach.

6. Assemble equipment on overbed table within reach.

7. Raise the bed to a comfortable working height. Stand on the patient's right side if you are right-handed, patient's left side if you are left-handed.

8. Put on disposable gloves. Assist the patient to dorsal recumbent position with knees flexed, feet about 2 feet apart, with her legs abducted. Drape patient. Alternately, use the Sims', or lateral, position. Place the patient's buttocks near the edge of the bed with her shoulders at the opposite edge and her knees drawn toward her chest. Slide waterproof drape under patient.

9. Put on clean gloves. Clean the perineal area with washcloth, skin cleanser, and warm water, using a different corner of the washcloth with each stroke. Wipe from above the orifice downward toward the sacrum (front to back). Rinse and dry. Remove gloves. Perform hand hygiene again.

10. Open sterile catheterization tray on a clean overbed table using sterile technique.

11. Put on sterile gloves. Grasp upper corners of drape and unfold drape without touching nonsterile areas. Fold back a corner on each side to make a cuff over gloved hands. Ask patient to lift her buttocks and slide sterile drape under her with gloves protected by cuff.

12. Place a fenestrated sterile drape over the perineal area, exposing the labia, if appropriate.

13. Place sterile tray on drape between patient's thighs.

14. Open all the supplies. Open package of antiseptic swabs. Alternately, fluff cotton balls in tray before pouring antiseptic solution over them. Open specimen container if specimen is to be obtained.

15. Lubricate 1 to 2 inches of catheter tip.

16. With thumb and one finger of nondominant hand, spread labia and identify meatus. If the patient is in the side-lying position, lift the upper buttock and labia to expose the urinary meatus. **Be prepared to maintain separation of labia with one hand until catheter is inserted and urine is flowing well and continuously.**

Intermittent Female Urethral Catheterization   *continued*

17. Use the dominant hand to pick up a cotton ball. **Clean one labial fold, top to bottom (from above the meatus down toward the rectum), then discard the cotton ball. Using a new cotton ball for each stroke, continue to clean the other labial fold, then directly over the meatus.**

18. With the noncontaminated, dominant hand, place drainage end of catheter in receptacle. If a specimen is required, place the end into the specimen container in the receptacle.

19. **Using the dominant hand, hold the catheter 2 to 3 inches from the tip and insert slowly into the urethra. Advance the catheter until there is a return of urine (approximately 2 to 3 inches [4.8 to 7.2 cm]). Do not force the catheter through the urethra into the bladder.** Ask the patient to breathe deeply, and rotate the catheter gently if slight resistance is met as the catheter reaches the external sphincter.

20. Hold the catheter securely at the meatus with the nondominant hand while the bladder empties. If a specimen is being collected, remove the drainage end of the tubing from the specimen container after required amount is obtained and allow urine to flow into the receptacle. Set specimen container aside and place lid on container.

21. Allow the bladder to empty. Withdraw catheter slowly and smoothly after urine has stopped flowing. Remove equipment and dispose of it according to facility policy. Discard syringe in sharps container to prevent reuse. Wash and dry the perineal area, as needed.

22. Remove gloves. Assist the patient to a comfortable position. Cover the patient with bed linens. Place the bed in the lowest position.

23. Put on clean gloves. Secure the container lid and label specimen. Send urine specimen to the laboratory promptly or refrigerate it.

24. Remove gloves and additional PPE, if used. Perform hand hygiene.

Note: Intermittent catheterization in the home is performed using clean technique. The bladder's natural resistance to the microorganisms normally found in the home makes sterile technique unnecessary. Catheters are washed, dried, and stored for repeated use. Clean technique involves the use of cleansed reusable catheters, washing hands with soap and water, and daily cleansing of the perineum or more often only when fecal or other wastes are present (Newman, 2008, as cited in Herter & Wallace, 2010). Cleansing the perineal area to decrease bacteria in the surrounding area is highly recommended (Herter & Wallace, 2010).

Removal of an indwelling catheter is performed using clean technique. Take care to prevent trauma to the urethra during the procedure. Completely deflate the catheter balloon before catheter removal to avoid irritation and damage to the urethra and meatus. The patient may experience burning or irritation the first few times he or she voids after removal, due to urethral irritation. If the catheter was in place for more than a few days, decreased bladder muscle tone and swelling of the urethra may cause the patient to experience difficulty voiding or an inability to void. Monitor the patient for urinary retention. It is important to encourage adequate oral fluid intake to promote adequate urinary output. Check facility policy regarding the length of time the patient is allowed to accomplish successful voiding after catheter removal.

DELEGATION CONSIDERATIONS

Removal of an indwelling catheter is not delegated to nursing assistive personnel (NAP) or to unlicensed assistive personnel (UAP). Depending on the state's nurse practice act and the organization's policies and procedures, removal of an indwelling catheter may be delegated to licensed practical/vocational nurses (LPN/LVNs). The decision to delegate must be based on careful analysis of the patient's needs and circumstances, as well as the qualifications of the person to whom the task is being delegated. Refer to the Delegation Guidelines in Appendix A.

EQUIPMENT

- Syringe sufficiently large to accommodate the volume of solution used to inflate the balloon (balloon size/inflation volume is printed on the balloon inflation valve on the catheter at the bifurcation)
- Waterproof, disposable pad
- Disposable gloves
- Additional PPE, as indicated
- Washcloth, skin cleanser, and warm water to perform perineal hygiene after catheter removal

ASSESSMENT

- Check the medical record for an order to remove the catheter.
- Assess for discharge or encrustation around the urethral meatus.
- Assess urine output, including color and current amount in drainage bag.

NURSING DIAGNOSIS

- Impaired Urinary Elimination
- Risk for Injury
- Urinary Retention

OUTCOME IDENTIFICATION AND PLANNING

- Catheter will be removed without difficulty and with minimal patient discomfort.
- Patient voids without discomfort after catheter removal.
- Patient voids a minimum of 250 mL of urine within 6 to 8 hours of catheter removal.
- Patient's skin remains clean, dry, and intact, without evidence of irritation or breakdown.
- Patient verbalizes an understanding of the need to maintain adequate fluid intake, as appropriate.

IMPLEMENTATION

ACTION	RATIONALE
1. Confirm the order for catheter removal in the medical record. Gather equipment.	Verifying the medical order ensures that the correct intervention is administered to the right patient. Assembling equipment provides for an organized approach to the task.
2. Perform hand hygiene and put on PPE, if indicated.	Hand hygiene and PPE prevent the spread of microorganisms. PPE is required based on transmission precautions.
3. Identify the patient.	Identifying the patient ensures the right patient receives the intervention and helps prevent errors.
4. Close the curtains around the bed and close the door to the room, if possible. Discuss the procedure with the patient and assess the patient's ability to assist with the procedure.	This ensures the patient's privacy. Discussion promotes reassurance and provides knowledge about the procedure. Dialogue encourages patient participation and allows for individualized nursing care.
5. Adjust the bed to a comfortable working height, usually elbow height of the caregiver (VISN 8 Patient Safety Center, 2009). Stand on the patient's right side if you are right-handed, patient's left side if you are left-handed.	Having the bed at the proper height prevents back and muscle strain. Positioning allows for ease of use of dominant hand for catheter removal.

ACTION	RATIONALE
6. Position the patient as for catheter insertion. Drape the patient so that only the area around the catheter is exposed. Slide waterproof pad between the female patient's legs or over the male patient's thighs.	Positioning allows access to site. Draping prevents unnecessary exposure and promotes warmth. The waterproof pad will protect bed linens from moisture and serve as a receptacle for the used catheter after removal.
7. Remove the leg strap, tape, or other device used to secure the catheter to the patient's thigh or abdomen.	This action permits removal of catheter.
8. Insert the syringe into the balloon inflation port. Allow water to come back by gravity. Alternately, aspirate the entire amount of sterile water used to inflate the balloon (Figure 1). Refer to manufacturer's instructions for deflation. **Do not cut the inflation port.**	Removal of sterile water deflates the balloon to allow for catheter removal. All of the sterile water must be removed to prevent injury to the patient. Aspiration by pulling on the syringe plunger may result in collapse of the inflation lumen; contribute to the formation of creases, ridges, or cuffing at the balloon area; and increase the catheter balloon diameter size on deflation, resulting in difficult removal and urethral trauma.

FIGURE 1 Removing fluid from balloon.

ACTION	RATIONALE
9. Ask the patient to take several slow deep breaths. **Slowly and gently remove the catheter.** Place it on the waterproof pad and wrap it in the pad.	Slow deep breathing helps to relax the sphincter muscles. Slow gentle removal prevents trauma to the urethra. Using a waterproof pad prevents contact with the catheter.
10. Wash and dry the perineal area, as needed.	Cleaning promotes comfort and appropriate personal hygiene.
11. Remove gloves. Assist the patient to a comfortable position. Cover the patient with bed linens. Place the bed in the lowest position.	These actions provide warmth and promote comfort and safety.

ACTION	RATIONALE
12. Put on clean gloves. Remove equipment and dispose of it according to facility policy. Note characteristics and amount of urine in drainage bag.	Proper disposal prevents the spread of microorganisms. Observing the characteristics ensures accurate documentation.
13. Remove gloves and additional PPE, if used. Perform hand hygiene.	Removing PPE properly reduces the risk for infection transmission and contamination of other items. Hand hygiene prevents the spread of microorganisms.

EVALUATION

- Catheter is removed without difficulty and with minimal patient discomfort.
- Patient voids without discomfort after catheter removal.
- Patient voids a minimum of 250 mL of urine within 6 to 8 hours of catheter removal.
- Patient's skin remains clean, dry, and intact, without evidence of irritation or breakdown.
- Patient verbalizes an understanding of the need to maintain adequate fluid intake, as appropriate.

DOCUMENTATION

- Document the type and size of catheter removed and the amount of fluid removed from the balloon. Also document the patient's tolerance of the procedure. Record the amount of urine in the drainage bag. Note the time the patient is due to void. Document any other assessments, such as unusual urine characteristics or alterations in the patient's skin. Also record urine amount on intake and output record, if appropriate.

SKILL 177   CATHETERIZING THE MALE URINARY BLADDER

Urinary catheterization is the introduction of a catheter (tube) through the urethra into the bladder for the purpose of withdrawing urine. Catheter-associated urinary tract infections are the most common hospital-acquired infection in the United States and is one reason catheterization should be avoided whenever possible. When it is deemed necessary, it should be performed using strict aseptic technique and left in place for the shortest length of time possible (Hooton et al., 2010). The duration of catheterization is the most important risk factor for the development of a UTI (Bernard et al., 2012).

Intermittent urethral catheters, or straight catheters, are used to drain the bladder for shorter periods. If a catheter is to remain in place for continuous drainage, an indwelling urethral catheter is used. Indwelling catheters are also called *retention* or *Foley* catheters. The indwelling urethral catheter is designed so that it does not slip out of the bladder. A balloon is inflated to ensure that the catheter remains in the bladder once it is inserted.

Intermittent catheterization should be considered as an alternative to short-term or long-term indwelling urethral catheterization to reduce catheter-associated urinary tract infections (Hooton et al., 2012). Intermittent catheterization is becoming the gold standard for the management of bladder-emptying dysfunctions and following surgical interventions. Certain advantages to intermittent catheterization, including the lower risks of catheter-associated UTI and complications, may make it a more desirable and safer option than indwelling catheterization (Herter & Wallace Kazer, 2010, p. 343–344).

The following procedure reviews insertion of an indwelling catheter into the male urinary bladder. The procedure for an intermittent catheter of a male bladder follows as a Skill Variation.

DELEGATION CONSIDERATIONS

The catheterization of the male urinary bladder is not delegated to nursing assistive personnel (NAP) or to unlicensed assistive personnel (UAP). Depending on the state's nurse practice act and the organization's policies and procedures, catheterization of the male urinary bladder may be delegated to licensed practical/vocational nurses (LPN/LVNs). The decision to delegate must be based on careful analysis of the patient's needs and circumstances, as well as the qualifications of the person to whom the task is being delegated. Refer to the Delegation Guidelines in Appendix A.

EQUIPMENT

- Sterile catheter kit that contains:
  - Sterile gloves
  - Sterile drapes (one of which is fenestrated)
  - Sterile catheter (Use the smallest appropriate-size catheter, usually a 14F to 16F catheter with a 5- to 10-mL balloon [Newman, 2008]).
- Antiseptic cleansing solution and cotton balls or gauze squares; antiseptic swabs
- Lubricant
- Forceps
- Prefilled syringe with sterile water (sufficient to inflate indwelling catheter balloon)
- Sterile basin (usually base of kit serves as this)
- Sterile specimen container (if specimen is required)
- Flashlight or lamp
- Waterproof, disposable pad

- Sterile, disposable urine collection bag and drainage tubing (may be connected to catheter in catheter kit)
- Velcro leg strap, catheter securing device, or tape

- Disposable gloves
- Additional PPE, as indicated
- Washcloth, skin cleanser, and warm water to perform perineal hygiene before and after catheterization

ASSESSMENT

- Assess the patient's normal elimination habits.
- Assess the patient's degree of limitations and ability to help with activity.
- Assess for activity limitations, such as hip surgery or spinal injury, which would contraindicate certain actions by the patient.
- Assess for the presence of any other conditions that may interfere with passage of the catheter or contraindicate insertion of the catheter, such as urethral strictures or bladder cancer.
- Check for the presence of drains, dressings, intravenous fluid infusion sites/equipment, traction, or any other devices that could interfere with the patient's ability to help with the procedure or that could become dislodged.
- Assess bladder fullness before performing the procedure, either by palpation or with a handheld bladder ultrasound device, and question the patient about any allergies, especially to latex and iodine.
- Ask the patient if he has ever been catheterized. If he had an indwelling catheter previously, ask why and for how long it was used. The patient may have urethral strictures, which may make catheter insertion more difficult.
- If the patient is 50 years of age or older, ask if he has had any prostate problems. Prostate enlargement typically is noted around the age of 50 years.
- Assess the characteristics of the urine and the patient's skin.

NURSING DIAGNOSIS

- Impaired Urinary Elimination
- Risk for Infection
- Urinary Retention

OUTCOME IDENTIFICATION AND PLANNING

- Patient's urinary elimination will be maintained, with a urine output of at least 30 mL/hour, and the patient's bladder will not be distended.
- Patient's skin remains clean, dry, and intact, without evidence of irritation or breakdown.
- Patient verbalizes an understanding of the purpose for, and care of, the catheter, as appropriate.

IMPLEMENTATION

ACTION	RATIONALE
1. Review chart for any limitations in physical activity. Confirm the medical order for indwelling catheter insertion.	Physical limitations may require adaptations in performing the skill. Verifying the medical order ensures that the correct intervention is administered to the right patient.
2. Gather equipment. Obtain assistance from another staff member, if necessary.	Assembling equipment provides for an organized approach to the task. Assistance from another person may be required to perform the intervention safely.
3. Perform hand hygiene and put on PPE, if indicated.	Hand hygiene and PPE prevent the spread of microorganisms. PPE is required based on transmission precautions.
4. Identify the patient.	Identifying the patient ensures the right patient receives the intervention and helps prevent errors.
5. Close the curtains around the bed and close the door to the room, if possible. Discuss the procedure with the patient and assess the patient's ability to assist with the procedure. Ask the patient if he has any allergies, especially to latex or iodine.	This ensures the patient's privacy. Discussion promotes reassurance and provides knowledge about the procedure. Dialogue encourages patient participation and allows for individualized nursing care. Some catheters and gloves in kits are made of latex. Some antiseptic solutions contain iodine.
6. Provide good lighting. Artificial light is recommended (use of a flashlight requires an assistant to hold and position it). Place a trash receptacle within easy reach.	Good lighting is necessary to see the meatus clearly. A readily available trash receptacle allows for prompt disposal of used supplies and reduces the risk of contaminating the sterile field.
7. Assemble equipment on overbed table within reach.	Arranging items nearby is convenient, saves time, and avoids unnecessary stretching and twisting of muscles on the part of the nurse.

ACTION	RATIONALE

8. Adjust the bed to a comfortable working height, usually elbow height of the caregiver (VISN 8 Patient Safety Center, 2009). Stand on the patient's right side if you are right-handed, patient's left side if you are left-handed.

Having the bed at the proper height prevents back and muscle strain. Positioning allows for ease of use of dominant hand for catheter insertion.

9. Position the patient on his back with thighs slightly apart. Drape the patient so that only the area around the penis is exposed. Slide waterproof pad under the patient.

This prevents unnecessary exposure and promotes warmth. The waterproof pad will protect bed linens from moisture.

10. Put on clean gloves. Clean the genital area with washcloth, skin cleanser, and warm water. Clean the tip of the penis first, moving the washcloth in a circular motion from the meatus outward. Wash the shaft of the penis using downward strokes toward the pubic area. Rinse and dry. Remove gloves. Perform hand hygiene.

Gloves reduce the risk of exposure to blood and body fluids. Cleaning the penis reduces microorganisms near the urethral meatus. Hand hygiene reduces the spread of microorganisms.

11. Prepare urine drainage setup if a separate urine collection system is to be used. Secure to bed frame according to manufacturer's directions.

This facilitates connection of the catheter to the drainage system and provides for easy access.

12. Open sterile catheterization tray on a clean overbed table, using sterile technique.

Placement of equipment near worksite increases efficiency. Sterile technique protects patient and prevents spread of microorganisms.

13. Put on sterile gloves. Open sterile drape and place on patient's thighs. Place fenestrated drape with opening over penis.

This maintains a sterile working area.

ACTION	RATIONALE
14. Place catheter setup on or next to patient's legs on sterile drape.	Sterile setup should be arranged so that the nurse's back is not turned to it, nor should it be out of the nurse's range of vision.
15. Open all the supplies. Open package of antiseptic swabs. Alternately, fluff cotton balls in tray before pouring antiseptic solution over them. Open specimen container if specimen is to be obtained. Remove cap from syringe prefilled with lubricant.	It is necessary to open all supplies and prepare for the procedure while both hands are sterile.
16. Place drainage end of catheter in receptacle. If the catheter is pre-attached to sterile tubing and drainage container (closed drainage system), position catheter and setup within easy reach on sterile field. Ensure that clamp on drainage bag is closed.	This facilitates drainage of urine and minimizes risk of contaminating sterile equipment.
17. Lift penis with nondominant hand. Retract foreskin in uncircumcised patient. **Be prepared to keep this hand in this position until the catheter is inserted and urine is flowing well and continuously. Use the dominant hand to pick up an antiseptic swab or use forceps to pick up a cotton ball. Using a circular motion, clean the penis, moving from the meatus down the glans of the penis. Repeat this cleansing motion two more times, using a new cotton ball/swab each time. Discard each cotton ball/swab after one use.**	The hand touching the penis becomes contaminated. Cleansing the area around the meatus and under the foreskin in the uncircumcised patient helps prevent infection. Moving from the meatus toward the base of the penis prevents bringing microorganisms to the meatus.

ACTION	RATIONALE

18. Hold penis with slight upward tension and perpendicular to patient's body. Use the dominant hand to pick up the lubricant syringe. **Gently insert tip of syringe with lubricant into urethra and instill the 10 mL of lubricant.**

The lubricant causes the urethra to distend slightly and facilitates passage of the catheter without traumatizing the lining of the urethra (Society of Urologic Nurses and Associates, 2005c). If the prepackaged kit does not contain a syringe with lubricant, the nurse may need assistance in filling a syringe while keeping the lubricant sterile. Some facilities use lidocaine jelly for lubrication before catheter insertion. The jelly comes prepackaged in a sterile syringe and serves a dual purpose of lubricating and numbing the urethra. A medical order is necessary for the use of lidocaine jelly.

19. Use the dominant hand to pick up the catheter and hold it an inch or two from the tip. Ask the patient to bear down as if voiding. **Insert catheter tip into meatus. Ask the patient to take deep breaths. Advance the catheter to the bifurcation or "Y" level of the ports. Do not use force to introduce the catheter.** If the catheter resists entry, ask the patient to breathe deeply and rotate the catheter slightly.

Bearing down eases the passage of the catheter through the urethra. The male urethra is about 20 cm long. Having the patient take deep breaths or twisting the catheter slightly may ease the catheter past resistance at the sphincters. Advancing an indwelling catheter to the bifurcation ensures its placement in the bladder and facilitates inflation of the balloon without damaging the urethra.

20. Hold the catheter securely at the meatus with your nondominant hand. Use your dominant hand to inflate the catheter balloon. **Inject the entire volume of sterile water supplied in the prefilled syringe. Once the balloon is inflated, the catheter may be gently pulled back into place. Replace foreskin over the catheter.** Lower penis.

Bladder or sphincter contraction could push the catheter out. The balloon anchors the catheter in place in the bladder. Manufacturer provides appropriate amount of solution for the size of catheter in the kit; as a result, use entire syringe provided in the kit.

ACTION	RATIONALE
21. Pull gently on the catheter after the balloon is inflated to feel resistance.	Improper inflation can cause patient discomfort and malpositioning of catheter.
22. Attach catheter to drainage system, if necessary.	Closed drainage system minimizes the risk for microorganisms being introduced into the bladder.
23. Remove equipment and dispose of it according to facility policy. Discard syringe in sharps container. Wash and dry the perineal area, as needed.	Proper disposal prevents the spread of microorganisms. Placing syringe in sharps container prevents reuse. Promotes comfort and appropriate personal hygiene.
24. Remove gloves. Secure catheter tubing to the patient's inner thigh or lower abdomen (with the penis directed toward the patient's chest) with Velcro leg strap, catheter securing device, or tape. Leave some slack in catheter for leg movement.	Proper attachment prevents trauma to the urethra and meatus from tension on the tubing. Whether to take the drainage tubing over or under the leg depends on gravity flow, patient's mobility, and comfort of the patient.
25. Assist the patient to a comfortable position. Cover the patient with bed linens. Place the bed in the lowest position.	Positioning and covering provide warmth and promote comfort.
26. Secure drainage bag below the level of the bladder. Check that drainage tubing is not kinked and that movement of side rails does not interfere with catheter or drainage bag.	This facilitates drainage of urine and prevents the backflow of urine.
27. Put on clean gloves. Obtain urine specimen immediately, if needed, from drainage bag. Label specimen. Send urine specimen to the laboratory promptly or refrigerate it.	Catheter system is sterile. Obtaining specimen immediately allows access to sterile system. Keeping urine at room temperature may cause microorganisms, if present, to grow and distort laboratory findings.
28. Remove gloves and additional PPE, if used. Perform hand hygiene.	Removing PPE properly reduces the risk for infection transmission and contamination of other items. Hand hygiene prevents the spread of microorganisms.

EVALUATION

• Catheter is inserted using sterile technique, results in the immediate flow of urine, and the bladder is not distended.
• Patient does not experience trauma, reports little to no pain on insertion, and the perineal area remains clean and dry.

DOCUMENTATION

• Document the type and size of catheter and balloon inserted, as well as the amount of fluid used to inflate the balloon. Document the patient's tolerance of the activity. Record the amount of urine obtained through the catheter and any specimen obtained. Document any other assessments, such as unusual urine characteristics or alterations in the patient's skin. Record urine amount on intake and output record, if appropriate.

SKILL VARIATION	Intermittent Male Urethral Catheterization

1. Check the medical record for the order for intermittent urethral catheterization. Review the patient's chart for any limitations in physical activity. Gather supplies. Obtain assistance from another staff member, if necessary.
2. Perform hand hygiene. Put on PPE, as indicated, based on transmission precautions.
3. Identify the patient. Discuss the procedure with the patient and assess the patient's ability to assist with the procedure. Ask the patient if he has any allergies, especially to latex or iodine.
4. Close the curtains around the bed and close the door to the room, if possible.
5. Provide good lighting. Artificial light is recommended (use of a flashlight requires an assistant to hold and position it). Place a trash receptacle within easy reach.
6. Assemble equipment on overbed table within reach.
7. Raise the bed to a comfortable working height. Stand on the patient's right side if you are right-handed, patient's left side if you are left-handed.
8. Position patient on his back with thighs slightly apart. Drape patient so that only the area around the penis is exposed. Slide waterproof pad under patient.
9. Put on clean gloves. Clean the genital area with washcloth, skin cleanser, and warm water. Clean the tip of the penis first, moving the washcloth in a circular

continued on page 942

Intermittent Male Urethral Catheterization *continued*

---

motion from the meatus outward. Wash the shaft of the penis using downward strokes toward the pubic area. Rinse and dry. Remove gloves. Perform hand hygiene again.

10. Open sterile catheterization tray on a clean overbed table using sterile technique.

11. Put on sterile gloves. Open sterile drape and place on patient's thighs. Place fenestrated drape with opening over penis.

12. Place catheter setup on or next to patient's legs on sterile drape.

13. Open all the supplies. Open package of antiseptic swabs. Alternately, fluff cotton balls in tray before pouring antiseptic solution over them. Open specimen container if specimen is to be obtained.

14. Remove cap from syringe prefilled with lubricant.

15. Lift penis with nondominant hand. Retract foreskin in uncircumcised patient. **Be prepared to keep this hand in this position until catheter is inserted and urine is flowing well and continuously.**

16. **Use the dominant hand to pick up an antiseptic swab or use forceps to pick up a cotton ball. Using a circular motion, clean the penis, moving from the meatus down the glans of the penis. Repeat this cleansing**

motion two more times, using a new cotton ball/swab each time. Discard each cotton ball/swab after one use.

17. Hold penis with slight upward tension and perpendicular to patient's body. Use the dominant hand to pick up the lubricant syringe. **Gently insert tip of syringe with lubricant into urethra and instill the 10 mL of lubricant.**

18. With the noncontaminated, dominant hand, place drainage end of catheter in receptacle. If a specimen is required, place the end into the specimen container in the receptacle.

19. Use the dominant hand to pick up the catheter and hold it an inch or two from the tip. Ask the patient to bear down as if voiding. Insert catheter tip into meatus. Ask the patient to take deep breaths as you advance the catheter 6 to 8 inches (14.4 to 19.2 cm) or until urine flows.

20. Hold the catheter securely at the meatus with the nondominant hand while the bladder empties. If a specimen is being collected, remove the drainage end of the tubing from the specimen container after the required amount is obtained and allow urine to flow into the receptacle. Set specimen container aside.

Intermittent Male Urethral Catheterization   *continued*

21. Allow the bladder to empty. Withdraw the catheter slowly and smoothly after urine has stopped flowing. Remove equipment and dispose of it according to facility policy. Discard syringe in sharps container to prevent reuse. Wash and dry the genital area, as needed. Replace foreskin in forward position, if necessary.

22. Remove gloves. Assist the patient to a comfortable position. Cover the patient with bed linens. Place the bed in the lowest position.

23. Put on clean gloves. Cover and label the specimen. Send the urine specimen to the laboratory promptly or refrigerate it.

24. Remove gloves and additional PPE, if used. Perform hand hygiene.

Note: Intermittent catheterization in the home is performed using clean technique. The bladder's natural resistance to the microorganisms normally found in the home makes sterile technique unnecessary. Catheters are washed, dried, and stored for repeated use. Clean technique involves the use of cleansed reusable catheters, washing hands with soap and water, and daily cleansing of the perineum or more often only when fecal or other wastes are present (Newman, 2008, as cited in Herter & Wallace Kazer, 2010). Cleansing the perineal area to decrease bacteria in the surrounding area is highly recommended (Herter & Wallace Kazer, 2010).

SKILL 178   CARING FOR A SUPRAPUBIC URINARY CATHETER

A suprapubic urinary catheter may be used for long-term continuous urinary drainage. This type of catheter is surgically inserted through a small incision above the pubic area. Suprapubic bladder drainage diverts urine from the urethra when injury, stricture, prostatic obstruction, or gynecologic or abdominal surgery has compromised the flow of urine through the urethra. A suprapubic catheter is often preferred over indwelling urethral catheters for long-term urinary drainage. Suprapubic catheters are associated with decreased risk of contamination with organisms from fecal material, elimination of damage to the urethra, a higher rate of patient satisfaction, and lower risk of catheter-associated urinary tract infections. The drainage tube is secured with sutures or tape. Care of the patient with a suprapubic catheter includes skin care around the insertion site; care of the drainage tubing and drainage bag is the same as for an indwelling catheter.

DELEGATION CONSIDERATIONS

The care of a suprapubic urinary catheter, in the postoperative period, is not delegated to nursing assistive personnel (NAP) or to unlicensed assistive personnel (UAP) in the acute care setting. The care of a healed suprapubic catheter site in some settings may be delegated to NAP or UAP who have received appropriate training, after assessment of the catheter by the registered nurse. Depending on the state's nurse practice act and the organization's policies and procedures, the care of a suprapubic urinary catheter may be delegated to licensed practical/vocational nurses (LPN/LVNs). The decision to delegate must be based on careful analysis of the patient's needs and circumstances, as well as the qualifications of the person to whom the task is being delegated. Refer to the Delegation Guidelines in Appendix A.

EQUIPMENT

- Washcloth
- Skin cleanser and water
- Disposable gloves
- Additional PPE, as indicated
- Velcro tube holder or tape to secure tube
- Drainage sponge (if necessary)
- Plastic trash bag
- Sterile cotton-tipped applicators and sterile saline solution (if the patient has a new suprapubic catheter)

ASSESSMENT

- Assess the suprapubic catheter and bag, observing the condition of the catheter and the drainage bag connected to the catheter, and the product style.
- If a dressing is in place at the insertion site, assess the dressing for drainage.
- Inspect the site around the suprapubic catheter, looking for drainage, erythema, or excoriation.
- Assess the method used to secure the catheter in place. If sutures are present, assess for intactness.
- Assess the characteristics of the urine in the drainage bag.
- Assess the patient's knowledge of caring for a suprapubic catheter.

NURSING DIAGNOSIS

- Impaired Urinary Elimination
- Risk for Infection
- Deficient Knowledge

OUTCOME IDENTIFICATION AND PLANNING

- Patient's skin remains clean, dry and intact, without evidence of irritation or breakdown.
- Patient verbalizes an understanding of the purpose for, and care of, the catheter, as appropriate.
- Patient's urinary elimination is maintained, with a urine output of at least 30 mL/hour, and the patient's bladder is not distended.

IMPLEMENTATION

ACTION	RATIONALE
1. Gather equipment.	Assembling equipment provides for an organized approach to the task.
2. Perform hand hygiene and put on PPE, if indicated.	Hand hygiene and PPE prevent the spread of microorganisms. PPE is required based on transmission precautions.
3. Identify the patient.	Identifying the patient ensures the right patient receives the intervention and helps prevent errors.
4. Close the curtains around the bed and close the door to the room, if possible. Explain what you are going to do, and why you are going to do it, to the patient. Encourage the patient to observe or participate, if possible.	This ensures the patient's privacy. Explanation relieves anxiety and facilitates cooperation. Discussion promotes cooperation and helps to minimize anxiety. Having the patient observe or assist encourages self-acceptance.
5. Assemble equipment on overbed table within reach.	Arranging items nearby is convenient, saves time, and avoids unnecessary stretching and twisting of muscles on the part of the nurse.
6. Adjust the bed to a comfortable working height, usually elbow height of the caregiver (VISN 8 Patient Safety Center, 2009). Assist the patient to a supine position. Place waterproof pad under the patient at the stoma site.	Having the bed at the proper height prevents back and muscle strain. The supine position is usually the best way to gain access to the suprapubic urinary catheter. A waterproof pad protects linens and patient from moisture.
7. Put on clean gloves. Gently remove old dressing, if one is in place. Place dressing in trash bag. Remove gloves. Perform hand hygiene.	Gloves protect the nurse from blood, body fluids, and microorganisms. Proper disposal of contaminated dressing and hand hygiene deter the spread of microorganisms.
8. Assess the insertion site and surrounding skin.	Any changes in assessment could indicate potential infection.

ACTION	RATIONALE

9. Wet washcloth with warm water and apply skin cleanser. **Gently cleanse around suprapubic exit site.** Remove any encrustations. If this is a new suprapubic catheter, use sterile cotton-tipped applicators and sterile saline to clean the site until the incision has healed. Moisten the applicators with the saline. **Clean in circular motion from the insertion site outward.**

Using a gentle skin cleanser helps to protect the skin. The exit site is the most common area of skin irritation with a suprapubic catheter. If encrustations are left on the skin, they provide a medium for bacteria and an area of skin irritation.

10. Rinse area of all cleanser. Pat dry.

The skin needs to be kept dry to prevent any irritation.

11. If the exit site has been draining, place a small drain sponge around the catheter to absorb any drainage. Be prepared to change this sponge throughout the day, depending on the amount of drainage. Do not cut a 4 × 4 gauze to make a drain sponge.

A small amount of drainage from the exit site is normal. The sponge needs to be changed when it becomes soiled to prevent skin irritation and breakdown. The fibers from a cut 4 × 4 gauze may enter the exit site and cause irritation or infection.

12. Remove gloves. Form a loop in the tubing and anchor it on the patient's abdomen.

Anchoring the catheter and tubing absorbs any tugging, preventing tension on, and irritation to, the skin or bladder.

13. Assist the patient to a comfortable position. Cover the patient with bed linens. Place the bed in the lowest position.

Positioning and covering provide warmth and promote comfort. Bed in lowest position promotes patient safety.

14. Put on clean gloves. Remove or discard equipment and assess the patient's response to the procedure.

Gloves prevent contact with blood and body fluids. The patient's response may indicate acceptance of the catheter or the need for health teaching.

15. Remove gloves and additional PPE, if used. Perform hand hygiene.

Removing PPE properly reduces the risk for infection transmission and contamination of other items. Hand hygiene prevents the spread of microorganisms.

EVALUATION

- Patient's skin remains clean, dry, and intact, without evidence of irritation or breakdown.
- Patient verbalizes an understanding of the purpose for, and care of, the catheter, as appropriate.
- Patient's urinary elimination is maintained, with a urine output of at least 30 mL/hour.
- Patient's bladder is not distended.

DOCUMENTATION

- Document the appearance of catheter exit site and surrounding skin, urine amount and characteristics, as well as patient's reaction to the procedure.

SKILL 179 — COLLECTING A URINE SPECIMEN (CLEAN CATCH, MIDSTREAM) FOR URINALYSIS AND CULTURE

Collecting a urine specimen for urinalysis and culture is an assessment measure to determine the characteristics of a patient's urine. A voided urine specimen for culture is collected midstream to provide a specimen that most closely reflects the characteristics of the urine being produced by the body. If the patient is able to understand and follow the procedure, the patient may collect the sample on his or her own, after explanation and instruction. The following procedure reviews collection of a clean catch, midstream urine specimen. The procedure to collect a bagged urine specimen from an infant or young child, as well as the procedure to obtain a urine specimen from a urinary diversion follow as Skill Variations.

DELEGATION CONSIDERATIONS

Obtaining a urine specimen by midstream collection may be delegated to nursing assistive personnel (NAP) or to unlicensed assistive personnel (UAP), as well as licensed practical/vocational nurses (LPN/LVNs). The decision to delegate must be based on careful analysis of the patient's needs and circumstances, as well as the qualifications of the person to whom the task is being delegated. Refer to the Delegation Guidelines in Appendix A.

EQUIPMENT

- Moist cleansing towelettes or skin cleanser, water, and washcloth
- Nonsterile gloves
- Additional PPE, as indicated
- Sterile specimen container; urine collection tubes, based on facility policy
- Biohazard bag
- Appropriate label for specimen, based on facility policy and procedure

ASSESSMENT

- Ask the patient about any medications that he or she is taking, because medications may affect the results of the test.
- Assess for any signs and symptoms of a urinary tract infection, such as burning, pain (dysuria), or frequency.
- Assess the patient's ability to cooperate with the collection process. Determine the need for assistance to obtain specimen correctly.

NURSING DIAGNOSIS

- Impaired Urinary Elimination
- Anxiety
- Deficient Knowledge

OUTCOME IDENTIFICATION AND PLANNING

- Adequate amount of urine is obtained from the patient without contamination.
- Patient exhibits minimal anxiety during specimen collection and demonstrates an ability to collect a clean urine specimen.

IMPLEMENTATION

ACTION	RATIONALE
1. Verify the order for a urine specimen collection in the medical record. Gather equipment.	Verifying the medical order is crucial to ensuring that the proper procedure is administered to the right patient. Assembling equipment provides for an organized approach to the task.
2. Perform hand hygiene and put on PPE, if indicated.	Hand hygiene and PPE prevent the transmission of microorganisms. PPE is required based on transmission precautions.
3. Identify the patient.	Identifying the patient ensures the right patient receives the intervention and helps prevent errors.
4. Explain the procedure to the patient. If the patient can perform the task without assistance after instruction, leave the container at bedside with instructions to call the	Explanation provides reassurance and promotes cooperation.

ACTION	RATIONALE

nurse as soon as a specimen is produced.

5. Check the specimen label with the patient's identification bracelet. Label should include the patient's name and identification number, time specimen was collected, route of collection, identification of the person obtaining the sample, and any other information required by facility policy.

Confirmation of patient identification information ensures the specimen is labeled correctly for the right patient.

6. Assemble equipment on overbed table within reach.

Arranging items nearby is convenient, saves time, and avoids unnecessary stretching and twisting of muscles on the part of the nurse.

7. Have the patient perform hand hygiene, if performing self-collection.

Hand hygiene prevents the transmission of microorganisms.

8. Close the curtains around the bed and close the door to the room, if possible.

Closing the door or curtain provides for patient privacy.

9. Put on nonsterile gloves. Assist the patient to the bathroom, or onto the bedside commode or bedpan. Instruct the patient not to defecate or discard toilet paper into the urine.

Gloves reduce the transmission of microorganisms. Stool and/or toilet paper may contaminate the specimen.

10. Instruct the female patient to separate the labia for cleaning of the area and during collection of urine. Female patients should use the towelettes or wet washcloth to clean each side of the urinary meatus, then the center over the meatus, from front to back, using a new wipe or a clean area of the washcloth for each stroke. Instruct the female patient to **keep the**

Cleaning the perineal area or penis reduces the risk for contamination of the specimen. Separation of labia avoids contamination by perineal skin and hair. Retraction of foreskin avoids contamination by skin.

ACTION	RATIONALE

labia separated after cleaning and during collection (Figure 1). Male patients should use a towelette to clean the tip of the penis, wiping in a circular motion away from the urethra. Instruct the uncircumcised male patient to retract the foreskin before cleaning and during collection (Figure 2).

FIGURE 1 Cleaning female perineum. Separating labia and cleansing from front to back.

FIGURE 2 Cleaning male perineum. Wiping in a circular motion away from urethra.

11. **Do not let the container touch the perineal skin or hair during collection. Do not touch the inside of the container or the lid. Have patient void a small amount (approx. 30 mL/1 oz.) of urine into the toilet, bedpan, or commode. The patient should then stop urinating briefly, and then continue voiding into the collection container. Collect the urine specimen (10 to 20 mL is**

Collecting a midstream specimen ensures that fresh urine is analyzed. Some urine may have collected in the urethra from the last void. By voiding a little before collecting the specimen, the specimen will contain only fresh urine.

ACTION	RATIONALE
sufficient), and then instruct the patient to finish voiding in the toilet, bedpan, or commode. Instruct the uncircumcised male patient to replace the foreskin after collection.	
12. Place lid on container. If necessary, transfer the specimen to appropriate containers/tubes for specific test ordered, according to facility policy.	Placing the lid on the container helps to keep the specimen clean and prevents spills.
13. Assist the patient from the bathroom, off the commode, or off the bedpan. Provide perineal care, if necessary.	Perineal care promotes patient comfort and hygiene.
14. Remove gloves and perform hand hygiene.	Removing gloves properly reduces the risk for infection transmission and contamination of other items. Hand hygiene reduces the transmission of microorganisms.
15. Place label on the container per facility policy. Note specimen collection method, according to facility policy. Place container in plastic, sealable biohazard bag.	Proper labeling ensures accurate reporting of results. Packaging the specimen in a biohazard bag prevents the person transporting the container from coming in contact with urine.
16. Remove other PPE, if used. Perform hand hygiene.	Removing PPE properly reduces the risk for infection transmission and contamination of other items. Hand hygiene reduces the transmission of microorganisms.
17. Transport the specimen to the laboratory as soon as possible. If unable to take the specimen to the laboratory immediately, refrigerate it.	If not refrigerated immediately, urine may act as a culture medium, allowing bacteria to multiply and skewing the results of testing. Refrigeration prevents the bacteria from multiplying.

EVALUATION

• Uncontaminated urine specimen is collected and sent to the laboratory promptly.

- Patient demonstrated the proper technique for specimen collection and stated that anxiety is lessened.

DOCUMENTATION

- Document that the specimen was sent to the laboratory. Note the specimen collection method. Note the characteristics of the urine, including odor, amount (if known), color, and clarity. Include any significant patient assessments, such as patient complaints of burning or pain on urination.

SKILL VARIATION	Obtaining a Bagged Urine Specimen for Urinalysis from an Infant or Young Child

1. Verify the order for a urine specimen collection in the medical record. Gather equipment
2. Perform hand hygiene and put on PPE, if indicated.
3. Identify the patient. Explain the steps to a young child, if old enough, and to the parents. Talk to the child at the child's level, stressing that no pain will be involved.
4. Check specimen label with the patient's identification bracelet. Label should include the patient's name and identification number, time specimen was collected, route of collection, identification of the person obtaining sample, and any other information required by facility policy.
5. Remove the diaper or underwear. Perform thorough perineal care with skin cleanser and water: for girls, spread labia and cleanse area; for boys,

retract foreskin if intact and cleanse glans of penis. Pat skin dry.
6. Remove paper backing from adhesive faceplate. Apply faceplate over labia or over penis. Gently push faceplate so that seal forms on skin (Figure A).

FIGURE A Applying infant urine collection bag.

7. Apply clean diaper or underwear over bag to help prevent dislodgement. Remove gloves and perform hand hygiene. **Check bag every 15 minutes to see whether the child has voided.**
8. As soon as the patient has voided, perform hand hygiene and put on nonsterile gloves. Gently remove

Obtaining a Bagged Urine Specimen for Urinalysis from an Infant or Young Child *continued*

bag by pushing skin away from bag. Transfer urine to appropriate containers/tubes for specific test ordered, according to facility policy.

9. Perform perineal care and reapply diaper or clothing.

10. Remove gloves. Perform hand hygiene.

11. Place label on the container per facility policy. Place container in plastic, sealable biohazard bag.

12. Remove other PPE, if used. Perform hand hygiene.

13. Transport the specimen to the laboratory as soon as possible. If unable to take the specimen to the laboratory immediately, refrigerate it.

14. If the collection bag falls off or does not adhere completely, remove the bag, perform perineal care, and apply a new collection bag.

SKILL VARIATION | Obtaining a Urine Specimen from a Urinary Diversion

Equipment: Cleansing solution, based on facility policy; sterile gauze; sterile water or saline, or cleansing solution for stoma site (povidone-iodine, chlorhexidine), based on facility policy; double lumen or straight catheter (8 to 16Fr); sterile water-based lubricant if catheter not self-lubricated; sterile specimen container and urine collection tubes, based on facility policy; sterile and nonsterile gloves; new ostomy appliance; skin cleanser; disposable washcloth or washcloth and towel

1. Verify the order for a urine specimen collection in the medical record. Gather equipment.

2. Perform hand hygiene and put on PPE, if indicated.

3. Identify the patient. Explain the procedure to the patient.

4. Check specimen label with the patient's identification bracelet. Label should include the patient's name and identification number, time specimen was collected, route of collection, identification of the person obtaining the sample, and any other information required by facility policy.

continued on page 954

5. Assemble equipment on overbed table within reach. Open supplies, maintaining sterility of sterile items.

6. Put on nonsterile gloves. Remove ostomy appliance. If one-piece system is in place, remove entire appliance. If two-piece system is in place, remove collection pouch only, leaving appliance pouch only, leaving faceplate wafer intact on skin.

7. Using a circular motion from stoma opening outward, clean the stoma site with the sterile water, sterile saline, or other cleansing solution, based on facility policy.

8. Remove gloves and put on sterile gloves. Blot stoma with sterile gauze.

9. Place open end of urinary catheter into specimen container. Lubricate the catheter with lubricant. If using straight catheter, gently insert the urinary catheter into the stoma site and advance 2 to 3 inches. If using a double-lumen catheter, gently insert catheter tip into stoma and advance the inner catheter approximately 1 to 2 inches. Hold the catheter in position until urine begins to drip. **If you meet resistance, rotate the catheter gently until it slides forward. Do not force the catheter. If you continue to meet**

resistance, do not force it any further. If urine does not flow into the catheter, ask the patient to shift position and/or cough to mobilize urine (Williams, 2012).

10. Collect approximately 5 to 10 mL of urine before removing catheter. This may take 5 to 15 minutes. Once catheter is removed, cap the specimen container. Clean and dry the stoma and peristomal skin. Replace ostomy appliance. Refer to Skill 156. If necessary, transfer the specimen to appropriate containers/tubes for specific test ordered, according to facility policy.

11. Remove gloves and perform hand hygiene.

12. Place label on the container per facility policy. Note specimen collection method, according to facility policy. Place container in plastic, sealable biohazard bag. Dispose of equipment according to facility policy.

13. Remove other PPE, if used. Perform hand hygiene.

14. Transport the specimen to the laboratory as soon as possible. If unable to take

the specimen to the laboratory immediately, refrigerate it.
15. Alternately, once appliance is removed and stoma cleansed, hold the sterile specimen cup under the stoma to collect urine (Mahoney et al., 2013; Williams, 2012).

SKILL 180 OBTAINING A URINE SPECIMEN FROM AN INDWELLING URINARY CATHETER

Indwelling catheter drainage tubes have special sampling ports in the tubing for removal of urine for testing. Most sampling ports are needleless systems. However, some ports require the use of a needle or blunt cannula to access the sampling port. The drainage tubing below the access port may be bent back on itself or clamped so that urine collects near the port, unless contraindicated, based on the patient's condition. **Do not open the drainage system to obtain urine specimens to avoid contamination of the system and bladder infection. Never take urine specimens from the catheter drainage bag because the urine is not fresh and bacteria may be present on the bag.**

DELEGATION CONSIDERATIONS

Obtaining a urine specimen from an indwelling catheter may be delegated to nursing assistive personnel (NAP) or to unlicensed assistive personnel (UAP), as well as licensed practical/vocational nurses (LPN/LVNs). The decision to delegate must be based on careful analysis of the patient's needs and circumstances, as well as the qualifications of the person to whom the task is being delegated. Refer to the Delegation Guidelines in Appendix A.

EQUIPMENT

- 10-mL sterile syringe
- Blunt cannula or 18-gauge needle, if needed, based on specific catheter in use
- Alcohol or other disinfectant wipes
- Nonsterile gloves
- Additional PPE, as indicated

- Sterile specimen container; urine collection tubes, based on facility policy
- Biohazard bag
- Appropriate label for specimen, based on facility policy and procedure

ASSESSMENT

- Verify the medical order for specimen collection.
- Review the medical record for information about any medications that the patient is taking, because medications may affect the results of the test.
- Assess the characteristics of the urine draining from the catheter.
- Inspect the catheter tubing to identify the type of sampling port present.

NURSING DIAGNOSIS

- Impaired Urinary Elimination
- Anxiety
- Deficient Knowledge

OUTCOME IDENTIFICATION AND PLANNING

- Adequate amount of urine is obtained from the patient without contamination or adverse effect.
- Patient experiences minimal anxiety during the collection process.
- Patient demonstrates an understanding of the reason for the specimen collection.

IMPLEMENTATION

ACTION	RATIONALE
1. Verify the order for a urine specimen collection in the medical record. Gather equipment.	Verifying the medical order is crucial to ensuring that the proper procedure is administered to the right patient. Assembling equipment provides for an organized approach to the task.
2. Perform hand hygiene and put on PPE, if indicated.	Hand hygiene and PPE prevent the transmission of microorganisms. PPE is required based on transmission precautions.
3. Identify the patient.	Identifying the patient ensures the right patient receives the intervention and helps prevent errors.
4. Explain the procedure to the patient.	Explanation provides reassurance and promotes cooperation.
5. Check the specimen label with the patient's identification	Confirmation of patient identification information ensures the

ACTION	RATIONALE
bracelet. Label should include the patient's name and identification number, time specimen was collected, route of collection, identification of person obtaining the sample, and any other information required by facility policy.	specimen is labeled correctly for the right patient.
6. Assemble equipment on overbed table within reach.	Arranging items nearby is convenient, saves time, and avoids unnecessary stretching and twisting of muscles on the part of the nurse.
7. Close the curtains around the bed and close the door to the room, if possible.	Closing curtain or door provides for patient privacy.
8. Put on nonsterile gloves.	Gloves reduce the transmission of microorganisms.
9. Clamp the catheter drainage tubing or bend it back on itself distal to the port. If an insufficient amount of urine is present in the tubing, allow the tubing to remain clamped up to 30 minutes, to collect a sufficient amount of urine, unless contraindicated. Remove lid from specimen container, keeping the inside of the container and lid free from contamination.	Clamping the tubing ensures the collection of an adequate amount of fresh urine. Clamping for an extended period of time leads to overdistention of the bladder. Clamping may be contraindicated based on the patient's condition (e.g., after bladder surgery). The container needs to remain sterile so as not to contaminate the urine.
10. **Cleanse aspiration port vigorously with alcohol or other disinfectant wipe and allow port to air dry.**	Cleaning with alcohol deters entry of microorganisms when the needle punctures the port.
11. Attach the syringe to the needleless port or insert the needle or blunt-tipped cannula into the port. Slowly aspirate enough urine for specimen (usually 10 mL is adequate; check facility	Using a leur-lock syringe or blunt-tipped needle prevents a needlestick. Collecting urine from the port ensures that the specimen will contain fresh urine. Unclamping catheter drainage tubing prevents

ACTION	RATIONALE

requirements) (Figure 1). Remove the syringe from the port. Engage the needle guard, if needle was used. **Unclamp the drainage tubing.**

overdistention of and injury to the patient's bladder.

FIGURE 1 Inserting the needle in aspiration port and slowly withdrawing urine specimen.

12. If a needle or blunt-tipped cannula was used on the syringe, remove from the syringe before emptying the urine from the syringe into the specimen cup. Place the needle into a sharps collection container. **Slowly inject urine into the specimen container. Take care to avoid touching the syringe tip to any surface. Do not touch the edge or inside of the collection container.**

Forcing urine through the needle breaks up cells and impedes accurate results of microscopic urinalysis. If the urine is injected quickly into the container, it may splash out of the container or into the nurse's eyes. Avoid touching edge or inside of container to avoid contamination.

13. Replace lid on container. If necessary, transfer the specimen to appropriate containers/ tubes for specific test ordered, according to facility policy. Dispose of syringe in a sharps collection container.

Proper disposal of equipment prevents injury and transmission of microorganisms. Safe disposal of sharps prevents accidental injury.

14. Remove gloves and perform hand hygiene.

Removing gloves properly reduces the risk for infection transmission and contamination of other items. Hand hygiene reduces the transmission of microorganisms.

15. Place label on the container per facility policy. Note

Proper labeling ensures accurate reporting of results. Packaging

ACTION	RATIONALE
specimen collection method, according to facility policy. Place container in plastic sealable biohazard bag.	the specimen in a biohazard bag prevents the person transporting the container from coming in contact with the specimen.
16. Remove other PPE, if used. Perform hand hygiene.	Removing PPE properly reduces the risk for infection transmission and contamination of other items. Hand hygiene reduces the transmission of microorganisms.
17. Transport the specimen to the laboratory as soon as possible. If unable to take the specimen to the laboratory immediately, refrigerate it.	If not refrigerated immediately, urine may act as a culture medium, allowing bacteria to multiply and skewing the results of testing. Refrigeration prevents the bacteria from multiplying.

EVALUATION

• Uncontaminated urine specimen is collected and sent to the laboratory without adverse effect.
• Patient does not experience increased anxiety during the collection process.

DOCUMENTATION

• Document the method used to obtain the specimen, type of specimen sent, and characteristics of urine. Note any significant patient assessments. Record urine volume on intake and output record, if appropriate.

SKILL 181 ADMINISTERING A VAGINAL CREAM

Creams, foams, and tablets can be applied intravaginally using a narrow, tubular applicator with an attached plunger. Suppositories that melt when exposed to body heat are also administered by vaginal insertion (see Skill Variation). Refrigerate suppositories for storage. Time administration to allow the patient to lie down afterward to retain the medication.

DELEGATION CONSIDERATIONS

The administration of medication as a vaginal cream is not delegated to nursing assistive personnel (NAP) or to unlicensed assistive personnel

(UAP). Depending on the state's nurse practice act and the organization's policies and procedures, administration of a vaginal cream may be delegated to licensed practical/vocational nurses (LPN/LVNs). The decision to delegate must be based on careful analysis of the patient's needs and circumstances, as well as the qualifications of the person to whom the task is being delegated. Refer to the Delegation Guidelines in Appendix A.

EQUIPMENT

- Medication with applicator, if appropriate
- Water-soluble lubricant
- Perineal pad
- Washcloth, skin cleanser, and warm water
- Gloves
- Additional PPE, as indicated
- Computer-generated Medication Administration Record (CMAR) or Medication Administration Record (MAR)

ASSESSMENT

- Assess the external genitalia and vaginal canal for redness, erythema, edema, drainage, or tenderness.
- Assess the patient for allergies.
- Verify patient name, dose, route, and time of administration.
- Assess the patient's knowledge of medication and procedure. If the patient has a knowledge deficit about the medication, this may be an appropriate time to begin education about the medication.
- Assess the patient's ability to cooperate with the procedure.

NURSING DIAGNOSIS

- Deficient Knowledge
- Risk for Allergy Response
- Anxiety

OUTCOME IDENTIFICATION AND PLANNING

- Medication is administered successfully into the vagina.
- Patient understands the rationale for the vaginal instillation.
- Patient experiences no allergy response.
- Patient's skin remains intact.
- Patient experiences no, or minimal, pain.
- Patient experiences minimal anxiety.

IMPLEMENTATION

ACTION	RATIONALE
1. Gather equipment. Check medication order against the original order in the medical record, according to facility	This comparison helps to identify errors that may have occurred when orders were transcribed. The primary care provider's

ACTION	RATIONALE
policy. Clarify any inconsistencies. Check the patient's chart for allergies.	order is the legal record of medication orders for each facility.
2. Know the actions, special nursing considerations, safe dose ranges, purpose of administration, and adverse effects of the medication to be administered. Consider the appropriateness of the medication for this patient.	This knowledge aids the nurse in evaluating the therapeutic effect of the medication in relation to the patient's disorder and can also be used to educate the patient about the medication.
3. Perform hand hygiene. 	Hand hygiene prevents the spread of microorganisms.
4. Move the medication cart to the outside of the patient's room or prepare for administration in the medication area.	Organization facilitates error-free administration and saves time.
5. Unlock the medication cart or drawer. Enter pass code and scan employee identification, if required.	Locking of the cart or drawer safeguards each patient's medication supply. Hospital accrediting organizations require medication carts to be locked when not in use. Entering pass code and scanning ID allows only authorized users into the system and identifies the user for documentation by the computer.
6. **Prepare medications for one patient at a time.**	This prevents errors in medication administration.
7. Read the CMAR/MAR and select the proper medication from unit stock or the patient's medication drawer.	This is the *first* check of the label.
8. Compare the label with the CMAR/MAR. Check expiration dates and perform calculations, if necessary. Scan the bar code on the package, if required.	This is the *second* check of the label. Verify calculations with another nurse to ensure safety, if necessary.

ACTION	RATIONALE
9. **Depending on facility policy, the third check of the label may occur at this point. If so, when all medications for one patient have been prepared, recheck the labels with the CMAR/MAR before taking the medications to the patient.**	This *third* check ensures accuracy and helps to prevent errors. *Note:* Many facilities require the *third* check to occur at the bedside, after identifying the patient and before administration.
10. Lock the medication cart before leaving it.	Locking the cart or drawer safeguards the patient's medication supply. Hospital accrediting organizations require medication carts to be locked when not in use.
11. Transport medications to the patient's bedside carefully, and keep the medications in sight at all times.	Careful handling and close observation prevent accidental or deliberate disarrangement of medications.
12. **Ensure that the patient receives the medications at the correct time.**	Check agency policy, which may allow for administration within a period of 30 minutes before or 30 minutes after the designated time.
13. Perform hand hygiene and put on PPE, if indicated.	Hand hygiene and PPE prevent the spread of microorganisms. PPE is required based on transmission precautions.
14. **Identify the patient. Compare the information with the CMAR/MAR. The patient should be identified using at least two methods** (The Joint Commission, 2013): a. Check the name on the patient's identification band. b. Check the identification number on the patient's identification band.	Identifying the patient ensures the right patient receives the medications and helps prevent errors. The patient's room number or physical location is not used as an identifier (The Joint Commission, 2013). Replace the identification band if it is missing or inaccurate in any way.

ACTION	RATIONALE
c. Check the birth date on the patient's identification band.	
d. Ask the patient to state his or her name and birth date, based on facility policy.	This requires a response from the patient, but illness and strange surroundings often cause patients to be confused.
15. **Complete necessary assessments before administering medications. Check the patient's allergy bracelet or ask the patient about allergies. Explain the purpose and action of each medication to the patient.**	Assessment is a prerequisite to administration of medications.
16. Scan the patient's bar code on the identification band, if required.	Provides an additional check to ensure that the medication is given to the right patient.
17. **Based on facility policy, the third check of the label may occur at this point. If so, recheck the labels with the CMAR/MAR before administering the medications to the patient.**	Many facilities require the *third* check to occur at the bedside, after identifying the patient and before administration. If facility policy directs the *third* check at this time, this *third* check ensures accuracy and helps to prevent errors.
18. Ask the patient to void before inserting the medication.	Empties the bladder and helps to minimize pressure and discomfort during administration.
19. Put on gloves.	Gloves protect the nurse from potential contact with contaminants and body fluids.
20. Position the patient so that she is lying on her back with the knees flexed. Maintain privacy with draping. Provide adequate light to visualize the vaginal opening.	Position provides access to vaginal canal and helps to retain medication in the canal. Draping limits exposure of the patient and promotes warmth and privacy. Adequate light facilitates ease of administration.
21. Spread labia with fingers, and cleanse area at vaginal orifice with washcloth and warm water, using a different corner of the washcloth with each stroke. Wipe from above the vaginal orifice	These techniques prevent contamination of the vaginal orifice with debris surrounding the anus.

ACTION	RATIONALE
downward toward the sacrum (front to back).	
22. Remove gloves and put on new gloves.	Prevents spread of microorganisms.
23. Fill vaginal applicator with prescribed amount of cream. (See the accompanying Skill Variation for administering a vaginal suppository.)	This ensures the correct dosage of medication will be administered.
24. Lubricate applicator with the lubricant, as necessary.	Ordinarily, lubrication is unnecessary, but it may be used to reduce friction while inserting the applicator.
25. Spread the labia with your nondominant hand and gently introduce the applicator with your dominant hand, in a rolling manner, while directing it downward and backward.	This follows the normal contour of the vagina for its full length.
26. After the applicator is properly positioned, labia may be allowed to fall in place if necessary to free the hand for manipulating the plunger. Push the plunger to its full length and then gently remove applicator with plunger depressed.	Pushing the plunger will gently deploy the cream into the vaginal orifice.
27. **Ask the patient to remain in the supine position for 5 to 10 minutes after insertion.** Offer the patient a perineal pad to collect drainage.	This gives the medication time to be absorbed in the vaginal cavity. As medication heats up, some medication may leak from the vaginal orifice.
28. Dispose of the applicator in an appropriate receptacle or clean the nondisposable applicator according to manufacturer's directions.	Disposal prevents transmission of microorganisms. Cleaning prepares the applicator for future use by same patient for continuing treatment.
29. Remove gloves and additional PPE, if used. Perform hand hygiene.	Removing PPE properly reduces the risk for infection transmission and contamination of other items. Hand hygiene prevents the spread of microorganisms.

ACTION	RATIONALE
30. Document the administration of the medication immediately after administration. See Documentation section below.	Timely documentation helps to ensure patient safety.
31. Evaluate the patient's response to the medication within an appropriate time frame.	The patient needs to be evaluated for therapeutic and adverse effects from the medication.

EVALUATION

- Patient receives the medication via the vagina.
- Patient understands the rationale for the medication administration.
- Patient experiences no allergy response.
- Patient experiences no or minimal discomfort.
- Patient experiences no or minimal anxiety.

DOCUMENTATION

- Document the administration of the medication immediately after administration, including date, time, dose, and route of administration on the CMAR/MAR or record using the required format. Prompt recording avoids the possibility of accidentally repeating the administration of the drug. If using a bar-code system, medication administration is automatically recorded when the bar code is scanned. PRN medications require documentation of the reason for administration. Document assessment, characteristics of any drainage, and the patient's response to the treatment, if appropriate. If the drug was refused or omitted, record this in the appropriate area on the medication record and notify the primary care provider. This verifies the reason medication was omitted and ensures that the primary care provider is aware of the patient's condition.

SKILL VARIATION | Administering a Vaginal Suppository

Prepare medication as outlined in steps 1–12 above (Skill 181).

1. Perform hand hygiene and put on PPE, if indicated.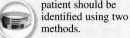

2. Identify the patient. The patient should be identified using two methods.

3. Close the door to the room or pull the bedside curtain.

continued on page 966

Administering a Vaginal Suppository *continued*

4. **Complete necessary assessments before administering medications. Check allergy bracelet or ask patient about allergies. Explain the purpose and action of the medication to the patient.**

5. Scan the patient's bar code on the identification band, if required.

6. Ask the patient to void before inserting the medication.

7. **Based on facility policy, the third check of the label may occur at this point. If so, recheck the labels with the CMAR/MAR before administering the medications to the patient.**

8. Put on gloves. Position the patient so that she is lying on her back with the knees flexed. Maintain privacy with draping. Adequate light should be available to visualize the vaginal opening.

9. Spread labia with fingers, and clean area at vaginal orifice with washcloth and warm water, using a different corner of the washcloth with each stroke. Wipe from above orifice downward toward sacrum (front to back).

10. Remove gloves and put on new gloves.

11. Remove the suppository from its wrapper and lubricate the round end with the water-soluble lubricant. Lubricate your gloved index finger on your dominant hand.

12. Spread the labia with your nondominant hand.

13. Insert the rounded end of the suppository along the posterior wall of the canal. Insert to the length of your finger.

14. Remove gloves.

15. **Ask the patient to remain in a supine position for 5 to 10 minutes after insertion.**

16. Offer the patient a perineal pad to collect drainage.

17. Remove additional PPE, if used. Perform hand hygiene.

18. Document administration of the medication on the CMAR/MAR immediately after administering the medication.

19. Evaluate the patient's response to the medication within an appropriate time frame.

20. Assist the patient to a comfortable position after the required 5 to 10 minutes in the supine position.

SKILL 182

Intracranial pressure (ICP), the pressure inside the cranium, is the result of blood, tissue, and cerebrospinal fluid circulating in the ventricles and subarachnoid space (Moreda et al., 2009). ICP monitoring is used to assess cerebral perfusion When ICP increases, as a result of conditions such as a mass (e.g., a tumor), bleeding into the brain or fluid around the brain, or swelling within the brain matter itself, neurologic consequences may range from minor to severe, including death (Hill et al., 2012). Normal ICP is less than 15 mm Hg. Elevated ICP, intracranial hypertension, is a sustained ICP of 20 mm Hg or more (Schimpf, 2012; Barker, 2008).

An external ventriculostomy is one method used to monitor ICP. It is part of a system that includes an external drainage system and an external transducer. This device is inserted into a ventricle of the brain, most commonly the nondominant lateral ventricle, through a hole drilled into the skull. The catheter is connected by a fluid-filled system to a transducer, which records the pressure in the form on an electrical impulse (Hinkle & Cheever, 2014). The ventriculostomy can be used to measure the ICP, to drain cerebrospinal fluid (CSF), such as removing excess fluid associated with hydrocephalus, or to decrease the volume in the cranial vault, thereby decreasing the ICP, and to instill medications. ICP and blood pressure measurements are used to calculate cerebral perfusion pressure (CPP), the pressure needed to perfuse the blood upward to the brain against gravity (Barker, 2008). ICP monitoring also provides information about intracranial compliance, the ability of the brain to tolerate stimulation or increase in intracranial volume without an increase in pressure through waveform assessment (AANN, 2011; Barker, 2008; Hinkle & Cheever, 2014).

DELEGATION CONSIDERATIONS

The care of a patient with an external ventriculostomy may not be delegated to nursing assistive personnel (NAP) or to unlicensed assistive personnel (UAP). Depending on the state's nurse practice act and the organization's policies and procedures, care for these patients may be delegated to licensed practical/vocational nurses (LPN/LVNs). The decision to delegate must be based on careful analysis of the patient's needs and circumstances, as well as the qualifications of the person to whom the task is being delegated. Refer to the Delegation Guidelines in Appendix A.

EQUIPMENT

- Ventriculostomy setup
- Carpenter level, bubble-line level, or laser level according to facility policy
- PPE, as indicated

ASSESSMENT

- Assess the color of the fluid draining from the ventriculostomy. Normal CSF is clear or straw colored. Cloudy CSF may suggest an infection. Red or pink CSF may indicate bleeding.
- Assess vital signs, because changes in vital signs can reflect a neurologic problem.
- Assess the patient's pain level. The patient may be experiencing pain at the ventriculostomy insertion site.
- Perform a neurologic assessment.
- Assess the patient's level of consciousness. If the patient is awake, assess for his or her orientation to person, place, and time. If the patient's level of consciousness is decreased, note the patient's ability to respond and to be aroused.
- Inspect pupil size and response to light. Pupils should be equal and round and should react to light bilaterally. Any changes in level of consciousness or pupillary response may suggest a neurologic problem.
- If the patient can move the extremities, assess strength of hands and feet. A change in strength or a difference in strength on one side compared with the other may indicate a neurologic problem.

NURSING DIAGNOSIS

- Risk for Injury
- Risk for Ineffective Cerebral Tissue Perfusion
- Pain
- Risk for Infection

OUTCOME IDENTIFICATION AND PLANNING

- Patient maintains intracranial pressure at less than 15 mm Hg and cerebral perfusion pressure at 60 to 90 mm Hg (Hickey, 2014).
- Patient is free from infection.
- Patient is free from pain.
- Patient/significant others understand the need for the ventriculostomy.

IMPLEMENTATION

ACTION	RATIONALE
1. Review the medical orders for specific information about ventriculostomy parameters.	The nurse needs to know the most recent order for the height of the ventriculostomy. For example, if the health care practitioner has ordered that the ventriculostomy is to be at 10 cm, this means the patient's ICP must rise above 10 cm before the ventriculostomy will drain CSF.

ACTION	RATIONALE
2. Gather the necessary supplies.	Preparation promotes efficient time management and an organized approach to the task.
3. Perform hand hygiene and put on PPE, if indicated.	Hand hygiene and PPE prevent the spread of microorganisms. PPE is required based on transmission precautions.
4. Identify the patient.	Identifying the patient ensures the right patient receives the intervention and helps prevent errors.
5. Close the curtains around the bed and close the door to the room, if possible. Explain what you are going to do and why you are going to do it to the patient.	This ensures the patient's privacy. Explanation relieves anxiety and facilitates cooperation.
6. Assemble equipment on overbed table within reach.	Arranging items nearby is convenient, saves time, and avoids unnecessary stretching and twisting of muscles on the part of the nurse.
7. Assess patient for any changes in neurologic status.	Patients with ventriculostomies are at risk for problems with the neurologic system.
8. Set the zero reference level. **Assess the height of the ventriculostomy system to ensure that the stopcock is at the appropriate reference point: the tragus of the ear, the outer canthus of the patient's eye or the patient's external auditory canal (AANN, 2011; Moreda et al., 2009), using carpenter level, bubble-line level, or laser level, according to facility policy.** Adjust the height of the system if needed.	For measurements to be accurate, the stopcock must be at a reference point to approximate the catheter tip at the level of the foramen of Monro. Use of the same reference point for all readings is critical to ensure accuracy (Moreda et al., 2009). Use of a carpenter level, bubble-line level, or laser level, ensures accuracy (Moreda et al., 2009). If the ventriculostomy is used just to measure the ICP and not to drain the CSF, the stopcock will be turned off to the drip chamber.
9. Set the pressure level, based on prescribed pressure.	When the ICP is higher than the prescribed pressure level,

ACTION	RATIONALE

Move the drip chamber to the ordered height. Assess the amount of CSF in the drip chamber if the ventriculostomy is draining.

cerebrospinal fluid will drain into the drip chamber. If the ventriculostomy is to drain CSF, the nurse must turn the stopcock off to the drip chamber to obtain a measurement of ICP. After the ICP value is obtained, remember to turn the stopcock back off to the transducer so that CSF is allowed to drain.

10. **Zero the transducer.** Turn the stopcock off to the patient. Remove the cap from the transducer, being careful not to touch the end of the cap. Press and hold the calibration button on the monitor until the monitor beeps. Return the cap to the transducer. **Turn the stopcock off to the drip chamber to obtain an ICP reading and waveform tracing. After obtaining a reading, turn the stopcock off to the transducer.**

The readings would not be considered accurate if the transducer had not been recently zeroed. If the stopcock is not turned off to the patient, when opened to room air, CSF will flow out of the stopcock. The end of the cap must remain sterile to prevent an infection. The stopcock must be off to the drip chamber (open to the transducer) to obtain an ICP. If the ventriculostomy is to drain CSF, the nurse must turn the stopcock off to the drip chamber. After the ICP value is obtained, remember to turn the stopcock back off to the transducer so that CSF is allowed to drain into the drip chamber.

11. **Adjust the ventriculostomy height to prevent too much drainage, too little drainage, or inaccurate ICP readings.**

If the patient's head is lower than the ventriculostomy, the drainage of CSF will slow or stop. If the patient's head is higher than the ventriculostomy, the drainage of CSF will increase. Any ICP readings taken when the ventriculostomy is not level with the outer canthus of the eye would be inaccurate.

12. Care for the insertion site according to the facility's policy. Maintain the system using strict sterile technique. Assess the site for any signs of infection, such as purulent drainage, redness, or

Site care varies, possibly ranging from leaving the site open to air to applying antibiotic ointment and gauze. Sterile technique helps to prevent infection (Barker, 2008). Securing the catheters after insertion prevents

ACTION	RATIONALE
warmth. Ensure the catheter is secured at the site per facility policy. If the catheter is sutured to the scalp, assess integrity of the sutures.	dislodgement and breakage of the device.
13. Calculate the cerebral perfusion pressure (CPP), if necessary. Calculate the difference between the systemic mean arterial pressure (MAP) and the ICP.	CPP is an estimate of the adequacy of the blood supply to the brain.
14. Remove PPE, if used. Perform hand hygiene.	Removing PPE properly reduces the risk for infection transmission and contamination of other items. Hand hygiene prevents the spread of microorganisms.
15. Assess ICP, MAP, and CPP at least hourly. Note drainage amount, color, clarity. If there is an increase in the ICP, the value should be obtained more often, as often as every 15 minutes (AANN, 2011).	Frequent assessment provides valuable indicators for identifying subtle trends that may suggest developing problems.
16. Assess ICP drainage system at least every 4 hours, checking the insertion site, all drainage system tubing and parts, for cracks in the system or leakage from insertion site or system. Label external ventriculostomy tubing and access ports clearly.	Frequent monitoring allows for early identification of problems and prompt intervention. Clear labeling prevents accidental use as an intravenous access (AANN, 2011).

EVALUATION

- Patient demonstrates a CPP and an ICP within identified parameters.
- Patient remains free from infection.
- Patient understands the need for the ventriculostomy.
- Patient reports little to no pain.

DOCUMENTATION

- Document the following information: amount and color of CSF, ICP, and CPP; pupil status; motor strength bilaterally; orientation to time, person, and place; level of consciousness; vital signs; pain; appearance of insertion site; and height of ventriculostomy.

SKILL 183 APPLYING A FORCED-WARM AIR DEVICE

Patients returning from surgery are often hypothermic. The application of a forced-air warming device is a more effective way of rewarming the patient compared to using warm blankets. This device circulates warm air around the patient.

DELEGATION CONSIDERATIONS

Application of a forced-warm air device is not delegated to nursing assistive personnel (NAP) or to unlicensed assistive personnel (UAP). Application of a forced-warm air device may be delegated to licensed practical/vocational nurses (LPN/LVNs). The decision to delegate must be based on careful analysis of the patient's needs and circumstances, as well as the qualifications of the person to whom the task is being delegated. Refer to the Delegation Guidelines in Appendix A.

EQUIPMENT

- Forced-warm air device
- Forced-air blanket
- Electronic thermometer
- PPE, as indicated

ASSESSMENT

- Assess patient's temperature and skin color and perfusion. Patients who are hypothermic are generally pale to dusky and cool to the touch and have decreased peripheral perfusion.
- Inspect nail beds and mucous membranes of patients with darker skin tones for signs of decreased perfusion.

NURSING DIAGNOSIS

- Risk for Imbalanced Body Temperature
- Hypothermia

OUTCOME IDENTIFICATION AND PLANNING

- Patient will return to and maintain a temperature of 97.7°F to 99.5°F (36.5°C to 37.5°C).
- Patient's skin will become warm, capillary refill will be less than 2 to 3 seconds, and patient will not experience shivering.

IMPLEMENTATION

ACTION	RATIONALE
1. Check the patient's medical record for the order for the use of a forced-air warming	Reviewing the order validates the correct patient and correct procedure. Organization facilitates

ACTION	RATIONALE
device. Gather the necessary supplies.	performance of the task. Preparation promotes efficient time management and an organized approach to the task.
2. Perform hand hygiene and put on PPE, if indicated.	Hand hygiene and PPE prevent the spread of microorganisms. PPE is required based on transmission precautions.
3. Identify the patient.	Identifying the patient ensures the right patient receives the intervention and helps prevent errors.
4. Close the curtains around the bed and close the door to the room, if possible. Explain what you are going to do and why you are going to do it to the patient or significant other. Place necessary supplies on the bedside stand or overbed table, within easy reach.	This ensures the patient's privacy. Explanation relieves anxiety and facilitates cooperation. Bringing everything to the bedside conserves time and energy. Arranging items nearby is convenient, saves time, and avoids unnecessary stretching and twisting of muscles on the part of the nurse.
5. **Assess the patient's temperature.**	Baseline temperature validates the need for use of the device and provides baseline information for future comparison.
6. Plug forced-air warming device into electrical outlet. Place forced-air blanket over patient, with plastic side up (Figure 1). Keep air-hose inlet at foot of bed.	Blanket should always be used with the device. To avoid causing burns, *do not* place air hose under cotton blankets with airflow blanket.

FIGURE 1 Forced-air blanket on patient, plastic side up, with air hose inlet at foot of bed. (The photograph is reproduced herein with permission. © 3M 2014. All rights reserved.)

ACTION	RATIONALE
7. Securely insert air hose into inlet. Place a lightweight fabric blanket over the forced-air blanket, according to manufacturer's instructions. Turn the machine on and adjust temperature of air to desired effect.	Air hose must be properly inserted to ensure that it will not fall out. Blanket will help keep warmed air near the patient. Adjust air temperature, depending on desired patient temperature. If blanket is being used to maintain an already stable temperature, it may be turned down lower than if needed to raise patient's temperature.
8. Remove PPE, if used. Perform hand hygiene.	Removing PPE properly reduces the risk for infection transmission and contamination of other items. Hand hygiene prevents transmission of microorganisms.
9. **Monitor the patient's temperature at least every 30 minutes while using the forced-air device. If rewarming a patient with hypothermia, do not raise the temperature more than 1°C/hour to prevent a rapid vasodilation effect.**	Monitoring the patient's temperature ensures that the patient does not experience too rapid a rise in body temperature, resulting in vasodilation.
10. Discontinue use of the forced-air device once patient's temperature is adequate and the patient can maintain the temperature without assistance.	Forced-air device is not needed once the patient is warm and stable enough to maintain temperature.
11. Remove device and clean according to agency policy and manufacturer's instructions.	Proper care of equipment helps to maintain function of the device.

EVALUATION
- Patient's temperature returns to the normal range of 97.7°F to 99.5°F (36.5°C to 37.5°C) and the patient is able to maintain this temperature.
- Patient's skin is warm.
- Patient is free from shivering.

DOCUMENTATION

- Document the patient's temperature and the route used for measurement. Record that the forced-air warming device was applied to the patient. Document appearance of the skin and that the patient did not experience any adverse effects from the warming device. Record that the patient's temperature was monitored every 30 minutes, as well as the actual temperature after 30 minutes.

SKILL 184   COLLECTING A WOUND CULTURE

A wound culture may be ordered to identify the causative organism of an infected wound. Identifying the invading microorganism will provide useful information for selecting the most appropriate therapy. A nurse or other primary care provider can perform a wound culture. Maintaining strict asepsis is crucial so that only the pathogen present in the wound is isolated. It is essential to use the correct swab, based on the tests ordered, for collection of a specimen to isolate aerobic and/or anaerobic organisms.

DELEGATION CONSIDERATIONS

Collection of a wound culture is not delegated to nursing assistive personnel (NAP) or to unlicensed assistive personnel (UAP). Depending on the state's nurse practice act and the organization's policies and procedures, collection of a wound culture may be delegated to licensed practical/vocational nurses (LPN/LVNs). The decision to delegate must be based on careful analysis of the patient's needs and circumstances, as well as the qualifications of the person to whom the task is being delegated. Refer to the Delegation Guidelines in Appendix A.

EQUIPMENT

- A sterile Culturette kit (aerobic or anaerobic) with swab, or a culture tube with individual sterile swabs
- Sterile gloves
- Clean, disposable gloves
- Additional PPE, as indicated
- Plastic bag or appropriate waste receptacle
- Patient label for the sample tube
- Biohazard specimen bag
- Bath blanket (if necessary to drape the patient)
- Supplies to clean the wound and reapply a sterile dressing after obtaining the culture

ASSESSMENT

- Assess the situation to determine the need for wound culture. Confirm any medical orders relevant to obtaining a wound culture,

as well as wound care, and/or any wound care included in the nursing plan of care.
- Assess the patient's level of comfort and the need for analgesics before obtaining the wound culture.
- Inspect the wound and the surrounding tissue. Assess the location, appearance of the wound, stage (if appropriate), drainage, and types of tissue present in the wound. Measure the wound. Note the stage of the healing process and characteristics of any drainage. Assess the surrounding skin for color, temperature, and edema, ecchymosis, or maceration.

NURSING DIAGNOSIS
- Impaired Skin Integrity
- Impaired Tissue Integrity
- Disturbed Body Image

OUTCOME IDENTIFICATION AND PLANNING
- Wound culture is obtained without evidence of contamination, exposing the patient to additional pathogens, or causing discomfort for the patient.

IMPLEMENTATION

ACTION	RATIONALE
1. Review the medical orders for obtaining a wound culture. Gather necessary supplies.	Reviewing the order and plan of care validates the correct patient and correct procedure. Preparation promotes efficient time management and an organized approach to the task.
2. Perform hand hygiene and put on PPE, if indicated.	Hand hygiene and PPE prevent the spread of microorganisms. PPE is required based on transmission precautions.
3. Identify the patient.	Identifying the patient ensures the right patient receives the intervention and helps prevent errors.
4. Assemble equipment on overbed table within reach.	Organization facilitates performance of the task.
5. Close the curtains around the bed and close the door to the room if possible. Explain	This ensures the patient's privacy. Explanation relieves anxiety and facilitates cooperation.

ACTION	RATIONALE

what you are going to do and why you are going to do it to the patient.

6. Assess the patient for possible need for nonpharmacologic pain-reducing interventions or analgesic medication before obtaining the wound culture. Administer appropriate prescribed analgesic. Allow enough time for the analgesic to achieve its effectiveness before beginning the procedure.

Pain is a subjective experience influenced by past experience. Wound care and dressing changes may cause pain for some patients.

7. Place an appropriate waste receptacle within easy reach for use during the procedure.

Having the waste container handy means that soiled materials may be discarded easily, without the spread of microorganisms.

8. Adjust bed to comfortable working height, usually elbow height of the caregiver (VISN 8, 2009).

Having the bed at the proper height prevents back and muscle strain.

9. Assist the patient to a comfortable position that provides easy access to the wound. If necessary, drape the patient with the bath blanket to expose only the wound area. Place a waterproof pad under the wound site. Check the culture label against the patient's identification bracelet.

Patient positioning and use of a bath blanket provide for comfort and warmth. Checking the culture label with the patient's identification ensures the correct patient and the correct procedure.

10. If there is a dressing in place on the wound, put on clean gloves. Carefully and gently remove the soiled dressings. If there is resistance, use a silicone-based adhesive remover to help remove the tape. If any part of the dressing sticks to the underlying skin, use small amounts of

Gloves protect the nurse from handling contaminated dressings. Cautious removal of the dressing is more comfortable for the patient and ensures that any drain present is not removed. A silicone-based adhesive remover allows for the easy, rapid, and painless removal without the associated problems of skin

ACTION	RATIONALE
sterile saline to help loosen and remove it.	stripping (Denyer, 2011; Benbow, 2011). Sterile saline moistens the dressing for easier removal and minimizes damage and pain.
11. After removing the dressing, note the presence, amount, type, color, and odor of any drainage on the dressings. Place soiled dressings in the appropriate waste receptacle.	The presence of drainage should be documented. Discarding dressings appropriately prevents the spread of microorganisms.
12. Assess the wound for appearance, stage, presence of eschar, granulation tissue, epithelialization, undermining, tunneling, necrosis, sinus tract, and drainage. Assess the appearance of the surrounding tissue. Measure the wound.	This information provides evidence about the wound healing process and/or the presence of infection.
13. Remove your gloves and put them in the receptacle.	Discarding gloves prevents the spread of microorganisms.
14. Set up a sterile field, if indicated, and wound cleaning supplies. Put on the sterile gloves. Alternately, clean gloves (clean technique) may be used when cleaning a chronic wound.	Sterile gloves maintain surgical asepsis. Clean technique is appropriate when cleaning chronic wounds.
15. Clean the wound. Refer to Skill 55. Alternately, irrigate the wound, as ordered or required (see Skill 185).	Cleaning the wound removes previous drainage and wound debris, which could introduce extraneous organisms into the collected specimen, resulting in inaccurate results.
16. Dry the surrounding skin with gauze dressings. Put on clean gloves.	Moisture provides a medium for growth of microorganisms. Excess moisture can contribute to skin irritation and breakdown. The use of a culture swab does not require immediate contact with the skin or wound, so clean gloves are appropriate to protect the nurse from contact with blood and/or body fluids.

ACTION	RATIONALE
17. Twist the cap to loosen the swab on the Culturette tube, or open the separate swab and remove the cap from the culture tube. **Keep the swab and inside of the culture tube sterile.**	Supplies are ready to use and within easy reach, and aseptic technique is maintained.
18. If contact with the wound is necessary to separate wound margins to permit insertion of the swab deep into the wound, put a sterile glove on one hand to manipulate the wound margins. Clean gloves may be appropriate for contact with pressure ulcers and chronic wounds.	If contact with the wound is necessary to collect the specimen, a sterile glove is necessary to prevent contamination of the wound.
19. **Carefully insert the swab into the wound. Press and rotate the swab several times over the wound surfaces. Avoid touching the swab to intact skin at the wound edges. Use another swab if collecting a specimen from another site.**	Cotton tip absorbs wound drainage. Contact with skin could introduce extraneous organisms into the collected specimen, resulting in inaccurate results. Using another swab at a different site prevents cross-contamination of the wound.
20. Place the swab back in the culture tube. **Do not touch the outside of the tube with the swab.** Secure the cap. Some swab containers have an ampule of medium at the bottom of the tube. It might be necessary to crush this ampule to activate. Follow the manufacturer's instructions for use.	The outside of the container is protected from contamination with microorganisms, and the sample is not contaminated with organisms not in the wound. Surrounding the swab with culture medium is necessary for accurate culture results.
21. Remove gloves and discard them accordingly.	Removing gloves properly reduces the risk for infection transmission and contamination of other items.
22. Put on gloves. Place a dressing on the wound, as appropriate, based on medical orders	Wound dressings protect, absorb drainage, provide a moist environment, and promote wound

ACTION	RATIONALE
and/or the nursing plan of care. Refer to Skills 55, 56, and 57. Remove gloves.	healing. Removing gloves properly reduces the risk for infection transmission and contamination of other items.
23. After securing the dressing, label dressing with date and time. Remove all remaining equipment; place the patient in a comfortable position, with side rails up and bed in the lowest position.	Recording date and time provides communication and demonstrates adherence to plan of care. Proper patient and bed positioning promotes safety and comfort.
24. Label the specimen according to your institution's guidelines and send it to the laboratory in a biohazard bag.	Proper labeling ensures proper identification of the specimen.
25. Remove PPE, if used. Perform hand hygiene.	Removing PPE properly reduces the risk for infection transmission and contamination of other items. Hand hygiene prevents the spread of microorganisms.

EVALUATION

• Patient's wound is cultured without contamination, and the patient remains free of exposure to additional pathogens.

DOCUMENTATION

• Document the location of the wound, the assessment of the wound, including type of tissue present, presence of necrotic tissue, stage (if appropriate), and characteristics of drainage. Include the appearance of the surrounding skin. Document cleansing of the wound and obtaining the culture. Record any skin care and/or dressing applied. Note pertinent patient and family education and any patient reaction to this procedure, including patient's pain level and effectiveness of nonpharmacologic interventions or analgesia, if administered.

SKILL 185 | PERFORMING IRRIGATION OF A WOUND

Irrigation is a directed flow of solution over tissues. Wound irrigations are ordered to clean the area of pathogens and other debris and to promote wound healing. Irrigation procedures may also be ordered to apply heat or antiseptics locally. If the wound edges are approximated, clean technique may be used; if the wound edges are not approximated, sterile equipment and solutions are used for irrigation. Normal saline is often the solution of choice when irrigating wounds.

DELEGATION CONSIDERATIONS

Irrigation of a wound and procedures requiring the use of a sterile field and other sterile items are not delegated to nursing assistive personnel (NAP) or to unlicensed assistive personnel (UAP). Depending on the state's nurse practice act and the organization's policies and procedures, these procedures may be delegated to licensed practical/vocational nurses (LPN/LVNs). The decision to delegate must be based on careful analysis of the patient's needs and circumstances, as well as the qualifications of the person to whom the task is being delegated. Refer to the Delegation Guidelines in Appendix A.

EQUIPMENT

- A sterile irrigation set, including a basin, irrigant container, and irrigation syringe
- Sterile irrigation solution as ordered, warmed to body temperature, commonly 0.9% normal saline solution
- Plastic bag or other waste container to dispose of soiled dressings
- Sterile gloves
- Sterile drape (may be optional)
- Clean, disposable gloves
- Moisture-proof gown, mask, and eye protection
- Additional PPE, as indicated
- Sterile dressing set or suture set (for the sterile scissors and forceps)
- Waterproof pad and bath blanket, as needed
- Sterile gauze dressings
- Sterile packing gauze, as needed
- Tape or ties
- Skin-protectant wipes

ASSESSMENT

- Assess the situation to determine the need for wound irrigation. Confirm any medical orders relevant to wound care and any wound care included in the nursing plan of care.
- Assess the current dressing to determine if it is intact.
- Assess the patient's level of comfort and the need for analgesics before wound care. Assess if the patient experienced any pain related to previous dressing changes and the effectiveness of interventions employed to minimize the patient's pain.
- Assess for excess drainage or bleeding or saturation of the dressing.

• Inspect the wound and the surrounding tissue. Assess the location, appearance of the wound, stage (if appropriate), drainage, and types of tissue present in the wound. Measure the wound. Note the stage of the healing process and characteristics of any drainage. Assess the surrounding skin for color, temperature, and edema, ecchymosis, or maceration.

NURSING DIAGNOSIS

• Risk for Infection
• Acute Pain
• Impaired Skin Integrity
• Impaired Tissue Integrity

OUTCOME IDENTIFICATION AND PLANNING

• Wound is cleaned without contamination or trauma and without causing the patient to experience pain or discomfort.
• Wound continues to show signs of progression of healing.
• Patient demonstrates an understanding of the need for wound irrigation.

IMPLEMENTATION

ACTION	RATIONALE
1. Review the medical orders for wound care or the nursing plan of care related to wound care. Gather necessary supplies.	Reviewing the order and plan of care validates the correct patient and correct procedure. Preparation promotes efficient time management and an organized approach to the task.
2. Perform hand hygiene and put on PPE, if indicated.	Hand hygiene and PPE prevent the spread of microorganisms. PPE is required based on transmission precautions.
3. Identify the patient.	Identifying the patient ensures the right patient receives the intervention and helps prevent errors.
4. Assemble equipment on overbed table within reach.	Organization facilitates performance of the task.
5. Close the curtains around the bed and close the door to the room if possible. Explain	This ensures the patient's privacy. Explanation relieves anxiety and facilitates cooperation.

ACTION	RATIONALE
what you are going to do and why you are going to do it to the patient.	
6. Assess the patient for possible need for nonpharmacologic pain-reducing interventions or analgesic medication before wound care and/or dressing change. Administer appropriate prescribed analgesic. Allow enough time for the analgesic to achieve its effectiveness before beginning the procedure.	Pain is a subjective experience influenced by past experience. Wound care and dressing changes may cause pain for some patients.
7. Place a waste receptacle or bag at a convenient location for use during the procedure.	Having a waste container handy means the soiled dressing may be discarded easily, without the spread of microorganisms.
8. Adjust the bed to a comfortable working height, usually elbow height of the caregiver (VISN 8, 2009).	Having the bed at the proper height prevents back and muscle strain.
9. Assist the patient to a comfortable position that provides easy access to the wound area. Position the patient so the irrigation solution will flow from the clean end of the wound toward the dirtier end. Use the bath blanket to cover any exposed area other than the wound. Place a waterproof pad under the wound site.	Patient positioning and use of a bath blanket provide for comfort and warmth. Gravity directs the flow of liquid from the least contaminated to the most contaminated area. Waterproof pad protects underlying surfaces.
10. Put on a gown, mask, and eye protection.	Using PPE, such as gowns, masks, and eye protection, is part of *Standard Precautions*. A gown protects clothes from contamination should splashing occur. Goggles protect mucous membranes of eyes from contact with irrigant fluid or wound drainage.

ACTION	RATIONALE
11. Put on clean gloves. Carefully and gently remove the soiled dressings. If there is resistance, use a silicone-based adhesive remover to help remove the tape. If any part of the dressing sticks to the underlying skin, use small amounts of sterile saline to help loosen and remove it.	Gloves protect the nurse from handling contaminated dressings. Cautious removal of the dressing is more comfortable for the patient and ensures that any drain present is not removed. A silicone-based adhesive remover allows for the easy, rapid, and painless removal without the associated problems of skin stripping (Denyer, 2011; Benbow, 2011). Sterile saline moistens the dressing for easier removal and minimizes damage and pain.
12. After removing the dressing, note the presence, amount, type, color, and odor of any drainage on the dressings. Place soiled dressings in the appropriate waste receptacle.	The presence of drainage should be documented. Discarding dressings appropriately prevents the spread of microorganisms.
13. Assess the wound for appearance, stage, presence of eschar, granulation tissue, epithelialization, undermining, tunneling, necrosis, sinus tract, and drainage. Assess the appearance of the surrounding tissue. Measure the wound.	This information provides evidence about the wound healing process and/or the presence of infection.
14. Remove your gloves and put them in the receptacle.	Discarding gloves prevents the spread of microorganisms.
15. Set up a sterile field, if indicated, and wound cleaning supplies. Pour warmed sterile irrigating solution into the sterile container. Put on the sterile gloves. Alternately, clean gloves (clean technique) may be used when irrigating a chronic wound or pressure ulcer.	Using warmed solution prevents chilling the patient and may minimize patient discomfort. Sterile technique and gloves maintain surgical asepsis. Clean technique is appropriate for irrigating chronic wounds or pressure ulcers.
16. Position the sterile basin below the wound to collect the irrigation fluid.	Patient and bed linens are protected from contaminated fluid.

ACTION	RATIONALE
17. Fill the irrigation syringe with solution. Using your non-dominant hand, gently apply pressure to the basin against the skin below the wound to form a seal with the skin.	The solution will collect in the basin and prevent the irrigant from running down the skin. Patient and bed linens are protected from contaminated fluid.
18. Gently direct a stream of solution into the wound. Keep the tip of the syringe at least 1 inch above the upper tip of the wound. When using a catheter tip, insert it gently into the wound until it meets resistance. Gently flush all wound areas.	Debris and contaminated solution flow from the least contaminated to most contaminated area. High-pressure irrigation flow may cause patient discomfort as well as damage granulation tissue. A catheter tip allows the introduction of irrigant into a wound with a small opening or one that is deep.
19. Watch for the solution to flow smoothly and evenly. When the solution from the wound flows out clear, discontinue irrigation.	Irrigation removes exudate and debris.
20. Dry the surrounding skin with gauze dressings.	Moisture provides a medium for growth of microorganisms. Excess moisture can contribute to skin irritation and breakdown.
21. Apply a skin protectant to the surrounding skin.	A skin protectant prevents skin irritation and breakdown.
22. Apply a new dressing to the wound (see Skills 55, 56, 57).	Dressings absorb drainage, protect the wound, and promote healing.
23. Remove and discard gloves. Apply tape, Montgomery straps, or roller gauze to secure the dressings. Alternately, many commercial wound products are self-adhesive and do not require additional tape.	Tape or other securing products are easier to apply after gloves have been removed. Proper disposal of gloves prevents the spread of microorganisms.
24. After securing the dressing, label it with date and time. Remove all remaining equipment; place the patient in a comfortable position, with side rails up and bed in the lowest position.	Recording date and time provides communication and demonstrates adherence to plan of care. Proper patient and bed positioning promotes safety and comfort.

ACTION	RATIONALE
25. Remove remaining PPE. Perform hand hygiene.	Removing PPE properly reduces the risk for infection transmission and contamination of other items. Hand hygiene prevents the spread of microorganisms.
26. Check all wound dressings every shift. More frequent checks may be needed if the wound is more complex or dressings become saturated quickly.	Checking dressings ensures the assessment of changes in patient condition and timely intervention to prevent complications.

EVALUATION

- Wound irrigation is completed without contamination and trauma.
- Patient verbalizes little to no pain or discomfort.
- Patient verbalizes understanding of the need for irrigation.
- Patient's wound continues to show signs of progression of healing.

DOCUMENTATION

- Document the location of the wound and that the dressing was removed. Record your assessment of the wound, including evidence of granulation tissue, presence of necrotic tissue, stage (if appropriate), and characteristics of drainage. Include the appearance of the surrounding skin. Document the irrigation of the wound and solution used. Record the type of dressing that was applied. Note pertinent patient and family education and any patient reaction to this procedure, including patient's pain level and effectiveness of nonpharmacologic interventions or analgesia if administered.

Appendix A

Guidelines for Delegation Decision Making

Delegation involves the transfer of responsibility for the performance of an activity to another individual while retaining accountability for the outcome. Used appropriately, delegation can result in safe and effective nursing care. Delegation can free the registered nurse (RN) to focus on assessment and development or revision of the nursing care plan (Trossman, 2012). Delegation allows the registered nurse to attend to more complex patient care needs, develops the skills of nursing assistive personnel, and promotes cost containment for the health care organization. The RN determines appropriate nursing practice by using nursing knowledge, professional judgment, and the legal authority to practice nursing (American Nurses Association [ANA], 2007).

In delegating, the registered nurse must ensure appropriate assessment, planning, implementation, and evaluation. Decision making about delegation is a continuous process. These guidelines provide quick reference for the delegation decision-making information found in each skill.

DELEGATION CRITERIA

There are three criteria to be considered by the registered nurse when deciding to delegate care activities (National Council of State Boards of Nursing [NCSBN], 2005):

1. The State Nursing Practice Act must permit delegation and outline the authorized task(s) to be delegated or authorize the registered nurse to decide delegation.
2. The person making the delegation has the appropriate qualifications: appropriate education, skills and experience, as well as current competency.
3. The person receiving the delegation must have the appropriate qualifications: appropriate education, training, skills and experience, as well as evidence of current competency.

In addition, according to the ANA and NCSBN (2006), the delegated task(s) must not require critical thinking or professional judgment.

DELEGATION PROCESS

Delegation is a multistep, continuous process.

1. The registered nurse must assess the situation, identifying the needs of the patient, considering the circumstances and setting, as well as the competence of the person to whom the task is being delegated.

987

The registered nurse may proceed with delegation if patient needs, circumstances, and available resources indicate patient safety will be maintained with delegated care.

2. The registered nurse plans for and communicates clearly the specific task(s) to be delegated. The registered nurse may proceed with delegation if the nature of the task, competence of the person receiving the delegation, and patient implications indicate patient safety will be maintained with delegated care.

3. The registered nurse assures accountability. The registered nurse may proceed with delegation if the registered nurse and person receiving the delegation accept the accountability for their respective roles in the delegated patient care.

4. The registered nurse supervises performance of the delegated task(s), providing directions and clear expectations of how the task(s) is to be performed. The registered nurse monitors performance, intervenes if necessary, and ensures the appropriate documentation.

5. The registered nurse must evaluate the entire delegation process, evaluating the patient, the performance of the task(s), and obtain and provide feedback.

6. The registered nurse must reassess and adjust the overall plan of care as needed.

FIVE RIGHTS OF DELEGATION

The Five Rights of Delegation provide a resource to facilitate decisions about delegation. The NCSBN (1995) identifies the Five Rights of Delegation as follows:

- **Right Task:** One that is delegable for a specific patient.
- **Right Circumstances:** Appropriate patient setting, available resources, and other relevant factors considered.
- **Right Person:** Right person is delegating the right task to the right person to be performed on the right person.
- **Right Direction/Communication:** Clear, concise description of the task, including its objective, limits, and expectations.
- **Right Supervision:** Appropriate monitoring, evaluation, intervention, as needed, and feedback.

"DO-NOT-DELEGATE" CARE

Nursing care or tasks that should never be delegated except to another RN include:

- The initial and ongoing nursing assessment of the patient and his or her nursing care needs
- The determination of the nursing diagnosis, nursing care plan, evaluation of the patient's progress in relation to the care plan, and evaluation of the nursing care delivered to the patient
- The supervision and education of nursing personnel; patient teaching that requires an assessment of the patient and his or her education needs

- Any other nursing intervention that requires professional nursing knowledge, judgment, and/or skill.

DELEGATION DECISION TREE

Using skills, knowledge, and professional judgment, the registered nurse determines appropriate nursing practice based on the state practice act and professional scope of practice, the standards and code of ethics, and the organization's policies and procedures related to delegation (ANA & NCSBN, 2006).

The Decision Tree for Delegation by Registered Nurses distributed by the American Nurses Association and the National Council of State Boards of Nursing can assist nurses with delegation decisions. The Decision Tree for Delegation can be found at https://www.ncsbn.org/Delegation_joint_statement_NCSBN-ANA.pdf.

TAYLOR SUITE RESOURCES

Explore these additional resources for more information on delegation:

- thePoint online resource, http://thepoint.lww.com/Lynn4E
- Fundamentals of Nursing: *Chapter 14, Implementing* and *Chapter 22, Nurse Leader, Manager, and Care Coordinator*

REFERENCES AND RESOURCES

American Nurses Association (ANA). (2012). Principles for delegation by registered nurses to unlicensed assistive personnel. Silver Spring, MD: Author.

American Nurses Association (ANA). (2007). Unlicensed assistive personnel. Position statement. Retrieved from http://www.nursingworld.org/MainMenuCategories/Policy-Advocacy/Positions-and-Resolutions/ANAPositionStatements/Position-Statements-Alphabetically/Registered-Nurses-Utilization-of-Nursing-Assistive-Personnel-in-All-Settings.html.

American Nurses Association (ANA) and National Council of State Boards of Nursing (NCSBN). (2006) Joint statement on delegation. Available https://www.ncsbn.org/Delegation_joint_statement_NCSBN-ANA.pdf.

Ayers, D. M., & Montgomery, M. (2008). Hospital Nursing. Delegating the "right" way: Learn five tips for delegating effectively and safely. *Nursing, 38*(4), 56hn1-2.

Daley, K. (2013). Helping nurses strengthen their delegation skills. *American Nurse Today, 8*(3), 18.

National Council of State Boards of Nursing (NCSBN). (2005). Working with others: a position paper. Available https://www.ncsbn.org/Working_with_Others.pdf

Trossman, S. (2012). Is it OK to delegate?: Revised principles, resources aim to help RNs answer the question. *The American Nurse, 44*(6), 1, 6.

Weydt, A. (2010). Developing delegation skills. *Online Journal of Issues in Nursing, 15*(2), Manuscript 1.

Bibliography

Adams, D. (2012). Needlestick and sharps injuries: practice update. *Nursing Standard, 26*(37), 49–57.

Ağaç, E., & Gűnes, Ú.Y. (2010). Effect on pain of changing the needle prior to administering medicine intramuscularly: a randomized controlled trial. *Journal of Advanced Nursing, 67*(3), 563–568.

Altschuler, V., & Diaz, L. (2006). Bladder ultrasound. *MEDSURG Nursing, 15*(5), 317–318.

American Association for Clinical Chemistry (AACC). (2013). *Lab tests online. Fecal occult blood test and fecal immunochemical test.* Available at http://labtestsonline.org/understanding/analytes/fecal-occult-blood/tab/glance.

American Association of Critical Care Nurses (AACN). (2011). Lynn-McHale Wiegand, D.J. (Ed.): *AACN procedure manual for critical care* (6th ed.). Philadelphia: Elsevier Saunders.

American Association of Critical Care Nurses. (2010). *Venous Thromboembolism prevention.* Available at http://www.aacn.org/WD/Practice/Docs/PracticeAlerts/VTE%20Prevention%2004–2010%20final.pdf.

American Association of Critical-Care Nurses (AACN). (2010). *Practice Alert: Oral care in the critically ill.* Available at http://aacn.org/WD/Practice/Content/practicealerts.content?menu=Practice.

American Association of Critical-Care Nurses (AACN). (2010b). *Practice alert: Verification of feeding tube placement.* Available at http://aacn.org/WD/Practice/Docs/PracticeAlerts/Verification_of_Feeding_Tube_Placement_05–2005.pdf.

American Association of Critical Care Nurses (AACN). (2010c). *Family presence during resuscitation and invasive procedures.* Available at http://www.aacn.org/wd/practice/docs/practicealerts/family%20presence%2004–2010%20final.pdf.

American Association of Diabetes Educators. (2008). *Insulin pump therapy: Guidelines for successful outcomes.* Available at http://www.diabeteseducator.org/export/sites/aade/_resources/pdf/Insulin_Pump_White_Paper.pdf.

American Association of Neuroscience Nurses (AANN). (2012). *Cervical spine surgery. A guide to preoperative and postoperative patient care.* Glenview, IL: Author.

American Association of Neuroscience Nurses (AANN). (2011). *Care of the patient undergoing intracranial pressure monitoring/external ventricular drainage or lumbar drainage.* Glenview, IL: Author.

American Diabetes Association. (2013). Standards of medical care in diabetes—2013. *Diabetes Care, 36*(Suppl. 1): S11–S66.

American Dietetic Association (ADA). (2008). Position of the American Dietetic Association: Ethical and legal issues in nutrition, hydration, and feeding. *Journal of the American Dietetic Association, 108*(5), 873–882.

American Geriatrics Society (AGS). (2012). *Aging & health A to Z.* Available at http://www.healthinaging.org/aging-and-health-a-to-z/topic:falls/.

American Geriatrics Society and British Geriatrics Society. (2010). *AGS/BGS Clinical practice guideline: Prevention of falls in older persons.* Available at http://www.medcats.com/FALLS/frameset.htm.

American Heart Association (AHA). (2011). *BLS for healthcare providers. Student manual. Professional.* Author.

American Heart Association (AHA). (2012). *CPR & ECC. Two steps to staying alive with Hands-only CPR.* Available at http://www.heart.org/HEARTORG/CPRAndECC/HandsOnlyCPR/Hands-Only-CPR_UCM_440559_SubHomePage.jsp.

American Society for Parenteral and Enteral Nutrition (A.S.P.E.N.). (2011). *Guidelines: Access for administration of nutrition support.* Available at http://www.

nutritioncare.org/Professional_Resources/Guidelines_and_Standards/Guidelines/ Access_for_Administration_of_Nutrition_Support/.

Ames, N.J., Sulima, P., Yates, J.M., McCullagh, L., Gollins, S.L., Soeken, K., & Wallen, G.R. (2011). Effects of systematic oral care in critically ill patients: A multicenter study. *American Journal of Critical Care, 20*(5), e103-e113. Available at http://ajcc. aacnjournals.org/content/20/5/e103.full.pdf+html.

Apold, J., & Rydrych, D. (2012). Preventing device-related pressure ulcers. *Journal of Nursing Care Quality, 27*(1), 28–34.

Arbique, J., & Arbique, D. (2007). I.V. rounds. Reducing the risk of nerve injuries. *Nursing, 37*(11), 20–21.

Arroyo-Novoa, C., Figueroa-Ramos, M., Puntillo, K., et al. (2008). Pain related to tracheal suctioning in awake acutely and critically ill adults: A descriptive study. *Intensive & Critical Care Nursing, 24*(1), 20–27.

Association of Perioperative Registered Nurses (AORN). (2012). *Perioperative standards and recommended practices.* Denver, CO: AORN, Inc.

Association for Professionals in Infection Control and Epidemiology (APIC). (2005). *Hand hygiene for healthcare workers.* Available at http://www.apic.org/Resource_/ EducationalBrochureForm/370c41f0–380f-4d4d-aa33–67ca4407f3ef/File/ Hand-Hygiene-Healthcare-Workers-Brochure.pdf.

Azubike, N., Bullard, D., Chrisman, J., et al. (2012). Navigating the nasopharyngeal culture. *Nursing Made Incredibly Easy, 10*(6), 9–12.

Baird Holmes, S., & Brown, S. (2005). National Association of Orthopaedic Nurses. Guidelines for orthopaedic nursing: Skeletal pin site care. *Orthopaedic Nursing, 24*(2), 99–107.

Ball, A., & Smith, K. (2008). Optimizing transdermal drug therapy. *American Journal of Health-System Pharmacy, 65*(14), 1337–1346.

Baranoski, S., & Ayello, E.A. (2012). *Wound care essentials. Practice Principles* (3rd ed.). Philadelphia: Wolters Kluwer Health/Lippincott Williams & Wilkins.

Barker, E. (2008). *Neuroscience nursing. A spectrum of care* (3rd ed.). St. Louis: Mosby Elsevier.

Bauman, M., & Handley, C. (2011). Chest-tube care: The more you know, the easier it gets. *American Nurse Today, 6*(9), 27–32. Available at http://www.americannursetoday. com/Article.aspx?id=8256&fid=8172.

Beckman Coulter. (2009a). *Hemoccult®. Product instructions.* Available at https:// www.beckmancoulter.com/wsrportal/bibliography?docname=HOII%20-%20 462478.EA%20.pdf.

Beckman Coulter. (2009b). *Developing and interpreting Hemoccult® ICT Tests.* Available https://www.beckmancoulter.com/wsrportal/bibliography?docname= IB-17781A+Laminated+Hemoccult+ICT+Test+Procedure.pdf.

Beckman Coulter. (2009c). *Hemoccult® ICT. Patient instructions.* Available https:// www.beckmancoulter.com/wsrportal/ajax/downloadDocument/395087AD. pdf?autonomyId=TP_DOC_118305&documentName=395087AD.pdf.

Benbow, M. (2011). Addressing pain in wound care and dressing removal. *Nursing & Residential Care, 13*(10), 474, 476, 478.

Berg, M.D., Schexnayder, S.M., Chameides, L., et al. 2010 American Heart Association guidelines for cardiopulmonary resuscitation and emergency cardiovascular care. Part 13: Pediatric basic life support. *Circulation, 122*(18 Suppl. 3), S862–S875.

Bernard, M.S., Hunter, K.F., & Moore, K.N. (2012). Decrease the duration of indwelling urethral catheters and potentially reduce the incidence of catheter-associated urinary tract infections. *Urologic Nursing, 32*(1), 29–37.

Bernardini, J., Bender, F., Florio, T., et al. (2005). Randomized, double-blind trial of antibiotic exit site cream for prevention of exit site infection in peritoneal dialysis patients. *Journal of the American Society of Nephrology, 16*(2), 539–545.

Best, C. (2005). Caring for the patient with a nasogastric tube. *Nursing Standard, 20*(3), 59–65.

Bourgault, A., Ipe, L., Weaver, J., et al. (2007). Development of evidence-based guidelines and critical care nurses' knowledge of enteral feeding. *Critical Care Nurse, 27*(4), 17–29.

Brennan, M. (2008). Review: Routine NG decompression after abdominal surgery delays return of bowel function and increases pulmonary complications. *Evidence-Based Nursing, 11*(2), 55.

Bucher, L., Buruschkink R., Kenyon, D.M., et al. (2012). Improving outcomes with therapeutic hypothermia. *Nursing2012CriticalCare, 7*(5), 22–27.

Bullman, S. (2011). Ins and outs of suprapubic catheters—a clinician's experience. *Urologic Nursing, 31*(5), 259–264.

Burn Foundation. (2012). Burn prevention. Safety facts on scald burns. Available at http://www.burnfoundation.org/programs/resource.cfm?c=1&a=3.

Capezuti, E., Brush, B., Won, R., et al. (2008). Least restrictive or least understood? Waist restraints, provider practices, and risk of harm. *Journal of Aging & Social Policy, 20*(3), 305–322.

Capnography: New standard of care for sedation? (2012). *OR Manager, 28*(3), 17–20.

Carlson, J., Mayrose, J., Krause, R., et al. (2007). Extubation force: Tape versus endotracheal tube holders. *Annals of Emergency Medicine, 50*(6), 686–691.

Castle, N. (2007). Resuscitation of patients during pregnancy. *Emergency Nurse, 15*(2), 20–22.

Cecil, S., Chen, P.M., Callaway, S.E., et al. (2011). Traumatic brain injury: Advance multimodal neuromonitoring from theory to clinical practice. *Critical Care Nurse, 31*(2), 25–37.

Centers for Disease Control and Prevention (CDC). (2012). *The pink book: Appendices. Epidemiology and prevention of vaccine preventable diseases* (11th ed.). Appendix D. Vaccine administration. Vaccine administration guidelines. Available at www.cdc.gov/vaccines/pubs/pinkbook/pink-appendx.htm#appd.

Centers for Disease Control and Prevention (CDC). (2012b). *Tuberculosis (TB). Core curriculum on tuberculosis: What the clinician should know. Chapter 4. Diagnosis of tuberculosis disease.* Available at http://www.cdc.gov/tb/education/corecurr/index.htm.

Centers for Disease Control and Prevention (CDC). (2011a). *Chronic disease prevention and health promotion. Oral health.* Available at http://www.cdc.gov/chronicdisease/resources/publications/AAG/doh.htm.

Centers for Disease Control and Prevention (CDC). (2011b). *Injection safety. Safe injection practices to prevent transmission of infections to patients.* Available at http://www.cdc.gov/injectionsafety/IP07_standardPrecaution.html.

Centers for Disease Control and Prevention (CDC). (2011c). *Healthcare-associated infections (HAIs). Staphylococcus aureus in healthcare settings.* Available at http://www.cdc.gov/HAI/organisms/staph.html.

Centers for Disease Control and Prevention (CDC). (2011d). *Pertussis (whooping cough). Specimen collection. Pertussis testing video: Collecting a nasopharyngeal swab clinical specimen.* Available at http://www.cdc.gov/pertussis/clinical/diagnostic-testing/specimen-collection.html.

Centers for Disease Control and Prevention (CDC). (2011e). *Epilepsy. First aid for seizures.* Available at http://www.cdc.gov/epilepsy/basics/first_aid.htm.

Centers for Disease Control and Prevention. (2010). (Updated 2011). *Healthcare-associated infections (HAIs). Tools for protecting healthcare personnel. Sequence for donning and removing personal protective equipment (PPE).* Poster. Available at http://www.cdc.gov/HAI/prevent/ppe.html.

Centers for Disease Control and Prevention. (2004). *Guidance for the selection and use of personal protective equipment (PPE) in healthcare settings.* (Slide presentation). Available at http://www.cdc.gov/HAI/pdfs/ppe/PPEslides6–29–04.pdf.

Centers for Disease Control and Prevention. (2002). Guidelines for hand hygiene in health-care settings. *Morbidity and Mortality Weekly Report, 51*(RR16), 1–45.

Centers for Medicare & Medicaid Services (CMS). (2006). Department of Health and Human Services. Federal Register. 42 CFR Part 482. Conditions of Participation: Patients' Rights. Final Rule. Available at http://www.cms.gov/Regulations-and-Guidance/Legislation/CFCsAndCoPs/downloads/finalpatientrightsrule.pdf.

Charous, S. (2008). Use of the ON-Q pain pump management system in the head and neck Preliminary report. *Otolaryngology-Head and Neck Surgery, 138*(1), 110–112.

Collins, C., & Anderson, C. (2007). Deceptive simpoicity: systemic oxygen delivery and pulse oximetry. *Journal of Paediartics & Child Health, 43*(7–8), 510–512.

Cranwell-Bruce, L.A. (2009). PCA delivery systems. *MEDSURGNursing, 18*(2), 127–129, 133.

Crawford, J., & Doherty, L. (2010). Ten steps to recording a standard 12-lead ECG. *Practice Nurse, 21*(12), 622–630.

Crawford, C.L., & Johnson, J.A. (2012). To aspirate or not: An integrative review of the evidence. *Nursing, 42*(3), 20–25.

Crawford, D. (2011). Care and nursing management of a child with a chest drain. *Nursing Children and Young People, 23*(10), 27–33.

D'Arcy, Y. (2011b). New thinking about postoperative pain management. *OR Nurse, 5*(6), 28–36.

D'Arcy, Y. (2012). Treating acute pain in the hospitalized patient. *The Nurse Practitioner, 37*(8), 22–30.

D'Arcy, Y. (2008). Keep your patient safe during PCA. *Nursing, 38*(1), 50–55.

D'Arcy, Y. (2007a). New pain management options: Delivery systems and techniques. *Nursing, 37*(2), 26–27.

D'Arcy, Y. (2007b). Eyeing capnography to improve PCA safety. *Nursing, 37*(9), 18–19.

Degelau, J., Belz, M., Bungum, L., et al. (2012). Institute for Clinical Systems Improvement (ICSI). Prevention of falls (acute care). Health care protocol. Bloomington (MN): Institute for Clinical Systems Improvement (ICSI). Agency for Healthcare Research and Quality (AHRQ). Available at http://guideline.gov/content.aspx?id=36906#Section420.

Del Monte, L. (2009). *Noninvasive pacing: What you should know.* Educational Series. Redmond, WA: Physio-Control, Inc.

DeMeulenaere, S. (2007). Pulse oximetry: uses and limitations. *Journal for Nurse Practitioners, 3*(5), 312–317.

Denyer, J. (2011). Reducing pain during the removal of adhesive and adherent products. *British Journal of Nursing, 20*(15) (Tissue Viability Supplement), S28–35.

Domiano, K.L., Hinck, S.M., Savinske, D.L., et al. (2008). Comparison of upper arm and forearm blood pressure. *Clinical Nursing Research, 17*(4), 241–250.

Dondelinger, R.M. (2010). The fundamentals of…Infant warmers. *Biomedical Instrumentation & Technology, 44*(6), 485–487.

Durand, C., Alhammad, A., & Willett, K.C. (2012). Practical considerations for optimal transdermal drug delivery. *American Journal of Health-System Pharmacy, 69*(2), 116–124.

Durgude, Y., & Cocks, N. (2011). Nurse's knowledge of the provision of oral care for patients with dysphagia. *British Journal of Community Nursing, 16*(12), 604–610.

Emergency Nurses Association (ENA). Agency for Healthcare Research and Quality. National Guideline Clearinghouse. (2009). *Family presence during invasive procedures and resuscitation in the emergency department.* Available at http://www.guideline.gov/content.aspx?id=32594.

Ertuğ, N., & Ülker, S. (2011). The effect of cold application on pain due to chest tube removal. *Journal of Clinical Nursing, 21*(5/6), 784–790.

Exergen. (2007). *Temporal scanner reference manual.* Watertown, MA: Author. Available at www.exergen.com/medical/TAT/TAT5000Manual5.pdf.

Feil, M. (2012). Pennsylvania Patient Safety Authority. Pennsylvania patient safety advisory. Reducing risk if air embolism associated with central venous access devices. Available at http://patientsafetyauthority.org/ADVISORIES/AdvisoryLibrary/2012/Jun;9(2)/Pages/58.aspx.

Ferguson, A. (2005). Blood glucose monitoring. *Nursing Times, 101*(38), 28–29.

Fernandez, M., Burns, K., Calhoun, B., et al. (2007). Evaluation of a new pulse oximeter sensor. *American Journal of Critical Care, 16*(2), 146–152.

Fischbach, F., & Dunning, M. (2009). *A manual of laboratory and diagnostic tests* (8th ed.). Philadelphia: Wolters Kluwer/Lippincott Williams & Wilkins.

Frese, E.M., Fick, A., & Sadowsky, H.S. (2011). Blood pressure measurement guidelines for physical therapists. *Cardiopulmonary Physical Therapy Journal, 22*(2), 5–12.

Gannon, R. (2007). Current strategies for preventing or ameliorating postoperative ileus: A multimodal approach. *American Journal of Health-System Pharmacy, 64*(20), S8–S12.

Gilbert, R.T., & Burns, S.M. (2012). Increasing the safety of blind gastric tube placement in pediatric patients: The design and testing of a procedure using a carbon dioxide detection device. *Journal of Pediatric Nursing, 27*(5), 528–532.

Gevirtz, C. (2010). Getting current with iontophoretic fentanyl. *Nursing, 40*(2), 65.

Goulette, C. (2008). Follow your heart. Wireless telemetry

Gray-Micelli, D. (2012). Hartford Institute for Geriatric Nursing. FALLS. Nursing standard of practice protocol: Fall Prevention. Available at www.consultgerirn.org/topics/falls/want_to_know_more.

Hadaway, L. (2006). 5 steps to preventing catheter-related bloodstream infections. *LPN2009, 2*(5), 50–55.

Hahn, M. (2010). 10 considerations for endotracheal suctioning. *The Journal for Respiratory Care Practitioners, 23*(7), 32–33.

Hain, D.J., & Chan, J. (2013). Best available evidence for peritoneal dialysis catheter exit-site care. *Nephrology Nursing Journal, 40*(1), 63–69.

Hendrich, A. (2007). Predicting patient falls. *American Journal of Nursing, 107*(11), 50–58.

Herter, R., & Wallace Kazer, M. (2010). Best practices in urinary catheter. *Home Healthcare Nurse, 28*(6), 342–349.

Hess, C. (2013). *Clinical guide to skin & wound care* (7th ed.). Philadelphia: Wolters Kluwer Health/Lippincott Williams & Wilkins.

Hess, D.R., MacIntyre, N.R., Mishoe, S.C., et al. (2012). *Respiratory Care. Principles and Practice* (2nd ed.). Sudbury, MA: Jones & Bartlett Learning.

Hickey, J. (2014). *The clinical practice of neurological and neurosurgical nursing* (7th ed.). Philadelphia: Wolters Kluwer Health/Lippincott Williams & Wilkins.

Hicks, R.W., Hernandez, J., & Wanzer, L.J. (2012). Perioperative pharmacology: Patient-controlled analgesia. *AORN Journal, 95*(2), 255–262.

Higgins, D. (2008). Specimen collection. Part 4: Obtaining a nasal swab. *Nursing Times, 104*(20), 26–27.

Hill, M., Baker, G., Carter, D., et al. (2012). A multidisciplinary approach to end external ventricular drain infections in the neurocritical care unit. *Journal of Neuroscience Nursing, 44*(4), 188–193.

Hinkle, J.L. & Cheever, K.H., (2014). *Brunner & Suddarth's textbook of medical-surgical nursing* (13th ed.). Philadelphia: Wolters Kluwer Health/Lippincott Williams & Wilkins.

Hogan-Quigley, B., Palm, M.L., & Bickley, L. (2012). *Bates' Nursing Guide to Physical Examination and History Taking*. Philadelphia: Wolters Kluwer Health/Lippincott Williams & Wilkins.

Holman, C., Roberts, S., & Nicol, M. (2005). Practice update: Clinical skills with older people. Promoting oral hygiene. *Nursing Older People, 16*(10), 37–38.

Hooton, T.M., Bradley, S.F., Cardenas, D.D., et al. (2010). Diagnosis, prevention, and treatment of catheter-associated urinary tract infection in adults: 2009 international clinical practice guidelines from the Infectious Diseases Society of America. *Clinical Infectious Diseases, 50*(5), 625–663. Available at http://www.idsociety.org/uploadedFiles/IDSA/Guidelines-Patient_Care/PDF_Library/Comp%20UTI.pdf.

Houston, P.A. (2013). Obtaining vascular access in the obese patient population. *Journal of Infusion Nursing, 36*(1), 52–56.

Hunter, J. (2008). Subcutaneous injection technique. *Nursing Standard, 22*(21), 41–44.

I-Flow Corporation. (2012). On-Q pain relief system. Patient guidelines. Available at http://www.iflo.com/pdf/products/1307136A.pdf.

I-Flow Corporation. (2010). *On-Q PainBuster postoperative pain relief system. Floor nurse guide.* Available at http://www.iflo.com/prod_onq_classic.php.

Infusion Nurses Society (INS). (2011). Infusion nursing standards of practice. *Journal of Infusion Nursing, 34*(Suppl: 1S).

Ingram, P., & Lavery, I. (2005). Peripheral intravenous therapy: key risks and implications for practice. *Nursing Standard, 19*(46), 55–64.

Institute for Healthcare Improvement (IHI). (2011). *How-to guide: Improving hand hygiene.* Available at http://www.IHI.org.

Ireton, J. (2007). Tracheostomy suction: a protocol for practice. *Paediatric Nursing, 19*(10), 14–18.

I.V. Rounds. Comparing short peripheral canula insertion sites. (2008). *Nursing, 38*(5), 60.

Jablonski, R.A., Therrien, B., & Kolanowski, A. (2011). No more fighting and biting during mouth care: Applying the theoretical constructs of threat perception to clinical practice. *Research and Theory for Nursing Practice: An International Journal, 25*(3), 163–175.

Jacobson, R.M., Peery, J., Thompson, W.O., et al. (2010). Serum electrolyte shifts following administration of sodium phosphates enema. *Gastroenterology Nursing, 33*(3), 191–201.

Jacobson, T., Tescher, A., Miers, A., et al. (2008). Improving practice: Efforts to reduce occipital pressure ulcers. *Journal of Nursing Care Quality, 23*(3), 283–288.

Jarvis, C. (2012). *Physical examination & health assessment* (6th ed.). St. Louis: Saunders/Elsevier.

Jarzyna, D., Jungquist, C.R., Pasero, C., et al. (2011). American Society for Pain Management nursing guidelines on monitoring for opioid-induced sedation and respiratory depression. *Pain Management Nursing, 12*(3), 118–145.

Jensen, S. (2011.) *Nursing Health Assessment. A best practice approach.* Philadelphia: Wolters Kluwer Health/Lippincott Williams & Wilkins.

Jevon, P. (2010). Procedure for recording a standard 12-lead electrocardiogram. *British Journal of Nursing, 19*(10), 649–651.

The Joanna Briggs Institute. (2004). Clinical effectiveness of different approaches to peritoneal dialysis catheter exit-site care. *BestPractice, 8*(1), 1–7.

Johnson, R.H. (2011). Practical care: creative strategies for bathing. *Nursing & Residential Care, 13*(8), 392–394.

Johnson, C.L., Anderson, M.A., & Hill, P.D. (2012). Comparison of pulse oximetry measures in a healthy population. *MEDSURGNursing, 21*(2), 70–76.

Johnson, A., Schweitzer, D., & Ahrens, T. (2011). Time to throw away your stethoscope? Capnography: Evidence-based patient monitoring technology. *Journal of Radiological Nursing, 30*(1), 25–34.

The Joint Commission (TJC). (2013). *National patient safety goals.* Available at http://www.jointcommission.org/standards_information/npsgs.aspx.

The Joint Commission. (2012). Sentinel event alert issue 49: Safe use of opioids in hospitals. Available at http://www.jointcommission.org/sea_issue_49/.

Jones, T., Springfield, T., Brudwich, M., et al. (2011). Fecal ostomies. Practical management for the home health clinician. *Home Healthcare Nurse, 29*(5), 306–317.

Katsma, D.L., & Katsma, R.P.E. (2000). The myth of the 90°-angle intramuscular injection. *Nurse Educator, 25*(1), 34–37.

Kee, J.L., Hayes, E.R., & McCuistion, L.E. (2012). *Pharmacology. A nursing process approach* (7th ed.). St. Louis: Elsevier/Saunders.

Kelly, T., Timmis, S., & Twelvetree, T. (2010). Review of the evidence to support oral hygiene in stroke patients. *Nursing Standard, 24*(37), 35–38.

Kessler, B., Claude-Gutekunst, M., Donchez, A.M., et al. (2012). The merry-go-round of patient rounding: Assure your patients get the brass ring. *MEDSURGNursing, 21*(4), 240–245.

Khair, J. (2005). Guidelines for testing the placing of nasogastric tubes. *Nursing Times, 101*(20), 26–27.

Kleinman, M.E., Chameides, L., Schexnayder, S.M., et al. (2010). 2010 American Heart Association guidelines for cardiopulmonary resuscitation and emergency cardiovascular care. Part 14: Pediatric advanced life support. *Circulation, 122*(18 Suppl. 3), S876–S908.

Kligfield, P., Gettes, L.S., Bailey, J.J., et al. (2007). Recommendations for the standardization and interpretation of the electrocardiogram. Part 1: The electrocardiogram and its technology. *Journal of the American College of Cardiology, 49*(10), 1109–1127.

Kwekkeboom, K., Hau, H., Wanta, B., et al. (2008). Patients' perceptions of the effectiveness of guided imagery and progressive muscle relaxation interventions used for cancer pain. *Complementary Therapies in Clinical Practice, 14*(3), 185–194.

Kyle, T., & Carman, S. (2013). *Essentials of pediatric nursing.* (2nd ed.). Philadelphia: Wolters Kluwer Health/Lippincott Williams & Wilkins.

Lagerquist, D., Dabrowski, M., Dock, C., et al. (2012). Clinical evidence review. Care of external fixator pin sites. *American Journal of Critical Care, 21*(4), 288–292.

Larson, T., & Brady, W. (2008). Electrocardiographic monitoring in the hospitalized patient: A diagnostic intervention of uncertain clinical impact. *American Journal of Emergency Medicine, 26*(9), 1047–1055.

Layzell, M. (2008). Current interventions and approaches to postoperative pain management. *British Journal of Nursing, 17*(7), 414–419.

Lee, A., & Park, Y. (2012). Reducing peritoneal dialysis catheter exit site infections by implementing a standardized postoperative dressing protocol. *Renal Society of Australasia Journal, 8*(1), 18–22.

LeFever Kee, J. (2013). *Pearson handbook of laboratory and diagnostic tests with nursing implications* (7th ed.). Upper Saddle River, NJ: Pearson.

Link, M.S., Atkins, D.L., Passman, R.S., et al. (2010). 2010 American Heart Association guidelines for cardiopulmonary resuscitation and emergency cardiovascular care. Part 6: Electrical therapies: automated external defibrillators, defibrillation, cardioversion, and pacing. *Circulation, 122*(18 Suppl. 3), S706–S719.

Lyman, T.P., & Vlahovic, T.C. (2010). Foot care from A to Z. *Dermatology Nursing, 22*(5), 2–8.

Mahoney, M., Baxter, K., Burgess, J., et al. (2013). Procedure for obtaining a urine sample from a urostomy, ileal conduit, and colon conduit. A best practice guideline for clinicians. *Journal of Wound, Ostomy & continence Nursing, 40*(3), 277–279.

Maiocco, G., & Coole, C. (2012). Use of ultrasound guidance for peripheral intravenous placement in difficult-to-access patients. Advancing practice with evidence. *Journal of Nursing Care Quality, 27*(1), 51–55.

Malarkey, L.M., & McMorrow, M.E. (2012). *Saunders nursing guide to laboratory and diagnostic tests* (2nd ed.). St. Louis: Elsevier Saunders.

Malkin, B., & Berridge, P. (2009). Guidance on maintaining personal hygiene in nail care. *Nursing Standard, 23*(41), 35–38.

Malli, S. (2005). Device safety. Keep a close eye on vacuum-assisted wound closure. *Nursing, 35*(7), 25.

Martindell, D. (2012). Safety monitor. The safe use of negative-pressure wound therapy. *American Journal of Nursing, 112*(6), 59–63.

Mayo Clinic. (2011). *How to choose and use a walker.* Available at http://www.mayoclinic.com/health/walker/HA00060.

Mayo Foundation for Medical Education and Research (MFMER). (2012). *Peripheral artery disease (PAD). Lifestyle and home remedies.* Available at http://www.mayoclinic.com/health/peripheral-arterial-disease/DS00537/DSECTION=lifestyle-and-home-remedies.

Mayo Foundation for Medical Education and Research (MFMER). (2011a). *Amputation and diabetes: How to protect your feet.* Available at http://www.mayoclinic.com/health/amputation-and-diabetes/DA00140.

Mayo Foundation for Medical Education and Research (MFMER). (2011c). *Finger-nails: Do's and don'ts for healthy nails.* Available at http://www.mayoclinic.com/health/nails/WO00020.

Mayo Foundation for Medical Education and Research (MFMER). (2011d). *Oral health: Brush up on dental care basics.* Available at http://www.mayoclinic.org/healthy-living/adult-health/in-depth/dental/art-20045536.

McNett, M.M., & Olson, D.M. (2013). Executive summary. Evidence to guide nursing interventions for critically ill neurologically impaired patients with ICP monitoring. *Journal of Neuroscience Nursing, 45*(3), 120–123.

Meade, C., Bursell, A., & Ketelsen, L. (2006). Effects of nursing rounds on patients' call light use, satisfaction and safety. *American Journal of Nursing, 106*(9), 58–71.

MedlinePlus. (2012). *Penis care (uncircumcised).* Available at http://www.nlm.nih.gov/medlineplus/ency/article/001917.htm.

Metheny, N. (2008). Residual volume measurement should be retained in enteral feeding protocols. *American Journal of Critical Care, 17*(1), 62–4.

Moreda, M.V., Wyatt, A.H., & Olson, D.M. (2009). Keeping the balance. Understanding intracranial pressure monitoring. *Nursing2009Critical Care, 4*(6), 42–47.

Morrison, L.J., Kierzek, G., Diekema, D.S., et al. (2010). 2010 American Heart Association guidelines for cardiopulmonary resuscitation and emergency cardiovascular care. Part 3: Ethics. *Circulation, 122*(18 Suppl. 3), S665–S675.

Morton, P.G., & Fontaine, D.K. (2013). *Essentials of critical care nursing. A holistic approach.* Philadelphia: Wolters Kluwer Health/Lippincott Williams & Wilkins.

Munera-Seeley, V., Ochoa, J., Brown, N., et al. (2008). Use of a colorimetric carbon dioxide sensor for nasoenteric feeding tube placement in critical care patients compared with clinical methods and radiography. *Nutrition in Clinical Practice, 23*(3), 318–321.

Myers III, F.E., & Reyes, C. (2011). Combating infection. Blood cultures: 5 steps to doing it right. *Nursing, 41*(3), 62–63.

National Cancer Institute (NCI). (2012). *Gastrointestinal complications (PDQ®). Constipation.* Available at http://www.cancer.gov/cancertopics/pdq/supportivecare/gastrointestinalcomplications/HealthProfessional/page2#top.

National Diabetes Information Clearinghouse (NDIC). (2012). *Continuous glucose monitoring.* Available at http://diabetes.niddk.nih.gov/dm/pubs/glucosemonitor/index.aspx#continue.

National Heart, Lung, and Blood Institute (NHLBI). National Institutes of Health (NIH). (2005). *The fourth report on the diagnosis, evaluation, and treatment of high blood pressure in children and adolescents.* (NIH Publication No. 05–5267). Washington, D.C.: U.S. Department of Health and Human Services.

National Institute on Aging (NIA). (2012). *Age page. Foot Care.* Available at http://www.nia.nih.gov/health/publication/foot-care.

National Kidney and Urologic Diseases Information Clearinghouse (NKUDIC). (2012). *Urodynamic testing.* NIH publication No. 12–5106. Available at http://kidney.niddk.nih.gov/KUDiseases/pubs/urodynamic/index.aspx.

Nelson, R., Edwards, S., & Tse, B. (2007). Prophylactic nasogastric decompression after abdominal surgery. *Cochrane Database Systematic Review,* Issue 3. Art. No.: DOI: 10.1002/14651858.CD004929.pub3.

Ness, W., Hibberts, F., & Miles, S. (2012). Royal College of Nursing. Management of lower bowel dysfunction, including DRE and DRF. RCN guidance for nurses. London, U.K.: Royal College of Nursing.

Neumar, R.W., Otto, C.W., Link, M.S., et al. (2010). 2010 American Heart Association guidelines for cardiopulmonary resuscitation and emergency cardiovascular care. Part 8: Adult advanced cardiovascular life support. *Circulation, 122*(18 Suppl. 3), S729–S767.

Newman, D. (2008). Internal and external urinary catheters: A primer for clinical practice. *Ostomy Wound Management, 54*(12), 18–20, 22–26, 28–38.

Nicoll, L., & Hesby, A. (2002). Intramuscular injection: An integrative research review and guideline for evidence-based practice. *Applied Nursing Research, 16*(2), 149–162.

Obokhare, I. (2012). Fecal impaction: A cause for concern? *Clinics in Colon and Rectal Surgery, 25*(1), 53–57.

Ogedegbe, G., & Pickering, T. (2010). Principles and techniques of blood pressure measurement. *Cardiology Clinics, 28*(4), 571–586.

O'Grady, N.P., Alexander, M., Burns, L.A., et al. (2011). Guidelines for the prevention of intravascular catheter-related infections. *American Journal of Infection Control, 39*(4 Supplement), S1–S34.

Olrich, T., Kalman, M., & Nigolian, C. (2012). Hourly rounding: A replication study. *MEDSURGNursing, 21*(1), 23–36.

O'Neil, B.J., Hoekstra, J., Pride, Y.B., et al. (2010). Incremental benefit of 80-lead electrocardiogram body surface mapping over the 12-lead electrocardiogram in the detection of acute coronary syndromes in patients without ST-elevation myocardial infarction: Results from the optimal cardiovascular diagnostic evaluation enabling faster treatment of myocardial infarction (OCCULT MI) trial. *Academic Emergency Medicine, 17*(9), 932–939.

Palatini, P., & Parati, G. (2011). Blood pressure measurement in very obese patients: A challenging problem. *Journal of Hypertension, 29*(3), 425–429.

Pankop, R., Chang, K., Thorlton, J., et al. (2013). Implemented family presence protocols. An integrative review. *Journal of Nursing Care Quality, 28*(3), 281–288.

Pasero, C. & McCaffery, M. (2011). *Pain assessment and pharmacological management.* St. Louis: Mosby Elsevier.

Pasero, C., & McCaffery, M. (2005). Authorized and unauthorized use of PCA pumps: Clarifying the use of patient-controlled analgesia, in light of recent alerts. *American Journal of Nursing, 105*(7), 30–32.

Patchen, S.J., Timyam, L., & Atherton, S. (2010). Jerome Medical. *Your life in a halo made easier. Patient information manual.* Available http://assets.ossur.com/lisalib/getfile.aspx?itemid=7127

Pate, M. (2004). Placement of endotracheal and tracheostomy tubes. *Critical Care Nurse, 24*(3), 13.

Pate, M. & Zapata, T. (2002). Ask the experts: How deeply should I go when I suction an endotracheal or tracheostomy tube? *Critical Care Nurse, 22*(2), 130–131.

Patraca, K. (2005). Measure bladder volume without catheterization. *Nursing, 35*(4), 46–47.

Perry, S.E., Hockenberry, M.J., Lowdermilk, D.L., et al. (2010). *Maternal child nursing care* (4th ed.). Maryland Heights, MO: Mosby/Elsevier.

Pickering, T., Hall, J., Appel, L., et al. (2004). American Heart Association Scientific Statement. Recommendations for blood pressure measurement in humans and experimental animals. Part 1: Blood pressure measurement in humans: A statement for professionals from the subcommittee of professional and public education of the American Heart Association Council on High Blood Pressure Research. Available at http://hyper.ahajournals.org/cgi/content/full/45/1/142.

Polovich, M., White, J., & Kelleher, L. (Eds). (2009). *Chemotherapy and biotherapy guidelines and recommendations for practice* (3rd ed.). Pittsburgh, PA: Oncology Nursing Society.

Preston, G. (2008). An overview of topical negative pressure therapy in wound care. *Nursing Standard, 23*(7), 62–8.

Puck, A.L., Oakeson, A.M., Morales-Clark, A., et al. (2012). Obstetric life support. *Journal of Perinatal & Neonatal Nursing, 26*(2), 126–135.

Pullen, R.L. (2010). Using pulse oximetry accurately. *Nursing, 40*(4), 63.

Rew, M., & Smith, R. (2011). Reducing infection through the use of suprapubic catheters. *British Journal of Neuroscience Nursing, 7*(5), S13–S16.

Ritz, J., Pashnik, B., Padula, C., et al. (2012). Effectiveness of 2 methods of chlorhexidine bathing. *Journal of Nursing Care Quality, 27*(2), 171–175.

Roman, M., & Cabaj, T. (2005). Epidural analgesia. *MEDSURG Nursing, 14*(4), 257–259.

Rubin, B.K. (2010). Air and soul: the science and application of aerosol therapy. *Respiratory Care, 55*(7), 911–921.

Rudoni, C. (2008). A service evaluation of the use of silicone-based adhesive remover. *British Journal of Nursing, Stoma Care Supplement, 17*(2), S4, S6, S8–S9.

Sarro, A., Anthony, T., Magtoto, R., et al. (2010). Developing a standard of care for halo vest and pin site care including patient and family education: A collaborative approach among three greater Toronto area teaching hospitals. *Journal of Neuroscience Nursing, 42*(3), 169–173.

Satryb, S.A., Wilson, T.J., & Patterson, J.M. (2011). Casting: All wrapped up. *Orthopaedic Nursing, 30*(1), 37–43.

Sawhney, M. (2012). Epidural analgesia: What nurses need to know. *Nursing, 42*(8), 36–42.

Scales, K. (2008). A practical guide to venepuncture and blood sampling. *Nursing Standard, 22*(29), 29–36.

Schimpf, M.M. (2012). Diagnosing increased intracranial pressure. *Journal of Trauma Nursing, 19*(3), 160–167.

Self, W., Mattu, A., Jartin, M., et al. (2006). Body surface mapping in the ED evaluation of the patient with chest pain: Use of the 80-lead electrocardiogram system. *American Journal of Emergency Medicine, 24*(1), 87–112.

Shimizu, T., Mizutani, T., Yamahita, S., et al. (2011). Endotracheal tube extubation force: Adhesive tape versus endotracheal tube holder. *Respiratory Care, 56*(11), 1825–1829.

Shippee-Rice, R.V., Fetzer, S.J., & Long, J.V. (2012). *Gerioperative nursing care.* New York: Springer.

Sievert, D., Armola, R., & Halm, M.A. (2011). Chlorhexidine gluconate bathing: Does it decrease hospital-acquired infections? *American Journal of Critical Care, 20*(2), 166–170.

Society for Cardiological Science & Technology (SCST). (2010). *Clinical guidelines by consensus. Recording a standard 12-lead electrocardiogram.* Available at http://www.scst.org.uk/pages/page_box_contents.asp?pageid=808.

Society of Urologic Nurses and Associates (SUNA). (2010). *Prevention & control of catheter-associated urinary tract infection (CAUTI). Clinical practice guideline.* Available at https://www.suna.org/sites/default/files/download/cautiGuideline.pdf.

Society of Urologic Nurses and Associates. (2005c). *Male urethral catheterization: Clinical practice guideline.* Available at http://suna.org/resources/maleCatheterization.pdf.

Sole, M.L., Penoyer, D.A., Bennett, M., et al. (2011). Oropharyngeal secretion volume in intubated patients: The importance of oral suctioning. *American Journal of Critical Care, 20*(6), e141–e145.

Stephen-Haynes, J. (2008). Skin integrity and silicone: APPEEL "no-sting" medical adhesive remover. *British Journal of Nursing, 17*(12), 792–795.

Sullivan, B. (2008). Nursing management of patients with a chest drain. *British Journal of Nursing, 17*(6), 388–393.

Sultan, P., Carvalho, B., Rose, B.O., et al. (2011). Endotracheal tube cuff pressure monitoring: A review of the evidence. *Journal of Perioperative Practice, 21*(11), 379–386.

Tada, A., & Miura, H. (2012). Prevention of aspiration pneumonia with oral care. *Archives of Gerontology & Geriatrics, 55*(1), 16–21.

Taylor, C., Lillis, C., & Lynn, P. (2015). *Fundamentals of nursing: The art and science of person-centered nursing care.* (8th ed.). Philadelphia: Wolters Kluwer Health/Lippincott Williams & Wilkins.

Thompson, G. (2008). An overview of negative pressure wound therapy (NPWT). *Wound Care, 13*(6), Wound Care: S23–4, S26, S28–30.

Timms, A., & Hugh, P. (2012). Pin site care: guidance and key recommendations. *Nursing Standard, 27*(1), 50–55.

Titler, M.G., Shever, L.L., Kanak, M.F., et al. (2011). Factors associated with falls during hospitalization in an older adult population. *Research and Theory for Nursing Practice: An International Journal, 25*(2), 127–152.

Tracey, D., & Patterson, G. (2006). Care of the gastrostomy tube in the home. *Home Healthcare Nurse, 24*(6), 381–386.

U.S. Food and Drug Administration (FDA). (2013). *Medical devices. Blood glucose monitoring devices.* Available at http://www.fda.gov/%20medicaldevices/productsandmedicalprocedures/invitrodiagnostics/glucosetestingdevices/default.htm.

University of Iowa Hospitals and Clinics. (2008). *Using crutches safely.* Iowa City, Iowa: Author. Available at www.uihealthcare.com/topics/bonesjointsmuscles/bone3458.html.

Usichenko, T., Pavlovic, D., Foellner, S., et al. (2004). Reducing venipuncture pain by a cough trick: A randomized crossover volunteer study. *Anesthesia & Analgesia, 98*(2), 343–345.

Vanden Hoek, T.L., Morrison, L.J., Shuster, M., et al. (2010). 2010 American Heart Association guidelines for cardiopulmonary resuscitation and emergency cardiovascular care. Part 12: Cardiac arrest in special situations. *Circulation, 122*(18 Suppl. 3), S829–S861.

Van Leeuwen, A.M., Poelhuis-Leth, D., & Bladh, M.L. (2011). *Davis's comprehensive handbook of laboratory & diagnostic tests with nursing implications* (4th ed.). Philadelphia: F.A. Davis.

VISN 8 Patient Safety Center. (2012). *Safe patient handling and movement algorithms.* Tampa, FL: Author. Available at http://www.visn8.va.gov/visn8/patientsafetycenter/safePtHandling/default.asp.

Viswanathan, P., & Kidd, M. (2010). Effect of continuous passive motion following total knee arthroplasty on knee range of motion and function: a systematic review. *New Zealand Journal of Physiotherapy, 38*(1), 14–22.

Voegeli, D. (2012). Moisture-associated skin damage: aetiology, prevention and treatment. *British Journal of Nursing, 21*(9), 517–521.

Walker, J. (2012). Pin site infection in orthopaedic external fixation devices. *British Journal of Nursing, 21*(3), 148–151.

Walker, L., & Lamont, S. (2008). Graduated compression stockings to prevent deep vein thrombosis. *Nursing Standard, 22*(40), 35–38.

Waters, T., Collins, J., Galinsky, T., et al. (2006). NIOSH research efforts to prevent musculoskeletal disorders in the healthcare industry. *Orthopaedic Nursing, 25*(6), 380–389.

Weisgram, B., & Raymond, S. (2008). Using evidence-based nursing rounds to improve patient outcomes. *MEDSURG Nursing, 17*(6), 429–430.

White, A., Lopez, F., & Stone, P. (2010). Developing and sustaining an ultrasound-guided peripheral intravenous access program for emergency nurses. *Advanced Emergency Nursing Journal, 32*(2), 173–188.

Williams, J. (2012). Stoma care: obtaining a urine specimen from a urostomy. *Gastrointestinal Nursing, 10*(5), 11–12.

Wound, Ostomy and Continence Nurses Society (WOCN). (2012). Clean vs. sterile dressing techniques for management of chronic wounds. A fact sheet. *Journal of Wound, Ostomy and Continence Nursing, 39*(2S) (Supplement), S30–S34.

Wuhrman, E., Cooney, M., Dunwoody, C., et al. (2007). Authorized and unauthorized ("PCA by proxy") dosing of analgesic infusion pumps: Position statement with clinical practice recommendations. *Pain Management Nursing, 8*(1), 4–11.

Wyatt, A.H., Moreda, M.V., & Olson, D.M. (2009). Keeping the balance. Understanding intracranial pressure. *Nursing2009CriticalCare, 4*(5), 18–23.

Zed, P.J., Agu-Laban, R.B., Shuster, M., Green, R.S., Slavik, R.S., & Travers, A.H. (2008). Update on cardiopulmonary resuscitation and emergency cardiovascular care guidelines. *American Journal of Health-System Pharmacy, 65*(24), 2337–2346.

Zimmerman, P.G. (2010). Revisiting IM injections. *American Journal of Nursing, 110*(2), 60–61.